with chapters by

John R. Blackmon, M.D.
Associate Professor of Medicine

Warren G. Guntheroth, M.D.
Professor of Pediatrics

Michel Nasser, M.D.
Senior Postdoctoral Fellow
Division of Bioengineering

D. E. Strandness, Jr., M.D.
Professor of Surgery

THE UNIVERSITY OF WASHINGTON SCHOOL OF MEDICINE

3rd edition

CARDIOVASCULAR DYNAMICS

Robert F. Rushmer, M.D.

Director, Center for Bioengineering;
Professor and Head, Division of Bioengineering,
School of Medicine; Professor of Bioengineering,
College of Engineering, University of Washington

W. B. SAUNDERS COMPANY
PHILADELPHIA LONDON TORONTO

W. B. Saunders Company: West Washington Square
Philadelphia, Pa. 19105

12 Dyott Street
London, WC1A 1DB

1835 Yonge Street
Toronto 7, Ontario

Cardiovascular Dynamics

SBN 0-7216-7846-7

Print No.:   2   3   4   5   6   7   8   9

*This book is dedicated to
students interested in the cardiovascular system.*

PREFACE

CARDIOVASCULAR DYNAMICS is an extensive revision, enlargement and reorganization of a book originally published under the title Cardiac Diagnosis: A Physiologic Approach. The components of the cardiovascular system are presented in terms of their structure, function and control under normal conditions, followed by consideration of the changes induced by common disease states. This text was designed for students of the cardiovascular system in the broadest sense —from first year medical students to experienced cardiologists. It is specifically intended for use in vertical teaching, i.e., as a supplemental text for courses in Physiology, Physical Diagnosis and Clinical Cardiology.

The most important forms of cardiovascular disease are included among the examples employed to elucidate the nature of abnormal cardiovascular function. However, the text is not intended as a handbook for the practice of cardiology since it was not considered appropriate to detail all forms of cardiovascular disease.

With the passage of years, the most significant deficiency of the second edition of *Cardiovascular Dynamics* appeared to reside in the treatment of the examples of cardiovascular diseases from the clinical point of view. Circumstances have caused me to become progressively divorced from the continuous contact with patients required to maintain clinical competence. Responsibility for preparing the chapters dealing with cardiovascular diagnosis and management has been delegated to some colleagues whose knowledge of these subjects is vastly greater than my own. We all trust that this step will render the third edition more authoritative and useful for the cardiologists than the previous ones.

Many of the same illustrations are utilized since the basic concepts of cardiovascular function, control and disease have not changed too much in the past few years. New illustrations have been prepared according to the same objectives and approaches as in previous editions wherever possible.

Important ideas in each chapter have been illustrated in order to facilitate discussion and aid visualization of concepts. The figures are intended to explain ideas rather than offer evidence for arguments. Realism in the schematic drawings has been retained as much as possible to provide visual images of physiologic and pathologic mechanisms in situ rather than abstractions. The legend for each figure is self-explanatory and the illustrations are thus rendered independent of the text. Cross references are made to figures rather than text pages in the belief that it is more efficient to refresh

vii

the memory by studying pictures than by re-reading the text.

Graphs and tables have been avoided for two reasons: (a) their interpretation is often difficult and tedious and (b) it seems more important to understand why certain phenomena occur rather than how much specific variables are altered under experimental conditions. Graphs tend to suggest cause-and-effect relations which may not exist. When experimental records are reproduced, a schematic representation of the experimental method is included in most instances.

At the risk of appearing excessively biased, I have tried to avoid exhaustive presentations of conflicting viewpoints. If a single hypothesis appeared adequate to explain a particular phenomenon, alternative explanations have not necessarily been included. Attention has been directed to many deficiencies in current knowledge which can be corrected only by further investigations.

ROBERT F. RUSHMER, M.D.

ACKNOWLEDGMENTS

A BOOK OF THIS SORT represents a small sample of facts and concepts selectively extracted from a vast store of material on the subject. The final content of this manuscript has been greatly influenced by a series of investigations accomplished in association with a closely knit research team representing several fields of interest. The ingenuity, persistence and technical competence of this group were indispensable to the successful completion of the studies summarized in this text. The various research projects were supported in part by grants from the National Heart Institute of the National Institutes of Health, United States Public Health Service; the Washington State Heart Association and the American Heart Association.

Sandy Ritz carried the heavy secretarial load and I gratefully acknowledge her interest, cooperation and patience in the preparation of the manuscript. I gratefully acknowledge the wholehearted cooperation of the W. B. Saunders Company in the production of the book.

Most of the illustrations from the first edition were designed and executed by the author although many were refined and labeled by Miss Jessie Phillips, Miss Virginia Brooks and Mrs. Mary Jane Owens. The relatively small number of signed drawings is no indication of the extent of their contribution to the illustrations in the book. Seventy-five illustrations for the second edition were prepared by Mrs. Helen Halsey from rough sketches.

Several of the original illustrations in this book first appeared in articles by the author and his associates in the following journals: *American Journal of Physiology* (Fig. 7-10); *Circulation* (Figs. 2-13, 2-14, 5-2); *Circulation Research* (Figs. 3-6, 5-13); *Handbook of Physiology, Section II, Vol. I* (Figs. 3-18, 6-13, 6-14); *Physiological Reviews* (Figs. 7-4, 7-5, 7-9). I wish to express my appreciation to the publishers of these journals for permission to reproduce the illustrations.

ROBERT F. RUSHMER, M.D.

CONTENTS

CHAPTER 7

CARDIOVASCULAR RESPONSES DURING EXERTION........................... 220

CHAPTER 8

DETECTION OF PERIPHERAL VASCULAR DISEASE 244

by D. E. Strandness, Jr.

CHAPTER 9

THE CORONARY SYSTEM 261

by Michel G. Nasser, M.D.

CHAPTER 1

PROPERTIES OF THE VASCULAR SYSTEM

Living cells possess many of the attributes of microscopic chemical factories, containing many complex chemical processes producing molecular transformations to perform various specialized functions. Unicellular organisms contain all the mechanisms required to sustain life within a single membranous cell boundary. Multicellular organisms are made up of cells serving many different functions through the evolutionary process of specialization. All cells survive only so long as the logistics of metabolism are successfully met by an influx of oxygen, metabolic fuels and chemical components involved in the physiochemical processing (Fig. 1–1). Waste products, including carbon dioxide and toxic excretions, must be carried away at a rate which limits their accumulation. Some cells release energy (i.e., electrical excitation processes), others can perform external work (i.e., skeletal muscles) and virtually all cells produce heat which must be eliminated into the external environment. Our ability to perform external work often appears to be limited by the rate of delivery of the material which is used at the fastest rate in relation to its storage capacity within the body, namely oxygen. Many other tissues produce no external work

(i.e., producing movement of masses) but perform other useful functions such as the elimination of heat by the skin, digestion and absorption of foodstuffs in the gut, secretion of waste products by the kidney and elaboration of hormones by endocrine glands. In most of these tissues, the levels of activity are not limited by the rate of oxygen delivery to the tissues under normal conditions. In all tissues, the logistics of metabolism are effectively carried on by the combined effects of convection (currents of fluids near cells) and of diffusion.

Unicellular organisms such as amoebae live in large expanses of water with which they exchange these substances continuously, primarily by the process of diffusion. Diffusion is the movement of particles from regions of high concentration into regions of lower concentration. If a drop of dye is placed in a beaker of motionless water, the molecules of dye will gradually disperse until finally they are uniformly distributed throughout the water (Fig. 1–2A). This dispersion results from thermal agitation producing random movement of molecules (Brownian movement) such that at any moment more molecules are moving away from the source of dye than are moving toward it. If dye, salt, sugar and urea are

1

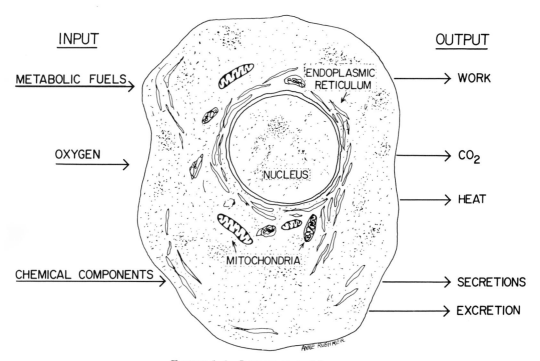

LOGISTICS OF METABOLISM

FIGURE 1–1   LOGISTICS OF METABOLISM

The nutrition of cells involves the delivery of oxygen, metabolic fuels and chemical constituents to the cells engaged in physicochemical processes to produce an output of work, CO_2 heat, secretions and excretions. The circulatory system of complex organisms must maintain an appropriate balance between the metabolic activity, the rate of delivery and the rate of removal of the chemical products from cellular activity.

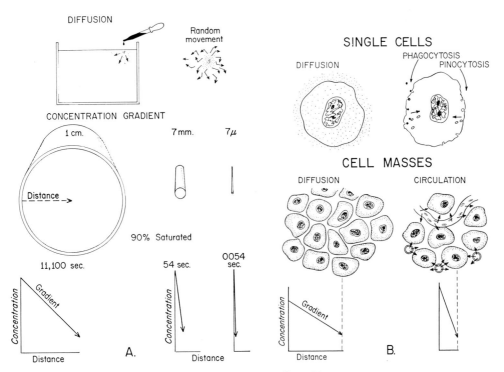

FIGURE 1–2 DIFFUSION AND CELL NUTRITION

A, The Process of Diffusion. Substances dissolved or suspended in a continuous fluid medium tend to become uniformly dispersed as the particles move from regions of higher concentration to regions of lower concentration through thermal agitation (Brownian movement). The rate of diffusion is determined by the steepness of the concentration gradient.

B, Nutrition of Cells. Many cells display active imbibition of solid particles (phagocytosis) and of droplets of fluid (pinocytosis) by envelopment or vesicle formation. Single cells may be nourished by diffusion alone. Small cell masses can also be nourished by diffusion. The concentration gradients are flattened and transport is slow. In large cell masses, steep concentration gradients are maintained by circulation of nutrient fluids or blood into the immediate vicinity of the individual cells in each tissue.

placed in four different regions of the water-filled beaker, they will all achieve uniform distribution by movement of each molecular species from the region of its high concentration into regions of its lower concentration.

By random movement, a molecule of water could theoretically pass from a man's head to his toe unassisted by circulation or flow currents, but this would require more than 100 years. The same molecule could cover a distance of 1.5 μ in approximately 0.003 second. In any particular continuous fluid phase the rate at which a substance diffuses depends primarily upon the steepness of the concentration gradient.

A cylinder of tissue 1 cm. in diameter, suddenly placed in an atmosphere of 100 per cent oxygen, would become 90 per cent saturated with oxygen after 11,100 seconds (about three hours). If the diameter of the cylinder were only 0.7 mm., the same degree of saturation would occur in 54 seconds (Fig. 1–2A). A single cell 7 μ in diameter would be saturated in .0054 second.[1] As the distance of diffusion from the surface to the center of the tissue is reduced the concentration gradient becomes very steep and diffusion occurs very rapidly. In general, a single cell, bathed in an expanse of nutrient fluid, can survive by diffusion alone (Fig. 1–2B). As the cell utilizes oxygen, its concentration drops in the protoplasm and other molecules of oxygen diffuse toward the cell from regions of higher concentration outside.

In addition, many different types of cells have the ability to engulf particles (phagocytosis) or to imbibe droplets of fluid in the form of vesicles which may move toward the center of the cell. This process of vesicle formation has long been known to occur in amoebae and has been called pinocytosis, i.e., "drinking" by cells. Infolding of the cell membrane produces a tiny pouch which envelops a droplet of extracellular fluid (Fig. 1–2B). This process is receiving greatly increased attention since electron micrographs of many different mammalian cells show circular rings which appear to be vesicles. Indeed, this process has been proposed as a mechanism for active transport of materials across the capillary endothelium (see Chapter 4).

As cells group together to form more complex organisms, the distance of diffusion to the center of the mass increases and the shallow diffusion gradient limits the rate of transfer of various substances (Fig. 1–2B). Such organisms must either subsist on low levels of metabolism or develop a circulatory system.

In a large complex mass of cells, like the mammalian body, rapid diffusion along steep concentration gradients is achieved by providing a continuous flow of blood in the vicinity of all cells. The streams of blood must be contained within channels which retard diffusion only minimally. These requirements are satisfied by hundreds of millions of thin-walled capillaries distributed profusely throughout every portion of the body. The capillary density (number of capillaries/volume of tissue) reflects the tissue's requirements for blood flow. With the specialization of cells and tissues into complex organisms, blood flow must not only supply metabolic needs but also serve other functions such as dissipation of heat, movement, secretion, absorption and excretion (see Chapter 4).

In mammalian forms, blood with high concentrations of oxygen and nutritive substances and with low concentrations of carbon dioxide and metabolites is brought into the vicinity of each cell in the body. In skeletal muscle, for example, each capillary serves tissue with a volume only about twelve times its own. Thus, the diffusion distances are very small and the concentration gradients are extremely steep so long as the capillary blood flow is not interrupted. When capillary flow ceases, the concentration gradients immediately begin to flatten and diffusion slows as the various substances approach uniform dispersion through the fluids. If the utilization of oxygen and metabolic fuels increases, their concentrations in the cells are reduced and the steeper concentration gradients accelerate diffusion. Faster capillary flow is then required to maintain maximally steep diffusion gradients.

Blood pumped by the heart is distributed to the billions of capillaries by a diffuse arborization of the arterial tree with a single artery giving off branches which divide and subdivide to produce a complicated ramification. In the same way, blood leaving the capillaries returns to the heart by way of venous channels which have similar ramifications. The functional properties of the circulatory system reflect this architectural arrangement.

THE SYSTEMIC CIRCULATION

The patterns of circulation in various tissues have been the subject of widespread investigation in many laboratories. Until recently, the caliber, length, volume and total cross-sectional area of various components of the systemic circulation have been based on data from dead and fixed material. Wiedeman[3] described geometrical relations of the microcirculation and the branching arterial and venous channels in live animals. (Fig. 1–3). In accordance with previous concepts, the cross-sectional area in-

creases at each branch point along the main arterial and venous trunks (Fig. 1–3A, C). The caliber of the veins is considerably greater than that of corresponding arterial channels. In the microcirculation, capillaries branch off arterioles (Fig. 1–3B) and frequently form branching networks such that the total cross section of venous capillaries and postcapillary venules is much greater than any other segment of the vascular tree (Fig. 1–3D). The volume of blood contained within the capillaries and arterioles is relatively small, particularly in comparison with postcapillary venules, venules and small veins (Fig. 1–3E). Thus, the capillaries contain a small and relatively fixed quantity of blood, the arterial system contains a larger but relatively constant quantity of blood and the veins contain a major portion of the total blood and can change their capacity to accommodate quite large variations in total and regional blood volume.

Visualization of the systemic circulation can be simplified by means of a schematic drawing in which all the capillaries are arranged in parallel (Fig. 1–4) and all arterial branches having the same caliber are arranged one above the other. Similarly, the corresponding branches of the venous system are vertically oriented. In this way it is possible to demonstrate the effects of the branching arterial and venous systems on the pressure and flow of blood in corresponding segments of the circulatory tree.

VOLUME FLOW THROUGH VARIOUS SEGMENTS OF THE CIRCULATORY SYSTEM

The anatomic complexity of the peripheral circulatory distribution tends to obscure some very basic principles which are obvious in a single tube. For example, if fluid flows into

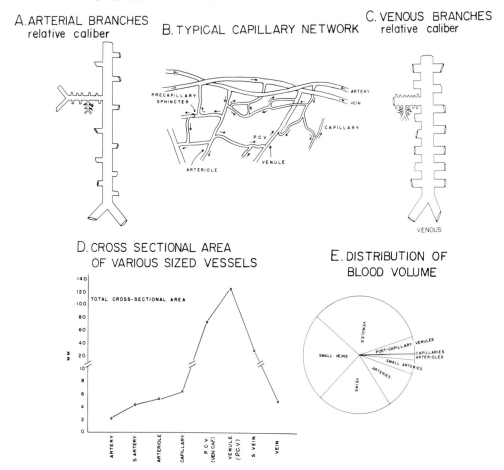

FIGURE 1–3   COMPONENTS OF THE SYSTEMIC CIRCULATION

A, The relative caliber of the aorta and its main branches are illustrated to show the increasing cross-sectional area with arborization.

B, Typical capillary networks are complex channels with flow regulated by arterioles and precapillary sphincters. (From Wiedeman, M. P., in Handbook of Physiology, Section 2: Circulation, Vol. II. W. F. Hamilton and P. Dow, eds. Washington, D. C., American Physiological Society, 1963.)

C, The relative caliber of the systemic veins is generally greater than the corresponding branches of the arterial system.

D, The cross-sectional area of the peripheral vessels increases gradually going from arteries to capillaries and then expands enormously at the postcapillary venule (more commonly known as venous capillaries) and even more at venules.

E, The total blood volume is distributed with the smallest amount in capillaries and the greatest amount on the venous side of the circulation, particularly the venules and small veins. (Presented through courtesy of Mary Wiedeman.[3])

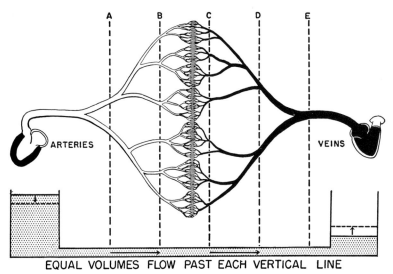

EQUAL VOLUMES FLOW PAST EACH VERTICAL LINE

FIGURE 1–4   VOLUME FLOW THROUGH THE SYSTEMIC CIRCULATION

Arborization of the systemic circulatory system is schematically represented with all vessels of the same caliber arranged vertically. This simplified illustration emphasizes the fact that the volume of fluid flowing past each vertical line in a unit time must be equal to the quantity entering and leaving the system, just as in a single tube.

the single straight tube at the bottom of Figure 1–4 at a rate of 5 liters per minute, the same quantity of fluid must flow out of the tube. Similarly, 5 liters must flow past each of the vertical lines (A, B, C, D, E) during each minute. The only possible exception to this rule would result from a net shift of fluid from one segment to another. Such a redistribution of fluid would produce transient and relatively insignificant differences in the flow past the various regions of the tube. A schematic representation such as Figure 1–4 shows the general applicability of this rule in the systemic circulation, namely; the quantity of blood flowing past each vertical line is exactly equal to the quantity pumped into the system and the quantity leaving the system per unit time, except for slight and transient differences due to redistribution of the fluid volumes within the system. It is true that the

flow may be greater through one parallel channel than through another, but the total flow through all corresponding segments must be essentially identical. This very simple principle is neglected in many discussions of circulatory dynamics.

CROSS-SECTIONAL AREA OF THE CIRCULATORY SYSTEM
(Fig. 1-5)

When an artery or vein bifurcates, the cross-sectional area of its branches exceeds that of the parent vessel. The number of vessels formed by this branching is so great that the estimated cross-sectional area of the capillaries is approximately 625 sq. cm. in a 13 kg. dog with an aortic area of only 0.8 sq. cm.[2] This peak value from Green[2] is retained in Figure 1–5, but the maximum cross-sectional area has been shifted toward the region of the post-

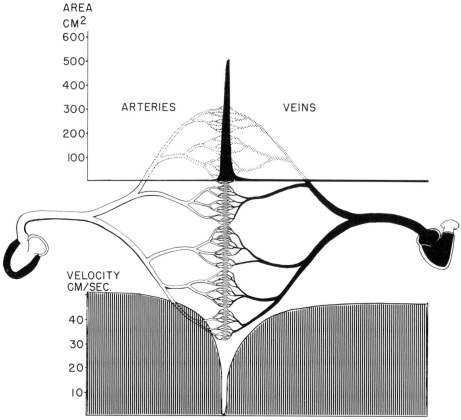

FIGURE 1–5 THE RELATION BETWEEN CROSS-SECTIONAL AREA AND THE VELOCITY OF FLOW IN THE SYSTEMIC CIRCULATION

Cross-sectional areas of various segments of the systemic circulation computed for a 13 kg. dog. Note the tremendous area in the arterioles, capillaries and venules. The velocity of blood flow is inversely proportional to the cross-sectional area so that blood flows through the capillaries at about 0.07 cm. per second (see reference 2).

capillary venule as suggested by Wiedeman's more recent data (see Fig. 1–3D). Since the volumes of blood flowing through corresponding segments of the system are equal, changes in cross-sectional area affect the velocity of blood flow.

VELOCITY OF BLOOD FLOW
(Fig. 1–5)

Just as water in a rushing stream slows down when it enters a broad pool, so the velocity of flow is reduced in regions of the circulation with large cross-sectional areas. In the aorta, blood travels at an average velocity of 40 to 50 cm. per second, and in the capillaries it moves at about 0.07 cm. per second.[2] Slow flow in the peripheral capillaries provides time for the exchange of materials across the capillary walls. After passing into the veins, the blood again accelerates as the cross-sectional area progressively decreases. However, the caliber of the veins exceeds that of corresponding arteries, so the velocity of venous blood only approaches and does not equal that of the arterial blood. It is obviously necessary to distinguish between volume flow and velocity of blood flow. The volume flow of blood through a particular tube depends upon the pressure gradient, the resistance to flow and the physical characteristics of blood.

RESISTANCE TO BLOOD FLOW IN THE CIRCULATION (Fig. 1–6)

Fluid flows through tubes in response to a gradient in pressure. The progressive reduction in the pressure of fluid passing through a tube of constant bore represents the energy which is lost as heat due to friction, i.e., heat lost in the collisions of the moving molecules composing the fluid. The difference between the pressures at the two ends of a tube is a measure of the frictional loss of energy or of the resistance to the flow of fluid. For example, consider a laminar flow of water through the horizontal tubes in Figure 1–6. The pressure gradient is indicated by the height of the columns of water in the vertical tubes. In a tube of constant bore, the pressure drop is directly proportional to the length of the tube. Thus, if the length of the tube is doubled, the magnitude of the pressure drop is also doubled. During passage of a homogeneous fluid through the segment labeled R, the pressure drop is given as 1 cm. of water. During

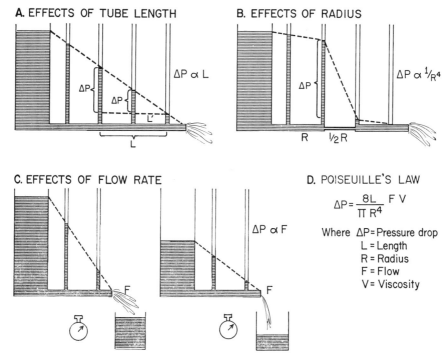

FIGURE 1–6 **FACTORS INFLUENCING THE PRESSURE DROP IN FLUIDS FLOWING THROUGH TUBES (POISEUILLE'S LAW)**

A, The drop in pressure (ΔP) during laminar flow of a homogeneous fluid through a rigid tube of constant caliber is directly proportional to the length of the tube.

B, Under the same conditions, the pressure drop is also inversely proportional to the reciprocal of the radius to the fourth power ($1/R^4$) and directly proportional to the volume flow (C) through the tube and to the viscosity (V) of the fluid. The relationships between these factors are included in the formula which is an expression of Poiseuille's law (D).

passage through the next segment, where the radius is only ½ R, the pressure drop is 16 cm. of water. The frictional resistance, as indicated by the pressure gradient, is proportional to $1/R^4$ (the reciprocal of the fourth power of the radius) so that reducing radius by one-half increases the pressure drop sixteenfold. The pressure drop is also directly proportional to the rate of flow. Finally, the pressure drop along a tube is directly proportional to the viscosity of the fluid. The interrelationships of these factors have been combined in a formula (Fig. 1–6) which summarizes Poiseuille's law for streamlined flow of viscous fluids through rigid tubes of constant caliber.

Poiseuille's law cannot be quantitatively applied to the circulatory system for several reasons: (a) Blood vessels are not rigid; they stretch in response to an increase in pressure. Elevated internal pressure may produce an increase in both radius and length. For this reason, the pressure and the dimensions of the tube are not independently variable. (b) Plasma is a truly viscous fluid, but whole blood is not. If plasma is perfused through an ordinary rigid tube, even the smallest differential pressure will produce some flow. On the contrary, when whole blood is perfused through the vascular system of an animal's extremity, no flow is produced until the pressure gradient from arteries to veins reaches 10 mm. Hg (even more in the presence of vasoconstriction). (c) Blood is not a homogeneous fluid since it contains large number of cellular elements which affect its flow through the vascular system.

PRESSURE GRADIENTS IN THE CIRCULATORY TREE

While Poiseuille's law is not entirely applicable to the circulatory

system, the factors illustrated in Figure 1–6 apply in a qualitative sense. As the arterial blood pressure and the length of the vessels tend to remain relatively fixed and the viscosity of the blood has limited variability from moment to moment, the caliber of the vessels unquestionably plays a predominant role in determining both the pressure gradients and the flow through various segments of the circulatory system (Fig. 1–7). The blood flows through the major arterial trunks with little frictional loss, as indicated by the very gradual drop in the mean arterial pressure. As the arteries divide and sub-

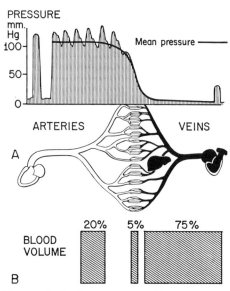

FIGURE 1–7   PRESSURES OF BLOOD IN THE SYSTEMIC CIRCULATION

A, The pressures in the arterial system are elevated and pulsatile. The mean arterial pressure declines very gradually as blood flows through the main branches of the arterial tree. In the small vessels, the pressure head diminishes rapidly and the fluctuations are damped out because of the high resistance to flow. In the major veins, the pressure gradient is again very shallow.

B, The volume of blood in the arteries is relatively fixed at about 20 per cent of the total. The veins contain about 75 per cent of the systemic blood volume but can alter their capacity over a wide range.

divide, the caliber of the vessels diminishes and the pressure gradients become correspondingly steeper. Some 80 per cent of the pressure drop along the arterial channels occurs in the terminal arteries and arterioles. Similarly, the confluence of veins is associated with a reduction in resistance as blood flows from the capillaries toward the heart. In the larger veins blood flows briskly in response to very shallow pressure gradients. The marked increase in resistance in the small vessels produces a precipitous fall in pressure which forms a functional line of demarcation between the arterial and the venous portions of the systemic circulation (Fig. 1-7).

THE RELATION BETWEEN CROSS-SECTIONAL AREA, FLOW VELOCITY AND FLOW RESISTANCE

The effects of the reduction in the caliber of a single vessel are quite different from those of a corresponding reduction in the caliber of many branching channels. The differences are presented schematically in Figure 1–8. A constricted section in a single tube (Fig. 1–8) results in a much greater resistance (pressure drop per unit length) and a much greater flow velocity. The same volume of fluid flowing through the large segment must rush through the smaller seg-

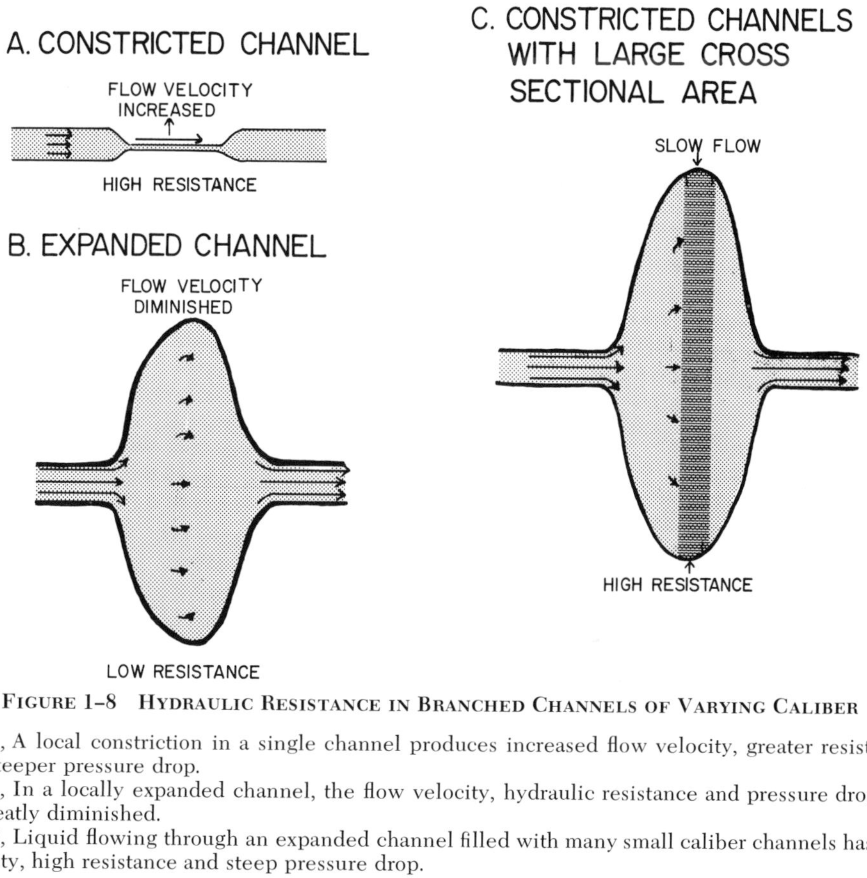

FIGURE 1–8 HYDRAULIC RESISTANCE IN BRANCHED CHANNELS OF VARYING CALIBER

A, A local constriction in a single channel produces increased flow velocity, greater resistance and steeper pressure drop.

B, In a locally expanded channel, the flow velocity, hydraulic resistance and pressure drop are all greatly diminished.

C, Liquid flowing through an expanded channel filled with many small caliber channels has low velocity, high resistance and steep pressure drop.

ment. In contrast, the flow velocity, resistance to flow and the pressure gradient per unit length are greatly reduced as liquid flows through a region of greatly increased cross-sectional area (Fig. 1–8B). Imagine the midportion of this expanded channel filled with tightly packed capillary tubes as suggested in Figure 1–8C. In this case, the flow velocity would still drop as the cross-sectional area expands, but the flow resistance and pressure drop would be greatly increased by the frictional resistance to flow of liquid through the short lengths of small caliber tubes. The same type of situation prevails in the branching arterial system and microcirculation as illustrated in Figure 1–5.

FUNCTIONS OF SYSTEMIC ARTERIES

The systemic arteries serve as a pressure reservoir by means of the elastic properties of the walls (Fig. 1–9A). The contracting left ventricle rapidly ejects blood into the aorta, which becomes distended as the arterial pressure rises. When the ventricle relaxes, the inflow ceases but the wall tension in the arteries continues to drive blood through the peripheral capillaries. The arterial pressure falls progressively until the next ventricular contraction. By this mechanism the systemic arterial pressure fluctuates above and below a mean pressure of about 90 mm. Hg and never falls to zero.

The aortic arch functions as a type of surge chamber immediately downstream from the left ventricle (Fig. 1–9A). Left ventricular ejection produces a very abrupt acceleration of blood into the arterial system which contains long columns of blood. If the arterial system were rigid, very high

pressures would develop throughout the system during contraction of the ventricles. The arterial perfusion pressure would drop to zero between ventricular contractions. The highly distensible aortic arch serves a function very much like the surge chamber often used to damp out large pressure surges produced by piston pumps as shown in Figure 1–9B. In this instance, the air is compressed during the ejection stroke and maintains pressure during the filling stroke. The function of arteries and the regulation of arterial pressure are discussed further in Chapter 5.

The pressure in an elastic tube is an expression of the tension exerted by its walls. Increased internal pressure can be attained by four mechanisms: (a) increased distention by accumulation of fluid, (b) active contraction of the walls without a change in contained volume, (c) external compression and (d) the hydrostatic effects of continuous columns of blood. If the arteries displayed purely elastic properties, the pressure-volume relations would be constant. In other words, so long as the mean arterial pressure remained the same, the mean volume of blood within the arterial system would also be constant. We know that the caliber of arteries *in situ* may be actively reduced by topically applied epinephrine.[4] The actual amount of significance of active constriction of the arteries is not known. In general, the arterial system is considered to have a relatively constant volume so long as the arterial pressure remains fixed.

Relatively small increments of volume change in the arteries produce large changes in pressure. For example, the arterial pulse wave at rest represents a large pressure fluctuation induced by the sudden injection of some 80 cc. of blood into the central end of the arterial system. In contrast,

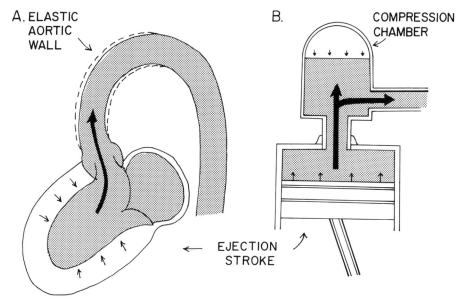

A. ELASTIC AORTIC WALL

B. COMPRESSION CHAMBER

← EJECTION STROKE

FIGURE 1–9   THE AORTIC ARCH AS A COMPRESSION CHAMBER

A, The elastic wall of the aorta distends during ejection of blood from the heart, storing pressure energy for gradual release during the interval between beats.

B, Air in a compression chamber attached to a piston pump is put under pressure during the ejection stroke and expands again during the filling stroke, damping violent fluctuations in pressure and flow.

a similar quantity of blood leaves the venous system at approximately equivalent rates during each cardiac cycle, but the venous pressure varies only a few millimeters of mercury during each cycle. This fact points up the principal differences between the relatively fixed-capacity arterial pressure reservoir and the variable-capacity, low pressure, venous volume reservoir.

THE TENSILE STRENGTH OF VASCULAR WALLS

The walls of the large arteries and veins are so thick and tough that their bursting pressure ranges in the thousands of millimeters of mercury. Interposed between the arteries and veins lie the capillaries which have exceedingly small diameters and very thin walls. Capillary walls are com- posed of a single layer of very thin endothelial cells. The wall thickness is of the order of a micron or less, very much smaller than the diameter of a red blood cell as illustrated in Figure 1–10. The endothelial cells are joined at their edges to form a flimsy cylin- drical channel. The capillary endo- thelium is very easily deformed and exhibits very little tensile strength. The junctions between the edges of the endothelial cells appear in electron micrographs as being even more delicate (Fig. 1–10B). Thin walls and small caliber are required in capillaries for the rapid diffusion of substances between the blood and tissues. The delicate capillary walls support pres- sure amounting to 20 to 30 mm. Hg at heart level and more than 100 mm. Hg in the lower extremities during stand- ing. At first sight, it is difficult to visualize how the fragile capillaries

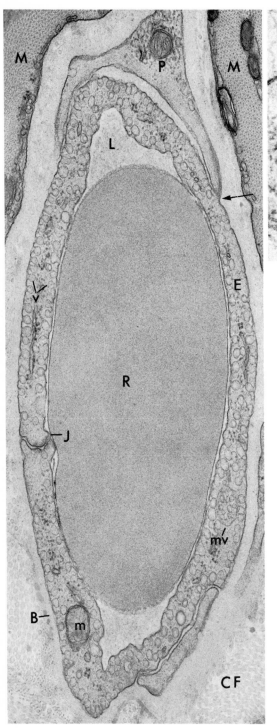

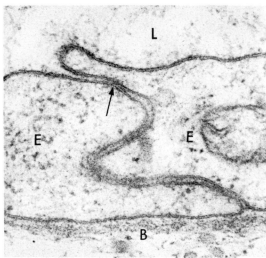

FIGURE 1–10   FINE STRUCTURE
OF CAPILLARIES

A, Capillaries are cylindrical channels formed of flat endothelial cells joined at their edges. The caliber of the capillary is about the same as the diameter of a red blood cell (R). Ring-like structures ("vesicles") are more abundant near both surfaces and have been assigned a role in transport of substances across the capillary walls.

B, The junction between adjacent endothelial cell edges appears to be tightly sealed, apparently lacking slits, pores or sieve-like structures postulated as necessary for the exchange of most constituents in the plasma. (Figs. 15–3 and 15–7 in R. S. Cotran, Fine structure of the microvasculature in relation to normal and altered permeability, in Physical Basic of Circulatory Transport, E. B. Reeve and A. C. Guyton, eds., Philadelphia: W. B. Saunders Co.).

can support such very high internal pressures. The explanation lies in the very small caliber of these vessels.

THE RELATION BETWEEN PRESSURE, WALL TENSION AND CALIBER OF VESSELS

This relationship is graphically illustrated by a partially inflated rubber balloon.[5] During inflation, the mid-portion of the balloon expands while the distal portion remains undistended (Fig. 1–11). The portion of the balloon with a large radius is very tense and resists indentation, indicating that the walls are under high tension. The pressure is equal throughout the inside of the balloon and yet in the undistended region the walls are relatively flaccid and can be easily compressed.[5] This commonplace example illustrates the law of Laplace ($T \propto p \times$

R), which states that the tension in the wall of a hollow cylinder is directly proportional to the product of the tube's radius and the pressure being supported by the wall. Burton,[6] applying this law to the vascular system, pointed out that an aorta with a radius of 1.3 cm. supports a pressure of 100 mm. Hg with a wall tension of 170,000 dynes per centimeter of length (Fig. 1–11). In contrast, capillaries with a radius of 4μ support a pressure of some 30 mm. Hg with a wall tension of only 16 dynes per centimeter of length. In other words, the pressure in the aorta is about three or four times as great as that in the capillaries while the radius is some three thousand times as great. Therefore, the wall tension in the aorta is about ten thousand times as great as that in the capillaries. In tubes of very small caliber, no great strength is required to support a high internal pressure. By the same token, the capillary walls can be very thin so that the distance of diffusion from the central portion of the capillary blood to the outside can be very short. These physical attributes of the capillaries are essential to their function.

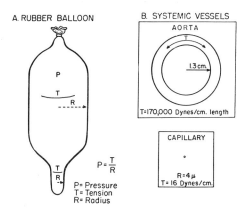

FIGURE 1–11   THE RELATION BETWEEN PRESSURE, WALL TENSION AND RADIUS IN HOLLOW ORGANS

A, In a partially expanded balloon, internal pressure is constant throughout, but the wall tension is very much greater in the distended portion than in the undistended tip because of the difference in radius. As the radius increases, the wall tension must also increase to support a given pressure.

B, Because of the tremendous differences in radius, the wall tension is approximately 10,000 times as great in the aorta as in a capillary, even though they support similar pressures.

THE STRUCTURE AND FUNCTION OF CAPILLARIES

A major portion of the pressure drop between the arteries and veins occurs at the points of controlled resistance at the entrance to the capillary channels (see Fig. 1–7). In addition, a fairly steep pressure gradient along the capillaries is required to maintain flow because of their small caliber. The velocity of blood flow is less in the capillaries than elsewhere because of their tremendous total cross-sectional area (Fig. 1-5). For the same reason, the total surface area of capillary walls is very extensive, particularly in relation to the quantity of blood within each capillary vessel and the total volume of the capillary beds (see Fig. 1–3E). All the blood in the capillaries comes very close to the extravascular tissue spaces, a condition essential for the rapid transfer of substances by diffusion.

Ions and small molecules diffuse across the capillary walls at a surprising rate. Flexner and his associates[7, 8] studied this problem with radioactive tracers and concluded that 60 per cent of the sodium in plasma was exchanged for extravascular sodium in one minute. Similarly, 64 per cent of the chloride in plasma and 140 per cent of the water were calculated to be exchanged each minute.[7] Using more quantitative techniques, Pappenheimer et al.[9] obtained evidence that the amount of water and lipid-insoluble molecules transferred is some two hundred times greater than the values calculated by Flexner and his group (see also Chapter 4). They found that the area of the capillary walls available for diffusion of a molecule the size of water is less than 0.2 per cent of the total wall surface. Ultramicroscopic holes or "pores" in the capillary wall with uniform diameters of 30 Angstrom units (A) account very well for the diffusion rates of fat-insoluble molecules ranging in size from that of sodium chloride to that of hemoglobin. The data could also be explained by a range of pore dimensions with a mean of 24 A and a standard deviation of 12 A. The total area of the "pores" is so small that they may be localized to the spaces between adjacent endothelial cells. Renkin[10] presented evidence that lipid-soluble substances may diffuse through the capillary endothelium so that capillary exchange of oxygen and carbon dioxide may utilize the entire capillary wall.

THE STRUCTURE OF CAPILLARY WALLS

The endothelial cells resemble fried eggs in shape and are only about 1μ thick except at the nucleus (Fig. 1–12). According to earlier studies these flat cells were believed to be joined at their edges by a substance called intercellular cement, which was visualized as composed of long chain molecules bridging the slit between adjacent cells. Interstices between these molecules have been considered responsible for the sieve-like properties of capillary walls and may correspond to the "pores" described previously.

The number and scale of capillaries defies the imagination. Krogh's oft quoted figures are believed to overestimate the numbers somewhat (see Majno[11]), but are still qualitatively revealing.

"It requires some mental effort to conceive how there can be room (on an area no larger than the cross section of an ordinary pin) for about 700 parallel tubes carrying blood, in addition to about 200 (skeletal) muscle fibers." Based on light microscopy, several pathways have been proposed to account for the movement of molecules and particles, large and small, to pass from the blood through the capillary wall and into the spaces between the cells in various tissues (Fig. 1–12). For example, penetration through endothelial cells has been widely accepted for small lipid-soluble molecules like oxygen and carbon dioxide and for water. Passage of other substances (including small inorganic and organic molecules and proteins) may be largely restricted by these cell membranes and occur only through the junctions between the edges of endothelial cells. The simplified schematic representation, as in Figure

STRUCTURE AND PERMEABILITY OF CAPILLARIES

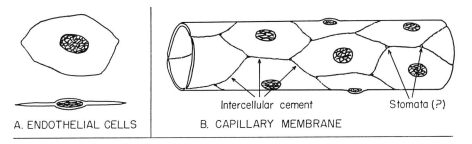

A. ENDOTHELIAL CELLS

Intercellular cement   Stomata (?)

B. CAPILLARY MEMBRANE

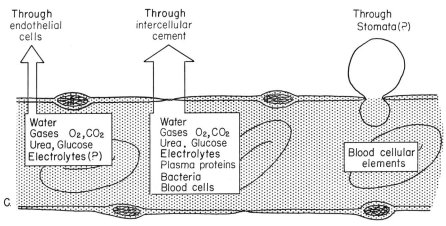

Through endothelial cells

Through intercellular cement

Through Stomata(?)

Water
Gases O_2, CO_2
Urea, Glucose
Electrolytes (?)

Water
Gases O_2, CO_2
Urea, Glucose
Electrolytes
Plasma proteins
Bacteria
Blood cells

Blood cellular elements

C.

FIGURE 1–12   STRUCTURE AND PERMEABILITY OF CAPILLARIES

Capillaries are formed of endothelial cells joined at their edges by "intercellular cement" to form tubes. It seems likely that water, gases, small organic molecules and possibly certain electrolytes can pass through the endothelial cells. Most of the capillary exchange probably occurs through the intercellular cement (see text). It has been postulated that blood cellular elements pass through orifices between endothelial cells, called stomata.

1–12, fails to take proper cognizance of the complexity of individual capillaries or the differences in anatomical and functional characteristics of capillaries in various tissues in the body. (See also Chapter 4 for further discussion.) The functional anatomy of capillaries has been studied intensively in recent years, particularly since electron microscopes became readily available. This body of knowledge has been ably reviewed by Majno[11] and by Contran,[12] while the functional aspects of capillary exchange have been summarized by Landis and Pappenheimer.[13]

In spite of the enormous surface area presented by the walls of millions of capillary tubes, these very thin endothelial membranes greatly retard the movement of most molecules involved in the capillary exchange processes. Water, ions and molecules in the plasma, which are relatively insoluble in lipids, are effectively retarded or blocked by the endothelial cell membranes, yet they are known to exchange rapidly between the blood and extravascular spaces. This discrepancy has been explained on the basis that the rapid capillary exchange of lipid insoluble substances must occur along the lines of junction where the edges of the endothelial cells are joined together (Fig. 1–12). For many years, the intercellular junctions were confidently regarded as the site of slits, pores or sieve-like structures through which most of the exchange took place.

This widely accepted concept was challenged when electron microscopes were employed to provide greatly increased magnification and resolution of the fine structure of capillaries. Electronmicrograms apparently failed to disclose the "pores, slits or sieves" and indicated that the lines of adhesion between the edges of endothelial cells were "anatomically tight junctions." (See Figure 1–10B.) In addition, the endothelial cells contained large numbers of circular shadows or "vesicles" which were interpreted as potential mechanisms for active transport directly through the endothelial cells by a process called "pinocytosis." According to this concept, a vacuole would form on the endothelial cell surface, enclosing a small globule of plasma or extravascular liquid, as the case may be. This vesicle would then move through the endothelial cell protoplasm to the opposite side of the cell and discharge its contents.

During the ensuing years, several pathways for transport of material were considered as illustrated in Figure 1–13A. These included (1) direct passage through endothelial cells, (2) migration of vesicles, (3) vesicles emptying from one to another, (4) passage along junctions (the dotted lines suggest diversion around tight junctions), (5) bypass of junction by diffusion through a thin layer of endothelial cells and (6) bypass of junction by vesicular transport.

This conceptual problem has now come nearly full circle with Karnovsky's[14] electron microscopic evidence that a readily identifiable peroxidase with a molecular weight of 40,000 passed directly through anatomically tight junctions and was distributed along their whole length. The passage of larger molecules (and particles) still suggests the need to postulate dispersed pores of 25 to 500 A, which might be visualized as transiently opening and closing or resealing. Alternatively the need to postulate such larger pores might be satisfied by active vesicular transport (Fig. 1–13), but this remains controversial.

In many tissues, capillaries are surrounded or enclosed by a sheath of cells or reticular fiber membranes (see also Chapter 4). This perivascular membrane forms a line of demarcation

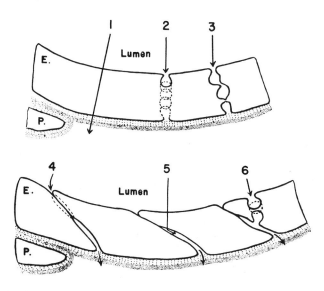

FIGURE 1–13 PREVIOUSLY POSTULATED PATHWAYS THROUGH CAPILLARY WALLS

Six possible pathways across a continuous capillary endothelium. 1. Direct pathway, mainly for gases, water and lipid-soluble substances. 2. Transport by vesicles. 3. Vesicles opening from one to another. 4. Passage along junctions, dotted lines indicate permanent sieve or intermittent opening. 5. Bypass of the junction by diffusion. 6. Bypass of the junction by vesicles. (Presented with permission of G. Majno, Ultrastructure of the vascular membrane, in Handbook of Physiology, Section 2: Circulation, Vol. 2, American Physiological Society, 1965).

between the perivascular space and the gelatinous matrix in the interstitial spaces.

The pericapillary sheath appears to give mechanical support to capillaries. Hyaluronidase applied to the frog mesentery abruptly produced microscopic petechial hemorrhages when liquefaction of the gels extended to the capilllaries, softening the supporting connective tissue sheath. It has long been recognized that increased "permeability" of capillaries may occur without increased fragility (characterized by the rupture of capillaries with the formation of petechial hemorrhages). It has been suggested that the capillary endothelium is responsible for permeability while the condition of the perivascular membrane determines the degree of capillary fragility.

Electron microscopy has demonstrated very distinctive differences in the structure of capillaries in various specialized tissues of the body. Luft and Hechter's[15] observations indicate a need for caution in basing morphologic and functional interpretations on electron micrographs of capillaries. When bovine adrenal glands were fixed one or two hours after the death of the animal, the capillary endothelium consistently exhibited fenestrations, but when adrenal glands prepared in a similar fashion were perfused with warm, oxygenated bovine blood for an hour or so, the capillaries were intact—no fenestrations could be seen. Thus, the structure of capillaries may be labile and may change under different conditions including the preparation of material for examination.

WATER BALANCE AT THE CAPILLARIES

Since water molecules move back and forth so rapidly between blood and tissues and since the pressure inside the capillaries is greater than extravascular pressure, why does water remain in the blood stream rather than pour out into the tissues? The fluid exchange across capillary walls was described by Starling[16] as follows:

In Lecture II, I called your attention to the fact that the non-diffusible constituents of the blood serum, chiefly proteins, were capable of exercising an osmotic pressure or osmotic attraction for water, which amounted to about 4 mm. Hg for every 1 per cent protein in the serum. Blood plasma with 6 to 8 per cent proteins would therefore exert an osmotic pressure of 25 to 30 mm. Hg as compared with an isotonic salt solution. The importance of these results lies in the fact that, although the osmotic pressure of the proteins of the plasma is so insignificant when contrasted with that of its saline constituents, it is of an order of magnitude comparable to that of the capillary blood pressure (see Figure 1-14); and whereas capillary pressure is the chief determining factor in the production of interstitial fluid, the osmotic difference of pressure dependent on the greater concentration of the fluid within as compared with that without the blood vessels might be sufficient to determine absorption. In fact the osmotic attraction of the serum, or plasma, for the extravascular fluid will be proportional to the forces expended in the production of the latter, so that at any given time there may be a balance between the hydrostatic pressure of the blood in the capillaries and the osmotic attraction of the blood for the surrounding fluids. With increased capillary pressure there must be increased transudation. The blood will become more concentrated until equilibrium is established at a somewhat higher point, when there is a more dilute fluid in the tissue spaces and therefore a higher absorbing force to balance the increased capillary pressure. With diminished capillary pressure there will be an osmotic absorption of salt solution from the extravascular fluid; this becomes richer in proteins, and the process will come to an end when the difference between its protein osmotic pressure and that of the intravascular plasma is equal to the diminished capillary pressure.

According to this hypothesis, the filtration or reabsorption of fluid across the capillary walls depends upon the net effect of four interdependent forces: (a) capillary pressure, (b) tissue pressure, (c) osmotic pressure of the plasma and (d) osmotic pressure of the tissue fluids. For sake of convenience, the difference between capillary pres-

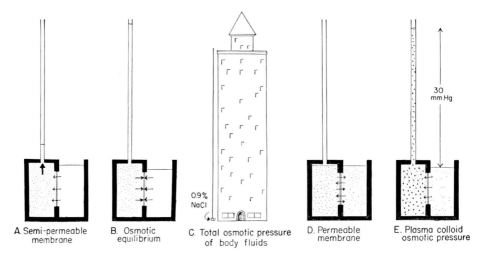

A. Semi-permeable   B. Osmotic   C. Total osmotic pressure   D. Permeable   E. Plasma colloid
   membrane   equilibrium   of body fluids   membrane   osmotic pressure

FIGURE 1–14   OSMOTIC PRESSURES IN BODY FLUID

A, When two solutions of different osmotic concentrations are separated by an appropriate semi-permeable membrane, fluid moves from the region of lower concentration through the membrane to dilute the solution with higher concentration.

B, Osmotic equilibrium is reached when the hydrostatic pressure in the vertical fluid column precisely balances the osmotic pressure exerted by the more concentrated solution.

C, The total osmotic pressure of any of the body fluids is about 7.9 atmospheres when equilibrated with pure water. This pressure is equivalent to the vertical column of 0.9 per cent saline solution extending to the top of a 20-story building.

D, If solutions of different osmotic concentration are separated by permeable membranes, no osmotic pressure is present at equilibrium because both the water and solutes diffuse to produce equal osmotic concentrations throughout the fluid phase. For this reason the tremendous potential osmotic pressure of body fluid (C) serves merely to maintain osmotic equilibrium throughout the fluid compartments of the body.

E, Since the capillary walls are highly permeable to solutes other than plasma proteins, the osmotic pressure of the plasma is determined by the difference in concentration of the proteins and amounts to only about 25 to 30 mm. Hg.

sure and tissue pressure will be called *effective capillary pressure* or *filtration pressure*. The difference between plasma and tissue osmotic pressure will be termed *effective plasma osmotic pressure*. The maximal effective plasma osmotic pressure ranges around 30 mm. Hg in regions where the capillaries are virtually impermeable to proteins. The average effective capillary pressure is in this range at heart level. Starling's hypothesis calls for a fairly complete balance of filtration and reabsorption in relatively impermeable capillaries at heart level when the mean capillary pressure approximates effective colloid osmotic pressure (Fig. 1–15). Under these con-

ditions, no filtrate or lymph would be formed.

VARIATIONS IN CAPILLARY PRESSURE

Most of the confirmatory evidence for Starling's hypothesis has been derived from experiments with capillaries at or near heart levels in small animals.[17] Clearly, filtration is most likely to predominate in regions where marked elevation in capillary pressure is not balanced by a corresponding increase in extravascular pressure.

Since fluid flows from regions of high pressure to regions of lower pressure, the pressure in peripheral veins

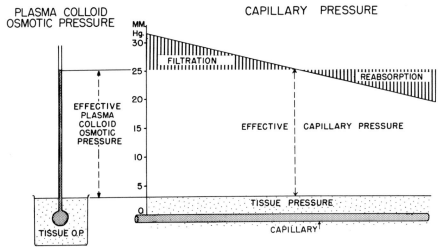

FIGURE 1–15   FACTORS DETERMINING FLUID EXCHANGE IN CAPILLARIES

The effective colloid osmotic pressure of the plasma is determined by the difference in protein concentration in tissues and in the plasma. The effective capillary pressure is the difference between capillary pressure and tissue pressure. The pressure gradient in capillaries under a specific set of conditions may produce filtration at the arteriolar end of the capillary and reabsorption in the venular end of the capillary with no net fluid exchange. Such complete fluid balance is the exception rather than the rule.

establishes the minimal capillary pressure in each capillary network. Similarly, the filling pressure of the right ventricle establishes the lower end of the shallow gradient in venous pressure (Fig. 1–7). Thus, the capillary pressure is affected by changes in either local venous pressure or the diastolic pressure in the right ventricle.

Some factors which affect capillary fluid balance are illustrated schematically in Figure 1–16. When a man stands up, the long hydrostatic columns of blood tend to produce great increases in capillary pressure without corresponding increases in effective osmotic pressure of the blood. This problem will be considered in Chapter 6.

CAPILLARY PERMEABILITY IN DIFFERENT REGIONS

The effective plasma osmotic pressure is markedly reduced in capillaries with greater permeability to protein.

Judged from the protein concentration of lymph from different regions, capillary permeability is not uniform throughout the body (Fig. 1–16). For example, lymph actively flowing from skin and connective tissues generally contains less than 1 per cent protein. Lymph from heart, lungs, intestines and kidney usually contains protein in concentrations between 3 and 4 per cent. Liver lymph carries as much as 6 per cent protein when the plasma concentration is only about 7 per cent, suggesting an effective colloid osmotic pressure of about 4 mm. Hg in the liver sinusoids. In tissues where protein escapes from capillaries in concentrations of 3 per cent or more, lymph flows continuously. However, lymph is not universally accepted as an example of tissue fluid.

THE LYMPHATIC SYSTEM

The filtrates from plasma which pass into the tissue spaces are either

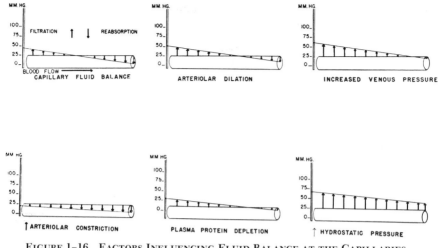

FIGURE 1-16　FACTORS INFLUENCING FLUID BALANCE AT THE CAPILLARIES

Filtration and reabsorption of fluid are balanced only when the effective plasma osmotic pressure precisely equals the mean effective capillary pressure. Dilatation of arterioles causes a steeper capillary pressure gradient with little change in venous pressure. Increased venous pressure and hydrostatic pressure in dependent parts elevates the pressures along the whole length of the capillary. Plasma protein depletion and increased capillary permeability reduce the tendency for reabsorption and foster excess filtration. Net reabsorption of fluid is aided by arteriolar constriction or by elevating the capillaries above heart level. (From Sodeman, W. A.: Pathologic Physiology: Mechanisms of Disease. Philadelphia, W. B. Saunders Co., 1956.)

reabsorbed into the blood or returned to the circulation by the lymphatic system. The lymphatic system is fundamentally a drainage system phylogenetically developed to return to the circulating blood fluids which have escaped from capillaries.[18] Although lymph flow appears to be rather sluggish, the amount of lymph returned to the blood stream in a day is roughly equivalent to the total plasma volume.

Lymphatic collecting vessels tend to travel in close anatomic relation to the veins and have a similar function, i.e., the return of blood elements from the tissues to the venous reservoirs near the heart (Fig. 1–17). The lymphatic and venous systems both have superficial and deep distributions. On the surface of the body, the superficial lymphatic collecting vessels usually accompany the superficial veins just beneath the skin. They also lie just beneath the mucous membrane throughout the whole length of the di-

gestive, respiratory and genito-urinary tracts. These networks of collecting lymphatics drain lymphatic capillaries abundantly distributed in the submucosa and in the dermis of the skin, forming a continuous network throughout all the internal and external linings of the body except the cornea of the eye.

The *deep* lymphatic vessels intertwine and anastomose around the veins which accompany the deep arteries in their regional distribution to the organs of the body (Fig. 1–17). Arteries, veins and deep lymphatics tend to share the same sheaths and are distributed to the same tissues and organs.

The lymphatic system has two transport functions: (*a*) the return of capillary filtrate to the circulation and (*b*) the removal of foreign particles and exudates from tissue spaces and serous cavities. Since the lymphatic capillary networks are distributed through the interstitial spaces along with the blood

LYMPHATIC SYSTEM PARALLELS THE VEINS

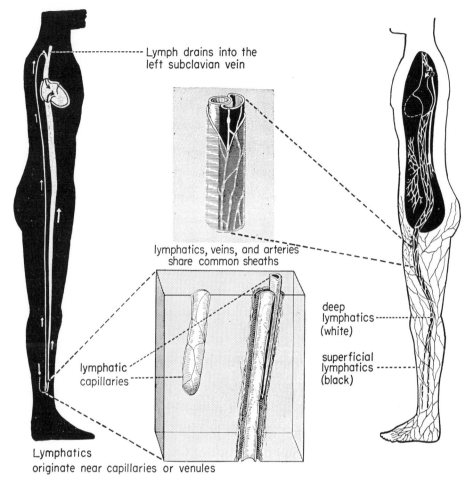

Lymph drains into the
left subclavian vein

lymphatics, veins, and arteries
share common sheaths

deep
lymphatics
(white)

superficial
lymphatics
(black)

lymphatic
capillaries

Lymphatics
originate near capillaries or venules

FIGURE 1–17   THE LYMPHATIC SYSTEM

The lymphatic system is essentially a "paravenous system" since the lymphatic capillaries lie in close association with the capillaries and veins of the blood vascular system; the collecting lymphatics tend to accompany veins and arteries and drain into the central veins. Like the veins, the lymphatic system consists of both deep and superficial distributions of vessels and carries constituents of the blood back to the region of the heart.

capillaries, the terminal vessels of the two systems must lie very near each other (Fig. 1–17). Most commonly, the lymphatic capillaries are believed to end blindly in interstitial spaces at varying distances from the capillaries of the blood vascular system. There is also evidence that lymphatic capillaries may develop along the perivascular spaces where growth appears to be less impeded. Lymphatic vessels which terminate within the pericapil-

lary spaces are ideally located for the transportation of filtrate from the capillary beds. Lymphatics lying free within the interstitial spaces may remove foreign particles and inflammatory exudates. Under certain conditions, apertures have been observed in lymphatic capillaries surrounded by inflammatory exudate.[19] When the tissues are clear of free fluid the lymphatic capillaries have continuous unbroken endothelial membranes.

There are many gaps in our knowledge of lymphatic function. The forces driving a fluid laden with protein and cellular elements through the continuous wall of a lymphatic capillary have not been clearly elucidated. This problem is most acute in the skin of a dependent extremity where vascular pressures are very high and the tissue pressures very low. The exact mechanisms elevating lymph from dependent extremities to the level of the subclavian vein are not universally agreed upon, although a number of possibilities exist. The lymphatic collecting vessels are intimately associated with the veins and are subject to the same muscular and abdominothoracic pumping actions (see Chapter 6). Confined within the same sheath as arteries and veins, the lymphatics would tend to be compressed by changes in the caliber of these vessels. Even the arterial pulse may act as an accessory pump, displacing lymph upward with each wave of distention. Irisawa[20] showed that both leg movements and weight bearing elevate lymphatic pressure propelling the lymph toward the heart. Finally, there is some evidence that certain lymphatics have independent contractility which could propel lymph by a peristaltic type of action. The lymphatic pressure in the thoracic duct must exceed the pressure in the subclavian veins into which it empties.

THE VENOUS SYSTEM

The veins not only act as conduits to channel blood from the capillaries to the heart, but they also adjust their total capacity to accommodate variations in total blood volume. The pressure at the point of outflow from a system of tubes establishes the lower end of the pressure gradient which promotes flow through the tubes. The point of outflow from the systemic veins is the right ventricle during each diastole. If the pressure in the right atrium fell below the pressure outside the wall of this vessel, the filling pressure of the right ventricle would be zero. Actually, the pressure within the right atrium and ventricle remains within a narrow range at very low levels in spite of changes in the total blood volume or the distribution of blood in the circulation. For example, the average normal adult can walk into a blood bank, give up 500 cc. of blood and, after a few minutes, walk out again.

The maintenance of a fairly constant right atrial and right ventricular pressure under varying conditions requires adjustments in the capacity of various portions of the venous system. Measurements on *isolated* segments of veins reveal smaller pressure increments with increasing volume than occur in arteries. The greater venous distensibility represents only part of the adaptability of the venous system. The venous system is of primary importance in its capacitance function since it contains 65 to 75 per cent of the total blood volume. In peripheral vascular beds, most of the blood is contained in the venules and small veins (see Fig. 1–3E) where relatively small changes in caliber of large numbers of small veins can greatly change the quantity of blood they contain. The variable capacity of the venous system is also vested in specialized venous reservoirs and in alterations in the caliber of venous channels through venoconstriction.

It has long been recognized that the spleen acts as a depot from which blood may be expressed in times of stress. This function is not well developed in the human spleen since it contains only some 200 to 250 cc. The subpapillary plexus of the skin has a potential role as a blood depot, but this function is intimately related to dissipation of heat. In other words, this blood is rarely released into the general circulation at the expense of temperature regulation. The pulmonary veins are generally believed to have a role in cushioning transient differences in the output of the right and left ventricles. Although measuring the capacity of internal organs is very difficult, there is some evidence that the capacity of the venous channels may also be controlled by "venomotor" activity. Variations in venous "tone" would contribute to adjustment in the capacity of the circulation in response to alteration in blood volume.

VENOUS RESISTANCE AND CAPACITANCE EFFECTS

The resistance to blood flow through the venules and veins is much less than that encountered in the precapillary resistance vessels (arterioles and precapillary sphincters). This fact is clearly shown in the steep pressure drop just upstream from the capillaries as illustrated schematically in Figure 1–8. However, the resistance to blood flow through postcapillary venules and small veins is not negligible because of their strategic position just downstream from the capillaries. For example, constriction of venules would elevate capillary pressure and promote increased filtration of fluid from the capillary blood. Conversely, venodilation accompanied by precapillary constriction could result in increased resorption of extravascular fluid into capillary blood, dehydrating the tissue and expanding the plasma volume. This kind of phenomenon is most obvious in the glomeruli of the kidney where a meshwork of capillaries is located between precapillary and postcapillary sphincters with extremely well developed control over the filtra-

tion rate. Folkow and Mellander[21] have stressed the importance of the changing ratio of precapillary and postcapillary resistance in other peripheral vascular beds. In skeletal muscle this factor plays an important role in the partititioning of fluid between the intravascular and extravascular spaces. Furthermore, contraction of skeletal muscles compresses the veins between the muscle bundles, expressing blood from the veins, propelling it toward the heart and reducing venous and capillary pressures in dependent extremities. The muscle pumping action on venous flow is discussed in greater detail in responses to arising (see Chapter 6). The capacity of the veins in the legs may be reflexly diminished by vasomotor reflexes when man stands. If so, this is a portion of the compensatory response to the erect stance.

Shepard[22] summarized evidence indicating that the output of the heart increased as the total peripheral resistance diminished (vasodilation) and the wall tension of the venous capacity vessels increased (venoconstriction). Among these conditions were exercise, hyperventilation, strong emotions, cold showers, severe anemia and the cardiovascular hormones epinephrine and isoproterenol. The stiffness and blood content of the peripheral venous channels is primarily controlled by autonomic reflexes involving pathways to the base of the brain and above, including the cerebral cortex as a part of complex neural control patterns as will be discussed in greater detail in many subsequent portions of this book, particularly Chapter 4.

PULMONARY CIRCULATION

The systemic and pulmonary vascular beds are connected in series to

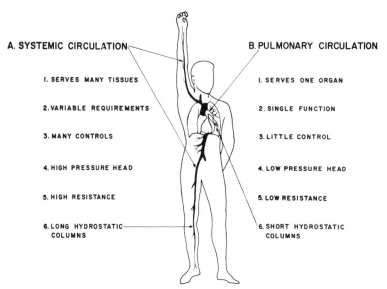

A. SYSTEMIC CIRCULATION

1. SERVES MANY TISSUES

2. VARIABLE REQUIREMENTS

3. MANY CONTROLS

4. HIGH PRESSURE HEAD

5. HIGH RESISTANCE

6. LONG HYDROSTATIC
   COLUMNS

B. PULMONARY CIRCULATION

1. SERVES ONE ORGAN

2. SINGLE FUNCTION

3. LITTLE CONTROL

4. LOW PRESSURE HEAD

5. LOW RESISTANCE

6. SHORT HYDROSTATIC
   COLUMNS

FIGURE 1–18   DIFFERENCES BETWEEN SYSTEMIC CIRCULATION AND PULMONARY CIRCULATION

The systemic circulation differs from the pulmonary circulation in a number of distinctive characteristics. These differences may be related to the differences in the functions, organization and environment of the two vascular beds.

form a continuous circuit. Although these two vascular systems are superficially similar, the following important differences between them are summarized in Figure 1–18. The systemic circulation is a high-resistance circuit with a large difference in pressure between the arteries and veins, while the pulmonary circuit normally offers very slight resistance to flow. The pulmonary vessels supply only one type of tissue (alveolar membranes), so the requirements for vasomotor control are not as great as those in the systemic circulation. The volume of blood in the pulmonary system is neither so great nor so variable as that in the systemic circulation. Since the lungs immediately enclose the heart, hydrostatic columns are fairly short even from the most distant portions of the pulmonary parenchyma. The pulmonary circulation is confined within the thoracic cage, so extravascular conditions are fairly uniform throughout.

ANATOMY OF THE PULMONARY CIRCULATION

The ramifications of the pulmonary arterial system closely parallel the arborization of the bronchial system. The mainstem bronchi give off lateral branches which divide and subdivide like the branches of a tree. At the tip of each terminal branch is a bronchiole which divides into two respiratory bronchioles. In turn, these divide into two branches, each of which gives off alveolar ducts. The alveolar ducts are connected through a variable number of atria to a tuft of alveolar sacs (air cells). A wax model of part of the bronchial tree of an infant, reconstructed by Boyden and Tompsett[23] is reproduced in Figure 1–19 to illustrate the complexity of the terminal airways and alveoli even at that early age. Gaseous interchange between the air and blood may occur in all divisions beyond the bronchioles.

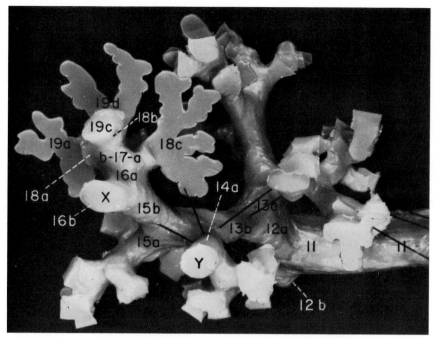

FIGURE 1–19   TERMINAL BRONCHIOLES AND ALVEOLI

A wax model of terminal respiratory airways of an infant. Ramus 16a, a respiratory bronchiole of the first order, gives rise to six terminal clusters of alveolar sacs. (Reproduced by the courtesy of Dr. Allen Boyden.[23])

Structurally, the main pulmonary arteries closely resemble the aorta. The walls of the main arteries and their branches remain essentially the same down to the intrapulmonary branches with outside diameters of about 1 mm., except that the amount of smooth muscle in the wall progressively increases in the smaller branches.[24] Muscular arteries ranging in diameter from 1 to 0.1 mm. have a prominent media of circularly arranged smooth muscle between the internal and external elastic laminae. The walls of arterial branches less than 0.1 mm. in diameter consist essentially of poorly supported endothelial tubes which abruptly break up into a profusely anastomotic capillary network. Thus, the pulmonary circulation does not contain any vessels corresponding to the muscular arterioles in the systemic circulation. The alveolar capillaries are the principal structural elements in the walls of the respiratory membranes (see Fig. 1–24A). The capillary network is so dense that in many alveoli the space between capillaries is less than their diameter.[25]

RESISTANCE TO BLOOD FLOW THROUGH THE PULMONARY CIRCUIT

For several reasons the normal intravascular pressures do not fall abruptly in the small vessels of the lung (Fig. 1–20): (a) There are no high-resistance muscular arterioles in the terminal ramifications of the vascular tree. (b) The pulmonary capillaries are extremely voluminous, diffusely anastomotic and of relatively large caliber. (c) The pulmonary vessels are passively distended in response to increased pulmonary blood flow. (d) There is a large reserve capacity in the lung which is not fully utilized except

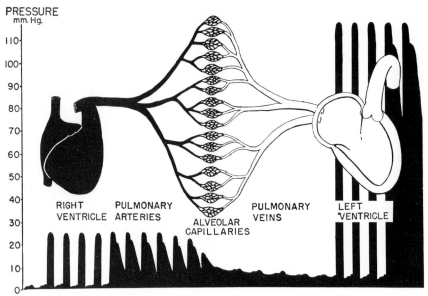

FIGURE 1–20   PRESSURES IN THE PULMONARY VASCULAR SYSTEM

Since the pulmonary arterial system offers slight resistance to blood flow, the mean pressure difference between pulmonary artery and left atrium amounts to only 4 to 6 mm. Hg. This low-pressure head drives the same volume of blood through the pulmonary circuit as flows through the systemic circulation with a gradient of some 90 mm. Hg.

under conditions of stress. For example, an entire lung with all its capillary bed can be removed without increasing the pulmonary arterial pressure. (e) Finally, all vessels in the pulmonary vascular tree have a somewhat larger caliber than corresponding vessels in the systemic circulation. The net effect is a total pulmonary resistance to flow only about one eighth of that in the systemic circulation.

During systole, the right ventricular pressure rises to about 22 mm. Hg. The pulmonary arterial pressures average about 22/8 mm. Hg with a mean arterial pressure of about 13 mm. Hg.[26] The pressure at the point of outflow from the pulmonary circuit (the left ventricular diastolic pressure) is about 7 mm. Hg (Fig. 1–20). Thus, a pressure gradient of only about 6 mm. Hg will force through the pulmonary circuit the same quantity of blood propelled through the systemic circuit by a gradient of 90 mm. Hg. Furthermore,

the pulmonary arterial pressure may remain unchanged or diminish slightly when the cardiac output increases threefold. One case has been described in which a pressure gradient of 4 mm. Hg propelled 15 liters of blood per minute through the pulmonary circuit.[27] The small pressure gradient between the pulmonary artery and the left atrium is the basis for the statement that the pulmonary circuit is a low resistance system.

FUNCTIONS OF THE PULMONARY CIRCULATION

The pulmonary circuit simultaneously performs three functions: (a) gaseous exchange of oxygen and carbon dioxide between the alveolar air and blood, (b) storage of blood in a variable volume reservoir and (c) blockade of foreign particles, thrombi and other types of emboli circulating in the systemic venous blood.

Gas Exchange: The Principal Function of the Lungs. Blood passing through the alveolar capillaries of the lungs is effectively spread into a layer about 10μ thick and 100 sq. m. in area. The alveolar air is separated from the hemoglobin in the blood by the alveolar epithelium, a thin basal membrane, the capillary endothelium, a layer of plasma and the red cell membrane. These barriers appear formidable when highly magnified in an electron microgram (Fig. 1–21), but these thin layers represent very slight obstacles to the rapid exchanges of alveolar gases with the blood. The oxygen tension is lower and the carbon dioxide tension is greater in blood

entering the alveolar capillaries than in the alveolar air. Blood traverses the alveolar capillaries in about 1 second. Propelled by their diffusion gradients, oxygen and carbon dioxide are exchanged so rapidly that blood leaving the alveolar capillaries is normally in virtual equilibrium with the alveolar air (Fig. 1–22A). The action of carbonic anhydrase in the erythrocytes and rapid dissociation of carbon dioxide from reduced hemoglobin as it is converted to oxyhemoglobin facilitate exchange of carbon dioxide. The gaseous exchange remains this rapid only when the diffusion distances are extremely small. Thus, very thin layers of fluid accumulating between the al-

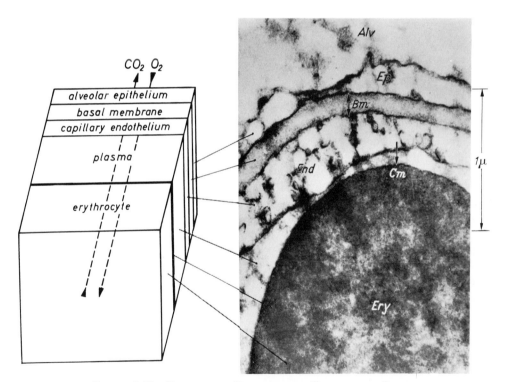

FIGURE 1–21   BARRIERS TO DIFFUSION OF GASES IN THE LUNGS

Interposed between the alveolar air and the hemoglobin in the blood are the alveolar epithelium, a basal membrane, the alveolar capillary endothelium, plasma, the red cell membrane and protoplasm. Despite these barriers, equilibrium is very rapidly established in blood flowing through the pulmonary capillaries despite their very short length. (From G. Thews, Gaseous diffusion in the lungs and tissues, in Physical Bases of Circulatory Transport: Regulation and Exchange, E. B. Reeve and A. C. Guyton, eds. Philadelphia. W. B. Saunders Co., 1967.)

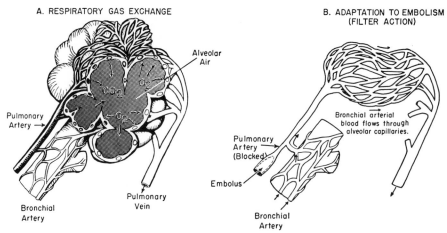

FIGURE 1–22   FUNCTIONS OF THE LUNG

A, Gas exchange, the principal function of the lungs, occurs because of the higher concentration of oxygen and lower concentration of carbon dioxide in the alveolar air than in the venous blood arriving at the pulmonary capillaries.

B, Embolic obstruction of pulmonary arteries does not produce necrosis of pulmonary parenchyma because bronchial arterial blood is diverted through dilated channels into the alveolar capillaries. Because of this dual blood supply, the lungs can serve as filters for emboli without self-destruction.

veolar air and the blood can seriously retard respiratory exchange.

Oxygen and carbon dioxide cannot be exchanged when the blood flows through collapsed alveoli because it does not come in close proximity to alveolar air. Thus, blood passing through non-aerated alveoli would retain the character of venous blood. However, resistance to flow increases markedly in atelectatic lung tissue, automatically shunting blood from non-aerated portions into the inflated regions of the lung.

Reservoir Function of the Lungs. Since the pulmonary vessels constitute a low-pressure, distensible system, any slight increase in outflow pressure at the left ventricle or relative increase in input from the right ventricle can cause considerable quantities of blood to accumulate within the lungs. Presumably, engorgement of the lungs will cause elevated pressure throughout the pulmonary circuit because the pressure gradient is so shallow. However, it seems likely that considerable distention may occur with little eleva-

tion in pressure. For example, there is evidence that substantial quantities of blood are displaced into the heart and lungs after reclining. Sjöstrand[28] reported that an average of more than 600 ml. of blood was shifted from the lower extremities to the rest of the body when standing subjects reclined. He concluded that more than half of this volume was accommodated in the lungs.

As much as 25 per cent of the blood in the thorax (heart and lungs) may be shifted to the legs. This reserve volume in the pulmonary circuit appears to be distributed diffusely through the lungs, where it is held "on tap" until drawn from in order to effect the rapid readjustment of the circulation required for larger cardiac output. Reserve blood in the lungs has been compared with water dammed up behind a sluice gate where it compensates for occasional variations in supply and output. On this basis, the lungs have an important reservoir function. This distensible vascular network may also serve to cushion transient differences in right and left ventricular output, e.g., at the onset of violent exercise.

Filter Action of the Lungs. If foreign bodies, thrombi, air bubbles or fat particles enter the systemic arterial system, they generally occlude a terminal artery within some organ. This reduces or eliminates circulation to the tissues supplied by that arterial branch, and the tissue cells frequently die. If it occurs in a vital organ such as the brain or heart, this is a serious event. Fortunately, most of the emboli enter the blood stream on the venous side of the circulation and lodge in the lungs. By virtue of a double circulation, the pulmonary vascular tree is particularly adapted to filtering out these circulating vascular plugs without self-destruction.

In parallel with the pulmonary arterial system, the bronchial arteries transmit oxygenated blood throughout the walls of the bronchial tree as far peripherally as the bronchioles.[25] Anastomotic connections between pulmonary and bronchial arteries are not believed to occur normally. However, anastomoses of small caliber exist in the walls of the bronchioles and alveolar ducts, where they share common capillary beds (Fig. 1–22B). The venous drainage from the bronchial arterial system is by way of the pulmonary vein except in the first two or three divisions of the bronchial tree. Obstruction or occlusion of a branch of the pulmonary artery does not affect the blood supply to the bronchial system. Dilatation of channels in the common capillary networks provides a mechanism for diverting oxygenated blood through the alveolar membranes when pulmonary arterial flow is arrested or reduced (Fig. 1–22B). Thus, lung tissue is rarely destroyed by obstruction of the pulmonary blood supply. The diffuse anastomotic connections between adjacent alveoli provide additional protection against occlusion of small peripheral branches of the pulmonary arterial system. The affected lung tissue survives while the embolus is resorbed or recanalized, after which the tissue resumes its activity. There is every reason to believe that this sequence of events occurs repeatedly during any person's lifetime without producing symptoms unless the embolus is very large or is located in a critical position.

SUMMARY

The systemic circulation consists of three functional divisions, the arterial pressure reservoir, the venous volume reservoir and the capillary networks. The precipitous drop of pressure due to high resistance to flow through the arterioles, capillaries and venules forms the functional region of demarcation between the arterial and venous systems. So long as the pressure difference between arteries and veins remains constant, the blood flow through the capillaries is determined by the resistance to flow through the minute vessels. The quantity of blood flowing per unit time through the arteries, capillaries and veins must be identical except for insignificant differences in flow involved in shifting blood from one region to another. The central arterial and venous pressures tend to remain fixed within relatively narrow ranges regardless of the total amount of blood flowing through the system per unit time (cardiac output). The average volume of blood in the arterial system tends to remain fairly constant so long as the mean arterial blood pressure is unchanged. In contrast, the central venous pressure tends to remain relatively constant in spite of variations in the total quantity and distribution of blood through adjustments in the capacity of venous reservoirs. Cardiovascular response to disease cannot be fully understood without consideration of the mechanisms by which the normal circulatory system adjusts to various conditions including changes in body posture, changes in regional blood flow and cardiac output.

REFERENCES

1. HILL, A. V. The diffusion of oxygen and lactic acid through tissues. *Proc. Roy. Soc.,* B104:39-96, 1928.
2. GREEN, H. D. Circulation: physical principles. Pp. 208-232 in *Medical Physics,* Vol. 1, O. Glasser, Ed. Chicago, Year Book Publishers, 1944.
3. WEIDEMAN, MARY P. Architecture of the terminal vascular bed. Chapter 18 in *Physical Bases of Circulatory Transport: Regulation and Exchange,* E. B. Reeve and A. C. Guyton, Eds. Philadelphia, W. B. Saunders Co., 1967.
4. HEYMANS, C., and VAN DEN HEUVAL-HEYMANS, G. New aspects of blood pressure regulation. *Circulation,* 4:581-586, 1951.
5. WOLF, A. V. Demonstrations concerning pressure-tension relations in various organs. *Science,* 115:243-244, 1952.
6. BURTON, A. C. On the physical equilibrium of small blood vessels. *Amer. J. Physiol.,* 164:319-329, 1951.
7. COWIE, D. B., FLEXNER, L. B., and WILDE, W. S. Capillary permeability, rate of transcapillary exchange of chloride in the guinea pig as determined with radiochloride. *Amer. J. Physiol.,* 158:231-236, 1949.
8. FLEXNER, L. B., COWIE, D. B., and VOSBURGH, G. J. Studies on capillary permeability with tracer substances. *Cold Spr. Harb. Symp. Quant. Biol.,* 13:88-98, 1948.
9. PAPPENHEIMER, J. R., RENKIN, E. M., and BORRERO, L. M. Filtration, diffusion and molecular sieving through peripheral capillary membranes. A contribution to the pore theory of capillary permeability. *Amer. J. Physiol.,* 167:13-46, 1951.
10. RENKIN, E. M. Capillary permeability to lipid-soluble molecules. *Amer. J. Physiol.,* 168:538-545, 1952.
11. MAJNO, G. Ultrastructure of the vascular membrane. Chapter 64 in *Handbook of Physiology, Section 2: Circulation,* Vol. 3, W. F. Hamilton and P. Dow, Eds. Washington, D.C., American Physiological Society, 1965.
12. COTRAN, R. S. The fine structure of microvasculature in relation to normal and abnormal permeability. Chapter 15 in *Physical Bases of Circulatory Transport: Regulation and Exchange,* E. B. Reeve and A. C. Guyton, Eds. Philadelphia, W. B. Saunders Co., 1967.
13. LANDIS, E. M., and PAPPENHEIMER, J. R. Exchange of substances through the capillary walls. Chapter 29 in *Handbook of Physiology, Section 2: Circulation,* Vol. 2, W. F. Hamilton and P. Dow, Eds. Washington, D.C., American Physiological Society, 1963.
14. KARNOVSKY, M. J. Ultrastructural basis of capillary permeability studied with peroxidase as a tracer. *J. Cell Biol.,* 35:213-236, 1967.
15. LUFT, J., and HECHTER, O. An electron microscopic correlation of structure with function in the isolated perfused cow adrenal, preliminary observations. *J. Biophys. Biochem. Cytol.,* 3:615-620, 1957.
16. STARLING, E. H. *The Fluids of the Body.* Chicago, W. T. Keener & Co. 1909, 186 pp.
17. LANDIS, E. M. Capillary permeability and factors affecting composition of capillary filtrate. *Ann. N. Y. Acad. Sci.,* 46:713-731, 1946.
18. MAYERSON, H. S. The physiologic importance of lymph. Chapter 30 in *Handbook of Physiology, Section 2: Circulation,* Vol. 2, W. F. Hamilton and P. Dow, Eds. Washington, D.C., American Physiological Society, 1963.
19. CLARK, E. R., and CLARK, E. L. Further observations on living lymphatic vessels in the transparent chamber in the rabbit's ear — their relation to the tissue spaces. *Amer. J. Anat.,* 52:273-305, 1933.
20. IRISAWA, A., and RUSHMER, R. F. Relationship between lymphatic and venous pressure in leg of dog. *Amer. J. Physiol.,* 196:495-498, 1959.
21. FOLKOW, B., MELLANDER, S., and SWEDEN, G. Veins and venous tone. *Amer. Heart J.,* 68:397-408, 1964.
22. SHEPHERD, J. T. Role of veins in the circulation. *Circulation,* 33:484-491, 1966.
23. BOYDEN, E. A., and TOMPSETT, D. H. The changing patterns in the developing lungs of infants. *Acta anat.,* 61:164-192, 1965.
24. BRENNER, O. Pathology of the vessels of the pulmonary circulation. *Arch. Int. Med.,* 56:211-237, 1935.
25. MILLER, W. S. *The Lung,* 2nd ed. Springfield, Illinois, Charles C Thomas, 1947, 222 pp.
26. COURNAND, A. Some aspects of the pulmonary circulation in normal man and in chronic cardiopulmonary diseases. *Circulation,* 2:641-657, 1952.
27. HICKAM, J. B. Atrial septal defect. A study of intracardiac shunts, ventricular outputs, and pulmonary pressure gradients. *Amer. Heart J.,* 38:801-812, 1949.
28. SJÖSTRAND, T.: Volume and distribution of blood and their significance in regulating the circulation. *Physiol. Rev.,* 33:202-228, 1953.

CHAPTER 2

FUNCTIONAL ANATOMY OF CARDIAC CONTRACTION

Blood is propelled along the branched vascular channels by the energy represented by pressure gradients, shallow in the arteries and veins and very steep at the sites of controlled resistance. As blood flows through the various series and parallel channels, pressure energy is dissipated in the form of heat due to friction. The energy lost during the circulation of the blood is restored by the contracting heart.

The two fundamental requirements of the cardiovascular system are (a) circulation of blood without interruption and (b) adjustment of blood flow in response to varying demands of the tissues. If the circulation is interrupted, even momentarily, survival of the individual is jeopardized because nervous tissue in the brain can suffer lasting damage from transient deprivation of oxygen. Thus, the heart must continue to beat repetitively and without a sustained interruption for a lifetime. Furthermore, the heart must adapt its output to balance the changing total flow through the billions of capillaries in the body.

The energy released during ventricular systole represents the com-bined output of the various bundles of myocardial fibers. The contribution of each bundle depends not only on its contractile power, but also on its anatomic orientation within the cardiac walls. This chapter is devoted to describing the functional anatomy of cardiac contraction as a background which is essential for an understanding of cardiac adaptability and control.

THE DEVELOPMENT OF THE NORMAL HEART

During embryologic development, the various tissues and organs rapidly pass through stages representing the evolutionary development of the species. For this reason, the extensive investigation of embryology in the chick is generally applicable to human embryos, but there is one important difference: the chick embyro is attached to the surface of an abundant yolk.

The heart develops from a pair of primordial tubes derived from clusters of endothelial cells which proliferate, become organized into strands of cells and acquire a lumen. These primitive tubes meet in the midline

33

and fuse into a single elongated chamber which will ultimately develop into the ventricles. From the simple cardiac tube, the endocardial primordia proliferate toward the head to form the aortic arch system. The caudal extensions of the primordial tubes become the omphalomesenteric veins. As the formation of gut proceeds caudally, fusion of the primordial tubes continues, forming the primitive atrium and finally the sinus venosus.

CONVOLUTION OF THE CARDIAC TUBE

The primitive cardiac tube grows longer more rapidly than either the investing pericardium or the surrounding somatic structures. It is anchored above by the arterial trunks and below by developing venous channels. Since the tube is fixed at both ends, its rapid elongation causes flexion, initially toward the right side of the embryo. As elongation continues, the cardiac tube becomes more tortuous (Fig. 2–1A). At the same time, constrictions develop which indicate the ultimate division of this single convoluted tube into atria and ventricles. As the ventricular region progressively expands and grows longer, it swings back toward the midline to cover the atrial region, which remains relatively fixed in position. In this process, the primitive atrium and arterial trunks, which were originally on opposite ends of the cardiac tube, are brought into apposition. Thus, the inflow tract and outflow tract are adjacent and all four valve rings ultimately merge into a single fibrous skeleton (see Fig 2–7). The developing atria expand laterally to form two extensive sacculations, the primitive right and left atria. These sacculations ultimately become the right and left auricles, while the main atrial chambers develop by progressive incorporation of the venous channels into the posterior wall (Fig. 2–1A, bottom).

THE INITIAL CARDIAC CONTRACTION

According to Patten,[1] the first signs of contraction of the heart in chick embryos appear while it is represented by only the ventricular portion of the cardiac tube (Fig. 2–1). Localized slow contractions usually are noted first on the right margin near the root of the primitive arterial trunks. However, the site and spread of these earliest undulations vary considerably. The initial contractions in the embryonic rat heart occur a few hours before the elaboration of fibrillae or cross striations.[2] About an hour after the first fibrillar contraction appears, the entire primitive ventricle contracts regularly and synchronously, but slowly. The nature of the contraction changes a few hours later as the atrium is formed. At this time, contractions originate in the atrial region and sweep over the ventricle like a peristaltic wave. The atrium assumes the role of pacemaker because its inherent rate of impulse formation is higher than that of the ventricle. The sinus venosus has an even faster inherent rhythm and assumes control as soon as it is formed. The sinus venosus ultimately forms the sinoatrial node, the normal pacemaker of the fully developed heart.

By the time the atrium and sinus venosus are formed, this primitive tubular heart is actively pumping blood through the developing circulatory system. During the peristaltic type of cardiac contraction, retrograde flow of blood is prevented by developing mounds of endocardial tissue which project into the lumen at the junction of the primitive atria and ventricles.[3] During each contraction

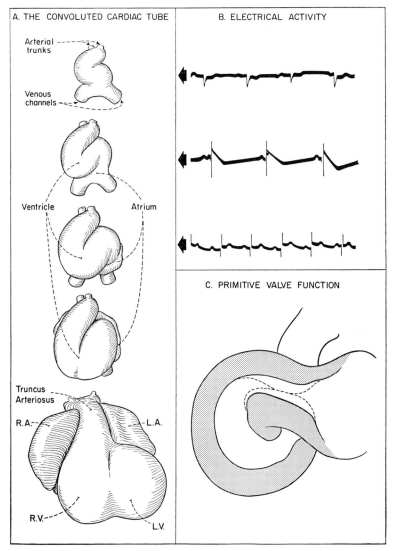

FIGURE 2–1   EMBRYOLOGIC DEVELOPMENT OF THE HEART

  A, The initial stage in the development of the heart is the formation of a single cardiac tube which will ultimately evolve into the ventricular portion of the heart. At this very early stage, contractions occur repetitively at a slow rate. Being anchored above by the developing arterial trunks and below by extensive venous channels, the cardiac tube, growing rapidly in length, is bent into a loop to the right of the midline. By progressive fusion of the cardiac primordia, the primitive atrium is formed and remains relatively fixed in position as the cardiac loop grows longer and swings back to the midline to cover the expanding atrial chambers. In this process the ventricle assumes a position anterior and caudal to the atria.

  B, Electrical activity can be recorded from the heart of the chick embryo at the very early stages of development, indicated by the first three drawings in part A. As the cardiac tube becomes convoluted, the electrocardiographic patterns produced by this electrical activity begin to resemble the patterns observed in fully developed hearts. (After Hoff *et al.*[4])

  C, Contraction of the cardiac tube is peristaltic in character, beginning in the atrial region and progressing toward the truncus arteriosus. During contraction at the atrioventricular junction, the endocardial surfaces come into apposition to prevent retrograde flow of blood. A similar valve action may be observed at the root of the truncus arteriosus. (After Patten *et al.*[3])

these endocardial cushions meet each other, completely blocking the channel (Fig. 2–1C). Thus, simple but effective atrioventricular valves are formed at this very early stage of development. Similar endocardial cushions develop in the outflow tract near the ventricular conus. This region ultimately becomes the conus of the right ventricle.

THE DEVELOPMENT OF THE ELECTROCARDIOGRAM

According to Hoff et al.,[4] electrical activity can be consistently recorded from chick embryos at the stage of development illustrated in Figure 2–1A. A few hours later a sharp downward deflection appears, which is interpreted as equivalent to a QRS complex. In the next three or four hours the atrium has become differentiated and the sinus venosus is formed. At about this time, downward deflections (P waves) can be recorded just preceding the QRS. As the primitive cardiac tube becomes convoluted, the electrocardiogram assumes a configuration similar to that of the adult (Fig. 2–1B). The fetal electrocardiogram in the human cannot be recorded by external electrodes on the maternal abdomen until about the twelfth week of gestation.

PARTITIONING OF THE ATRIOVENTRICULAR CANAL

At six weeks of age, the major components of the human heart can be readily identified. A shallow, interventricular groove forms a line of demarcation between the future right and left ventricles.

In spite of the apparent separation of the atria from the ventricles at the atrioventricular junction (Fig. 2–2A,

arrow), the heart actually consists of a common atrioventricular canal which empties into a single arterial trunk. A four-chambered heart is developed from this convoluted, dilated tube by the formation of three partitions separating the atria, the ventricles and the two main arteries.

The first step in the separation of the atrial and ventricular chambers begins with the growth of endocardial cushions from the dorsal and ventral portions of the atrioventricular groove. These masses of endocardial tissue later fuse to form a column which splits the stream of blood flowing from atrium to ventricle (Fig. 2–2C). At the same time a muscular septum develops from the interventricular groove toward the base of the heart, separating the right and left ventricles.

In the atrium, a crescentic ridge (septum primum) appears on the dorsocephalic part of the atrium and rapidly grows down toward the ventricle. As this septum grows across the common atrial chamber, the aperture between the right and left atria (foramen primum) is progressively constricted (Fig. 2–2D). However, before the foramen primum is completely closed, a new opening (foramen secundum) appears high on septum primum (Fig. 2–2E). The timely development of the foramen secundum prevents interruption in the shunting of blood from the right atrium into the left.

Another septum (secundum) develops just to the right of the septum primum and extends like a curtain down over the aperture in the septum primum (Fig. 2–2F). The septum secundum grows beside the septum primum to become a second atrial partition which is complete except for a persistent aperture adjacent to the foramen secundum. The thickened

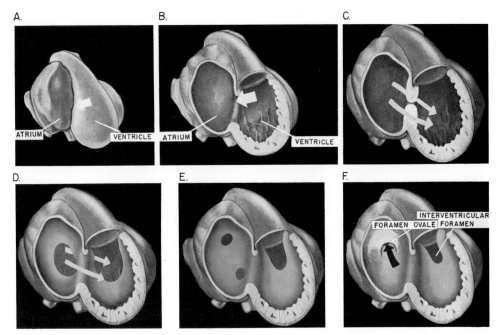

FIGURE 2–2   PARTITIONING OF THE HEART

A, When the cardiac tube illustrated in Figure 2–1*A* is observed in a lateral view, the atrium and ventricles appear to be divided by a deep atrioventricular invagination.

B, Actually, this groove is merely a constriction at the atrioventricular junction. The embryonic heart at this stage is still a simple tube which has become convoluted and expanded into primitive chambers. A four-chambered heart with corresponding arterial trunks is formed by the elaboration of three septa dividing the atria, ventricles and truncus arteriosus.

C, First, the atrioventricular channel is divided at its waist by proliferating endocardial cushions which fuse into a column.

D, Septa dividing the atrium and ventricle grow simultaneously toward the atrioventricular grooves. If either of these partitions fails to form, the fully developed heart has only a single atrium or a single ventricle.

E, An aperture in the developing atrial septum persists near its junction with the endocardial cushions (the foramen primum). Before foramen primum is closed, a new aperture appears high on the interventricular septum (foramen secundum). These two embryonic apertures are the most common sites of interatrial septal defects.

F, The foramen secundum is covered by the developing septum secundum which grows down over the aperture. Its advancing edge becomes thickened to produce the foramen ovale, which acts as a unidirectional flutter valve. Closure of the interventricular foramen awaits the development of a complex spiral septum dividing the truncus arteriosus and conus region of the primtive ventricle (see Fig. 2–3).

edge of this aperture forms the margin of the foramen ovale. The thin septum primum acts as a unidirectional flutter valve, permitting blood to flow only from the right atrium into the left. The functional significance of this unidirectional valve is considered later in relation to circulatory adjustments after birth (see Chapter 13). Closure of the interventricular foramen awaits the partitioning of the conus and truncus arteriosus.

THE SPIRAL AORTIC PULMONARY SEPTUM

The truncus arteriosus resembles a cylinder (Fig. 2–3*A*), extending from the conus region just above the partially divided ventricular chambers to its bifurcation into the aorta and pulmonary arteries. A pair of ridges appearing at the bifurcation and on opposite sides of the truncus arteriosus pursue a spiral course toward the ventricles (Fig. 2–3*B*). These ridges

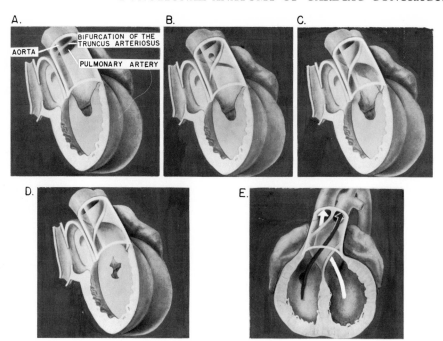

FIGURE 2–3   PARTITIONING OF THE ARTERIAL TRUNKS

A, The truncus arteriosus is illustrated as a transparent cylinder with the heart viewed in the right anterior oblique position.

B, A pair of spiral ridges develop in the internal surface of the truncus arteriosus, beginning at the bifurcation of the truncus arteriosus into the fourth and sixth aortic arches. Retaining their positions on opposite sides of the cylinder, the ridges pursue a spiral course toward the ventricles.

C, The ridges grow into the lumen and fuse to produce a spiral septum which extends into the conus region of the ventricles where they swing into line with the upper margin of the interventricular septum.

D, The interventricular foramen is normally obliterated by masses of endocardial tissue growing from the ventricular septum, the endocardial cushions and the spiral aortic pulmonary septum. This mass of endocardial tissue thins out to form the membranous portion of the interventricular septum just below the origin of the aorta and pulmonary artery. This is the most common site of interventricular septal defects.

E, The significance of the spiral aortic septum is more readily appreciated in a frontal view of the heart. The aortic pulmonary septum executes a spiral of about 180 degrees and swings into line with the superior margin of the interventricular septum. This process accounts for the manner in which the aortic and pulmonary trunks are entwined in the fully developed heart. Blood from the left ventricle enters the aorta, which passes to the right behind the pulmonary artery. The pulmonary artery passes in front of the aorta and turns posteriorly on the left side of the mediastinum.

grow toward the axis of the cylinder and fuse to form a continuous spiral septum which twists 180 degrees and swings into line with the advancing edge of the interventricular septum (Fig. 2–3C). The spiral form of the aortic pulmonary septum accounts for the manner in which the pulmonary artery and aorta intertwine in the fully developed heart (Fig. 2–3E).

The remaining interventricular foramen is closed by developing endocardial tissue from the atrioventricular cushions, the interventricular septum and the spiral aortic pulmonary septum (Fig. 2–3D). The connective tissue which occludes the interventricular foramen gradually thins out to form the membranous portion of the interventricular septum.

THE FORMATION OF CARDIAC VALVES

The semilunar valves begin to form during the division of the truncus arteriosus into the aorta and pulmonary artery (Fig. 2–4A). At the junction of the ventricular conus and the truncus arteriosus, the spiral ridges on opposite sides of the channel develop localized pads of embryonic connective tissue (Fig. 2–4B). As the spiral ridges grow across the lumen, these endocardial cushions form two projections into each vessel and a third pad of tissue grows into each vessel from a point opposite the line of fusion of the spiral septum (Fig. 2–4B). In this way, three pads of connective tissue project into the lumens of the vessels and are gradually excavated and molded into valve cusps forming semilunar valves (Fig. 2–4C). The formation of the atrioventricular valves cannot be visualized so easily. Thick flaps of tissue proliferate from the region of the atrioventricular junction down into the ventricular chamber. The exact mechanism by which these crude flaps are converted into beautifully formed valve cusps, intricately guyed by chordae tendineae arising from the appropriate papillary muscles, is not clear.

THE DUCTUS ARTERIOSUS

Both the pulmonary arteries and the ductus arteriosus are remnants of the sixth pair of aortic arches. Like all the other pairs of aortic arches, the sixth connects the ventral and the dorsal aorta and corresponds to the gill arches in fishes. Branching vessels arise from both the right and left limbs of the sixth aortic arch to supply the developing lungs. As the pulmonary branches from the right aortic arch develop, communication with the

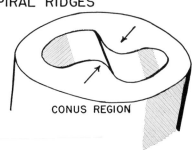

A. SPIRAL RIDGES

CONUS REGION

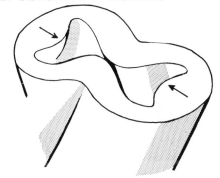

B. SECONDARY MOUNDS

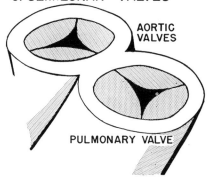

C. SEMILUNAR VALVES

AORTIC VALVES

PULMONARY VALVE

FIGURE 2–4 FORMATION OF THE SEMILUNAR VALVES

A, The semilunar valves develop during the separation of the truncus arteriosus by the spiral aortic pulmonary septum (see Fig. 2–3).

B, Pads of endocardial tissue develop at the sites of the valves. These pads originate from the spiral aortic pulmonary septum and as secondary mounds on opposite sides of the channel.

C, When partitioning of the truncus arteriosus is complete, three pads of endocardial tissue appear in the aorta and in the pulmonary artery. These pads are shaped and thinned out to produce the semilunar aortic and pulmonary valves.

dorsal aorta regresses and ultimately disappears. The remnant of the sixth aortic arch between the pulmonary artery and the left aortic arch persists as the ductus arteriosus. During fetal life, blood ejected by the right ventricle can bypass the pulmonary circuit and enter the descending aorta. The functional significance of this short circuit is more clearly visualized in relation to the fetal circulation as a whole. (See Chapter 13.)

CONCEPTS OF MUSCULAR CONTRACTION

The walls of the heart are composed of bundles and sheets of myocardial fibers intertwined in a very complex fashion. Electron micrographs show that myofibrils are made up of still smaller filaments, each about 50 to 100 Å in diameter (Fig. 2–5). Huxley[5] has clearly demonstrated that there are two types of myofilaments, one being almost twice as thick as the other. These thick and thin filaments are linked together by an intricate system of cross bridges which project from the thick fibers at fairly regular intervals. He proposed a sliding model concept of muscular contraction, summarized schematically in Figure 2–5. This concept rapidly achieved wide acceptance because it was consistent with much other evidence and supported by crisp, detailed electron micrographs.[6] The two types of myofilaments have been identified in association with the cross bands of muscle. The thin filaments extend in both directions from the Z band. The dark A band is occupied by the thick filaments, which are partially overlapped by the thin filaments. The central light area (H zone) of the A band represents the region occupied only by the thicker filaments. Over a wide range of muscle lengths, the A bands remain of constant length during both contraction and stretching. The I bands shorten in relation to the shortening of the muscle. As the width of the I band diminishes, the H zone shrinks as these two sets of filaments slide past each other. Actually, the tips of filaments may meet and deform at extreme degrees of shortening, and the expected new sets of bands appear at the points of contact.

Ample evidence indicates that the thin filaments are indeed actin and the thick filaments are myosin. The nature of the cross bridges is not known, but they have been assigned an important role in a theory proposed by Huxley.[6] According to this scheme, the cross bridges oscillate and are able to form attachments at specific sites on the thin actin filaments and draw them a short distance.

THE RELATION OF MYOCARDIUM TO OTHER TYPES OF MUSCLE

Since the contractile mechanisms are similar in the various kinds of muscle, the principle differences in their function arise from differences in the mechanisms for excitation and control. Because myocardium superficially resembles skeletal muscle in its cross striation, in color and in the speed, vigor and duration of its contraction, the common tendency is to assume that cardiac muscle is only slightly different from skeletal muscle. On the contrary, myocardium more closely resembles visceral smooth muscle with respect to its functional characteristics and control (Fig. 2–6). Bozler[7, 8] has classified smooth muscle into two main divisions, (a) multiunit smooth muscle and (b) visceral smooth muscle. Multiunit smooth muscle, in the peripheral vascular

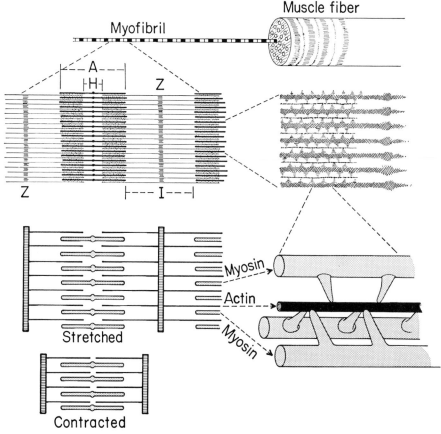

FIGURE 2–5   MUSCULAR CONTRACTION

The myofibrils are composed of overlapping thick myosin filaments and thin actin filaments. The amount of overlap is diminished during stretching and increased during contraction. Many cross bridges are observed at regular intervals between the actin and myosin filaments. These cross bridges have been visualized as forming linkages at specific sites on the actin fibers and drawing them onward during contraction. (After Huxley.[6])

system and the bladder, is directly innervated by motor nerves originating in the autonomic nervous system and resembles skeletal muscle in many aspects of its excitation and control.

In contrast, visceral smooth muscle, in the ureter, uterus and gastrointestinal tract, is not directly innervated by motor nerves (Fig. 2–6). Waves of excitation originate in the muscle fibers and are conducted throughout the contiguous cells. Although protoplasmic continuity between adjacent cells cannot be

demonstrated, a mass of visceral smooth muscle functions like a syncytium, so that excitation originating at one site may spread to all other portions. In the ureter, pacemaker activity is well developed at a point near the hilus of the kidney. Waves of excitation originate at this point at fairly regular intervals and proceed in an orderly fashion down the length of the tube. Thus, the electrical activity of visceral smooth muscle is similar to that of the myocardium but very different from that of skeletal muscle (Fig. 2–6). Visceral smooth muscle is

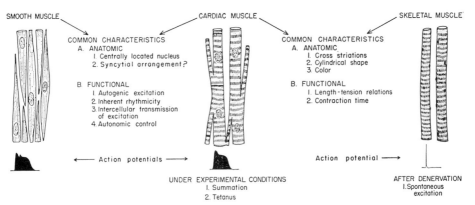

FIGURE 2–6   ANATOMIC AND FUNCTIONAL SIMILARITY BETWEEN DIFFERENT TYPES OF MUSCLE

Properties common to visceral smooth muscle and myocardium are listed between schematic drawings of these fibers. Functional characteristics shared by myocardium and skeletal muscle are similarly indicated between drawings. These different types of fibers are distinguished by their controlling mechanisms, the fundamental contractile process being very similar in each type. As far as control is concerned, myocardium is more closely related to visceral smooth muscle than to skeletal muscle. Schematic representations of action potentials from three types of muscle are indicated at the bottom of respective drawings. Smooth muscle has a rapid depolarization which is sustained for an extended period and may have multiple superimposed spikes (after Bozler[7,8]). Myocardium tends to remain depolarized for a period approximately equal to the duration of contraction. In contrast, skeletal muscle rapidly recovers its polarization after excitation and responds to repetitive stimulation to produce sustained contractions. Under experimental conditions summation and tetanus can be produced in myocardial fibers, even though such a response is usually considered typical of skeletal muscle. Denervated skeletal muscle exhibits spontaneous autogenic excitation (fibrillation), which is the typical form of excitation in myocardium and visceral smooth muscle.

controlled by the autonomic nervous system principally through the release of hormonal substances rather than through direct motor innervation. Thus, visceral smooth muscle is closely related to myocardium so far as its excitation and control are concerned. If the completeness of contraction or relaxation can vary in smooth muscle, there is no *a priori* reason for discarding this possibility in the myocardium.

The similarity of the basic contractile mechanisms is emphasized by the fact that apparent differences among the various types of muscle can be largely eliminated under specific conditions. For example, tetanus can be produced in papillary muscle from a mammalian heart maintained at 27° C. and electrically stimulated at a rapid rate.[9] A skeletal muscle deprived of its motor nerve supply exhibits

fibrillation due to myogenic impulses which spread along the individual fibers to produce asynchronous contractions. This phenomenon can be directly observed on the surface of the tongue after degeneration of its motor nerves.

ANATOMIC COMPONENTS OF THE HEART

Four rings of dense connective tissue are joined to form a single fibrous "skeleton" of the heart. The atria, ventricles, valves and arterial trunks are all firmly attached to this skeleton (Fig. 2–7). The two atria resemble a thin-walled, shallow cup of myocardium divided by a partition down the center. Each atrium has an atrial appendage, the functional significance of which is completely un-

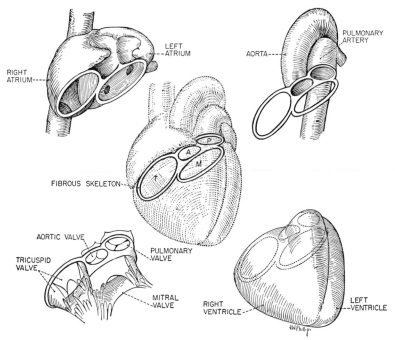

FIGURE 2–7   ANATOMIC COMPONENTS OF THE HEART

The fibrous skeleton of the heart consists of four valve rings joined together. To these dense connective tissue annuli fibrosi are fastened the two major arterial trunks and all four cardiac chambers. The atria and arterial trunks are attached to the superior surface of this fibrous skeleton and the ventricles and atrioventricular valve leaflets are fastened to its inferior aspect.

known. The margins of the atrial shell are fastened to the superior surface of the mitral and tricuspid valve rings.

The aorta and the pulmonary artery originate at the superior surface of the corresponding semilunar valve rings. Thus, the atrial chambers and the arterial trunks are anchored to the superior surface of the fibrous skeleton. The inflow and outflow channels of each ventricle lie side by side. The atrioventricular (A-V) valves are fastened to the inferior surface of the mitral and tricuspid valve rings, with the fibrous connective tissue at the root of each valve leaflet merging with that of the corresponding valvular ring. Chordae tendineae, extending from the inferior margins of each leaflet of the A-V valves, are fastened directly to the internal surface of the

ventricular walls and to papillary muscles projecting from the endocardial surface of the ventricular chambers.

The right and left ventricles are fastened to the entire circumference of the fibrous skeleton of the heart. The upper margin of the interventricular septum is attached along the line of fusion between the mitral and tricuspid valve rings. The membranous portion of the septum is fused at the junction of the pulmonary and aortic valve rings.

THE ANATOMY OF THE VENTRICULAR WALLS

The ventricles serve as the major source of energy for the circulation of blood and are composed of sheets of myocardial fibers encircling the ventricular chambers in a complex fashion[10, 11] reminiscent of the windings of a turban. The various muscular layers in the ventricles are so tightly bound together that they are very difficult to dissect into individual components. According to Robb and Robb,[11] the ventricular walls are composed of four different muscles: the superficial sinospiral and bulbospiral muscles and the deep sinospiral and bulbospiral muscles (Fig. 2–8). This traditional view of ventricular anatomy was based on a special technique of dissection by a kind of unrolling process of hearts which had been prepared by prolonged soaking in strong chemicals to release binding between layers. This method was challenged by Grant,[12] and the concept tested by Streeter and Bassett[13] who measured the angles subtended by the myocardial fibers measured at 1 mm. intervals from endocardium to epicardium in pigs' hearts. The successive layers of myocardium displayed a progressive change in orientation like an open Japanese fan, without abrupt changes in fiber orientation (Fig. 2–9). The same kind of pattern was described for the interventricular septum and the anterior, posterior and free walls of the left ventricle, except at the root of papillary muscles. These measurements do not reveal discrete layers or sheets of myocardium in the ventricular walls.

Comparing myocardial orientation in the distended and contracted state, Streeter *et al.*[14] observed that, despite an increase in wall thickness as the chamber was compressed, the fiber orientation was not apparently rearranged, except at the apical portion of the lateral wall. These observations indicate that minimal tension should develop between successive layers of myocardium during contraction, contrary to my views expressed in previous publications[17, 18] and in the previous edition of this book. It would now appear that the concept of tension or force stored in the form of "interfascicular tension" between myocardial layers during systole and released during diastole should be reevaluated, perhaps abandoned.

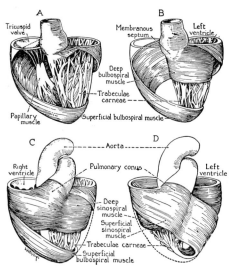

FIGURE 2–8 ANATOMY OF THE
VENTRICULAR WALLS

A, The superficial bulbospiral muscle bundles arise principally from the mitral ring and form the external investment for portions of the left and right ventricles as they spiral toward the apex. Emerging from the vortex on the inside of the chambers, these muscle bundles spiral back toward the valve rings either as trabeculae carneae or as papillary muscles which are joined to the valves through chordae tendineae.

B, The deep bulbospiral muscle fibers encircle the basilar portions of the left ventricle.

C, The deep sinospiral muscle encircles both the right and the left ventricular chambers.

D, The superficial spinospiral muscle is a counterpart of the superficial bulbospiral muscle. The anatomic distinction between the superficial sinospiral and bulbospiral muscles is arbitrary and functionally unimportant. (After Robb and Robb.[11])

THE FUNCTIONAL ANATOMY
OF HEART VALVES

The heart valves are so simple and effective that the best available man-

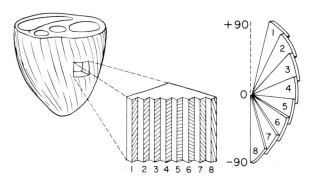

**FIGURE 2–9   ORIENTATION OF THE
MYOCARDIAL FIBERS**

The orientation of myocardial
fibers in the left ventricular wall of a
pig's heart displays a progressive
angular displacement when examined
at 1 mm intervals. Abrupt changes in
fiber orientation representing discrete
layers (as in Fig. 2–8) were not found.
(From Streeter.[13])

made substitutes are gross caricatures
by comparison. Not only do they open
and close rapidly and seal completely
against high pressures, but their
delicate-appearing cusps may endure
the ravages of repetitive closure for
more than 80 years.

Semilunar Valves.   The aortic and
pulmonary valves are similar, each
consisting of three symmetrical valve
cusps. Two cusps of equal size could
close tightly but would not open completely without considerable elastic
stretch. Three cusps can theoretically
open to the full dimensions of the valve
ring and yet produce a perfect seal
when closed. Behind the aortic valve
cusps are three outpouchings, the
sinuses of Valsalva, which help prevent obstruction of the coronary ostia.
If a valve leaflet came in contact with
the coronary orifice, shutting off the
flow of blood from the aorta, coronary
pressure would fall rapidly as blood
left the coronary arterial system, and
the valve cusp would be sealed against
the coronary ostium by a high differential pressure. This unfortunate accident is presumably prevented by the
presence of adequate space behind
the open valve cusps.

Atrioventricular Valves.   The tricuspid and mitral valves are larger and
much more complicated than the semilunar valves. The anatomic distinction
between the mitral valve and the tricuspid valve is largely artificial since
both valves consist fundamentally of
two large opposing cusps and small
intermediary cusps at each end. However, the chordae tendineae of the
tricuspid valve usually insert on three
fairly distinct groups of papillary
muscles, while only two principal
papillary muscles serve the mitral
valve. The anatomy of the papillary
muscles is subject to considerable
individual variability, some being
deeply notched, grooved or separated into multiple heads. Since the
structure and function of the mitral
and tricuspid valves are similar,
only the former will be described
in detail.

THE MITRAL VALVE.   The mitral
valve is interposed between the low-
pressure left atrium and high-pressure
left ventricle. The two valve cusps are
unequal in size. The large anterome-
dial (aortic) cusp hangs down like a
curtain between the mitral and aortic
orifices, while the shorter postero-
lateral cusp originates from the lateral
portions of the mitral ring. The combined surface area of the two valve
cusps is nearly twice as great as the
area of the mitral orifice which they
must occlude. The mitral valve orifice
is considerably smaller than the mitral
ring because the valve cusps are joined
at the commissures so the upper portion of the mitral valve resembles a
funnel.

The chordae tendineae correspond
to multiple guy lines extending from
the papillary muscles into the struc-

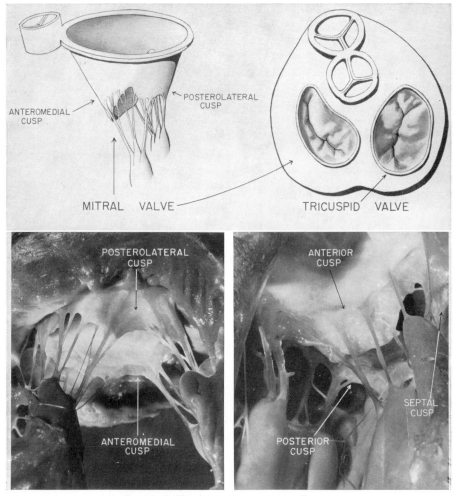

FIGURE 2–10   ATRIOVENTRICULAR VALVES

A, The mitral valve is shaped like a funnel when open and is closed by the approximation of two broad, membranous cusps. The chordae tendineae originate from the tips of two sets of papillary muscles and prevent eversion of the valve cusps into the left atrium during ventricular systole. The major chordae merge into the edge of the short leaf, but may insert several millimeters back from the edge of the larger aortic leaf.

B, The mitral and tricuspid valves are similar in both structure and function. They both consist primarily of two broad, opposing valve cusps with smaller intermediate cusps situated at each end. The tricuspid valve has a somewhat larger intermediate cusp and a total of three separate papillary muscles. (After Spalteholz, W.: Hand Atlas of Human Anatomy. Philadelphia, J. B. Lippincott Co., 1933.)

C, In a normal heart specimen, the walls of the left ventricle were excised to illustrate the postero-lateral aspect of the mitral valves, chordae tendineae and papillary muscles. Transillumination reveals that fibers of the chordae tendineae extend long distances within the valve cusps.

D, The three papillary muscles and corresponding valve cusps of the tricuspid valve were photo-graphed as viewed from within the right ventricular cavity.

ture of the valve cusps (see Fig. 2–10). It is important to recognize that the chordae tendineae from adjacent regions of the two valve cusps insert upon the same or adjacent papillary muscles (Fig. 2–10). Thus, tension ex-erted through the chordae tends to draw the two valve cusps together. If the papillary muscles begin their contraction early in ventricular systole, traction on the valve cusps should facilitate apposition of the valves.

COORDINATION OF THE HEART BEAT

To produce efficient pumping, the complex mass of myocardial fibers must contract more or less simultaneously. The effectiveness of the ventricles is lost if the individual myocardial bundles contract in a random fashion, e.g., in ventricular fibrillation. Coordinated contraction of the complex pattern of myocardial bundles stems from the functional continuity of the myocardial fibers; excitation beginning at one site spreads to all other contiguous areas. Excitation of the thick ventricular walls is facilitated by a rapidly conducting system of Purkinje fibers. The conduction system is responsible for periodic initiation of excitation (pacemaker activity), a delay between atrial and ventricular contraction (A-V nodal delay) and the rapid spread of excitation to all portions of the ventricular walls so that their contraction is sufficiently simultaneous to produce effective pumping action. When the conduction system is operating normally, this stereotyped sequence of events is repeated during each successive cardiac cycle.

THE CONDUCTION SYSTEM OF THE HEART

The sino-atrial (S-A) node is a small mass of specialized myocardial tissues embedded in the atrial wall near the entrance of the superior vena cava (Fig. 2–11). This node consists of an accumulation of modified myocardial cells. Shaped like an Indian war club, it has a fringe of delicate fibers merging with surrounding myocardial fibers. The S-A node is the normal pacemaker, spontaneously originating the spreading waves of excitation at a more rapid rate than any other part of the heart. A large number of fibers from the parasympathetic and sympathetic nervous systems terminate in the vicinity of the S-A node. Discharge of the vagal fibers releases acetylcholine, which tends to slow the rate of impulse formation, and the sympathetic fibers release epinephrine-like substances, which act to accelerate the frequency of impulse formation. If it were iso-

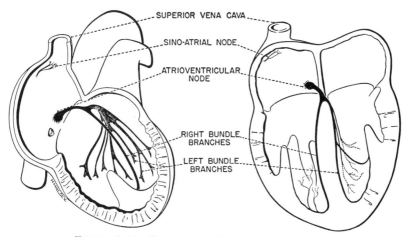

SUPERIOR VENA CAVA

SINO-ATRIAL NODE

ATRIOVENTRICULAR NODE

RIGHT BUNDLE BRANCHES

LEFT BUNDLE BRANCHES

FIGURE 2–11   CONDUCTION SYSTEM OF THE HEART

The sino-atrial node is the normal pacemaker of the heart. No specialized conduction system has been described in the atria. The A-V node, common bundle and bundle branches conduct the wave of excitation from the atrium to the ventricular myocardium.

lated from all neural and hormonal control, the S-A node would probably generate impulses at a rate in excess of 100 per minute. Since the vagal influence generally predominates, the "normal" heart rate ranges between 60 and 100 impulses per minute. The S-A node retains its position as pacemaker for the entire heart so long as it generates impulses at a faster rate than any other region of the myocardial syncytium and so long as the spreading wave of excitation is rapidly conducted from the atria into the ventricles.

THE SEQUENCE OF EXCITATION

Apparently no conduction system serves the atria, so a wave of excitation originating in the S-A node spreads in all directions like the concentric wave produced by dropping a pebble into a pool of water. It travels at a rate of about 1 meter per second and reaches the most distant portions of the atrium in about 0.08 second. As it approaches the interatrial septum, the wave of excitation reaches another mass of specialized conducting tissue, the atrioventricular (A-V) node.

The A-V node is located on the right side of the interatrial septum close to the entrance of the coronary sinus (Fig. 2–12). When the wave of excitation reaches the A-V node, it does not proceed directly to the ventricles but is delayed there for intervals ranging around 0.08 to 0.12 second. It has been suggested that this delay is due to slow conduction along delicate fibers connecting the atrial myocardium with A-V nodal tissue. During the A-V nodal delay, atrial contraction is largely completed. The A-V node is the bulbous end of a bundle of Purkinje fibers—the bundle of His—which passes forward along the right side of the interatrial septum before plunging downward across the A-V junction to the upper margin of the muscular interventricular septum. There the bundle divides into two branches—the right and left bundles—which descend on opposite sides of the interventricular septum. The bundle branches ramify into a network of Purkinje fibers which are distributed over the inner surface of the ventricular chambers.

After leaving the A-V node, the wave of excitation passes rapidly (4 to 5 meters per second) along the Pur-

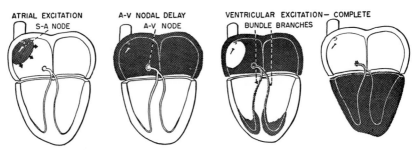

FIGURE 2–12   SEQUENCE OF CARDIAC EXCITATION

Excitation of the heart is normally initiated by an impulse which is generated by the S-A node and which spreads rapidly in all directions through the atrial musculature. After a slight delay at the A-V node, impulses are conducted by the Purkinje system into the ventricles where a wave of excitation spreads from the endocardial surfaces through the ventricular musculature.

kinje fibers of the common bundle and the bundle branches.[15] The endocardial surfaces of the ventricular chambers are excited early, and the endocardial layers (trabeculae carneae and papillary muscles) are first to contract. Thus, the wave of excitation probably penetrates the ventricular walls from the endocardial to the epicardial surface. The rapid spread of excitation through the ventricles produces more or less simultaneous contraction of the ventricular musculature.

THE SEQUENCE OF EVENTS DURING THE CARDIAC CYCLE

So long as the heart receives excitation along the normal pathways and the heart rate remains constant, each successive cardiac cycle tends to follow the same pattern of contraction and relaxation. A clear picture of the mechanical events of the cardiac cycle is required for logical interpretation of many physiologic events, e.g., timing of heart murmurs and analysis of electrocardiograms or arterial and venous pulse contours.

THE CARDIAC CYCLE: CINEFLUOROGRAPHIC ANGIOCARDIOGRAPHY

X-rays penetrating the body of a dog illuminate a fluorescent screen, producing an image of the cardiac silhouette. Motion pictures of these images record changes in the size and shape of the heart. If a radiopaque substance such as Diodrast is rapidly injected into the jugular vein, the course of the opacified blood can be followed through the heart and great vessels.[16] The changes in size and configuration of the individual cardiac chambers can be visualized as a two-dimensional projection or silhouette.

For purposes of orientation, the anatomic relations of the great vessels and cardiac chambers in the heart of the dog are indicated in Figure 2–13 as viewed from the right side. Note that the right ventricle does not extend to the apex of the heart in the dog. Further, the configuration of the ventricular chambers is not the same in dogs and in man. Although the fundamental principles of cardiac contraction in dogs probably resemble those in humans, caution must be exercised in applying the discussion which follows to cardiac function in man.

The typical sequence of events which occurs during filling and contraction of the right atrium and right ventricle of a dog is illustrated in Figure 2–14. Diodrast flowed along the superior vena cava during the eight frames in column A and entered the right atrium in the third frame of column B (B-3). In frame B-5, the tricuspid valves everted into the right atrium and blood gushed into the right ventricle (B-6). The variations in density of the right ventricular shadow in frames B-7 and B-8 represent the mixing of the incoming blood with the residual blood remaining in the ventricle after the preceding systole. The next contraction began in frames C-5 and C-6, as indicated by the protrusion of the right atrial appendage associated with atrial systole. In frame C-6, the right ventricle began to contract and in the next three frames was reduced to a small triangular area with its base at the tricuspid valves. Between frames C-8 and D-1 (1/15 second), the right ventricle was filled and apparently remained unchanged in size until the succeeding contraction (D-8). During the remainder of this cycle, Diodrast passed through the right atrium and flowed into the inferior vena cava down to the level of the diaphragm against the oncoming

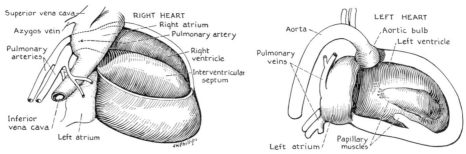

FIGURE 2–13 ROENTGENOGRAPHIC ANATOMY OF DOG HEART

The anatomic relations of the cardiac chambers and arterial trunks in the dog as viewed from the right side for comparison with angiocardiograms presented in subsequent figures. The right atrium lies above the left atrium on the posterior aspect of the heart. The interventricular septum presents a convex surface to the right ventricular cavity. Thus, the right ventricular cavity has a crescentic transverse section and partially encircles the left ventricular cavity.

stream of blood. The opacified blood in the inferior vena cava returned to the heart during the next filling period. The right ventricle did not distend noticeably during the latter part of diastole even when there was sufficient pressure to force Diodrast against the stream of blood into the inferior vena cava. Diastolic filling appears to be largely complete very early in the diastolic interval.

Filling of the Right Ventricle. Diastolic filling of the right ventricle can be studied by injecting Lipiodol into a systemic vein. Lipiodol is a radiopaque, viscous oil which is very cohesive and tends to flow along with the stream of blood as a long ribbon or as multiple globules, depending upon how it is injected. The course of one Lipiodol streamer ascending the inferior vena cava is indicated by serial tracings in Figure 2–15. The movement was relatively slow during systole. At the beginning of the rapid filling in early diastole the Lipiodol streamer accelerated rapidly, passing along the inferior vena cava, through the atrium and into the right ventricle. Thus, the blood which fills the right ventricle comes not only from the atrium but also from a considerable distance down the inferior vena cava.

Blood streams from the superior and inferior venae cavae converge at the right atrium. Streamers of Lipiodol and Diodrast moving down the superior vena cava frequently exhibit a spiral flow as they enter the ventricle (Fig. 2–15). This is attributed to a swirling motion of the blood produced by the confluence of the two streams. These currents tend to mix the venous blood within the right ventricle.

Contraction of the Right Ventricle. Cinefluorographic films indicate that a longitudinal section of the right ventricular chamber is roughly triangular. It is bounded by a convex septal wall and the concave free wall, which enclose a crescent-shaped slit between them (Fig. 2–13). The action of the right ventricle resembles that of the old-fashioned bellows used to kindle fires. Since the sides of the bellows are large compared to the space between them, their very slight movement toward each other causes displacement of a large volume from within. In the right ventricular cavity, a relatively narrow space is confined between two broad surfaces so that the surface area of the chamber is very great in relation to the volume.[17, 18]

Blood is ejected from the right ventricle by three separate mechanisms occurring more or less simultaneously (Fig. 2–16): (*a*) Contraction

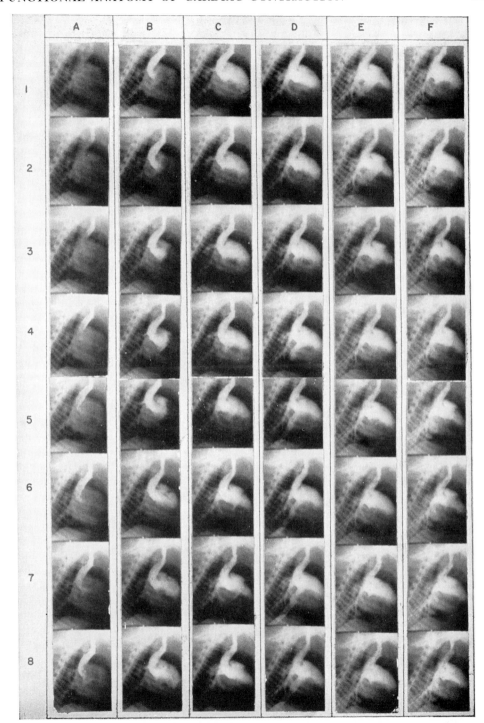

FIGURE 2–14   CHANGES IN SIZE AND SHAPE OF THE RIGHT ATRIUM AND VENTRICLE

Successive frames from a cinefluorographic film exposed at 15 frames per second illustrate the filling and contraction of the right atrium and right ventricle during 3.2 seconds following the injection of contrast medium. Examine each column in succession from above downward to observe the sequence of events.

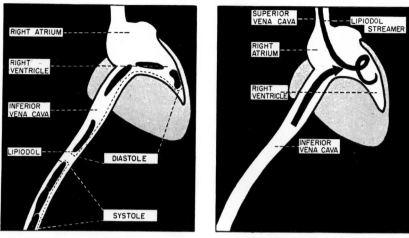

FIGURE 2-15 FILLING OF THE RIGHT VENTRICLE

Lipiodol streamers, floating freely in the blood, move relatively slowly during one phase of the cardiac cycle, then suddenly accelerate and move without hesitation into the right ventricular cavity, presumably during the rapid filling phase of ventricular diastole (see text). Similar streamers of Lipiodol descending along the superior vena cava frequently display a swirling motion which may be due to the convergence of the two currents of blood flowing into the atrium.

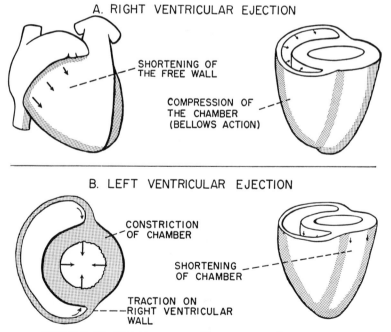

FIGURE 2-16 COMPONENTS OF VENTRICULAR CONTRACTION

A, Blood is ejected from the right ventricle by shortening of the free wall with downward displacement of the tricuspid valve ring and movement of the free wall toward the interventricular septum by myocardial shortening. Compression of the right ventricular cavity may be supplemented by traction exerted on the free wall by left ventricular contraction.

B, Left ventricular ejection is accomplished primarily by a reduction in the diameter of the chamber with some additional shortening of the longitudinal axis.

of the spiral muscles draws the tricuspid valve ring toward the apex of the heart and shortens the longitudinal axis of the chamber. This shortening is the most obvious movement but is much less effective than the bellows action in ejecting blood. (*b*) The free wall of the right ventricle moves toward the convex surface of the interventricular septum. This movement is very slight but extremely effective in ejecting blood. (*c*) Contraction of the deep circular fibers enclosing the left ventricular cavity must produce a greater curvature of the interventricular septum (Fig. 2–16), although the midportion (central axis) of this septum remains remarkably fixed in both position and length. Since the free wall of the right ventricle is attached to the left ventricle along the interventricular groove, traction on this wall will also contribute to the bellows action on the right ventricular cavity. This effect is so slight that it cannot be readily demonstrated on cinefluorographic films. It has been clearly shown, however, that the free wall of the right ventricle can be almost completely destroyed by cauterization in dogs[19] or by coronary occlusion in man[20] without obvious effects on the circulatory efficiency.

Clearly, the configuration of the right ventricle is ideally suited to the ejection of large volumes of blood with minimal amounts of myocardial shortening. On the other hand, this architectural design is not conducive to the development of high intraventricular pressure.[17] If the normal right ventricle were suddenly required to provide the intraventricular pressures normally developed in the left ventricle, the right ventricular myocardium would have to develop tension many times as great as that in the left ventricle. Thus, we see that the right ventricle is specifically adapted to the task of pumping large or widely varying volumes of blood against a very low outflow pressure. Since the pulmonary vascular tree normally offers slight resistance to flow, the right ventricle normally ejects blood at relatively low pressure into the pulmonary artery. A sudden increase in pulmonary arterial pressure (massive pulmonary embolism) frequently leads to sudden death because the right ventricular myocardium cannot sustain the higher pressures needed to provide adequate flow through the lungs.

Contraction of the Left Ventricle. Contraction of the left ventricle involves both a reduction in the diameter of the cylindrical portion and a shortening along the longitudinal axis of the chamber. Contraction of the circumferential muscle bundles acts to reduce the diameter of the chamber (see Fig. 2–16). This action accounts for most of the power and volume of the ejection, since the volume contained decreases with the square of the radius in a cylinder. Shortening of the longitudinal axis is less prominent and less effective in ejecting blood because the volume displacement is directly proportional to the change in length.

Shortening of the chamber involves movement of the mitral valve ring toward the apex of the heart. During diastole, the A-V junction rapidly ascends toward the left atrium. Since the interventricular septum shortens very little, the distance between the root of the aorta and the apex of the heart changes very little.

In contrast to the right ventricle, the left ventricular cavity has a small surface area in relation to the contained volume by virtue of its cylindrical contour. The thick cuff of deep myocardial bundles is ideally situated to develop a very high internal pressure during contraction. Thus, the left ventricle is architecturally designed as a high-pressure pump, which is consistent with its role of supplying energy for the flow of blood through the high-pressure, high-resistance, systemic circulation. The normal left ventricle has less adaptability than the right ventricle in ejecting large volumes of blood. When the left ventricle is exposed to an excessive volume load for extended periods of time, e.g., in aortic insufficiency, the chambers often become tremendously dilated so that the surface area per unit volume is increased. In other words, the left ventricle assumes some of the characteristics of the right ventricle when large volumes must be ejected during each stroke.

Clearly, the anatomic and architectural features of the ventricular chambers reflect the type of work which each must perform. By the same token, the functional characteristics of the circulatory trees which they serve establish the nature of the load or the working conditions for each ventricular chamber.

Continuous measurements of the various ventricular dimensions provide an opportunity to synthesize a description of the changes in the volume.

Techniques for Recording Cardiac Performance in Intact Dogs. Although it has not been possible to measure directly the absolute ventricular volume in intact animals, new techniques have been devised[21, 22] for continuously recording the circumference, diameter and length of the left ventricular chamber. The left ventricular pressure and the flow of blood through the aorta have also been measured in intact dogs, and records of all these parameters of ventricular function have been obtained during a wide range of activities for periods of days or weeks. These methods are described here briefly because they are recent developments which are not generally familiar; much of the data

discussed in the remainder of this section have been obtained by these means.

Left ventricular diameter has been measured by variable inductance gauges installed within that chamber and connected to a recorder by wires on the outside. The gauge comprises a coil, anchored at one end to the free wall of the left ventricle, and a stylus, anchored to the midportion of the interventricular wall and free to move within the coil. The position of the stylus within the coil can be recorded to a fraction of a millimeter by recording changes in inductance of the coil (see Fig. 2–17A).

Left ventricular length can also be determined with a variable inductance gauge. For this measurement the gauge is installed between the root of the aorta and the apex of the chamber (Fig. 2–17C).

Left ventricular circumference has been measured by a variable resistance gauge (a mercury-filled rubber tube) encircling the chamber; a wire from one end of the gauge passes into the right ventricular cavity to follow the contour of the interventricular septum. The absolute circumference of the gauge is determined from roentgenograms exposed perpendicular to the long axis of the ventricle (see Fig. 2–17C).

SONOCARDIOMETERY.[21, 22] Alternatively, a ventricular dimension may be measured in the intact dog with the sonocardiometer. With this instrument, the distance across the ventricular cavity is determined as the transit time of bursts of ultrasonic vibrations passing between barium titanate crystals installed on its walls. These sound waves travel through blood and the ventricular walls at 1.5 mm./msec., so that this transit time can be continuously recorded and calibrated as ventricular diameter.

The internal diameters and in-

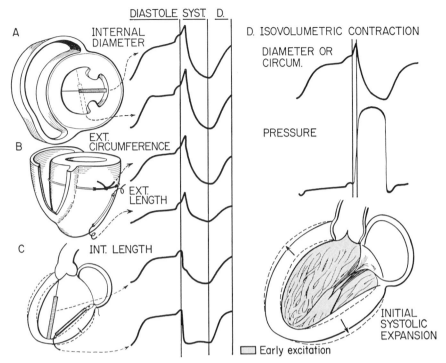

DIASTOLE SYST. D.

A   INTERNAL DIAMETER

B   EXT. CIRCUMFERENCE

    EXT. LENGTH

C   INT. LENGTH

D. ISOVOLUMETRIC CONTRACTION

DIAMETER OR CIRCUM.

PRESSURE

INITIAL SYSTOLIC EXPANSION

☐ Early excitation

FIGURE 2–17   CYCLIC CHANGES IN LEFT VENTRICULAR DIMENSIONS

A, During ventricular diastole, all dimensions increase, rapidly at first and more gradually during the latter part of the filling interval. Atrial contraction adds a slight additional increment of blood. At the onset of ventricular systole, the internal diameters (A), external circumference and length (B) abruptly increase because the internal length (C) shortens during this interval which is called the isovolumetric contraction (D). The external length increases during this interval when the internal length is abruptly diminishing because of the outward bending of the thick-walled ventricle.

ternal length of the left ventricle have been measured by variable induct-ance coils (Fig. 2–17A,C). The external circumference and the length of the left and right ventricles have been meas-ured by variable resistance gauges (delicate rubber tubes filled with mercury). These records illustrate the following characteristics of the filling and emptying of the ventricles. At the beginning of the diastolic interval, all dimensions of the ventricular cham-ber increase rapidly. This phase of rapid diastolic filling is very brief and merges abruptly or gradually into the phase of slow filling which persists until atrial contraction ensues. When the ventricles are maximally dis-tended, the dimensions reach a plateau

at the end of the rapid filling phase and do not increase further during the remainder of diastole. Such an interval of unchanging ventricular volume is termed *the period of diastasis.* The diastolic interval normally ends with the onset of atrial contraction, which begins as the wave of excitation spreads over the atrium. Contraction of the atrial musculature reduces the capac-ity of the atrial chambers and displaces blood forward into the ventricles or backward into the great veins, de-pending on which course offers the least resistance.

   The Isovolumic Phase of Ventri-cular Systole. As the wave of excita-tion extends rapidly along the Purkinje system (Fig. 2–12) and spreads over the endocardial surface of the ventricles, the trabeculae carneae and the papillary muscles are excited and begin to contract. The shortening papillary muscles exert traction on the chordae tendineae, drawing the atrioventricular valves into apposition, and the rising ventricular pressure seals them tight. The contracting papillary muscles draw the antrioventricular valve edges toward the apex,[23, 24] and the shortening endocardial layers draw the atrioventricular valve rings toward the apex of the heart. Since all four valves are closed, the contracting muscles elevate the pressure within the ventricle but do not change the volume they contain. Thus, the interval during which ventricular pressure rises to a level sufficient to open the semilunar valves has been called the period of isovolumic contraction. At the onset of systole, the length of the ventricles is abruptly shortened as the atrioventricular diaphragm rapidly descends. The other dimensions (diameter, circumference and external length) of the ventricle simultaneously expand. The sudden lengthening of the circumferentially oriented constrictor muscles in the ventricle, just before they contract, may increase the effectiveness of their contraction.

Ventricular Systole. As the full thickness of the ventricular wall becomes excited, pressure in the ventricles exceeds corresponding arterial pressure and blood is very rapidly ejected from the ventricles. The rapidity of ventricular emptying is indicated by the reduction in the ventricular dimensions, rapid during early systole and slowing during the last part of systole. The various dimensional changes illustrated in Figure 2–17 are applicable to ventricular systole when the heart is normally well filled at the end of diastole. If the ventricular chambers are not well filled during diastole, the circumference is reduced at the onset of systole and systolic ejection is accomplished primarily by shortening of the longitudinal ventricular axis. This type of ejection occurs when cardiac size is below the normal range as a result of extremely fast heart rates, positive radial acceleration or exposure of the heart for experimental purposes.

THE MECHANICAL EFFECTS OF CARDIAC CONTRACTION

The cyclic changes in the various dimensions of the ventricles combine to produce alternating expansion and contraction of total ventricular volume. Such changes in volume have been recorded by inserting the exposed hearts of animals into rigid chambers called cardiometers. (See Fig. 2–18.)

Myocardial contraction produces a sequence of changes in the pressure and volume of blood in the ventricles which is traditionally described in terms of the atrial, ventricular and arterial pressures and of the variations in the combined volume of both ventricles measured by a cardiometer as illustrated schematically in Figure 2–18.

During the later portion of diastole, the ventricular pressure equals the atrial pressure because the two chambers are connected through the wide A-V orifices and little or no blood is flowing between them. The wave of excitation spreading over the atrium is followed by atrial contraction. The contraction slightly increases both intra-atrial and intraventricular pressures because it suddenly compresses this portion of the venous volume reservoir. As the atrium contracts, blood may be displaced into the ventricular chambers or back into the large venous

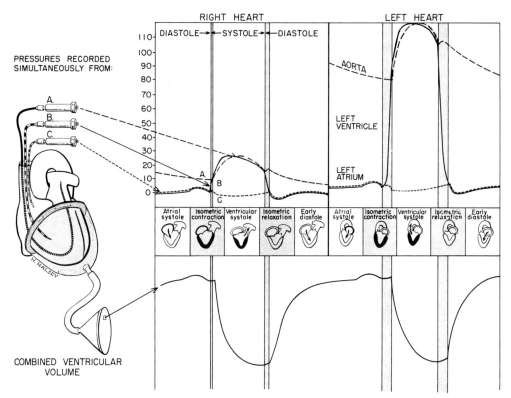

FIGURE 2–18   MECHANICAL EFFECTS OF CARDIAC CONTRACTION

Simultaneous changes in atrial, ventricular and arterial pressures in the right and left ventricles are illustrated schematically along with fluctuations in combined ventricular volume to indicate the sequence of events during a single cardiac cycle. Note that ventricular pressure exceeds corresponding arterial pressure only during the first portion of systole (see text). The great difference in pressure developed by the two ventricles is consistent with the differences in their architecture (see Fig. 2–16).

channels, depending upon which course offers the least resistance. The quantity of blood which enters the ventricle in response to atrial contraction is quite variable.

Excitation of the ventricles begins as atrial contraction is being completed, and ventricular contraction begins about 0.075 second later.[25] Ventricular pressure rises to exceed arterial pressure during the period of isometric contraction, which lasts about 0.013 second in the right ventricle[26] and about 0.06 second in the left ventricle (Fig. 2–18).

During this period the ventricular volume is unchanged except for the movement of blood required to

close and displace the valves. This period of isovolumic contraction is characterized by a slight reduction in recorded ventricular volume and a slight increase in atrial pressure due to ballooning of the A-V valves. The atria relax and begin to refill during ventricular systole. Isovolumic contraction of the ventricle ends when ventricular pressure exceeds the arterial pressure and is followed by rapid ejection of blood into the arterial system. Thus, the arterial pressure is elevated while the ventricular volume is abruptly diminished.

During the initial portion of systolic ejection, the ventricular pressures rise well above the pressure in the arterial channels into which they discharge. This transient, steep pressure gradient (somewhat exaggerated in Fig. 2–18) produces rapid acceleration of outflowing blood to produce a peak flow rate early in systole. During the later portion of systole, pressure in the ventricles actually drops slightly below the pressure in the corresponding artery, even though the ventricular volume continues to diminish, indicating persistent outflow of blood. These changes in pressure gradient and volume changes in the ventricles find important functional significance in the performance of the heart in terms of blood flow rates.

The intraventricular and arterial pressures tend to level off and descend as the rate of ejection from the ventricles drops below the rate at which blood leaves the arterial system through the capillaries. The onset of ventricular relaxation is associated with a rapid drop in ventricular pressures below arterial pressure. The semilunar valves become approximated by a retrograde surge of blood in the root of the aorta, which produces the dicrotic notch in the arterial pressure wave. During isovolumic relaxation, ventricular pressure rapidly drops below atrial pressure. The A-V valves swing open before a gush of blood from the atrium. The ventricles rapidly refill with blood from the thoracic veins and atria, as indicated by the abrupt upswing in the ventricular volume curve. The slope of the volume curve indicates that early filling of the ventricles is more rapid than the ejection of blood by ventricular contraction. Ventricular filling is largely complete very soon after the onset of ventricular relaxation and, if the diastolic interval is sufficiently long, ventricular volume reaches a plateau during which no more blood enters from the atrium—the period of

diastasis. The length of the diastolic interval is determined largely by the time required for the pacemaker to discharge the new wave of excitation which initiates another cardiac cycle.

BLOOD FLOW: METHODS OF MEASUREMENT

The rate of ventricular ejection can be estimated from the systolic downslope on cardiometer records. Obviously, the rate of change of ventricular volume is related to the flow velocity and volume flow rates of blood leaving the ventricles. A clear picture of ventricular ejection cannot be obtained from measurements of changing dimensions and pressures. Detailed information regarding the blood flow out of each ventricle and at various key arteries and veins is absolutely essential for a comprehensive understanding of cardiovascular function and control. A wide variety of flow measuring devices have been employed in physiological and clinical studies. Extensive discussion of methodology is not appropriate in this type of discussion. However, some representatives examples of flow detecting devices are presented schematically in Figure 2–19 as representative examples, divided into five rather arbitrary categories.

Some Volume Sensors. If fluid flow is defined as the change of volume or displacement of a volume per unit time, (dV/dt), a most direct approach would utilize sensors responding to changes in volume, such as the cardiometer illustrated in Figure 2–18. Each of the methods illustrated in the left hand column of Figure 2–19 has been employed in physiological investigations, and many other techniques in the same category have been described in other publications.[27–29] A volumetric container and a timer

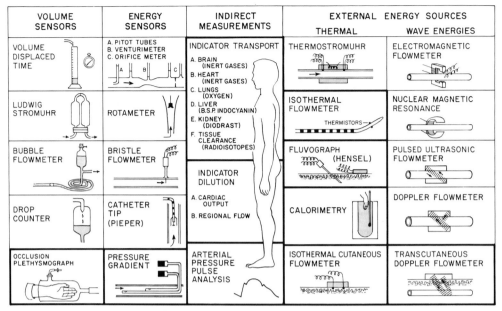

VOLUME SENSORS	ENERGY SENSORS	INDIRECT MEASUREMENTS	EXTERNAL ENERGY SOURCES	
			THERMAL	WAVE ENERGIES
VOLUME DISPLACED TIME	A. PITOT TUBES B. VENTURIMETER C. ORIFICE METER	INDICATOR TRANSPORT A. BRAIN (INERT GASES) B. HEART (INERT GASES) C. LUNGS (OXYGEN) D. LIVER (B.S.P. INDOCYANIN) E. KIDNEY (DIODRAST) F. TISSUE CLEARANCE (RADIOISOTOPES)	THERMOSTROMUHR	ELECTROMAGNETIC FLOWMETER
LUDWIG STROMUHR	ROTAMETER		ISOTHERMAL FLOWMETER THERMISTORS	NUCLEAR MAGNETIC RESONANCE
BUBBLE FLOWMETER	BRISTLE FLOWMETER	INDICATOR DILUTION A. CARDIAC OUTPUT B. REGIONAL FLOW	FLUVOGRAPH (HENSEL)	PULSED ULTRASONIC FLOWMETER
DROP COUNTER	CATHETER TIP (PIEPER)		CALORIMETRY	DOPPLER FLOWMETER
OCCLUSION PLETHYSMOGRAPH	PRESSURE GRADIENT	ARTERIAL PRESSURE PULSE ANALYSIS	ISOTHERMAL CUTANEOUS FLOWMETER	TRANSCUTANEOUS DOPPLER FLOWMETER

FIGURE 2–19 BLOOD FLOW DETECTING AND MEASURING DEVICES

Various types of flow detecting and measuring devices are illustrated schematically to indicate the diversity of methods that have been used in the past. The indirect techniques have found common use in clinical diagnosis and are described in greater detail in Chapter 3, Section 2.

serve as a standard for calibrating flowmeters just as a mercury column is a common standard for calibrating pressure gauges. The Ludwig strohmuhr, bubble flowmeter and drop counter and plethysmograph all monitor changes in volume which can be calibrated in terms of flow rates of blood. To directly measure volumetric blood flow requires gaining access to the entire volume of blood flowing through a blood vessel, which generally requires undesirably preliminary steps such as cannulation or exposure under surgical conditions. A notable exception is the venous occlusion plethysmograph by which arterial inflow is collected within the veins and measured by a volume sensor; it is applicable only to accessible peripheral vascular beds.

Some Energy Sensors. The energy content of moving blood may be used to activate sensors such as Pitot tubes, venturimeters, orifice meters, rotameters and bristle flowmeters as illustrated schematically in Figure 2–19. These have been described in considerable detail elsewhere.[27–29] The catheter tip flowmeter of Pieper[30] responds to the momentum of flowing blood impinging upon a very small plate exposed to the blood streaming along a channel. The flow rate along an artery can be continuously computed from the pressure gradient measured at two sites at known distances along a vascular channel by means of double lumen catheters and carefully matched pressure transducers in accordance with a technique described by Fry and his associates.[31] All of these techniques have provided information of value in controlled experiments on experimental animals. Pieper's catheter has been employed to provide information about dynamic changes in flow rates in intact healthy animals, and the pressure gradient technique has been employed in both animals and man.

Some Indirect Measurements. Most of our available information about blood flow in man has come from various techniques by which blood flow is estimated by measurement of the concentration of substances in blood or tissue.[32] In this connection, the term indirect is used to imply that the recorded variable is distinctly dissimilar to the target variable, a distinction which is sometimes quite arbitrary Clearly, the estimation of blood flow by measuring the changing concentrations of dyes or radioisotopes or dissolved gases conforms to this definition. The quantity of blood required to transport the oxygen taken into the lungs per minute can be calculated by means of the Fick formula.[33] This and other techniques applicable to man are described in Section 2 of Chapter 3. Blood flows computed from oxygen transport or indicator dilution are very useful but share two common deficiencies: flow rates can be estimated only at low sampling rates so that rapid changes cannot be followed and the sampling requires withdrawal of samples which can be obtained only by inserting needles or catheters through the skin into the blood vessels. Estimation of blood flow from a continuous record of central aortic pressure has theoretical and practical limitations.[34]

External Energy Sensors. The rate at which heat is carried away from a heat source is an indirect method of estimating flow which has been widely used in both engineering and basic medical science. The hot-wire anemometer is practically a standard for fluid dynamics of gases, but its application to liquid poses serious problems. The thermostromuhr of Rein had a distinguished place in physiological research but rapidly faded into obscurity after a critical evaluation by Shipley, Gregg and Warn.[35] Since heat can be so easily generated and controlled by electronic circuitry, and since temperatures can be precisely measured by thermocouples or thermistors, many thermal flowmeters have been proposed for application to the body surface or to internal structures.[36-38] However, these devices all have a common source of uncertainty due to the fact that heat flows so readily between continuous media of all sorts. In other words, it is very difficult to confine induced thermal energy to the blood or to a single tissue.

Electromagnetic and ultrasonic wave energies have produced a growing selection of new types of flow detecting devices applicable to physiological experiments on healthy animals and man.[39] They are capable of responding rapidly to dynamic responses. Since they have contributed greatly to our knowledge in the past decade, these techniques are described in somewhat greater detail.

Two main types of flow detecting devices have been developed to the point that the transducers could be chronically implanted on the outside of arteries or veins during aseptic surgery so that cardiovascular responses could be studied during spontaneous and experimentally induced changes in activity for days, weeks or months after recovery.

Electromagnetic Flowmeters. If a strip of metal moved through the magnetic field between the poles of a magnet at right angles to the lines of force, a voltage or potential difference is generated in the metal strip in accordance with Faraday's induction law (Fig. 2–19). The induced voltage could be registered using electrodes in contact with the metal strip. An ionic solution, such as blood plasma, is also an electrical conductor. If blood flows between the poles of a magnet, a potential difference can be registered between electrodes making electrical contact with the fluid. To avoid polarization of electrodes and artifacts from extraneous electrical currents (i.e., electrocardiogram), fluctuating magnetic fields have been used by energizing the magnet with fluctuating currents (sine wave, square wave, trapezoidal and so forth). Since 1936 Kolin's early application of the Faraday principle[40] has been followed by extensive development, notably by Denison and Spencer[41] and many others, including industrial concerns. As a result, electromagnetic flowmeters with good stability, rapid response and reliable calibrations are available commercially. The principles and characteristics of these devices are covered in greater detail in other publications.[42, 43]

Pulsed-Ultrasonic Flow Sensor. A flow detecting device has been developed in the laboratory utilizing bursts of ultrasound and based on the simple principle that sound travels faster in fluid when moving with the stream than against the stream.[44] In other words, sound will take longer to travel upstream between two points than to travel downstream between the same two points. If the separation of the two points and the velocity of the sound in the still medium are known, then the velocity of the medium may be calculated or recorded based on the difference in the transit times upstream and downstream.

Two ultrasonic transmitting crystals are mounted diagonally at opposite ends of a plastic cylinder which is bivalved and fitted on the outside of an artery. Bursts of ultrasound (i.e., 5 megacycles/second) are transmitted diagonally across the stream of blood, alternately upstream and downstream. The transit time of these paired bursts are compared, amplified and recorded to represent the velocity of blood flow, averaged across the channel.

Ultrasonic Doppler Shift Blood Flow Detection. Everyone is familiar with the Doppler shift in frequency which causes the change in pitch in a railroad whistle as it passes a stationary observer. If a continuous beam of ultrasound is transmitted diagonally into a column of blood, a small fraction of the sound energy backscatters from particles in the blood to reach a receiver on the opposite side of the channel.[45] If the blood is stationary, the ultrasonic frequency at the receiver is the same as the transmitter frequency. If the blood is moving, however, a Doppler shift in frequency occurs such that the ultrasound reaching the receiver differs from the transmitted frequency by the amount dependent in part upon the velocity with which the backscattering particles are moving. By mixing the transmitted frequency with the backscattered frequency, a beat frequency is generated which is audible (0 to 10,000 c.p.s.) under normal blood flow conditions and can be recorded to indicate dynamic changes in blood flow velocity in arteries or veins. In its simplest form, this device does not distinguish forward from backward flow. The ultrasonic flowmeters are less accurate than the electromagnetic flowmeters on both theoretical and practical grounds. However, these and other flow detecting devices have potential value in various applications to basic medical science or clinical diagnosis.[46]

DYNAMIC PROPERTIES OF LEFT VENTRICULAR EJECTION

The availability of sensors which can be chronically implanted in animals has provided opportunities to study changes in pressures, dimensions and flows in strategic locations in the cardiovascular system during spontaneous and induced responses in intact healthy animals after recovery from the surgery (Fig. 2–20A). Since the sampling rates of these techniques are very rapid, they can accurately follow rapid changes in aortic flow, left ventricular diameter and arterial pressure (Fig. 2–20B). The recorded wave forms contain a great deal more

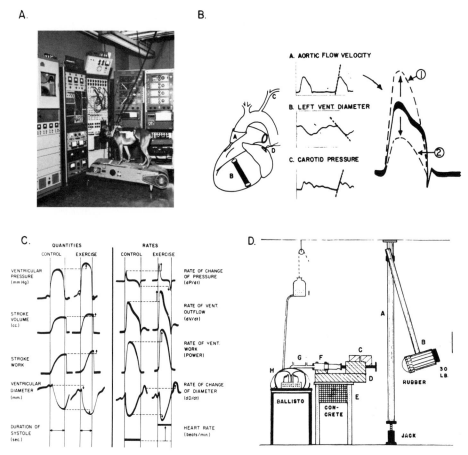

FIGURE 2–20   LEFT VENTRICULAR EJECTION CHARACTERISTICS

A, Chronically indwelling flow sensors, catheters and dimensional gauges provide an opportunity to study spontaneous cardiovascular responses in healthy dogs fully recovered from the surgery.

B, Typical wave forms of aortic flow rates, ventricle diameter and systemic arterial pressure all reveal very steep slopes during the initial stages of ventricular ejection when blood is being rapidly propelled out of the left ventricle.

C, Many characteristics of ventricular performance can be derived from direct measurements of pressure dimensions and flow.

D, To simulate the rapid acceleration of blood accomplished by the normal left ventricle in cadavers required blows by a 30 pound mass on a 8 foot lever arm striking a piston to drive blood into the aorta. (After Starr et al.[48])

information than is apparent from merely measuring either the mean values or the magnitudes at the peaks and valleys of the deflections. For example, the upslope of the aortic flow velocity recording is very steep, indicating that ventricular myocardium not only develops very high pressures very quickly, but also accelerates the blood very rapidly to high peak flow velocity very early during the ejection period. The downslope on the left ventricular diameter record confirms reduction in chamber diameter as the ventricle rapidly ejects blood into the aorta. As blood rapidly enters the root of the aorta, the pressure abruptly rises, inducing a pulse wave which spreads rapidly through the arterial tree. From direct recordings of aortic flow rate and left ventricular pressure and diameter, additional information can be derived using simple analogue computers and ratemeters as illustrated in Figures 2–20 and 2–22. The most significant features of left ventricular ejection are very steep slopes on the records of ventricular pressure, ventricular outflow rate (aortic flow) and ventricular diameter during the initial phases of left ventricular systole. These steep slopes indicate exceedingly rapid rates of increase in ventricular pressure and ventricular ejection velocity.

One might imagine that the muscular ventricular walls squeeze down on the contained blood much as one would milk a cow or squeeze a lemon in a clenched fist. According to Spencer and Greiss,[47] blood accelerates in the aorta exceedingly rapidly (averaging 4650 cm./sec.^{2}) to the peak velocity early in systole. To produce such rapid acceleration of blood, the ventricle must develop forces some five times the force of gravity.

Thus, the contracting myocardium propels outflowing blood with a sudden impulse like a piston struck with a mallet. For example, everyone is aware of the fact that every heart beat causes the whole body to recoil slightly, a phenomenon which can be directly observed while standing quietly on a sensitive scale. This phenomenon has been utilized in the development of a "ballistocardiograph" for studying cardiac function (see Fig. 3–25). When Starr and his associates[48] attempted to reproduce in a cadaver a recoil sufficient to simulate the normal ballistocardiographic record, they found that no available pumps could discharge blood into the aorta with sufficient acceleration to equal that of the normal heart. They finally found it necessary to use a 30 pound mass on an eight foot lever arm, striking a piston and driving blood into the cadaver's aorta (Fig. 2–20D) to produce ballistocardiographic deflections of an amplitude approaching that of normal men of equivalent size. The functional importance of these dynamic characteristics will be discussed in more detail in Chapter 3.

RIGHT VENTRICULAR EJECTION

The pattern of ejection from the normal right ventricle differs from that described for the left ventricle. The velocity of ejection increases more gradually and reaches its peak near mid systole. Flow from the ventricle also decelerates more gradually, and ejection persists longer. The retrograde flow usually associated with the closure of the semilunar valves at the end of systole occurs later. The average acceleration is lower (i.e., 2480 cm/sec.^{2}), and the pressure reversal occurs later.

These differences in the ejection patterns of the two ventricles may be attributed to their architecture and

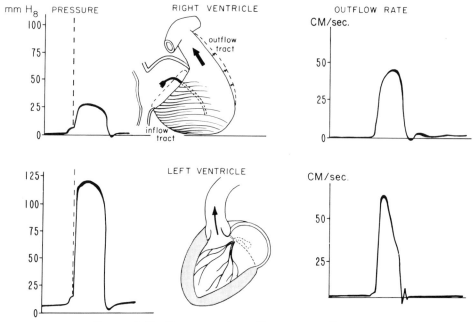

FIGURE 2–21   RIGHT AND LEFT VENTRICULAR EJECTION

In contrast with the left ventricle, right ventricular ejection produces a much more gradual pressure rise to a lower peak ventricular pressure and more gradual fall in pressure at the end of systole. Similarly, right ventricular outflow begins earlier, accelerates more gradually to a lower peak velocity occuring near mid-systole and decelerates more gradually than left ventricular outflow.

function. The rapid acceleration of blood and early peak flow velocity from the left ventricle suggest a powerful and effective mechanism for pumping against a high pressure. The thick walls of myocardium must contract very nearly synchronously to generate such a powerful impulse. In contrast, the right ventricular chamber can be likened to a crevice between two broad surfaces which exert a bellows type of action in ejecting blood. Further, a substantial body of evidence indicates that the inflow tract of the right ventricle contracts early and displaces the blood into the outflow tract. The conus region contracts last. Since the pressure in the pulmonary artery is very low at the onset of right ventricular systole, ejection begins as soon as right ventricular pressure rises only 8 to 10 mm. Hg. These factors

appear to account, at least in part, for the early onset of pulmonary flow, the gradual increase in outflow velocity from the right ventricle and the longer duration of ejection.

This description of right ventricular ejection patterns has been based on records obtained from indwelling gauges in healthy dogs with minimal intrathoracic pathology. In a few dogs with atelectasis and hydrothorax persisting after the surgical implantation of the gauges, the right ventricular ejection pattern closely resembled the normal left ventricular ejection pattern. A high peak flow velocity developed very early in systole, implying a greatly increased right ventricular impulse. Apparently, the right ventricle responds to an increase in outflow pressure by assuming the ejection properties of the left ventricle. This finding is not entirely surprising in view of the fact that during chronic pulmonary hypertension the right ventricle changes into a thick-walled chamber, very much like the left ventricle in form. Thus, the right ventricle is capable of conversion into a high-impulse pump like the normal left ventricle.

LEFT VENTRICULAR PERFORMANCE IN QUANTITATIVE PHYSICAL TERMS

A description of ventricular function solely in terms of absolute values of pressures, dimensions and flows is incomplete because a great deal of valuable information is contained within the waveforms, produced by recording systems capable of faithfully reproducing rapid changes. A more comprehensive description of cardiac function can be obtained[49] by extracting additional derived information using relatively simple analogue computers. For example, the signals from a pulsed ultrasonic flow sensor implanted on the aorta, along with ventricular pressure and diameter recordings, can be stored on magnetic tape and subsequently analyzed to provide 11 important variables as illustrated in Figure 2–22.

The pulsed ultrasonic flow sensor (or an electromagnetic flowmeter) inscribes a characteristic flow velocity wave indicating the rate at which blood is flowing from the left ventricle through the root of the aorta. This flow signal can be recorded directly without modification as at the top of the right hand column (Fig. 2–22). At the end of the experiment, known flows may be passed through the flow section in place on the aorta to provide a calibration for the system in terms of instantaneous volume flow rates (ml./sec.). The aortic flow signals can also be processed by a simple integrator that adds up to the flow occurring during each successive cardiac cycle to provide a deflection proportional to stroke volume. This process is equivalent to measuring the area under the original flow curve and calibrating it in terms of volume flow per stroke. Similarly, the aortic flow signal can be integrated by a circuit that adds up the flow over a set period of time (i.e., each 2.5 seconds). The height of each successive series of steps indicates the volume flow per unit time and can be calibrated as cardiac output (ml./min. or liters/min.). The slope of aortic flow wave form indicates the rate of change of velocity or acceleration of the blood. During the initial steep upslope on the flow record, a sharp spike is inscribed in the acceleration record indicating that the steepest slope and maximal increase in velocity occurs very early in systole.

The acceleration record, which was obtained by differentiating the flow waveform, indicates the rate at which the flow was increasing or decreasing. Since the flowmeter samples the average flow velocity across the vascular lumen, a reliable value for the peak linear velocity cannot be derived unless the profile of the flow velocity is known. The estimated peak acceleration is very high, e.g., 3000 cm./sec.^{2} during exercise on these records. Values reported by Noble (see Ref. 63, Chapter 3) are even higher (5000 to 10,000 cm./sec.^{2}). During the latter portions of systole, the acceleration record drops below the baseline, indicating the progressive slowing of ventricular outflow after the early peak flow velocity is attained.

The left ventricular pressure can be recorded directly from an indwelling catheter extending from the left ventricle to a high fidelity pressure gauge either just outside the heart or outside the body. The form of the ven-

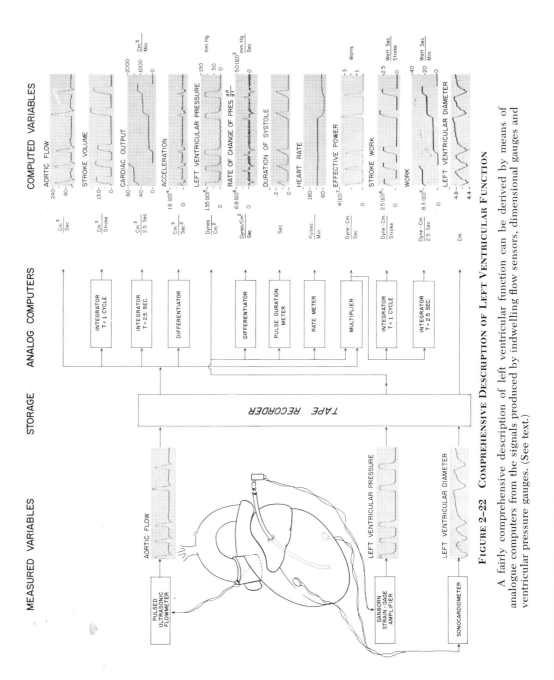

FIGURE 2–22 COMPREHENSIVE DESCRIPTION OF LEFT VENTRICULAR FUNCTION

A fairly comprehensive description of left ventricular function can be derived by means of analogue computers from the signals produced by indwelling flow sensors, dimensional gauges and ventricular pressure gauges. (See text.)

tricular pressure pulse is generally familiar, although attention is usually directed to the peak amplitude rather than to the details of the waveform. Tracings of the systolic pressure frequently exhibit a rounded dome shape, but the pressure may peak early in systole when ventricular ejection is exceptionally rapid and peripheral resistance is less than normal. The steep upslope and downslope of the ventricular record represents the rapid rate of rise and fall of pressure in the ventricle. This rate of change of pressure can be directly inscribed by passing the signal through a differentiating circuit to provide deflections, an upward spike followed by a downward spike, representing the slopes on the ventricular pressure record. The amplitudes of these spikes reflect the maximum rates of rise or fall (slope) of the ventricular pressure pulses. These amplitudes are very labile, indicating that the rate at which the ventricular pressure changes is readily altered under such conditions as spontaneous changes in heart rate, exercise, sympathetic stimulation and administration of catecholamines. The rate of change of pressure must be influenced by the degree of synchronization in the activation of the myocardial bundles and in the rate at which tension develops in these fibers.

The duration of ventricular systole in seconds can be indicated by the height of a ramp which begins as the ventricular pressure rises above some low level and is terminated when the pressure returns to the low level. The heart rate can be indicated in terms of the reciprocal of the interval between each pair of successive beats. The recorded heart rate refers to the heart rate represented by the duration of the preceding cycle (Fig. 2–22).

In a mechanical pump, the duration of the stroke is determined by the r.p.m. of the crankshaft. Similarly, there is an inverse relationship between the duration of systole and the heart rate. This relationship tends to be preserved under many different conditions, although the reasons are not so apparent in the heart as they are in a mechanical pump.

Effective power indicates the rate at which the ventricle was performing work and was derived by continuously multiplying the aortic flow rate by the ventricular pressure. This deflection continuously indicates the rate of effective energy conversion by the contracting ventricle calibrated in terms of dyne-cm./sec. or watts. Effective power is not a measure of the total rate of energy liberation because the viscous losses within the myocardium are not measured. Instead, the power record is interpreted as a measure of the rate at which energy is transferred from the left heart to the peripheral vasculature. Since peak outflow occurs early in systole when the pressure is achieving its maximum levels, power is also attaining its peak at this time. The stroke work record, derived by the integration of the power record for each successive cycle, is a measure of the total energy transferred to the peripheral vasculature during the cardiac cycle. Again, this process is similar to a manual measurement of the area under the waveform on the effective power record. Work per unit time (i.e., 2.5 seconds) can be recorded as a series of steps very much as the cardiac output was recorded in the third record from the top.

Finally, the changing ventricular diameter can be recorded directly to indicate the changing dimensions of the chamber. A much more appropriate dimension for completeness would be the changing volume of the left ventricle but we are not able to make this measurement at sampling rates approaching those of the other recorded variables in Figure 2–22.

REFERENCES

1. PATTEN, B. M. The first heart beats and the beginning of the embryonic circulation. *Amer. Scien.*, 39:225–243, 1951.
2. GOSS, C. M. First contractions of the heart without cytological differentiation. *Anat. Rec.*, 76:19–27, 1940.
3. PATTEN, B. M., KRAMER, T. C., and BARRY, A. Valvular action in the embryonic chick heart by localized apposition of endocardial masses. *Anat. Rec.*, 102:299–311, 1948.
4. HOFF, E. C., KRAMER, T. C., DuBOIS, D., and PATTEN, B. M. The development of the electrocardiogram of the embryonic heart. *Amer. Heart J.*, 17:470–488, 1939.
5. HUXLEY, H. E. The double array of filaments in cross-striated muscle. *J. Biophys. Biochem. Cystol.*, 3:631–648, 1957.
6. HUXLEY, H. E. The contraction of muscle. *Sci. Amer.*, 199:66–82, 1958.
7. BOZLER, E. An analysis of the properties of smooth muscle. *Cold Spr. Harb. Symp.*, 4:260–266, 1936.
8. BOZLER, E. Action potentials and conduction of excitation in muscle. *Biol. Symp.*, 3:95–110, 1941.
9. DiPALMA, J. R., and MASCATELLO, A. V. Excitability and refractory period of isolated heart muscle of the cat. *Amer. J. Physiol.*, 164:589–600, 1951.
10. MALL, F. P. On the muscular architecture of the ventricles of the human heart. *Amer. J. Anat.*, 11:211–266, 1911.
11. ROBB, J. S., and ROBB, R. C. The normal heart. *Amer. Heart J.*, 23:455–467, 1942.
12. GRANT, R. P. Notes on muscular architecture of the left ventricle. *Circulation*, 32:301–308, 1965.
13. STREETER, D. D., JR., and BASSETT, D. L. An engineering analysis of myocardial fiber orientation in pig's left ventricle in systole. *Anat. Rec.*, 155:503–512, 1966.
14. STREETER, D. D., JR., SPOTNITZ, H. M., PATEL, D. J., ROSS, J., JR., and SONNENBLICK, E. H. Fiber orientation in the canine left ventricle during diastole and systole. *Circulat. Res.*, 24:339–347, 1969.
15. CURTIS, H. J., and TRAVIS, D. M. Conduction in Purkinje tissue of the ox heart. *Amer. J. Physiol.*, 165:173–178, 1951.
16. RUSHMER, R. F., and CRYSTAL, D. K. Changes in configuration of the ventricular chambers during the cardiac cycle. *Circulation*, 4:211–218, 1951.
17. RUSHMER, R. F., and THAL, N. The mechanics of ventricular contraction: a cinefluorographic study. *Circulation*, 4:219–228, 1951.
18. RUSHMER, R. F., and THAL, N. Factors influencing stroke volume: a cinefluorographic study of angiocardiography. *Amer. J. Physiol.*, 168:509–521, 1952.
19. KAGAN, A. Dynamic responses of the right ventricle following extensive damage by cauterization. *Circulation*, 5:816–823, 1952.
20. ZAUS, E. A., and KEARNS, W. M., JR. Massive infarction of the right ventricle and atrium. *Circulation*, 6:593–598, 1952.
21. BAKER, D., ELLIS, R. M., FRANKLIN, D. L., and RUSHMER, R. F. Some engineering aspects of modern cardiovascular research. *Proc. Inst. Radio Engrs.*, 47:1917–1924, 1959.
22. RUSHMER, R. F., FRANKLIN, D. L., and ELLIS, R. M. Left ventricular dimensions recorded by sonocardiometry. *Circulat. Res.*, 4:684–688, 1956.
23. RUSHMER, R. F. Initial phase of ventricular systole: Asynchronous contraction. *Amer. J. Physiol.*, 184:188–194, 1956.
24. RUSHMER, R. F., FINLAYSON, B. L., and NASH, A. A. Movements of the mitral valve. *Circulat. Res.*, 4:337–342, 1956.
25. WIGGERS, C. J., and KATZ, L. N. The contour of the ventricular volume curves under different conditions. *Amer. J. Physiol.*, 58:439–475, 1921–22.
26. COBLENTZ, B., HARVEY, R. M., FERRER, M. I., COURNAND, A., and RICHARD, D. W., JR. The relationship between electrical and mechanical events in the cardiac cycle of man. *Brit. Heart J.*, 11:1–22, 1949.
27. BRUNER, H. D. Peripheral blood flow measurement. P. 222 in *Methods in Medical Research*, Sect. 3, Vol. 8, W. S. Root, Ed. Chicago, Year Book Publishers, 1960.
28. BURTON, A. C. A critical survey of methods available for the measurement of human peripheral blood flow. *Ciba Found. Symp. Peripheral Circulation in Man*, 1954.
29. GREEN, H. D. Circulation blood flow measurement. P. 66 in *Methods in Medical Research*, Sect. 2, Vol. 1, V. R. Potter, Ed. Chicago, Year Book Publishers, 1948.
30. PIEPER, H. P. Catheter-tip blood flowmeter for measurement of pulmonary arterial blood flow in closed-chest dogs. *Rev. Sci. Instrum.*, 34:908–910, 1963.
31. GREENFIELD, J. C., JR., and FRY, D. L. Measurement errors in estimating aortic blood velocity by pressure gradient. *J. Appl. Physiol.*, 17:1013–1019, 1962.
32. KETY, S. S. Theory and applications of the exchange of inert gas at the lungs and tissues. *Pharmacol. Rev.*, 3:1–41, 1951.
33. VISSCHER, M. B., and JOHNSON, J. A. The Fick principle: Analysis of a potential error in its conventional application. *J. Appl. Physiol.*, 5:635–638, 1953.
34. VAN CITTERS, R. L., and BARNETT, G. O. Computation of blood flow velocity from the pressure pulse compared with direct measurement by the ultrasonic flowmeter. *Proc. San Diego Symp. Biomed. Engrs.*, pp. 79–86, 1963.
35. SHIPLEY, R. E., GREGG, D. E., and WARN, J. T. Operative mechanism of some errors

in the application of the thermostromuhr method to the measurement of blood flow. *Amer. J. Physiol.*, 136:263–274, 1942.

36. HENSEL, H. Messkopf zur Durchblutungsregistrierung an Oberflächen. *Arch. Ges. Physiol.*, 268:604–606, 1959.

37. HARDING, D. C., BAKER, D. W., and RUSHMER, R. F. Isothermal cutaneous blood flowmeter. *Proc. Ann. Conf. Engr. Med. Biol., 17th*, 6:77, 1964.

38. KATSURA, S., WEISS, R., BAKER, D. W., and RUSHMER, R. F. Isothermal blood flow velocity probe. *IRE Trans. Med. Electron.*, ME6:283–285, 1959.

39. WATSON, N. W., and RUSHMER, R. F. Ultrasonic blood flowmeter transducers. *Proc. San Diego Symp. Biomed. Engrs.*, pp. 87–91, 1963.

40. KOLIN, A. An electromagnetic flowmeter: Principles of the method and its application to blood flow measurements. *Proc. Soc. Exp. Biol. Med.*, 35:53–56, 1936.

41. DENISON, A. B., and SPENCER, M. P. Magnetic flowmeters. P. 178 in *Medical Physics*, Vol. 3. Chicago, Year Book Publishers, 1960.

42. SPENCER, M. P., and DENISON, A. B. Square-wave electromagnetic flowmeter for surgical experimental application. Pp. 321–341 in *Methods in Medical Research*, Vol. 8. Chicago, Year Book Publishers, 1960.

43. WETTERER, E. Flowmeters: Their theory, construction and operation. Pp. 1294–1324 in *Handbook of Physiology, Section 2: Circulation*, Vol. 2, W. F. Hamilton and P. Dow, Eds. Washington, D. C., American Physiological Society, 1963.

44. FRANKLIN, D. L., BAKER, D. W., ELLIS, R. M., and RUSHMER, R. F. A pulsed ultrasonic flowmeter. *IRE Trans. Med. Electron.*, ME6:204–206, 1959.

45. FRANKLIN, D. L., SCHLEGEL, W., and RUSHMER, R. F. Blood flow measured by Doppler frequency shift of back-scattered ultrasound. *Science*, 134:564–565, 1961.

46. RUSHMER, R. F., BAKER, D. W., and STEGALL, H. F. Transcutaneous Doppler flow detection as a nondestructive technique. *J. Appl. Physiol.*, 21:554–566, 1966.

47. SPENCER, M. P., and GREISS, F. S. Dynamics of ventricular ejection. *Circulat. Res.*, 10:274–279, 1962.

48. STARR, I., SCHNABEL, T. G., JR., and MAYOCK, R. L. Studies made by simulating systole at necropsy. II. Experiments on the relation of cardiac and peripheral factors to the genesis of the pulse wave and ballistrocardigram. *Circulation*, 8:44–61, 1953.

49. FRANKLIN, D. L., VAN CITTERS, R. L., and RUSHMER, R. F. Left ventricular function described in physical terms. *Circulat. Res.*, 11:702–711, 1962.

CHAPTER 3

THE CARDIAC OUTPUT

I. FACTORS AFFECTING CARDIAC OUTPUT

An understanding of the principles governing cardiovascular responses in the normal person is a prerequisite for interpreting changes induced by disease. The five basic mechanisms by which cardiac output can be adjusted are indicated in Figure 3–1. The cardiac output is determined by the product of the heart rate and stroke volume. Stroke volume is the diastolic volume of the ventricle minus the volume of blood in the ventricle at the end of systole. Diastolic filling is determined by the effective filling pressure and the resistance to distension offered by the ventricular wall. The degree of systolic ejection depends upon the degree of shortening which the ventricular myocardium can attain while working against the arterial pressure. The changes in contractile properties of the myocardium are manifest in many different ways, affecting the rate, amount and duration of tension development, shortening and relaxation. All or parts of these changes in ventricular performance have been included rather indiscriminately under the general term "contractility." Cardiac control clearly involves all five major factors: (1) heart rate, (2) ventricular filling or distending pressure, (3) ventricular "distensibility," (4) contractile proper-

ties of the myocardium and (5) arterial pressure. A comprehensive discussion would include the contributing factors to each and the interactions of all the mechanisms, a most complex and perplexing problem.

The following discussion will be devoted to a consideration of the control of the heart rate and some of the

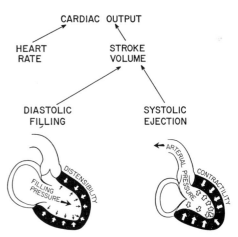

FIGURE 3–1 FACTORS AFFECTING STROKE VOLUME

The cardiac output is influenced by at least five different factors which include changes in heart rate and by four mechanisms which influence the stroke volume, namely (a) filling pressure, (b) ventricular distensibility, (c) arterial pressure and (s) contractility. Distensibility and contractility are terms which may in fact cover a number of additional independent factors.

70

factors affecting contraction and distention of the cardiac chambers. Some mechanical and architectural features of the ventricles will receive attention because they also may affect the function of the heart as a pump.

CONTROL OF HEART RATE

Normally the heart rate is determined by the frequency with which the sinoatrial (S-A) node generates the impulses which spread over the atrium and ultimately activate the heart in the sequence illustrated in Figure 2–12. Given suitable conditions, any myocardial fiber is capable of generating a conducted impulse, but the S-A node retains its role as a pacemaker of the heart (1) so long as it generates impulses more rapidly than any other part of the heart and (2) so long as the conduction system functions normally (see Chapter 12). During the embryonic development of the heart, the ventricle forms first; initially it contracts very slowly and irregularly (see Fig. 2–1). As the atrium develops, its faster inherent rate of impulse formation becomes manifest. The atrium takes over the pacemaker role, and the embryonic heart rate quickens. The sinus venosus, the last portion of the heart to appear, has the highest rate of impulse formation and takes over the role of pacemaker. The S-A node is a vestigial remnant of the sinus venosus and is the pacemaker of the fully developed heart.

THE NATURE OF PACEMAKER ACTIVITY

The heart is only one example of a structure with an autogenic pacemaker. The ureter displays contraction waves that originate at a point near the pelvis of the kidney and descend at regular intervals toward the urinary bladder.

The point where these conducted waves of excitation originate is also called a *pacemaker*, capable of spontaneously generating conducted impulses at regular intervals. The electrical potentials associated with this wave of excitation can be readily recorded. During the interval between the action potentials representing waves of excitation, the recorded potentials along the ureter remain steady at a low level. At the site of the pacemaker, however, the cellular potentials rise progressively until they reach the threshold of excitability which sets off a conducted impulse (Fig. 3–2A). This gradual rise in potential between action potentials is called a *prepotential* and apparently represents a spontaneous phasic swing in the potential on the membranes of cells which establishes the rate at which contraction waves descend the ureter.[1] If the ureter is transected below the normal pacemaker, a new pacemaker site becomes established in the lower segment. This new pacemaker displays a prepotential but generates impulses at a slower rate than the normal site. The inherent rate of pacemaker activity is progressively slower at greater and greater distances below the pelvis of the kidney.

The correspondence between the pacemakers of the ureter and of the heart is obvious. The specialized myocardial fibers in the S-A node generate spontaneous swings in membrane potential, recorded as prepotentials within those myocardial cells which serve as pacemakers. When the membrane potential reaches the critical threshold level, a conducted impulse spreads in all directions over the atrial musculature. No prepotentials are visible in recordings from within other atrial myocardial cells; the resting membrane potentials remain steady between each period of excitation.

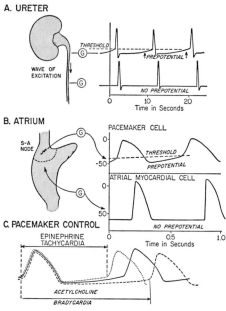

FIGURE 3–2   PACEMAKER ACTIVITY

A, Waves of excitation periodically pass down the ureter from a "pacemaker" site at which the membrane potentials of the cells spontaneously change (prepotentials) until threshold is reached to produce a propagated impulse spreading from cell to cell down the ureter.

B, Pacemaker cells in the sinus node normally exhibit spontaneous changes in membrane potentials (prepotentials) which lead to waves of excitation spreading centripetally from this site over the atrium.

C, Changes in heart rate induced by epinephrine or acetylcholine, acting at the pacemaker site, result from changes in the rate of membrane depolarization (slope of the prepotential) with very little alteration in the level of the threshold of excitability.

The heart rate is normally adjusted through a change in the discharge rate of the S-A node. If the slope of the prepotential is altered, the interval required to reach the threshold level would change. West et al.[2] inserted very fine ultramicroelectrodes into individual S-A nodal cells which were apparently acting as pacemaker. When epinephrine was applied to the site, the rate of discharge was accelerated and prepotential slope became much steeper (Fig. 3–2C). In contrast, administration of acetylcholine produced slowing of the heart rate, associated with a much more gradual prepotential slope and a smaller action potential. Although changes in discharge rate could theoretically be achieved by alterations in threshold, this mechanism apparently is not as significant as the prepotential slope (Fig. 3–2C). Acetylcholine is the transmitter substance released from the parasympathetic nerves to the heart and norepinephrine is generally regarded as the transmitter substance released by sympathetic nerves distributed to the heart. Thus, the influences of these substances applied directly to pacemaker sites are believed to mimic the action of the sympathetic and parasympathetic nerves in the control of heart rate.

AUTONOMIC CONTROL OF HEART RATE

In 1899, Hunt[3] concluded that the accelerator (sympathetic) nerves of the heart are almost always in tonic activity. The action potentials arriving at the region of sinus node are believed to trigger the release of an epinephrine-like substance at the nerve endings. At the base of the brain, in the medulla oblongata, is the region where electrical stimulation produces large effects on both the heart rate and peripheral vascular resistance.[4] The term *cardio-regulatory center* for such poorly localized sites is somewhat misleading, but is common usage. From the "medullary centers," nerve fibers descend to the intermediolateral columns of the spinal cord (see Chapter 4). The fibers course out to the sympathetic trunk through T_1, T_2, T_3, T_4 and sometimes T_5 and pass up to the stellate ganglion and to the heart through the cardiac nerves (Fig. 3–4). Although the accelerator nerves cannot be dissociated from the other sympathetic nerves to the heart, the sympathetic accelerator fibers appear to be more prominent on the right than on the left.[5]

The motor nucleus of the vagus nerve lies not far from the medullary sites where electrical stimulation produces tachycardia. However, the vagal nerve endings distributed to the S-A node produce a profound slowing of the heart by the mechanism illustrated in Figure 3–2C.

The actions of acetylcholine and the sympathetic transmitter substance are mutually antagonistic. For example, if the vagus nerve is stimulated, the heart rate promptly slows.[6] If sympathetic accelerator fibers are simultaneously stimulated at an appropriate frequency, the heart rate can be brought back to the control levels (Fig. 3–3A). Then if the vagal stimulation is discontinued so that the sympathetic stimulation is unopposed, the heart rate promptly accelerates. An acceleration of the heart rate alone is not a very effective mechanism for increasing cardiac output without additional mechanisms to maintain or to increase the stroke volume (Fig. 3–3B).

The heart rate can be precisely adjusted by balancing the retarding effects of vagal discharge against the accelerating effects of sympathetic stimulation. This is a form of reciprocal innervation at the effector organ, the S-A node. In addition, reciprocal innervation is also prominent in the central control over heart rate (i.e., at the medullary center). For example, the neural connections are so organized that activation of the motor nucleus of the vagus is associated with simultaneous inhibition of the medullary accelerator centers. The medullary centers of cardiac and peripheral vascular control are important in the control of blood pressure.[7] However, these control centers are influenced

by nerves converging from a wide variety of sites and sources (Fig. 3–4).

ORIGINS OF AFFERENT NERVES CONVERGING ON THE CARDIOREGULATORY CENTERS

The vagus and sympathetic nerves conduct impulses which result from a more or less continuous bombardment of the cardioaccelerator and cardioinhibitor centers by afferent nerves from all over the body. The cardioregulatory centers are influenced by afferent fibers corresponding to those which play upon the vasomotor centers (see Chapter 4).

Impulses from the cerebral cortex impinge upon the cardioaccelerator and cardioinhibitor centers, as evidenced by many common experiences. Excitement, anxiety, fear and depression[8, 9] affect the heart rate without any direct relation to metabolic activity. Cardioacceleration occurs in anticipation of physical exertion before there is any significant increase in metabolism. An occasional individual can voluntarily alter his heart rate.[10] Clearly, the influence of higher centers on cardiovascular regulation cannot be ignored.

Stretch receptors in the carotid sinus and aortic arch exert a powerful influence on the cardioregulatory centers. A change in arterial blood pressure is reflected in a corresponding change in the frequency of impulses from the baroceptors which in turn influences the cardioregulatory centers and the heart rate. In general a drop in arterial blood pressure induces an acceleration of the heart and vice versa.

Digital pressure on a hypersensitive carotid sinus promptly produces bradycardia, reduced peripheral resistance, a severe drop in arterial

A. AUTONOMIC BALANCE IN HEART RATE CONTROL

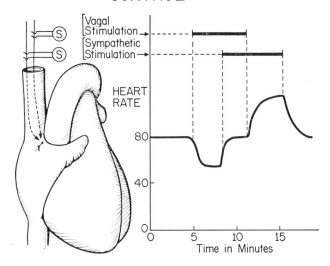

B. STROKE VOLUME DURING ARTIFICIAL TACHYCARDIA

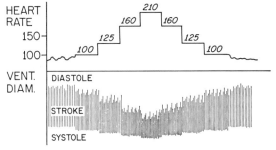

FIGURE 3–3   HEART RATE

A, Impulses descending the vagus nerve to the sinus node tend to produce slowing of the heart which can be precisely countered by activity of the sympathetic nerves to this site. Thus, the heart rate is regulated in terms of the balance between the sympathetic and vagal effects on the pacemaker.

B, An artificially induced tachycardia produces a progressive reduction in ventricular dimensions and in stroke deflection indicating that tachycardia alone is not an efficient mechanism for increasing cardiac output unless other mechanisms act to maintain or increase stroke volume.

blood pressure and syncope.[11] Insertion of a needle into the brachial artery of subjects in the erect position frequently produces a very similar response.[12] Such syncopal reactions, termed *vago-vagal reactions*, may be produced by many conditions.[13, 14] Since sensory fibers from virtually all parts of the body influence heart rate and peripheral resistance, only a few

of the more prominent examples can be mentioned.

Stimulation of internal organs may produce drastic cardiac inhibition. For example, stimulation of nerve endings in the upper portion of the respiratory tract may produce intense vagal depression of the heart rate. Thus, anesthetists must be extremely careful during intubation of the trachea be-

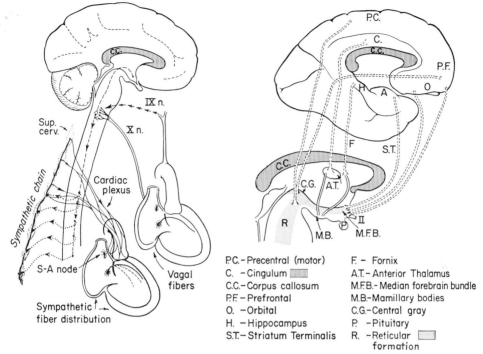

IX n.
Sup. cerv.
X n.
Sympathetic chain
Cardiac plexus
S-A node
Vagal fibers
Sympathetic fiber distribution

P.C.
C.
P.F.
O
A
H
F
S.T.
C.C.
C.G.
A.T.
R
P
II
M.B.
M.F.B.

P.C. – Precentral (motor)
C. – Cingulum
C.C. – Corpus callosum
P.F. – Prefrontal
O. – Orbital
H. – Hippocampus
S.T. – Striatum Terminalis

F. – Fornix
A.T. – Anterior Thalamus
M.F.B. – Median forebrain bundle
M.B. – Mamillary bodies
C.G. – Central gray
P. – Pituitary
R. – Reticular formation

FIGURE 3–4   NEURAL CONTROL OF THE HEART

A, The vagus nerve endings are concentrated in the region of the sinus node and atrioventricular node and are more diffusely distributed over the atrium. They do not extend to the ventricular myocardium. Sympathetic fibers from $T_1 - T_5$ are distributed to all parts of the atrium and ventricles. Impulses traveling along the vagus and sympathetic nerves to the heart come from the medulla or the diencephalon.

B, Neural pathways from many parts of the brain converge on the diencephalic region to influence autonomic outflow to the heart and other visceral structures.

cause increased vagal activity may lead to cardiac standstill and death. Inhalation of irritant gases may intensely affect the heart rate. Phasic changes in heart rate (sinus arrhythmia) occur during normal respiratory cycles.

The gastrointestinal tract is supplied with afferent nerve fibers which travel along the vagus to the medulla. Nausea and vomiting are commonly associated with slowing of the heart whether they are due to digital stimulation of the pharynx or to ingestion of toxic substances. Visceral pain fibers are widely distributed and have a powerful slowing effect on heart rate. Painful stimulation of skeletal muscles may produce a similar autonomic

response. Pressure on the eyeball may produce a profound slowing of the heart through the "oculocardiac reflex." In general, visceral afferent nerves, originating in nearly all tissues and organs except the skin, produce bradycardia. In contrast, somatic pain from the skin generally produces tachycardia along with some increase in arterial blood pressure. Additional details concerning the origins of nerve impulses which influence both heart rate and contractile properties of the heart are presented in Figure 3–4.

If a stepwise increase in heart rate is produced by stimulating electrodes installed upon the right atrium near the S-A node, a progressive reduction in the diastolic dimensions – and in stroke volume — is seen (Fig. 3–3*B*). An increase in heart rate accompanied by a diminution in stroke volume is not an efficient mechanism for increasing total cardiac output. Thus, it is important to consider the factors which influence the quantity of blood ejected during each systole (the stroke volume).

CONTROL OF STROKE VOLUME

Most mechanical or piston pumps with which we are familiar have a constant displacement and eject precisely the same quantity of liquid during each successive stroke. The output of such a pump is regulated merely by speeding or slowing the repetition rate with no change in the quantity of liquid discharged with each stroke. The heart is remarkable in its ability to compensate to changing conditions by adjustments in heart rate, in the volume at the end of the filling period (diastolic volume) and in the volume remaining in the ventricles at the end of ejection (systolic volume). A wide variety of different factors may influence the stroke volume under various conditions which may be grouped for convenience under such headings as geometry, intrinsic properties of myocardium and external control mechanisms.

GEOMETRICAL FACTORS
AFFECTING STROKE VOLUME

The architectural features of the right and left ventricles were described in Chapter 2. Neither ventricle conforms to a simple geometrical shape. In spite of the gross differences in their shape, wall thickness and outflow resistance, the two ventricles must expel precisely the same volumes averaged over any significant period of

time; otherwise large volumes of blood would be transferred between the systemic and pulmonary vascular beds.

The absolute volume of blood contained within the individual ventricular chambers can be estimated by several techniques but their results are not entirely consistent or absolute. A symposium devoted to measurement of left ventricular volume in 1966 revealed discrepancies of significant magnitude between roentgenographic and indicator-dilution techniques of measurement.[15] According to Dodge *et al.*,[16] the left ventricles of normal subjects contain some 70 to 80 ml. $\pm$ 10 to 20 ml. per square meter of body surface at the end of diastole with 60 to 75 per cent of that volume ejected during systole. In contrast, Rapaport[17] reported ventricular volumes estimated by thermodilution in man at about 100 ml./M^2 in normal man and about 50 per cent of the diastolic volume ejected during systole. All agree that the ventricles may fill to varying degrees during diastole and empty to varying degrees during systolic ejection. A substantial, but variable, amount of blood remains in the ventricular chambers at the end of systole.

THE DEGREE OF MYOCARDIAL SHORTENING IN DIFFERENT MUSCLES OF THE HEART. The various myocardial bundles in the ventricles are oriented in different directions (see Fig. 2–9) and describe circles of different diameters, so the degree of myocardial shortening must vary widely in different layers. In Figure 3–5*B*, the relative wall thickness and the radius of the left ventricular chamber at a particular size are represented by volume I. Volume II represents the same cross section with the ventricular volume reduced by half. In both cases it is obvious that the radius and

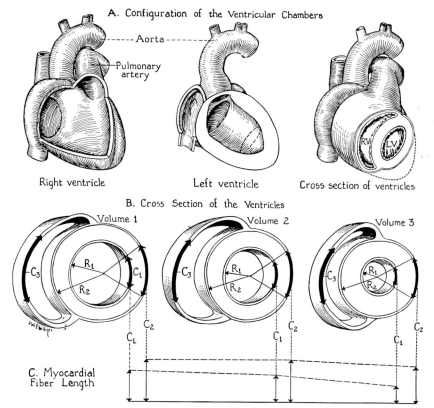

A. Configuration of the Ventricular Chambers

------ Aorta ------

Pulmonary artery

Right ventricle   Left ventricle   Cross section of ventricles

B. Cross Section of the Ventricles

Volume 1   Volume 2   Volume 3

C. Myocardial Fiber Length

FIGURE 3–5   THE DEGREE OF MYOCARDIAL SHORTENING IN THE VENTRICULAR WALLS

The right ventricular cavity is enclosed by the convex interventricular septum and the concave free wall, which may be considered a segment of a very large sphere. Very slight shortening of the fibers in the free wall of the right ventricle (C_3) will eject very large volumes (see Fig. 3–6).

The left ventricle has been compared to a very thick-walled cylinder with a conoid segment at the apex. The circumferentially arranged fibers account for most of the wall thickness which encloses the cylindrical portion of the chamber. The circles described by the inner layers have a much smaller radius (R_1) and circumference (C_1) than those described by the outer layers (R_2 and C_2). As the left ventricle contracts, the inner layers must shorten to a greater degree than the outer layers in ejecting a particular volume. On the basis of this analysis, during any normal systolic ejection the outer layers of myocardium shorten to a lesser extent and the superficial spiral muscles shorten least of all. It is possible that no two layers of myocardial fibers shorten to exactly the same extent during ejection.

circumference of the inner layers of myocardium (R_1 and C_1) are less than those of the outer layer (R_2, C_2). During contraction from volume I to volume II, the radius and circumference of the inner layer are reduced much more than those of the outer layers. This means that the inner layer of myocardium must shorten more than the outer layers. If this analysis is correct, the thickness of the ventricular walls should increase during systole and decrease during diastole.

It is apparent that during any particular ventricular contraction, the inner layers of circumferential myocardium may shorten to the greatest extent. The relative degree of myocardial shortening in the inner lining of spiral muscle (trabeculae carneae) and papillary muscles cannot be assessed by this type of analysis. The difference in degrees of shortening by various myocardial layers is diminished when the diastolic and systolic volumes remain large; the maximum difference between the shortening of the superficial spiral muscle and that of the inner layer of deep constrictor fibers would occur when the left ventricle empties maximally (see volume III in Fig. 3–5).

Relation of Diastolic Volume to the Degree of Myocardial Shortening. The degree of myocardial shortening can be reduced without changing the stroke volume if the diastolic distention of the ventricles is increased.[18]

A very slight reduction in circumference of a large sphere would eject a very much greater volume than the same reduction in circumference of a small sphere. The superficial muscles tend to conform most closely to a spherical shape, and this analysis applies within limits to these myocardial fibers (Fig. 3–6).

Deep muscles in the left ventricle are arranged circumferentially around a roughly cylindrical cavity. Here again, the reduction in volume produced by a reduction in circumference is much greater when the original circumference is large than when it is small. Thus, the degree of myocardial shortening required to eject a particular stroke volume is much less if the initial fiber length (diastolic volume) is great (Fig. 3–6).

The anatomical arrangement and orientation of the myocardial fibers in the ventricular walls was presented in Chapter 2 (Figs. 2–8 and 2–9). Close inspection revealed that virtually all fibers described helical courses conforming to neither purely longitudinal nor circumferential orientation (Fig. 2–9). A clear or concise description of contribution of the various layers to the circumferential contraction or shortening of the chambers is not yet possible. However, we may regard the deep fibers in the midportion of the ventricular wall as being roughly circumferential and the inner and outer layers as being oriented obliquely, pro-

viding a strong longitudinal pull in addition to a circumferential constriction. The layers in between appear to progressively change in orientation in intermediate stages. In subsequent discussion, the implication that the deep fibers are circumferentially oriented must be tempered with the knowledge that this is an oversimplification.

Evidence has been presented that under normal conditions, ventricular contraction generally corresponds to a reduction in the chamber from volume I to volume II in Figure 3–5. Although the same stroke volume can be ejected by a change from volume II to volume III (Fig. 3–5), the relative degree of myocardial shortening would be much greater. When the diastolic volume is large, a relatively large stroke volume can be ejected with small degrees of myocardial shortening.

Since the free wall of the right ventricle corresponds to a segment of a large sphere while the left ventricle resembles a cylinder, equal myocardial shortening in the two chambers would produce much larger stroke volumes from the right ventricle than from the left (Fig. 3–6). The right and left ventricles must eject roughly equal quantities, so the degree of myocardial shortening cannot be equal in the two ventricles.

FACTORS OPPOSING COMPLETE VENTRICULAR EMPTYING

Muscle fibers cannot shorten to an infinitely small length. If all the myocardial fibers constricted 20 per cent of their initial length, the inner layer of circumferential fibers would have attained this value and ceased contributing any tension, while the outer layers might be able to contract still more. From this point on, further shortening by the outer layers would

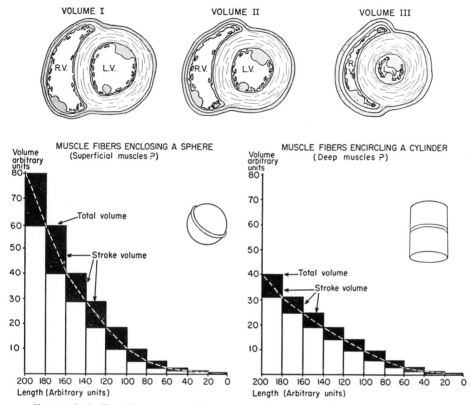

FIGURE 3–6   THE RELATION OF MYOCARDIAL LENGTH TO VENTRICULAR VOLUME

The volume of blood ejected by a ventricle (stroke volume) depends upon two factors: (*a*) the diastolic volume and (*b*) the amount of myocardial shortening. Normally, the ventricles are well distended with blood during diastole (volume I) and eject only a portion of the blood within the chambers during systole (volume II). Similar volumes of blood could theoretically be ejected from less distended ventricles (such as volume II) by much more complete systolic emptying (volume III).

The superficial spiral muscles encircle a large volume which is roughly spherical in shape. Under these conditions, very slight degrees of myocardial shortening will eject very large volumes. The larger the initial volume, the greater the volume ejected for a particular degree of myocardial shortening as indicated by the black areas on the left.

The deep constrictor muscles encircle the cylindrical portion of the left ventrical chamber. The change in volume produced by a reduction in the circumference of a cylinder is much smaller (black areas on the right) than is produced by the same reduction in circumference of a sphere (black areas on the left). Furthermore, the circumference of the left ventricle is much smaller than the circumference of the entire heart. Thus, the superficial spiral layers of myocardial fibers have a much greater initial length and enclose a sphere, so very slight shortening ejects large volumes. The deep constrictor muscles describe circles of small circumference around a cylinder, so they must shorten a great deal more to eject the same volume.

require an expenditure of energy in wrinkling and deforming the inner layers (Fig. 3–7).

The trabeculae carneae represent preformed wrinkles and combine with the papillary muscles to occupy space in the ventricles. This permits more complete systolic ejection than would be possible if the inner walls of the ventricular chamber were smooth (see Fig. 3–7). Because of the space occupied by papillary muscles and tra-

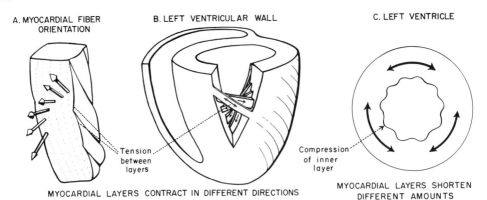

A. MYOCARDIAL FIBER ORIENTATION

B. LEFT VENTRICULAR WALL

C. LEFT VENTRICLE

Tension between layers

Compression of inner layer

MYOCARDIAL LAYERS CONTRACT IN DIFFERENT DIRECTIONS

MYOCARDIAL LAYERS SHORTEN DIFFERENT AMOUNTS

FIGURE 3–7   TENSION DEVELOPED BETWEEN MYOCARDIAL LAYERS (INTERFASCICULAR TENSION)

A, Although the right ventricular wall is quite thin, it contains myocardial fibers oriented in three different directions. Simultaneous contraction of these fibers must create tension in the fibrous and myocardial connections between the different layers (interfascicular tension).

B, The left ventricular wall is also composed of at least three layers of muscle, oriented primarily in three different directions (see Chapter 2). Interfascicular tension must develop in the connections between these layers during contraction.

C, The different layers of the thick-walled left ventricles must contract to different degrees in ejecting a particular volume of blood (see Fig. 3–5). This presumably causes tensions between layers of circularly arranged fibers, as well as compressing the inner layers.

beculae carneae, even the inner layers of circumferential fibers in the left ventricle can describe circles of reasonable diameter when the left ventricle is virtually empied. This mechanism is less important in the right ventricle because of (*a*) its thin wall, (*b*) the very long fibers which enclose the cavity and (*c*) the large circles described by these fibers.

The Law of Laplace. According to the Laplace formula ($P = T/R$), the pressure (*P*) developed by a particular level of wall tension (*T*) is inversely proportional to the radius of the chamber. This law was invoked to explain the difference between the wall thicknesses of the aorta and the systemic capillaries when these widely different structures sustain pressures of the same magnitude (see Fig. 1–11).

Applied to the contracting ventricle, the law of Laplace indicates that the myocardial tension required to sustain a particular level of intraventricular pressure diminishes as the radius of the chamber is reduced by ejection. In

other words, this factor would tend to compensate to some extent for the loss of myocardial tension through myocardial viscosity and interfascicular tension. On the other hand, if the diastolic volume is increased, greater myocardial tension is needed to develop a particular level of intraventricular pressure.

Diastolic Recoil. The ventricular walls are composed of myocardial fibers oriented in different directions (see Fig. 2–9). Although adjacent layers appear to maintain relative orientation during systolic ejection, some fraction of the contractile tension developed by the fibers may be expended in developing tension between adjacent fibers or by producing wrinkling, distortion and compression of the inner layers of muscle (Fig. 3–7C). This tension would be stored during the systolic ejection period and released in the form of diastolic recoil when the myocardial fibers suddenly relax. At the very onset of the diastolic interval, the ventricular walls appear to spring outward to produce abrupt filling; so rapid that the ventricular pressure drops to its lowest point in the cycle. This extremely rapid filling in early diastole has important functional significance particularly in the presence of rapid heart rates with brief diastolic filling intervals. A major portion of total ventricular filling occurs during a small fraction of a second in early diastole. Rapid heart rate usually is accompanied by more complete ejection. The more complete the systolic ejection, the greater should be the amount and speed of the diastolic recoil.

After the initial rapid filling phase, the ventricle distends much more gradually until the next atrial contraction signals another cycle is beginning. The contribution of atrial systole to ventricular filling depends in large measure on the degree of ventricular distension at the time. If the ventricles approach their maximal dimensions before atrial excitation, the contracting atrial myocardium adds very little to the ventricular volume (Fig. 3–8A). This phenomenon is believed to occur in man or animals resting quietly in the recumbent position. Under these conditions, heart rate is slow; filling pressure is ample and the ventricles may be maximally distended early in the diastolic filling period. This phenomenon is illustrated schematically in Figure 3–8 and discussed in greater detail in Chapter 6. Both the systolic and diastolic dimensions are diminished in the standing position (Fig. 3–8B), and in general the diastolic filling interval is shortened, ventricular volume progressively expands during the filling period and atrial contraction adds a significant additional increment to ventricular volume just before ventricular contraction begins. During exertion, stroke volume may remain about the same or increase slightly (see Chapter 7), in which case diastolic volume may increase slightly, systolic ejection may be slightly more complete or both. However, the changes in stroke volume during exertion are not nearly so pronounced as are the changes in the rates of ventricular performance (see Figs. 3–14, 3–17 and 3–18).

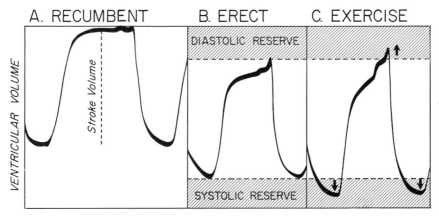

FIGURE 3–8   RESERVE CARDIAC OUTPUT

Changes in ventricular volume are represented schematically. In the supine position, the diastolic volume is approximately maximal and the stroke volume is relatively large. On standing, diastolic ventricular volume and stroke volume diminish to provide potential diastolic and systolic reserve capacity. During exertion, any increase in stroke volume may be attained by either greater diastolic filling, more complete systolic ejection or both.

Ventricular Distensibility. The architecture and geometry of the ventricular walls complicates the problem of assigning meaningful values or definitions to the term distensibility. For example, the diastolic recoil is sufficient to provide a rapid inrush of blood into the left ventricle — at effectively zero distending pressure. Under these conditions, ventricular distension is active rather than passive. The factors which terminate ventricular filling at some level below the maximal under various conditions (Fig. 3–8*B*, *C*.) have not been well elucidated. Furthermore, widely different ventricular volumes can be observed at the same or similar ventricular diastolic pressures in different "normal" subjects (i.e., comparing sedentary with athletic individuals) and patients with different forms of heart disease. Dodge *et al.*[16] reported ventricular volumes ranging from 100 to 400 ml. among 176 patients without consistent changes in ventricular pressure. However, in a particular normal individual, an increase in transmural pressure (intraventricular pressure minus extracardiac pressure) generally increased ventricular filling unless the heart was maximally distended as in Fig. 3–8*A*.

SHRINKAGE OF THE HEART DURING THORACOTOMY

Most profound changes in ventricular size and function occur during the administration of anesthesia and incision of the thorax as required to expose the heart.[19] This phenomenon was first noted during the recovery period following the application of various ventricular dimensional gauges to the heart of animals (see Figure 2–17). Immediately after installation of these gauges during aseptic surgery, the ventricular chambers were functioning near their minimal size even after the chest incision had been repaired and the lungs reinflated. During the succeeding hours or days, the recorded dimensions expanded and stabilized for many days at a much larger size. Stimulated by this observation, the changes in dimensions of the ventricular chambers were studied by cinefluorographic pictures taken sequentially during anesthesia, thoracotomy and application of a cardiometer (Fig. 3–9). These studies demonstrated that under such experimental conditions, the ventricular chambers were reduced in size to levels well below those observed under any other condition or stress. These observations have extremely important significance in the interpretation of experiments on exposed hearts of animals. Investigators must constantly keep in mind that when they first expose a heart of a mammal, like a dog, the heart may have already been rendered so abnormal that its function may be outside the normal range before any experimental procedure is undertaken. Despite these reservations, observations and concepts of value can be obtained from exposed hearts and even from isolated samples of tissue. Their application to the function of organs in intact, healthy man and animals must be extrapolated with extreme caution.

INTRINSIC PROPERTIES OF MYOCARDIUM

The mechanical properties of muscle can be studied most readily and quantitatively by excising a strip and testing it under rigidly controlled experimental conditions. Such studies have demonstrated similar features in common between skeletal muscle and myocardium. If the tension exerted by a strip of resting or relaxed muscle is recorded as it is progres-

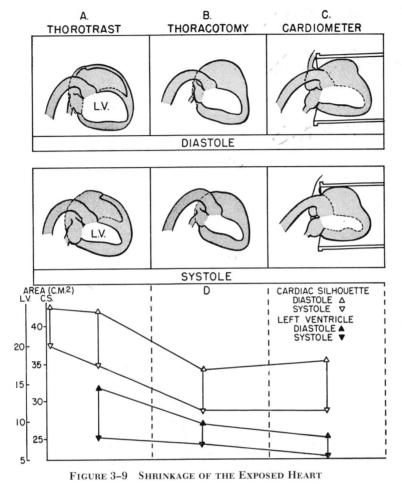

FIGURE 3–9   SHRINKAGE OF THE EXPOSED HEART

A, Thorotrast was injected into a normal unanesthetized dog and its course through the heart was recorded cinefluorographically. The area of the cardiac silhouette and of the left ventricle during both systole and diastole are indicated in the graph, D.

B, After anesthesia and thoracotomy, the heart definitely became smaller.

C, The cardiac silhouette changed in configuration when the heart was placed in a loose-fitting cardiometer, but its area was not diminished. The left ventricular area was further reduced by this procedure. The left ventricle emptied almost completely at the end of systole, a situation which never was encountered among intact dogs.

sively stretched, no tension is recorded until a certain length is reached. The length at which a muscle first begins to develop tension is the "resting length." Further elongation of the muscle produces increasing resting tension, slight at first and increasing more steeply at greater lengths as illustrated schematically in Figure 3–10. If skeletal muscle is stimulated to contract without shortening (isometric contrac-

tion), it develops slight contractile tension at resting length. If the same strip is stretched and stimulated to contract at a succession of increased lengths, the contractile tension becomes very much greater, up to about 145 per cent of resting length.[20] Skeletal muscle fibers develop maximal tension at lengths about the same as they had in the animal's body, but a glance at Figures 3–5, 3–6 and 3–8 indicates

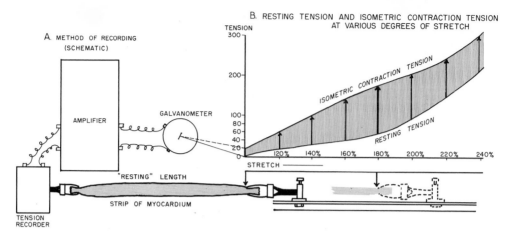

FIGURE 3–10   MECHANICAL PROPERTIES OF MYOCARDIAL BUNDLES (FROG)

A, Schematic diagram of experimental conditions employed by Lundin.[24]
B, Tension developed by a strip of frog myocardium was recorded as it was stretched from its "resting length" to 240 per cent of resting length with isometric contraction tension recorded at various degrees of stretch. The maximum contractile tension occurred at about 180 per cent of "resting length."

the difficulty of deciding what ventricular volume or dimension represents the "resting length" of myocardium.

The history of the basic concepts of cardiac function and control has been reviewed by Wiggers.[21] In 1895, Otto Frank recorded the isometric and isotonic contractions of frog myocardium and established that, within limits, myocardium resembles skeletal muscle in developing greater tension as its resting length is increased (Fig. 3–11B). Patterson, Piper and Starling[22] used the heart-lung preparation (Fig. 3–11A) to study the influence on cardiac function of variations in venous inflow, outflow resistance and heart rate.

VENTRICULAR RESPONSES IN THE HEART-LUNG PREPARATION

In the heart-lung preparation, the quantity of blood entering the ventricles could be increased by elevating the reservoir illustrated in Figure 3–11A. Experimentally induced elevation in "venous return" resulted in a higher filling pressure, a slight in-

crease in arterial blood pressure and greater diastolic and systolic ventricular volumes. Records of this type were interpreted as follows: (a) When the reservoir is elevated, the venous pressure rises and diastolic filling is increased. (b) The myocardial fibers fail to eject as much blood as entered during diastole, so an additional increment of blood remains within the ventricle. (c) The succeeding diastolic filling is even greater, but the volume ejected remains less than that which entered. (d) The diastolic filling exceeds the systolic ejection until the ventricles become distended to a point where the energy release by the myocardium is sufficiently increased to bring the inflow and outflow into balance. (e) The equilibrium between inflow and outflow is maintained with the ventricles at their new larger diastolic and systolic size until the volume load is reduced. (f) As the reservoir is lowered, the energy released by the myocardium is excessive for the volume of inflow and the quantity ejected exceeds the volume which entered. For a few beats, outflow exceeds in-

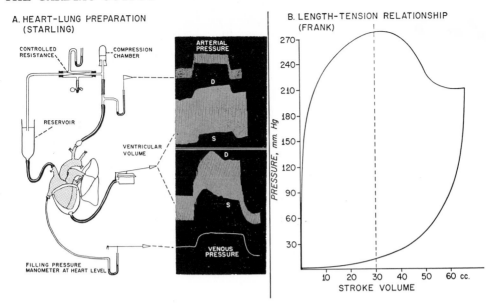

FIGURE 3–11   THE LENGTH-TENSION RELATIONSHIP OF MYOCARDIUM

A, The ventricles in a heart-lung preparation adapt to an increased work load (either increased arterial pressure or increased stroke volume) by an increase in diastolic distention. Such experiments led Starling and his associates to postulate that the energy released by the contracting myocardium was determined by the initial length of the myocardial fibers as indicated by the end diastolic ventricular volume. (After Patterson, Piper and Starling.[22])

B, The length-tension relationship of myocardium resembles that of skeletal muscle. Progressive stretch of relaxed myocardium is attended by a progressive increase in isometric contractile tension up to some level. This length-tension diagram, derived by Otto Frank from studies of frog myocardium, was employed by Starling to illustrate his concept of the "law of the heart" by applying values of pressure and stroke volume on the ordinate and abscissa which he regarded as representative of human subjects. The use of an isometric tension curve is not appropriate for illustrating changes which would occur with ejection of stroke volumes (see Fig. 3–12).

flow until the systolic and diastolic ventricular volumes return to a lower level, actually smaller than during the control period in Figure 3–11.

The increased distention of the ventricles in response to a sudden increase in outflow pressure was explained as follows: The systolic increase in intraventricular pressure is not sufficient to eject all the blood that entered during the previous diastole (Fig. 3–11A). The succeeding diastolic filling remains the same, so an additional increment of blood remains within the ventricle. The systolic and diastolic volumes expand until the energy released by the lengthened myocardial fibers is sufficient to

meet the greater requirements for intraventricular pressure during each cycle.

THE FRANK-STARLING MECHANISM

Starling and his associates[22] confirmed Frank's general conclusions except for one crucial point, namely, that an increased diastolic volume was usually, but not always, associated with a corresponding increase in filling pressure. They stated, "We thus find no constant connection between the diastolic tension and the succeeding contraction, though as a rule these two quantities will be altered together.

But we do find a direct proportion between the diastolic volume of the heart (i.e., the length of its muscle fibers) and the energy set free in the following systole.

"The law of the heart is therefore the same as that of skeletal muscle, namely that the mechanical energy set free on passage from the resting to the contracted state depends on the area of 'chemically active surfaces,' i.e., on the length of the muscle fibres."[22]

According to these data, the normal response to either a greater volume load or a greater pressure load is an increase in both the diastolic and systolic ventricular volumes. A heart which becomes distended with a small or normal load is considered fatigued or depressed even though it may maintain a "normal" output while operating at this larger size.

Wiggers and Katz (see Ref. 21) repeated these experiments using improved techniques. Their results confirmed those of Starling and his associates that an increase in stroke volume was attended by an increase in diastolic volume (greater initial length of myocardial fibers). However, they concluded that "such changes were never dissociated from changes in initial intraventricular pressures." Apparently, Starling was not convinced by this evidence because in subsequent publications he restated his belief that diastolic volume may change without corresponding alterations in filling pressure.[23]

For half a century variations in stroke volume were most frequently explained by a few fundamental rules which were generally held to apply so long as the functional condition of the myocardium remains within physiologic limits: (a) The *cardiac output* is determined by the venous return. (b) If the heart rate is constant, the *stroke volume* is determined by the

venous return. (c) *Stroke volume* of the ventricles depends directly on the diastolic filling. (d) The *tension* of resting myocardial fibers depends upon their length. (e) *Diastolic filling* (and diastolic volume) of the ventricles is determined by effective filling pressure. (f) *The mechanical energy set free on passage from the resting to the contracted state depends on the length of the myocardial fibers.*

A number of these concepts were derived from Starling's experiments, and most of them have been erroneously cited at one time or another as "Starling's law of the heart." A far more realistic notation would have been the Frank-Starling application of the length-tension relation of myocardium. The concept that the diastolic volume is always determined by the effective pressure (e) is contrary to both the results and the conclusions of Starling and his associates. By the same token, belief in a constant relation between length and tension of resting myocardial fibers (d) cannot be attributed to these investigators.

Assumptions Implicit in the Frank-Starling Mechanism. In retrospect, the unquestioning acceptance and durability of the Frank-Starling mechanism as the "law of the heart" seems difficult to reconcile with certain obvious weaknesses. It is now clear that the ventricles are normally maximally distended in the resting recumbent individual and become smaller on standing or during virtually any other cardiac compensation. In contrast, the exposed heart of the anesthetized dog approaches its minimal diastolic and systolic dimensions. It seems quite possible that the ventricles of the heart-lung preparation became distended in response to volume or pressure loads in part because they were about as small as they could get during the "control" periods.

One very significant conceptual

deficiency in the Frank-Starling approach is the assumption that the relation between muscle fiber length and *isometric* contractile tension would permit prediction of changes in stroke volume, stroke work or external energy release by the contracting myocardium. By definition, isometric contraction means that shortening of the muscle is prevented, a situation which precludes ejection of blood or accomplishing external work. For this reason, the responses of ventricular chambers and muscle strips must also be studied under conditions in which shortening can occur.

Loss of Myocardial Tension During Shortening

To study the dynamic properties of contracting myocardium, Lundin[24] utilized a strip of myocardium arranged as indicated in Figure 3–12 but equipped with a release mechanism which permitted the muscle to shorten during its contraction period. The loss of tension during shortening by 20 per cent was represented schematically by the downward slanting arrows. The maximum tension developed when shortening was prevented as completely as possible. If the muscle was permitted to shorten slowly, the loss of tension was slight. Rapid shortening was accompanied by profound reduction in contractile tension. This reciprocal relation between the contractile force and the velocity of shortening has been known for many years. Such a velocity dependent relationship might be ascribed to a form of "viscosity" by which much of the applied force is dissipated as heat due to friction. Greatly increased forces are required to displace or propel a viscous fluid at higher and higher velocities. Imagine for a moment, the amount of force required to propel a paddle through water as compared to thick paint or molasses. In a contract-

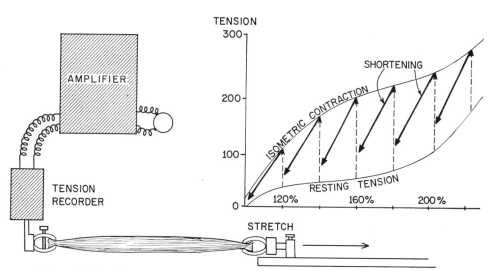

FIGURE 3–12   EFFECTS OF SHORTENING ON MYOCARDIAL CONTRACTILE TENSION

The increase in tension above resting tension developed by myocardial strips contracting under isometric conditions increased progressively from resting length to about 160 to 180 per cent of resting length, then diminished. If the myocardial strips shorten by 20 per cent during contraction, the contractile tension falls off sharply. (After Lundin.[24])

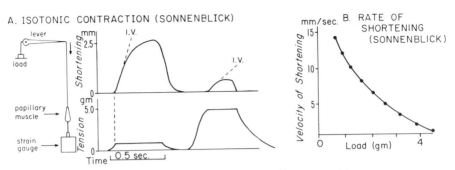

FIGURE 3-13   CONTRACTION OF EXCISED PAPILLARY MUSCLES

Isolated papillary muscles, contracting isotonically, begin to shorten after they have developed sufficient tension to elevate the load. The rate of shortening is greatest at the onset. The rate of shortening is diminished with an increasing load. (After Sonnenblick.[26])

ing muscle, internal viscosity might be visualized in terms of the forces developed by the contractile mechanism which fail to appear as external work because of dissipation of energy producing internal rearrangement within the muscle fiber. This is an attractive concept, but measurements of heat produced during muscular contraction indicate that the velocity of contraction is not limited by a passive internal viscosity in the muscle.[25] An alternative proposal is that the force on the muscle directly or indirectly influences the chemical reactions which produce the contractive forces.

Sonnenblick and his collaborators[26, 27] studied contraction of excised papillary muscles during shortening against a constant load as indicated in Figure 3-13. The rate of shortening is indicated by the slope of the shortening curve occurring under large and small load conditions. The initial portion of the curve is always steepest, indicating that the initial rate of shortening is the greatest during an isotonic contraction. By progressively increasing the load in a stepwise manner and noting the maximal velocity of shortening (steepest slope for each contraction), a curve can be drawn like that shown in Figure 3-13B. This graph demonstrates how

myocardial fibers shorten at their maximal rate and to a maximal extent under minimal load. By varying the rate of shortening, the load, the time elapsing between the onset of contraction and shortening and the initial length of the muscle, one can obtain a bewildering array of curves. Clearly, myocardial performance cannot be judged from studies of isometric contraction alone. The myocardial strips (i.e., in Figs. 3-12 and 3-13) were necessarily deprived of their blood supply. It is of importance to determine whether similar force-velocity relationships are apparent during contraction of the intact ventricles. For example, Fry *et al.*[28] conducted studies on a whole animal preparation in which left ventricular flow and pressure were varied independently. They reported that the velocity relationships in cardiac muscle appear to be much more dependent upon muscle length than is the case for skeletal muscle. A complex three-dimensional relationship between tension velocity and length was proposed as a preferred graphical method for analyzing myocardial function.

Functional Significance of Intrinsic Myocardial Properties. The applicability of concepts derived from observations under abnormal experimental conditions must ultimately be confirmed by appropriate measurements on intact animals and man functioning as nearly normally as possible. The Frank-Starling length-tension relationship appears to be manifest during certain spontaneous adaptations in intact, healthy animals (and apparently in man as well). For example, studies on the heart-lung preparation suggest that an increase in diastolic volume would be accompanied by increased energy release as expressed by increased outflow and increased stroke work. (See Fig. 3–14A). When a dog reclines from the sitting position, the ventricular diameter increases over a few beats until it appears to plateau at a maximum level. During the increase in diastolic diameter, the aortic outflow rate increases and the stroke volume (area under the flow curve) also increases. In a resting dog with spontaneously fluctuating heart rate (sinus arrhythmia), acceleration of the heart is accompanied by smaller diastolic dimensions and smaller stroke volume; slowing of the heart rate is associated with an increase in diastolic diameter and increased stroke volume (see also Fig. 3–27).

In contrast, certain other cardiovascular responses in normal animals and man do not apparently conform to the predictions implicit in the Frank-Starling length-tension relationship. For example, the left ventricular response to exercise (Fig. 3–14) reveals that when the animal stood up, the expected response occurred. However, rather drastic changes in many of the cardiac performance characteristics occurred during the period of exercise that do not appear to conform to any simple intrinsic control mechanism. The nature of these changes will be considered further in Chapter 8. The exercise response is one of many normal and pathological responses which do not conform to predictions from the Frank-Starling length-tension relationship. This suggests that external mechanisms can override or modify the intrinsic properties of the myocardial fibers. The most common and most extensive functional changes are induced by stimulation of the sympathetic nerves which are distributed to the ventricular myocardium (see Fig. 3–4).

Extrinsic Control of Cardiac Function. The heart is strongly influenced by the powerful controls exerted by the autonomic nervous system. The heart rate is influenced by the balance between the slowing effects of the parasympathetic nerves in the vagus and the accelerating effects of the sympathetic nerves. Stimulation of the vagus nerves to the heart have little effect on ventricular function if changes in heart rate are prevented. In fact, there is little direct evidence that parasympathetic nerves are distributed to the ventricular myocardium (see Fig. 3–4). Sympathetic nerves distributed throughout the heart act by the release of a chemical transmitter (norepinephrine) at the nerve endings. When the adrenal gland is stimulated, it secretes a combination of norepinephrine (20 per cent) and l-epinephrine (80 per cent) into the blood stream. Although intravascular injection of these substances was utilized for many years as a substitute for direct stimulation of sympathetic nerves to the heart, it is now generally recognized that circulating neurohormones are probably of little significance in normal cardiovascular control. Thus, the most important external control mechanisms affecting cardiac function are the parasympathetic and sympathetic effects on the myocardium.

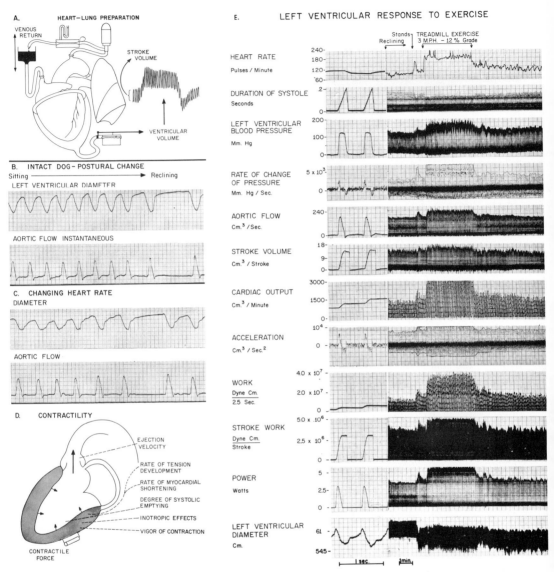

FIGURE 3–14   VENTRICULAR ADAPTATIONS DURING SPONTANEOUS ACTIVITY

A, In the heart-lung preparation, the ventricle responds to an increase in either volume load or pressure load by diastolic distension and increased energy release (Frank-Starling mechanism).

B, In intact dogs, the Frank-Starling mechanism is readily demonstrable in the increase in energy release associated with increased diastolic distension as the animal reclines.

C, This mechanism also occurs during spontaneous changes in heart rate (i.e., sinus arrhythmia) which represent variations in vagal discharge.

D, Changes in ventricular performance which do not conform to the Frank-Starling mechanism are commonly attributed to changes in "contractility," a term which has so many connotations that it is relatively meaningless.

E, The ventricular responses to exercise by healthy active dogs correspond to the changes induced by sympathetic stimulation. (From Rushmer *et al., Circulation,* 1963, *17*:118–141.)

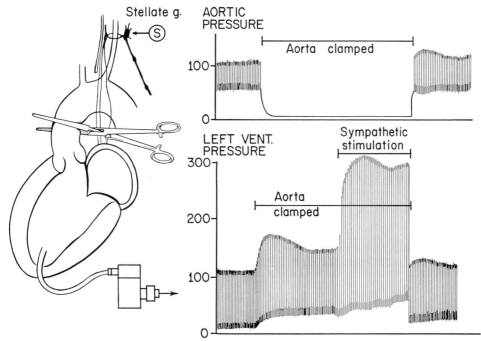

FIGURE 3–15   VENTRICULAR CONTRACTILE TENSION DURING SYMPATHETIC STIMULATION

Ventricular pressure is elevated during each systolic contraction by clamping the aorta so that the myocardium contracts more nearly isometrically. A very large additional increase in contractile tension can be produced by stimulating sympathetic cardiac nerves. This observation demonstrates a direct effect of the sympathetic nerve activity on myocardial contractile force, independent of any peripheral vascular effects of such stimulation.

Effects of Sympathetic Cardiac Nerves. The effects of the sympathetic nerve discharge to the heart are dramatically demonstrated by restricting the degree of myocardial shortening (see Fig. 3–15). Clamping of the aorta restricts ejection to the coronary outflow so that the myocardium contracts almost isometrically. The intraventricular pressure rises as aortic pressure rapidly drops toward zero. Ventricular systolic pressure is almost doubled when the ventricular contraction is rendered almost isometric (Fig. 3–15). If the sympathetic cardiac nerves on the left are stimulated when the ventricles are contracting almost isometrically, the ventricular pressure rises to extremely high levels, reaching 300 mm. Hg as in

Figure 3–15 and up to 500 mm. Hg in other experiments. The cardiac sympathetic nerves on the left side profoundly affect the maximum tension which can be developed by the ventricular myocardium. The cardiac nerves descending on the right side generally produce a greater change in the heart rate and a smaller increase in contractile tension. The sympathetic nerves to the heart on the right apparently converge on the S-A node to act on the pacemaker, while the left sympathetic nerves are more widely distributed to the atrial and ventricular myocardium (see Fig. 3–4).

Although the sympathetic innervation of the heart apparently induces changes more closely resembling those observed during spontaneous cardiovascular responses, such conclusions can be based only on more direct comparisons than can be achieved in the anesthetized, thoracotomized dog. Instead, the changes in cardiac performance must be studied continuously during various kinds of activity in healthy unanesthetized dogs (i.e., Fig. 3–14).

EFFECTS OF SYMPATHETIC NERVES ON VENTRICULAR EJECTION

The very great increase in ventricular systolic pressure accomplished during sympathetic discharge to an almost isometrically contracting myocardium is superimposed upon the intrinsic isometric length-tension relation of the muscle. In addition, sympathetic nerve activity also affects profoundly the velocity of shortening

of myocardium and the resulting ejection rates. A flowmeter mounted on the aorta consistently demonstrates the marked increase in peak outflow rate from the ventricle with the steep initial upslope indicating a characteristic increase in the acceleration of the blood during the powerful impulse produced by the contracting ventricular myocardium (Fig. 3–16). The same type of phenomenon is readily observed during spontaneous cardiac adaptations like exercise (see also Fig. 3–14). The typical response to sympathetic stimulation also includes a more rapid deceleration of outflow and a shorter systolic interval so that the stroke volume may be increased but little or not at all, in spite of transiently higher peak outflow rates during each cycle.

A comprehensive description of the effects of sympathetic discharge to the heart involves numerous aspects of

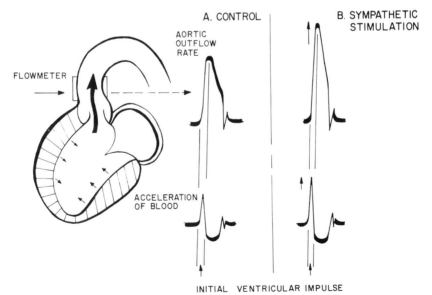

FIGURE 3–16   EJECTION VELOCITY AND ACCELERATION OF BLOOD

An ultrasonic or electromagnetic flowmeter mounted on the root of the aorta indicates the typical changes in ejection velocity, reaching a high peak flow early in systole. The steep initial upslope indicates very high acceleration of outflow. Sympathetic stimulation increases peak acceleration and elevates peak flow rates with reduced period of ejection to provide about the same stroke volume ejected in shorter time.

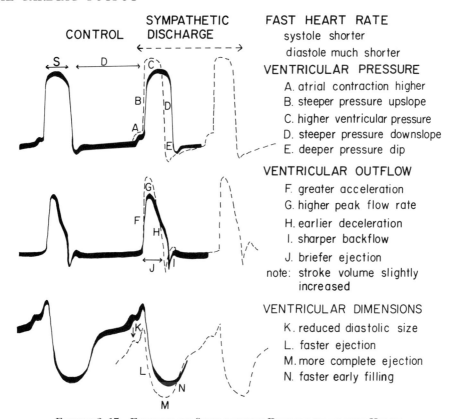

FAST HEART RATE
  systole shorter
  diastole much shorter
VENTRICULAR PRESSURE
  A. atrial contraction higher
  B. steeper pressure upslope
  C. higher ventricular pressure
  D. steeper pressure downslope
  E. deeper pressure dip

VENTRICULAR OUTFLOW
  F. greater acceleration
  G. higher peak flow rate
  H. earlier deceleration
  I. sharper backflow
  J. briefer ejection
  note: stroke volume slightly increased

VENTRICULAR DIMENSIONS
  K. reduced diastolic size
  L. faster ejection
  M. more complete ejection
  N. faster early filling

FIGURE 3–17   EFFECTS OF SYMPATHETIC DISCHARGE TO THE HEART

The many changes in left ventricular function produced by sympathetic discharge to the heart are indicated in relation to heart rate, ventricular pressure, outflow and dimensions. The principal effects are on the *rates* of ventricular function, including heart *rate*, *rate* of rise and *rate* of fall of ventricular pressure, ejection *velocity*, *rate* of change of velocity (acceleration), *rate* of deceleration and *rate* of change of dimensions.

the pressure, flow and dimensional changes during the cardiac cycle (Fig. 3–17). The faster heart rate signifies a reduced duration of each cardiac cycle accomplished by a moderate reduction in the duration of systolic interval and a much greater shortening of the diastolic filling interval. The ventricular pressure record exhibits a larger pressure effect from atrial contraction, a much steeper upslope at the onset of ventricular systole. The peak ventricular pressure is somewhat increased. The downslope of the pressure record is very steep, terminating in a deeper early diastolic trough associated with the diastolic recoil, followed by more

rapid rise in diastolic ventricular pressure. Manifestations of greater acceleration to a higher peak outflow rate, earlier deceleration of flow and shorter ejection period are all found in records from both the flow sensors and the dimensional gauges. This array of changes in ventricular performance has an important unifying feature which is summarized in Figure 3–18. The most significant effect of sympathetic discharge is to cause the myocardium to function more rapidly. For example, the *rate* of rise and the *rate* of fall of pressure are increased to a greater extent than the absolute value of peak pressure. The heart *rate* in-

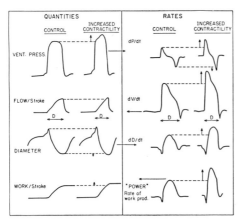

FIGURE 3-18 COMPONENTS OF INCREASED
CONTRACTILITY

The changes in ventricular performance induced by administration of *l*-epinephrine demonstrate that the increased "contractility" involved predominantly increased in the rates at which the variables change (dP/dt, dV/dt, dD/dt, and "power") without necessarily increasing the quantities (ventricular pressure, flow/stroke, diameter or work/stroke). The increase in systolic ventricular pressure is primarily the result of increased ejection velocity (dV/dt).

creased; the duration of systole decreased. The peak outflow *rate* or ejection velocity is greatly increased but the volume flow per stroke (stroke volume) is increased but slightly if at all. The *rate* of change of velocity (acceleration) is greatly and consistently increased. The *rate* of change of dimensions is increased while the absolute dimensions remain about the same or diminish. The net effect of all these changes is to eject about the same stroke volume in a shorter systolic interval, permitting an increase in heart rate with a sustained or increased stroke volume and greater cardiac output.

The changes in ventricular performance illustrated in Figures 3-17 and 3-18 can be consistently induced experimentally by direct stimulation of sympathetic nerves to the heart in dogs[29, 30] and by reflex stimulation of these nerves in man.[31] Of even greater

interest is the fact that changes of the same kind can be produced by selective stimulation of discretely localized sites at the base of the brain, in the diencephalon. In fact, it is possible to reproduce quite accurately the left ventricular responses to exertion without body movement by stimulating electrically very small diencephalic areas in the unanesthetized dog (see also Chapter 8).

DIENCEPHALIC INFLUENCES ON VENTRICULAR PERFORMANCE

Neural pathways pass from the hypothalamus and subthalamus to and through the medullary region to terminate at the intermediolateral cell columns of the spinal cord (see Fig. 3-4). The hypothalamus has long been regarded as the font of the autonomic nervous system and has been repeatedly explored by neurophysiologists using changes in arterial pressure as their principal criterion of sites of cardiovascular control. Thus, various regions in the diencephalon have been labeled "pressor" or "depressor areas" on the basis of elevation or reduction of systemic arterial pressure.[32] Although the anterior hypothalamus is generally regarded as being the site of predominantly depressor areas and the posterior hypothalamus as being largely pressor in its influence, recent exploration of these areas[33, 34] has demonstrated that powerful depressor responses can be induced easily and consistently from many locations (Fig. 3-19). For example, a very pronounced reduction in heart rate and systolic ventricular pressure and reduced rates of change in pressure and cumulative aortic flow were produced by stimulation in the ventral nuclear group of the thalamus. After the electrode tip was

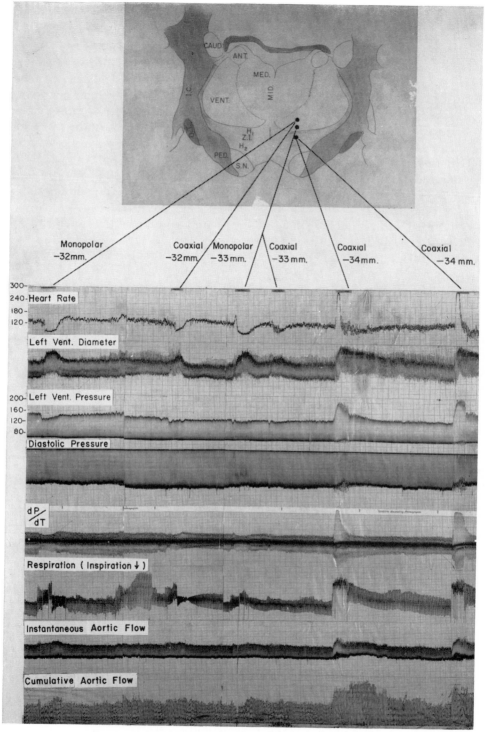

FIGURE 3–19 EFFECTS OF DIENCEPHALIC STIMULATION

Changes in ventricular performance in terms of the multiple variables. At the upper point, stimulation produced reduction in heart rate, increased ventricular diameter, reduced ventricular systolic pressure, diminished rate of change of pressure (dP/dt), altered respiration and little change in aortic flow. Two millimeters lower, the electrode was in the zona incerta and stimulation produced an extremely high transient tachycardia, increased diameter, increased ventricular systolic pressure, increased diastolic pressure, greatly increased rate of change of pressure and increased aortic flow. The sites producing these profound changes are apparently discretely localized in the diencephalon.

95

moved 2 mm. ventrad in the H_2 field of Forel, stimulation resulted in a very powerful pressor response (Fig. 3–19). This response included a transient, explosive acceleration in heart rate, greatly elevated systolic ventricular pressure and rate of change of pressure and augmented aortic peak flow rates and accumulated flow (cardiac output). Marked changes in respiratory patterns —panting—accompanied these cardiovascular changes.

Stimulation of selected areas of the brain stem quite easily produced cardiovascular changes much greater than any seen during spontaneous activity in these dogs.[35] Moreover, a very wide variety of cardiac responses has been produced by stimulation at different sites during exploration of these central regions (Fig. 3–20). At the sites indicated by the histologic sections, virtually every conceivable response was elicited and could be repeatedly induced. Of considerable interest was the fact that by selecting records from a rather large collection, examples could be found in which the changes were almost completely restricted to a single feature of cardiac function: heart rate, left ventricular diameter or left ventricular systolic pressure and left ventricular diastolic pressure. Despite the variation in the kinds of cardiovascular responses which are apparently embodied in the diencephalic mechanisms, stimulation of the same site in different animals consistently produced the same pattern of response. In fact, a cardiac response closely simulating the changes typically observed during treadmill exercise can be quite consistently reproduced by electrical stimulation in the H_2 field of Forel (see Chapter 8).

HYPOTHALAMIC FUNCTION IN CARDIAC CONTROL

A wide variety of different autonomic functions are represented in the base of the brain. For example, the

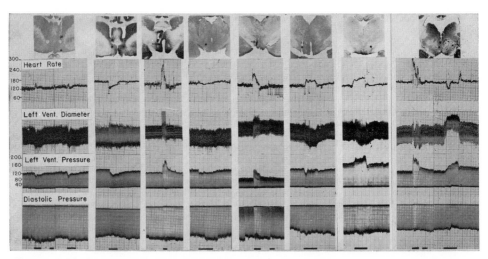

FIGURE 3–20   VARIABLE EFFECTS FROM DIFFERENT DIENCEPHALIC STIMULATION POINTS

Exploration of various sites in the diencephalon with stimulating electrodes demonstrated that many distinctive patterns of ventricular response can be elicited from different regions. Note that in some sites more or less isolated changes occur in one variable with little change in the others. However, repeated stimulation of a particular site consistently produces similar responses in the same or in different animals.

hypothalamus plays an extremely important role in the regulation of body temperature in both animals and man. Heat loss mechanisms (panting and sweating) can be induced by local heating of the preoptic and supraoptic regions in cats. The hypothalamus is apparently involved in sleep and waking; decreased activity of the hypothalamus results in somnolence and increased activity in this region leads to increased bodily activity. Somatic movements, including changes in posture and even running movements, can be produced by stimulating certain regions in the diencephalon. Many forms of overt sexual activity involve stereotyped behavior of a sort which may be influenced by the hypothalamus. This region also serves outward expressions suggesting rage. Each of these responses involves compensatory adjustments in the peripheral blood flow and also in cardiac function. Thus, it is not surprising to find that different portions of the hypothalamic region can induce such varied cardiovascular responses as are illustrated in Figure 3–20.

CEREBRAL CONTROL OF CARDIAC FUNCTION

Activity of portions of the cerebral cortex induces changes in overt behavior, and stimulation in these areas also results in some form of cardiovascular response. Thus, motor areas of the cerebral cortex, from which voluntary motion apparently stems, can also induce changes in the distribution of blood flow and increased cardiac activity. Excision of orbital surface of the frontal lobe produces extreme hyperactivity, including continuous pacing. Stimulation of this region has often been reported to induce pressor responses.[32] The cingulate gyrus has been implicated in the control of emotional behavior and apparently is a potent autonomic effector area. These few examples serve to emphasize the general principle that those portions of the central nervous system in which stimulation produces behavioral responses are also capable of causing cardiovascular effects.[35] This statement does not imply that the cardiovascular responses are necessarily appropriate for the type of behavior produced, because this correlation has not been demonstrated. However, the incorporation of nervous pathways capable of influencing autonomic function appears to represent an important feature of the organization of the central nervous areas controlling behavior. This type of architecture represents a potential mechanism by which patterns of autonomic adjustment may be automatically associated with particular types of behavior.

SUMMARY

The quantity of blood pumped by the heart per unit time (cardiac output) is determined by two main factors: (1) the heart rate and (2) the stroke volume. Normally each heart beat is initiated by a conducted wave of excitation generated by pacemaker cells in the S-A node. The frequency of discharge of the pacemaker is determined by the balance between the retarding effect of nerve impulses descending the vagus nerve and the acclerating effect of the sympathetic nerve impulses reaching this region. If the heart rate is increased experimentally by an artificial pacemaker directly exciting the atrium at a progressively greater rate, the stroke output of the ventricles diminishes and the cardiac output may not increase. Thus, acceleration of the heart rate alone is not necessarily an effective means of increasing cardiac output.

The quantity of blood ejected by the ventricles is represented by the difference between the volume at the end of diastolic filling and the volume at the end of systolic ejection. An increase in the diastolic distention of the ventricles produces an increase in the energy released during the subsequent systole in accordance with the Frank-Starling concept, derived and confirmed by studying the isolated or exposed hearts of dogs under rigid experimental conditions in which the investigator assumed complete control. The ventricular myocardium derives several advantages from function at large diastolic dimensions in addition to the well known increase in isometric contractile tension attained through the increased elongation of the muscle fibers. The tension developed by myocardium contracting without a change in length falls off sharply as the muscle is permitted to shorten (during systolic ejection). The contractile tension is more depleted by either a greater amount of shortening or a faster rate of shortening. To eject a particular volume the amount of myocardial shortening is greatly reduced when the ventricles function at large diastolic and systolic dimensions. The contractile tension which is lost and stored in the form of tension between layers of muscle fibers is also diminished by a reduction in relative myocardial shortening. On the other hand, the contraction tension required to elevate ventricular pressure to a particular level is increased by diastolic distention in accordance with the law of Laplace. Thus, the dimensions at which the ventricles function must represent the resultant of several interacting factors.

In addition to the functional and architectural factors indicated previously, the contractile properties of the myocardium can be greatly influenced by the stimulation of sympathetic nerves to the heart. Under the influence of these nerves, the ventricles develop tension more rapidly, shorten more rapidly, eject blood more rapidly, develop more power and can attain a much higher maximum contractile tension. The duration of systole is shortened so that, in spite of greatly accelerated ejection, the volume ejected may be not greater than during the control period. On the other hand, increased stroke volume may be produced by greater systolic ejection, by more diastolic distention or by a combination of both factors. Changes in ventricular performance are achieved by variations in sympathetic, but not by parasympathetic, discharge to the ventricles.

The cardioregulatory areas in the medulla influence the autonomic discharge to the heart as a portion of the pressoreceptor mechanism for maintaining systemic arterial pressure (see Chapter 6). The diencephalic and hypothalamic regions contain cardiovascular controls in complex neural mechanisms involved in temperature regulation, the intake of food and fluid, emotional and sexual behavior and many other patterns of behavior. It follows, then, that a wide variety of cardiovascular responses can be induced by electrical stimulation at various sites in the brain stem. Also areas of the cerebral cortex where stimulation induces changes in overt behavior also induce cardiovascular adaptations of one sort or another. Thus, there exists the possibility that the architecture of the central nervous system provides for combined patterns of somatic and autonomic adaptations.

II. CLINICAL ESTIMATION OF CARDIAC OUTPUT

Since the maximum capability of the heart can be evaluated only by determining the cardiovascular response to a load, a method for directly measuring cardiac output during exertion would be very valuable in cardiac diagnosis and prognosis. Unfortunately, direct measurements of cardiac function in man, although desirable, are virtually impossible because the heart is quite inaccessible for the determination of either stroke volume or absolute volume. Perhaps the most direct method is the calculation of changes in cardiac volume from the cardiac silhouette on roentgenographic plates (see Chapter 11). In recent years, a wide variety of techniques has been proposed to determine cardiac output by indirect methods. The basic principles and limitations of some of the techniques currently in vogue will be described.

From the foregoing discussion, it is clear that measurement of either cardiac output or stroke volume may not be sufficient to permit adequate evaluation of ventricular performance. Profound changes in the rates of change of various features of ventricular function may occur with little or no influence in stroke volume (see Figs. 3–17 and 3–18). In addition to techniques for measuring cardiac output, efforts must be directed toward devising methods of assessing the dynamic properties of ventricular performance. Some of the methods which are currently available will be presented along with some predictions for the future.

THE FICK PRINCIPLE

Blood flow through an organ can be determined if a substance is removed from or added to the blood during its flow through the organ. Applied to the lungs, the Fick principle is used to calculate the volume of blood required to transport the oxygen taken up from the alveoli per unit time. The fundamental concept is deceptively simple and can be illustrated schematically by representing the oxygen-carrying capacity of the blood as beakers on a conveyer belt (Fig. 3–21).

MEASUREMENT OF OXYGEN CONSUMPTION

Of necessity, the oxygen consumption is generally measured over a period of several minutes. The accuracy of oxygen uptake determinations from the clinical B.M.R. apparatus is generally inadequate for this purpose. A preferred technique consists of collecting in a spirometer all the air expired during carefully timed intervals and analyzing samples for oxygen content (Fig. 3–22). Comparing the oxygen content of the total exhaled volume with a similar volume of ambient air provides the data required to compute the oxygen uptake accurately.

THE ARTERIOVENOUS OXYGEN DIFFERENCE

The arterial blood throughout the body normally has a uniform oxygen content. However, to determine a significant A-V oxygen difference, it is necessary to obtain samples of *mixed* venous blood. The quantity of oxygen contained in venous blood depends upon the vascular bed from which it is returning. For example, blood from the kidneys and skin remains well satu-

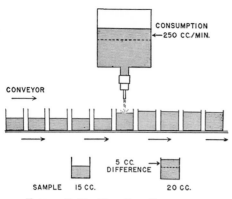

FIGURE 3–21   THE FICK PRINCIPLE

If each beaker on a conveyer belt receives 5 cc. of fluid as it passes under a dispenser delivering 250 cc. per minute, the beakers must pass the dispenser at a rate of 50 per minute (250/5) to carry that quantity of fluid. Similarly, if each 100 cc. of blood takes up 5 cc. of oxygen from the lungs (A-V oxygen difference) and 250 cc. of oxygen are consumed each minute, 50 increments of 100 cc. (5000 cc.) of blood must have passed through the lungs each minute. This is the Fick principle as it is applied to the calculation of cardiac output (see Fig. 3–22).

rated with oxygen while blood from the coronary vessels and exercising muscle is largely depleted of oxygen. The oxygen contents of venous blood from other tissues vary between these extremes. Due to laminar flow in the venous channels, currents of blood with a relatively high oxygen content may accompany streams with lower values in the same vein. The oxygen saturation of blood in the superior vena cava differs from that in the inferior vena cava and these two streams of blood do not mix completely within the right atrium. The Lipiodol streamers in Figure 2–15 graphically illustrate this fact. Mixing of blood does occur in the right ventricle and is almost complete by the time the blood has entered the pulmonary arteries. The oxygen content of a sample of blood obtained from the pulmonary artery represents an average value for

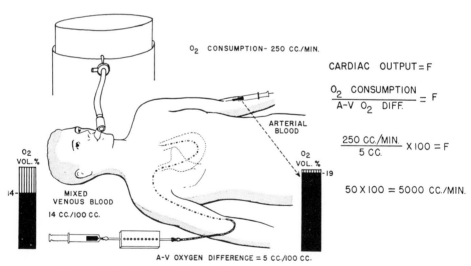

FIGURE 3–22   CARDIAC OUTPUT DETERMINED BY THE FICK PRINCIPLE

Computing cardiac output according to the Fick principle requires simultaneous determination of oxygen consumption and the arteriovenous oxygen difference. Exhaled air is collected to measure oxygen consumption per minute. Blood is withdrawn from the pulmonary artery through a catheter into a cuvette oximeter, so that the oxygen content of mixed venous blood can be read from a galvanometer. Arterial oxygen content is measured in a sample of blood from any systemic artery. The A-V oxygen difference in cubic centimeters of oxygen per 100 cc. of blood is obtained by subtracting the oxygen content of the mixed venous sample from the arterial oxygen content.

venous blood which can be used to establish the arteriovenous oxygen difference for calculating cardiac output by the Fick principle.

Cardiac Catheterization. In 1929, Forssmann[36] demonstrated that a catheter can be passed through the venous channels into the right chambers of the human heart (Fig. 3–22). Cournand and his associates[37, 38] established the safety of the procedure and stimulated widespread utilization of the method. The technique of cardiac catheterization and its sources of error have been described in detail by Cournand,[39] Warren,[40] Visscher[41] and Stow.[42]

Measurement of Blood Oxygen Content. Arterial and venous oxygen content can be directly measured with the Van Slyke apparatus, which is a time-consuming but accurate procedure in the hands of highly qualified technicians. For rapid determinations of blood oxygen content, a photoelectric method has been developed and compares favorably with Van Slyke determinations. Blood for analysis is drawn through a cuvette oximeter (Fig. 3–22), where it is transilluminated by a constant intensity light source, and the transmitted light is registered simultaneously in two spectral regions: approximately 750 to 900 millimicrons and 600 to 750 millimicrons, respectively. The former is near infra-red light in wave length and is transmitted by both oxyhemoglobin and reduced hemoglobin to approximately equal degrees. The other photocell responds to red light, which is transmitted well by oxyhemoglobin and to a very slight degree by reduced hemoglobin. The ratio between the light intensities recorded from the two wave lengths can be read in terms of absolute percentage of oxygen saturation after the apparatus has been satisfactorily calibrated by means of

Van Slyke analysis. Various spectrophotometric techniques have been successfully employed for the measurement of blood oxygen content. In experienced hands, these devices more than make up for the slight reduction in accuracy through the ease with which serial determinations can be obtained in rapid sequence while the patient is being studied.

Objective determinations of cardiac output have been of great value in advancing our knowledge of circulatory dynamics, with particular reference to pulmonary function in health and disease. However, the search for an objective test of cardiac reserve was not ended by the development of cardiac catheterization, because the procedure is too complicated for routine clinical use and is not entirely suitable for use during strenuous exertion. A normal value for cardiac output at rest is often obtained even when the cardiac reserve is seriously depleted. If cardiac catheterization provided no information beyond the resting cardiac output, its utilization would be largely limited to fundamental investigation. However, several additional types of information can be gained from catheterization which are particularly useful in the diagnosis of congenital malformations of the heart.

THE STEWART PRINCIPLE

The volume of fluid in a container can be calculated by adding a known quantity of dye and measuring the concentration of the material after it has become evenly dispersed through the fluid (Fig. 3–23A). The volume is calculated according to the formula $V = A/C$, where V is the volume of fluid, A is the amount of dye added and C is the concentration of the dye in

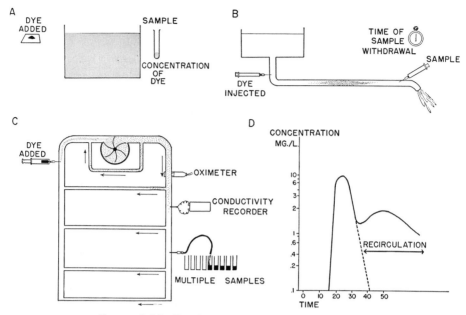

FIGURE 3–23   THE INDICATOR DILUTION TECHNIQUE

A, The volume of stationary fluid in a reservoir can be determined by completely mixing a known amount of dye and analyzing a sample for the concentration of the dye.

B, The volume flow through a simple tube can be estimated by injecting a known quantity of dye, withdrawing a sample at constant rate during the passage of the dye-containing fluid and determining the mean concentration of the sample.

C, A hydraulic model simulating the circulatory system illustrates the fact that an indicator substance may pass through short circuits and begin to recirculate before the mass of dye has passed the sampling point. Therefore it is necessary to devise means by which the amount of recirculating dye can be separated from the amount of dye sampled during its initial passage to arrive at a reliable mean concentration.

D, If the concentration of the dye passing a sampling point is plotted on semi-log paper, the descending limb after the peak can be extended to the baseline as a straight line. The area under the initial curve can be used to derive the mean concentration of the dye during its first circulation.

each cubic centimeter of the fluid. Stewart[43, 44] demonstrated that his method can also be applied to fluids in motion. Hamilton and his associates[45, 46] verified the usefulness of the method in calculating the flow through glass models and in the circulation.

GENERAL PRINCIPLES

The computation of a volume of stationary fluid by determining the dilution of a known quantity of dye is perfectly straightforward (Fig. 3–23). Similarly, the volume flow through a simple tubular system can theoretically

be determined with considerable accuracy by determining the average concentration of a known quantity of dye and the time during sampling according to the formula $F = A/Ct$, where F is flow, A is quantity of dye injected, C is the average concentration of dye in the sample and t is the duration of sample withdrawal (Fig. 3–23A). Under these conditions, the Stewart principle is quite as accurate as the Fick principle. However, conditions in the human circulation are more complex, as indicated by the hydraulic model in Figure 3–23C. Part of the dye injected at one point in this model has completely traversed the short circuits and begun to recirculate before the material has reached the more distant regions. The average concentration of the indicator substance can be measured by (1) collecting multiple samples in rapid succession, (2) continuously recording blood conductivity after saline injections or (3) making oximeter or densitometer recordings when dyes are injected. In any case, the concentration of indicator flowing past the point of recording reaches a peak, begins to descend and then increases again owing to recirculation. If the once-circulated dye can be separated from the recirculated dye, cardiac output can be computed with considerable accuracy.

The fundamental requirements for this method are (1) the injection of a material which can be accurately analyzed and which does not leave the blood during the test and (2) a sample of arterial blood which indicates the average concentration of the material during its first circulation through the arterial tree. Various dyes as well as saline solutions have been used with varying degrees of success and the average concentration has been determined either by repetitive sampling or by continuous recording.

BALLISTOCARDIOGRAPHY

The concept that a sudden motion of the blood in one direction must produce a recoil of the body in the opposite direction is not a new idea. In 1887, Gordon[47] compared the ballistic forces of the body to the recoil of a gun. In 1905 Henderson[48] used a "swinging table" to record the movements along the longitudinal axis of a patient reclining on its surface. The changing velocity of the moving blood within the circulatory system caused the table to oscillate during each successive cardiac cycle.

GENERAL PRINCIPLES

The recoil of a rifle is frequently employed as an analogy to explain the basic principles of ballistocardiography. If a rifle is rigidly fastened on a spring-mounted table, a discharging cartridge propels the bullet out of the barrel and displaces the rifle in the opposite direction (Fig. 3–24A). Recording the movements of the table in these circumstances might provide information concerning the magnitude of the powder charge (energy release) if other conditions are known. If the magnitude of the powder charge and the muzzle velocity were unknown, the weight of the bullet (mass ejected) could not be computed from the recorded deflections. The analysis would be seriously complicated if, during the recoil of the rifle, the speeding bullet struck a steel plate mounted on the same table. Since the blood does not leave the system, the recoil of the heart and body from ejection of blood into the arteries is even more complex. For example, the blood ejected from the two ventricles moves simultaneously in several directions after leaving the heart. Its energy is imparted to the body at every turn. Routine ballistocardiograms indicate movements of the body in only one direction. Simultaneous recordings in three dimensions are extremely difficult to analyze. Finally, the records may be seriously distorted by such factors as the coupling between the body and the table. The elasticity of the skin acts as a spring interposed between the moving body and the table top and may profoundly influence the recorded deflections.

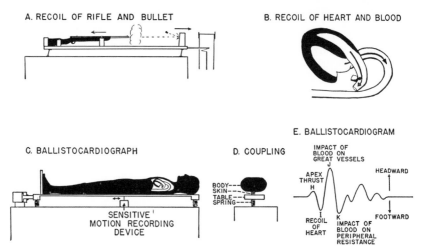

FIGURE 3–24   BALLISTOCARDIOGRAPHY

A, The recoil of a rifle during discharge of a cartridge can be recorded by attaching it rigidly to a spring-mounted table. The record would become seriously distorted if the bullet ricocheted from a barrier on the table during the recoil of the rifle.

B, The blood ejected by the ventricles travels in several directions simultaneously, imparting its energy to the body at every turn. For this reason, measurements of the recoil of the body in one direction only are inadequate.

C, A low-frequency spring-mounted table which has been critically damped has been recommended for ballistocardiography because the body cannot be rigidly fastened to the table. The tissues in contact with the table have an elasticity which is equivalent to interposing a spring between the body and the table top.

D, If the springs supporting the table are stiff in relation to the elasticity of the tissues, the recorded patterns tend to reflect the elastic properties of the tissues supporting the body as the forces are imparted by the heart and blood.

E, Ballistocardiographic records consist of a series of deflections which have been related to the events of the cardiac cycle. Although the forces developed by the heart and blood affect the recorded patterns, a consistent relationship between these deflections and stroke volume is probably fortuitous for the most part.

EVALUATION OF BALLISTOCARDIOGRAPHY

Starr and his associates[49] extended Henderson's observations and reawakened interest in the recoil phenomena by stating that the size of the initial waves, I and J, is related to the cardiac output, and that the form of the ballistic curve is determined by the shape of the curve of blood velocity in the great vessels.[50] Actually, the size of the initial deflection is determined by the acceleration of the fluid (the rate at which velocity of ejection is built up) and not by the total stroke output. The recorded oscillations are the resultant of vascular and body movements as they may be in phase and reinforce one another or be out of phase and cancel each other. Reconstruction of the ballistocardiographic records led to the following description of the causes of the various oscillations. The H wave begins with movements that take place during isometric contraction and are the most variable. The I wave is the result of a partly cancelled footward thrust developed as blood is ejected from the heart into the ascending aorta and pulmonary artery. The J wave has a complex origin, including the deceleration of blood in the heart, ascending aorta and pulmonary artery and the acceleration of blood in the descending aorta.

The obvious limitations of the method do not preclude the recognition of empirical relationships between various types of cardiac dysfunction and characteristic ballistocardiographic patterns. Since the amplitude of the deflections is influenced by the rate at which blood is accelerated, variations in the pattern should reveal alterations in the force of ventricular ejection. It may have value as a source of information about the dynamic performance of the heart (see Fig. 3–26).

PRESSURE PULSE CONTOUR METHOD

THE RELATION OF PULSE PRESSURE TO STROKE VOLUME

Erlanger and Hooker[51] recognized that the product of the pulse pressure and the heart rate indicated cardiac output, with the following reservations: "In order to be able to obtain a knowledge of the absolute velocity of blood flow from a knowledge of the pulse-pressure and pulse rate, it is necessary to know:

"1. The rate of systolic output. For if a given amount of blood be driven into the aorta with different rates the maximum pressure would be higher when this rate is rapid than when it is slow.

"2. The rate of flow from the arteries into the veins. For this flow continues during cardiac systole and consequently variations in the rate of this flow would vary the height to which the force of the heart would raise the systolic pressure.

"3. The distensibility of human arteries at different pressures. The distensibility diminishes as the pressure increases; consequently at a high pressure it would require a smaller systolic output to produce a pulse-pressure of a given magnitude than at a low pressure.

"4. The amount of blood in the systemic arteries under various conditions. The fall of pressure during diastole depends upon the relative amount of blood that escapes into the veins, not upon the absolute amount.

"We do not know how large any one of these factors is, but it seems probable that, under more or less normal conditions, none of them would produce a very large error. Upon this assumption we are perhaps justified in using the product of the pulse-pressure by the pulse rate as an index to the relative velocity of blood flow."

Clearly the stroke volume would be directly proportional to arterial pulse pressure only if the pressure-volume relations of the arterial system were not only constant and uniform among individuals, but linear from high pressure to low. Remington[52] presented a set of volume factors from known stroke volumes and pulse pressures, corrected for body size and distensibility curves. From this table, stroke volume/sq. m. body surface could be predicted with an error of about 25 per cent. According to Hamilton and Remington[53] pulse pressure correlates roughly with stroke volume determined by the dye dilution technique ($r = 0.88$). Over the normal pressure range, a pressure rise of 1 mm. Hg was equivalent to about 1 cc. of stroke volume/sq. m. For some purposes, this degree of accuracy might be quite sufficient. However, a great deal of effort has been expended in attempts to increase the precision with which stroke volume is derived from the pressure-pulse contour. This is no simple matter, considering the complexity of the situation.

ANALYSIS OF PULSE CONTOURS

If fluid is injected into a distensible container with fixed volume elasticity, the volume in the system can be calibrated in terms of the internal pressure (Fig. 3–25A). Once the volume-pressure relations are established, the volume contained can be determined by noting the pressure in the system. However, if fluid can escape from the system (Fig. 3–25B), the elastic chamber will remain distended only if fluid is pumped in at the same average rate as it leaks out. Under these circumstances, the pressure will increase as the chamber is distended and will decrease between pumping strokes as the fluid leaves the system. The difference between the maximal and minimal pressures indicates the amount of fluid injected at each stroke less the amount which left the system during the ejection period. If the distensible chamber is a long, narrow cylinder with elastic

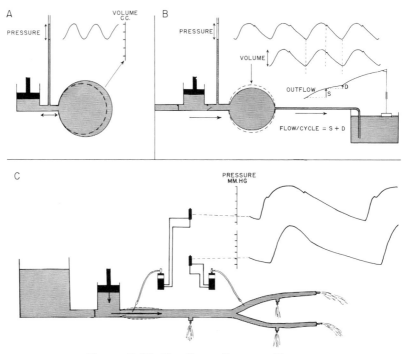

FIGURE 3–25   THE PULSE CONTOUR METHOD

A, The changes in the volume of the balloon can be determined by measuring the pressure if the pressure-volume relations are constant.

B, If fluid is pumped into a balloon and flows out through a tube offering some resistance, the flow through the system can be estimated from the pressure fluctuations. The volume and pressure within the balloon increase during ejection from the pump, but outflow occurs throughout the entire cycle. If pressure fluctuations are used to indicate changes in volume, the flow from the system can be estimated by determining the flow out of the system during diastole (D) and adding a computed value for outflow from the system during the stroke (S).

C, In the circulatory system, the pulse of pressure does not reach all parts of the elastic pressure reservoir simultaneously and its contour changes as it passes through the system (see also Fig. 5–3). Under these conditions, the volumes entering and leaving various portions of the system must be considered individually to reach maximum accuracy. Since this is not practical in intact animals or man, the computation of cardiac output from pressure pulses has been greatly simplified. However, each step toward simplification of the method involves sacrifice of accuracy.

walls, the fluid ejected by the pump is not instantaneously distributed through the system and the recorded pressure will be distorted by reflected waves. A similar situation obtains within the arterial system of the body.

Hamilton and Remington[53] recognized that prediction of stroke volume from pressure pulses must depend upon evaluation of the "individual arterial distensibility, knowledge of the pulse pressure in the arterial tree and its several parts, and the estimation of arteriolar drainage." They developed a table indicating the capacity of the various portions of the arterial tree at different pressures and another showing the pulse wave transmission times to the parts of the arterial tree at various diastolic pressures. These data were employed in the analysis of pressure pulses. Remington *et al.*[54] and Warner[55] subsequently reported a simplified technique which facilitates analysis of the pressure pulse with little increase in the error. The pulse contour method has one very important potential advantage. It permits computation of the stroke volume of individual cycles even though its accuracy may be limited.

COMPUTED AORTIC FLOW VELOCITY FROM THE PRESSURE GRADIENT

The mathematical relationship between pressure, viscosity and density expressed by the Navier Stokes equation is a fundamental and general expression describing fluid flow. Fry and his associates[56, 57] developed a modification of this relationship, which with suitable restrictions can be expressed as

$$-\mathrm{d}p/\mathrm{d}z = 1.1 \; (\rho/g) \; (\mathrm{d}\omega/\mathrm{d}t) + a\omega$$

where p is the lateral pressure in cm. H_2O, z is the distance between the pressure points in cm., ρ is the blood density in g/cm.^{3}, g is the acceleration of gravity in cm./sec.^{2}, t is time in seconds, 1.1 is an experimentally determined constant taking into account the nonuniform velocity distribution across the lumen and a is a frictional coefficient. By feeding into a computer the pressure difference between two points along the stream, the solution of the equation indicates the blood velocity from the pressure gradient continuously measured between two points a known distance apart. For this purpose, a double lumen catheter was fitted to a pair of carefully matched pressure gauges so that a very accurate recording of the instantaneous pressure difference between two points some 4 to 5 cm. apart was continuously registered. This pressure difference was fed into an analogue computer continuously solving the simplified equation to provide a flow velocity waveform, basically similar in shape to those recorded by other techniques (i.e., Fig. 3–16), often with superimposed high frequency noise. Practical difficulties result in part from the fact that the pressure difference at two points 5 cm. apart in the aorta rarely exceeds 1 or 2 mm. Hg even at high flow rates. For example, a 1 per cent error in estimating one of the two pressures would produce an error in the range of 10 per cent error in estimating the pressure gradient. High frequency "noise" often appears as spikes on an otherwise smooth flow wave form. Other problems related to drift of the baseline of the pressure gauges can produce gross distortion of the computed flow contour. Designation of zero flow is a problem except at the aortic arch where it is assumed that flow is zero at the end of diastole. Despite these technical difficulties, the pressure-gradient technique merits serious consideration because it represents one of the few methods by which instantaneous flow velocity can be estimated in man.

Jones[58] has advocated a further simplification of the basic flow formulae by substituting the time derivative of pressure (dp/dt) at a single site rather than the pressure gradient (dp/dz) described previously. Although waveforms resembling directly recorded flow records can be obtained, the theoretical validity of the method remains questionable despite reports of reasonably high correlation coefficients in comparisons with results from Fick or dye dilution techniques.[59]

Cardiac Evaluation from Dynamic Performance. Patients with very severe heart disease may have perfectly normal cardiac output and stroke at rest. The comprehensive recording of many simultaneous variables during spontaneous and induced cardiovascular responses (see Fig. 3–14, 3–17, and 3–18) have demonstrated that the most sensitive indicators of performance are the *rates* of change, including the rate of change of pressure (dp/dt), rate of ejection (outflow velocity) and rate of change of velocity (acceleration). During normal everyday stress, which provokes sympathetic discharge to the heart, the acceleration of outflow and the peak ejection velocity of both ventricles are accentuated. This is a primary mechanism for autonomic control of the heart. On the contrary, experimental procedures believed to depress ventricular function were also found to reduce peak ejection velocity and acceleration of the blood out of the ventricles. For example, experimental coronary occlusion was followed within 15 to 20 beats by increased heart rate and reduced peak flow velocity curve with more gradual upslope (Fig. 3–26). Similar changes were noted during experimental exsanguination severe enough to depress

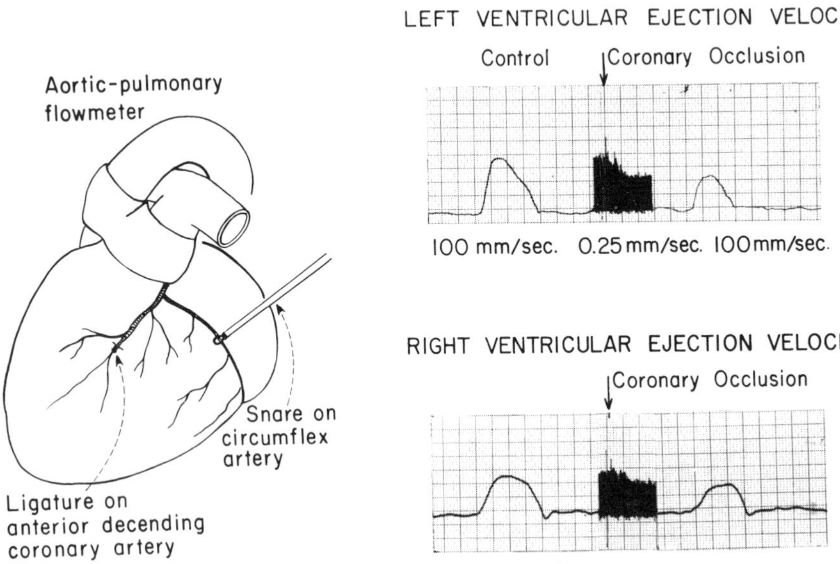

FIGURE 3–26   ACUTE CORONARY OCCLUSION

Acute ligation of the circumflex coronary artery by tightening a snare in a conscious dog with a previously ligated anterior descending coronary artery is promptly followed by a rapid reduction in the initial upslope in ejection velocity of both left and right ventricles. Peak outflow rate is depressed, and stroke volume is diminished. (From Rushmer.[60])

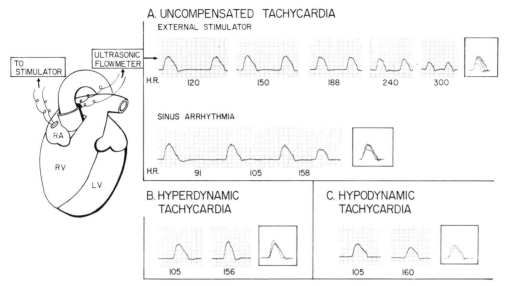

FIGURE 3–27   EJECTION VELOCITY AND ACCELERATION (SLOPE) WITH TACHYCARDIA

A, Increased heart rate, occurring spontaneously or from external stimulation, produces lower peak flow rates and smaller stroke volumes, but the initial upslope (maximal acceleration) is changed little or not at all.

B, Sympathetic stimulation produces increased acceleration, higher peak flow and shorter ejection.

C, Conditions depressing ventricular function characteristically produce marked reduction in maximal acceleration along with reduced peak flow and stroke volume. Such observations suggest that maximal acceleration may be a most valuable indicator of cardiac performance. (From Rushmer.[61])

the systemic arterial pressure. General anesthesia induced by pentobarbital or halothane produces corresponding effects.

If these experimental techniques are applicable to the appraisal of cardiac function in man, they require recording techniques which are sensitive to changes in dynamic events which transpire during the rapid acceleration of blood out of the ventricles at the onset of systole.[61] The rates of rise of ventricular and central aortic pressure are becoming widely recognized as important criteria of ventricular performance and capability. Acceleration of the blood out of the ventricles may prove to be an even better indicator of ventricular function. Changes in stroke volume and peak outflow rate can be observed during spontaneous and experimentally induced changes in heart rate (Fig. 3–27). When these waveforms are superimposed, the ini-

tial upslope appears to be unaffected. Stimulation of sympathetic nerves produces tachycardia accompanied by much higher peak outflow rate and steeper initial upslope on the flow records as indicated previously. In contrast, many conditions that depress ventricular performance, such as coronary obstruction (Fig. 3–26), produce tachycardia, lower peak outflow rate and more gradual upslope (diminished acceleration). These phenomena have also been observed by Noble, Trenchard and Guz,[62, 63] who concluded that maximum acceleration was closely associated with the maximum force in early systole and to the maximum initial velocity of shortening. They concur in the view that maximum acceleration is little affected by changes in posture or heart rate.[63] All these observations indicate the potential utility of directly measuring the dynamic properties of ventricular performance as criteria for evaluating the state of the ventricular myocardium. Information of potential value is embodied in several indicators employed in the past—the initial rate of rise of ventricular or central aortic pressure, the apex cardiogram and the ballistocardiogram. However, none of these has achieved general use for cardiac evaluation. The maximum acceleration of outflow from the ventricles may be the most important basis for cardiac evaluation proposed thus far.

PROJECTIONS FOR THE FUTURE OF CARDIAC EVALUATION

Outflow acceleration can be detected only by a flow sensing device. Among all the flow detectors presented in Figure 2–19, the techniques adaptable for use on man are the pressure gradient technique, the arterial pressure pulse analysis and the transcutaneous Doppler flow velocity sensor. In its simplest form, this device has provided useful clinical information regarding flow velocities in peripheral arteries. The newly developed pulse Doppler technique[64] permits sampling of flow velocity from a designated distance below the skin. This means that peak flow velocity and acceleration may well be sensed by a transducer positioned on the skin and receiving signals only from the axial stream in the aortic arch. If this prospect materializes, ventricular performance may be critically and objectively evaluated, without pain or hazard, directly through the skin of the thorax on normal subjects and patients alike.

SUMMARY

Cardiac output can be determined through the use of cardiac catheterization according to the Fick principle. The theory is basically sound. The accuracy of the determinations depends upon the cumulative errors caused by deviations from the "steady state" conditions required for application of this theory. Very significant errors result whenever respiratory or circulatory conditions are inconstant.

The indicator-dilution technique is also basically sound for computing flow through simple tubular systems. In the circulatory system, application of the Stewart principle is complicated by problems related to recirculation of the indicator. With proper precautions, this technique affords values comparable to those derived from cardiac catheterization.

Theoretically, stroke volume can be determined from an analysis of the arterial pulse contour. However, many sources of error are present, including intangible factors such as differences in arterial distensibility among individuals. If the pulse contour method can be calibrated by the Fick principle in a particular subject, it becomes much more reliable. If the magnitude of the potential errors is recognized, the pulse contour method has considerable practical value since stroke volume of individual cycles can be estimated.

Ballistocardiography has been widely used to compute values presumed to represent stroke volume or cardiac output. Reliable recordings of body movements in response to ballistic forces during the cardiac cycle may be related to the rate or force of ventricular ejection, but even the basic principles of the method fail to reveal any direct relationship between the magnitude of the deflections and the volume of blood ejected. This fact does not preclude the establishment of empirical relations between specific ballistocardiographic patterns and certain forms of cardiovascular disease.

REFERENCES

1. BOZLER, E. The activity of the pacemaker previous to the discharge of a muscular impulse. *Amer. J. Physiol.*, 136:543–552, 1942.

2. WEST, T. C., FALK, G., and CERVONI, P. Drug alteration of transmembrane potentials in atrial pacemaker cells. *J. Pharmacol. Exp. Ther.*, 117:245–252, 1956.

3. HUNT, R. Direct and reflex acceleration of the mammalian heart with some observations on the relations of the inhibitory and accelerator nerves. *Amer. J. Physiol.*, 2:395–470, 1899.

4. ALEXANDER, R. S. Tonic and reflex functions of medullary sympathetic cardiovascular centers. *J. Neurophysiol.*, 9:205–217, 1946.

5. RANDALL, W. C., MCNALLY, H., COWAN, J., CALIGUIRI, L., and ROHSE, W. G. Functional analysis of the cardioaugmentor and cardioaccelerator pathways in the dog. *Amer. J. Physiol.*, 191:213–217, 1957.

6. RUSHMER, R. F. Autonomic balance in cardiac control. *Amer. J. Physiol.*, 192:631–634, 1958.

7. BRONK, D. W., PITTS, R. I., and LARRABEE, M. G. Role of hypothalamus in cardiovascular regulation. *Res. Publ. Ass. Res. Nerv. & Ment. Dis.*, 20:323–341, 1940.

8. STEVENSON, I. P., and DUNCAN, C. H. Alterations in cardiac function and circulatory efficiency during periods of life stress as shown by changes in the rate, rhythm, electrocardiographic pattern and output of the heart in those with cardiovascular disease. *Res. Publ. Ass. Res. Nerv. & Ment. Dis.*, 29:799–817, 1950.

9. HICKAM, J. B., CARGILL, W. H., and GOLDEN, A. Cardiovascular reactions to emotional stimuli; effect on the cardiac output, arteriovenous oxygen difference, arterial pressure, and peripheral resistance. *J. Clin. Invest.*, 27:290–298, 1948.

10. FEIL, H., GREEN, H. D., and EIBER, D. Voluntary acceleration of heart in a subject showing the Wolff-Parkinson-White syndrome. *Amer. Heart J.*, 34:334–348, 1947.

11. DOWLING, C. V., SMITH, W. W., BERGER, A. R., and ALBERT, R. E. The effect on blood pressure in the right heart, pulmonary artery and systemic artery of cardiac standstill produced by carotid sinus stimulation. *Circulation*, 5:742–746, 1952.

12. RUSHMER, R. F. Circulatory collapse following mechanical stimulation of arteries. *Amer. J. Physiol.*, 141:722–729, 1944.

13. LEWIS, T. Lecture on vasovagal syncope and carotid sinus mechanism with comments on Gowers' and Nothnagel's syndrome. *Brit. Med. J.*, 1:873–876, 1932.

14. BAZETT, H. C., and MCGLONE, B. Note on pain sensations which accompany deep punctures. *Brain*, 51:18–23, 1928.

15. DAVILA, J. C. Measurement of left ventricular volume; a symposium. *Amer. J. Cardiol.*, 18:1–47, 208–252, 566–593, 1966.

16. DODGE, H. T., SANDLER, H., BAXLEY, W. A., and HAWLEY, R. R. Usefulness and limitations of radiographic methods for determining left ventricular volume. *Amer. J. Cardiol.*, 18:10–24, 1966.

17. RAPAPORT, E. Usefulness and limitation of thermal washout technics in ventricular volume measurement. *Amer. J. Cardiol.*, 18:226–230, 1966.

18. RUSHMER, R. F., CRYSTAL, D. K., and WAGNER, C. The functional anatomy of ventricular contraction. *Circulat. Res.*, 1:162–170, 1953.

19. RUSHMER, R. F., FINLAYSON, B. L., and NASH, A. A. Shrinkage of the heart in anesthetized, thoracotomized dogs. *Circulat. Res.*, 2:22–27, 1954.

20. WILKIE, D. R. The mechanical properties of muscle. *Brit. Med. Bull.*, 12:177–182, 1956.

21. WIGGERS, C. J. Determinants of cardiac performance. *Circulation*, 4:485–495, 1951.

22. PATTERSON, S. W., PIPER, H., and STARLING, E. H. The regulation of the heart beat. *J. Physiol.*, 48:465–513, 1914.

23. STARLING, E. H. *Principles of Human Physiology*, 3rd ed. Philadelphia, Lea & Febiger, 1920, 315 pp.

24. LUNDIN, G. Mechanical properties of cardiac muscle. *Acta physiol. scand.*, 7 (Suppl. 20): 7–86, 1944.

25. HILL, A. V. The heat of shortening and the dynamic constants of muscle. *Proc. Roy. Soc.*, 126:136–195, 1938.

26. SONNENBLICK, E. H. Force-velocity relations in mammalian heart muscle. *Amer. J. Physiol.*, 202:931–939, 1962.

27. DOWNING, S. E., and SONNENBLICK, E. H. Cardiac muscle mechanics and ventricular performance; force and time parameters. *Amer. J. Physiol.*, 207:705–715, 1964.

28. FRY, D. L., GRIGGS, D. M., and GREENFIELD, F. C. Myocardial mechanics: tension-velocity-length relationships in heart muscle. *Circulat. Res.*, 14:73–85, 1964.

29. SHIPLEY, R. E., and GREGG, D. E. The cardiac response to stimulation of the stellate ganglion and cardiac nerves. *Amer. J. Physiol.*, 143:396–401, 1945.

30. KELSO, A. F., and RANDALL, W. C. Ventricular changes associated with sympathetic augmentation of cardiovascular pressure pulses. *Amer. J. Physiol.*, 196:731–734, 1959.

31. KJELLBERG, S. R., RUDHE, U., and SJÖSTRAND, T. The influence of the autonomic nervous system on the contraction of the human heart under normal circulatory conditions. *Acta physiol. scand.*, 24:350–360, 1952.

32. FULTON, J. F., RANSON, S. W., and FRANTZ, A. M. The hypothalamus and central levels of autonomic function. *Res. Publ. Ass. Nerv. & Ment. Dis.*, 20:1–980, 1940.

33. SMITH, O. A., JR., JABBUR, S. J., RUSHMER, R. F., and LASHER, E. P. Role of hypothalamic structures in cardiac control. *Physiol. Rev.*, 40 (Suppl. 4): 136–145, 1960.

34. SMITH, O. A., JR., RUSHMER, R. F., and LASHER, E. P. Similarity of cardiovascular responses to exercise and diencephalic stimulation. *Amer. J. Physiol.*, 198:1139–1142, 1960.

35. RUSHMER, R. F., and SMITH, O. A. Cardiac control. *Physiol. Rev.*, 39:41–68, 1959.

36. FORSSMANN, W. Probing of the right heart *Klin. Wschr.*, 8:2085–2087, 1929.

37. COURNAND, A., and RANGES, H. A. Catheterization of right auricle in man. *Proc. Soc. Exp. Biol. Med.*, 46:462–466, 1941.

38. COURNAND, A., RILEY, R. L., BREED, E. S., BALDWIN, DEF., and RICHARDS, D. W. Measurement of cardiac output in man using technique of catheterization of right auricle or ventricle. *J. Clin. Invest.*, 24:106–116, 1945.

39. COURNAND, A., BALDWIN, J. S., and HIMMELSTEIN, A. *Cardiac Catheterization in Congenital Heart Disease.* New York, The Commonwealth Fund, 1949.

40. WARREN, J. V. Determination of cardiac output in man by right heart catheterization. *Meth. Med. Res.*, 1:224–232, 1948.

41. VISSCHER, M. B., and JOHNSON, J. A. The Fick principle: analysis of potential errors in its conventional application. *J. Appl. Physiol.*, 5:635–638, 1953.

42. STOW, R. W. Systematic errors in flow determinations by the Fick method. *Minnesota Med.*, 37:30–35, 1954.

43. STEWART, G. N. Researches on the circulation time and on the influences which affect it. *J. Physiol.*, 22:159–183, 1897.

44. STEWART, G. N. The output of the heart in dogs. *Amer. J. Physiol.*, 57:27–50, 1921.

45. HAMILTON, W. F., and REMINGTON, J. W. Comparison of the time concentration curves in arterial blood of diffusible and nondiffusible substances when injected at a constant rate and when injected instantaneously. *Amer. J. Physiol.*, 148:35–39, 1948.

46. KINSMAN, J. M., MOORE, J. W., and HAMILTON, W. F. Studies on the circulation: injection method: physical and mathematical considerations. *Amer. J. Physiol.*, 89:321–330, 1929.

47. GORDON, J. W. On certain molar movements of the human body produced by the circulation of the blood. *J. Anat., Lond.*, 11:533–536, 1877.

48. HENDERSON, Y. The mass-movements of the circulation as shown by a recoil curve. *Amer. J. Physiol.*, 14:287–298, 1905.

49. STARR, I., RAWSON, A. J., SCHROEDER, H. A., and JOSEPH, N. R. Studies on the estimation of cardiac output in man, and of abnormalities in cardiac function, from the heart's recoil and the blood's impacts; the ballistocardiogram. *Amer. J. Physiol.*, 127:1–28, 1939.

50. STARR, I., and SCHROEDER, H. A. Ballistocardiogram. II. Normal standards, abnormalities commonly found in diseases of the heart and circulation, and their significance. *J. Clin. Invest.*, 19:437–450, 1940.

51. ERLANGER, J., and HOOKER, D. R. An experimental study of blood-pressure and of pulse-pressure in man. *Johns Hopk. Hosp. Rep.*, 12:145–378, 1904.

52. REMINGTON, J. W. The relation between the stroke volume and the pulse pressure. *Minnesota Med.*, 37:105–110, 1954.

53. HAMILTON, W. F., and REMINGTON, J. W. The measurement of the stroke volume from the pressure pulse. *Amer. J. Physiol.*, 148:14–24, 1947.

54. REMINGTON, J. W., HAMILTON, W. F., WHEELER, N. C., and HAMILTON, W. F., JR. Validity of pulse contour method for calculating cardiac output of the dog, with notes on effects of various anesthetics. *Amer. J. Physiol.*, 159:379–384, 1949.

55. WARNER, H. R. Quantitation of stroke volume changes in man from the central pressure pulse. *Minnesota Med.*, 37:111–115, 1954.

56. FRY, D. L. The measurement of pulsatile flow by the computed pressure gradient technique. *IRE Trans. Med. Electron.*, ME6:259–264, 1959.

57. GREENFIELD, J. C. Pressure gradient technique. Pp. 83–93 in *Methods of Medical Research*, Vol. 11, R. F. Rushmer, Ed. Chicago, Yearbook Medical Publishers, Inc., 1966.

58. JONES, W. B., HEFNER, L. L. BANCROFT, W. H., and KLIP, W. Velocity of blood flow and stroke volume obtained from the pressure pulse. *J. Clin. Invest.*, 38:2087–2090, 1959.

59. JONES, W. B., RUSSELL, R. O., and DALTON, D. H. An evaluation of computed stroke volume in man. *Amer. Heart. J.*, 72:746–750, 1966.

60. RUSHMER, R. F. Initial ventricular impulse; a potential key to cardiac evaluation. *Circulation*, 29:268–283, 1964.

61. RUSHMER, R. F. Recent advances in cardiovascular physiology. *Anesthesia and Analgesia*, 45:383–389, 1966.

62. NOBLE, M. I. M., TRENCHARD, D., and GUZ, A. Left ventricular ejection in conscious dogs; measurement and significance of the maximum acceleration of blood from the left ventricle. *Circulat. Res.*, 19:139–147, 1966.

63. NOBLE, M. I. M., TRENCHARD, D., and GUZ, A. Effect of changing heart rate on cardiovascular function in the conscious dog. *Circulat. Res.*, 19:206–213, 1966.

64. RUSHMER, R. F., BAKER, D. W., and STEGALL, H. F. Transcutaneous Doppler flow detection as a nondestructive technique. *J. Appl. Physiol.*, 21:554–566, 1966.

CHAPTER 4

PERIPHERAL VASCULAR CONTROL

The human body is composed of billions of cells, variously specialized, grouped and organized to perform many different functions. They can survive and function only so long as their immediate environment contains an adequate supply of essential nutrient materials and a limited concentration of waste products.

The capillaries permeate every tissue of the body, and the blood is rarely more than 0.1 mm. from any cell. The capillaries are only about 0.017 mm. in diameter, but their total length is almost 60,000 miles.[1] Thus the blood and tissue fluids are exposed to a tremendous expanse of capillary surface through which materials may be exchanged. Cells which consume essential materials rapidly must either be situated near capillaries or operate effectively at low concentrations of the various vital materials.

The Circulations of the Body. Blood flows through the systemic and pulmonary circulations of the body, impelled by the pumping action of the heart in an amount of about 5000 cc./min. in an average man at rest. (Cardiac output in Figure 4-1). This is not the only circulation involved in the delivery of oxygen and nutrients to the

body cells. Filtration through the capillary walls occurs at rates ranging around 14 cc./min. of which about 11 cc./min. is resorbed back into the venous capillary blood in accordance with the Starling Hypothesis (see Chapter 1). The unresorbed fluid (about 3 cc./min.) is transported by the lymphatic system and restored to blood in the systemic veins near the heart. The process of diffusion is far more important to the circulatory process than the bulk filtration process as illustrated in Figure 4-1. For example, the exchange of water by diffusion back and forth across the capillary membrane actually exceeds the cardiac output. It amounts to more than 5000 cc./min., but how much more no one is certain. Similarly, the transfer of electrolytes, small organic molecules and gases occurs rapidly and in large quantity over the very small distances across endothelial barriers and between tissue cells (see Fig. 1-2A).

In tissues with very great or variable metabolic demands, the capillaries are arranged in close proximity to every tissue cell. For example, the number of capillaries in skeletal muscle is reported to be related to the

113

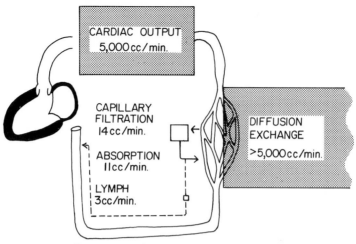

FIGURE 4-1   CIRCULATIONS IN THE BODY

The blood circulation delivers nutrients to the vicinity of the body cells in the microcirculation where local circulation involves filtration-reabsorption through capillary walls with lymphatic return of the residue and a very large exchange of water by diffusion.

oxidative activity of the individual fibers,[2] but only a fraction of the available capillaries in the myocardium is perfused at rest.[3] The high metabolic rate of tissues in small animals requires a higher rate of oxygen delivery than in larger animals; this rate of oxygen delivery accomplished by both a higher capillary density and higher unloading tension for oxygen in small animals.[4]

Oxygen Diffusion in Tissues. Each capillary subserves a volume of tissue immediately surrounding it since oxygen and other nutrient materials have highest concentration in blood and move outward along concentration gradients. Adjacent parallel capillaries (e.g., in striated muscle) supply cylindrical volumes of tissue around each capillary (Fig. 4-2A). As oxygen moves outward from the capillaries, the gas tension in the blood diminishes in the capillary blood flowing toward the venules, diminishing the unloading tension along the capillary. Theoretically the lowest oxygen

tension in the vicinity of a particular cylinder occurs at the periphery of the cylinder near the venule, sometimes called the "lethal corner" (Fig. 4-2A). Two adjoining tissue cylinders (e.g., in the brain) are illustrated with corresponding oxygen tension values in the capillaries and tissues shown in relief below (Fig. 4-2B). The oxygen partial pressure decreases from the arterial to the venous end of the cylinder and from the center to the periphery so that at the "lethal corner" the tension in the tissue is only about 17 mm. Hg or even somewhat less.[5] In exercising muscle and myocardium, the oxygen tension at its lower point apparently approaches the vanishing point since the venous oxygen tension is very low (see Figure 4-3). The consequences of diminished blood oxygen are illustrated in Figure 4-2C. Three levels may be distinguished below the normal. Reaction threshold occurs when vasodilation results from lowered venous oxygen pressures of 25 to 28 mm. Hg, and a "lethal level" is illustrated at 12 mm. Hg since the oxygen tension drops to 0 (Fig. 4-2C).

Thus, tissues with high metabolic rates (brain, muscle, kidney, and so forth) characteristically have dense capillary networks through which blood flows rapidly. By this mechanism, high concentrations of essential substances are maintained near the capillary walls, providing steep gradients for diffusion. Cells with lower requirements lie farther from the capillaries and are less affected by cessation of blood flow (Fig. 4-3A). Elimination of waste products proceeds in the reverse direction propelled by diffusion gradients with maximum concentrations at the site of production in the cells.

The delivery of substances to the tissues thus involves two steps: transportation by the blood to the capillary beds and local delivery by diffusion. The efficiency of the circulatory apparatus depends upon the success with which it provides adequate diffusion gradients within the tissues.

If, for example, the metabolic activity of skeletal muscle suddenly increased without a change in blood flow, the concentration of oxygen in and around the cells would drop, the diffusion gradient would steepen, the rate of diffusion would accelerate and the arteriovenous oxygen difference would widen (Fig. 4-3B). On the other hand, if an increased blood flow completely compensated for the increased oxygen utilization, oxygen delivery would be increased without a change in the arteriovenous oxygen difference and with little drop in tissue oxygen tension. Circulatory adjustment to the varying metabolic demands of skeletal muscle is never adequate to prevent a reduction in the oxygen content of venous blood, i.e., an increase in the arteriovenous difference.

Influenced by common personal experience, we are inclined to view peripheral vascular control primarily in terms of delivery of oxygen to the tissues, as is implied by Figure 4-3. When the circulation is restored after occluding the arterial supply to the arm or leg for a few minutes, the flushing of the skin, the throbbing of the limb and the return of the power of contraction all attest to the essential role of the blood supply in the function of muscles and skin.

Functional Anatomy of Peripheral Vascular Control. Zweifach[6] has described two distinct types of capillaries: arteriovenous capillaries and "true" capillaries. The A-V capillaries are "thoroughfare" channels with fairly direct courses from the arterioles to the venules. In general, blood flows continuously through the A-V capillaries, the rate of flow being varied through the changes in the caliber of the muscular arterioles and of the A-V capillaries themselves. A-V capillaries are invested with smooth muscle, which is abundant at the arteriolar end and more diffusely distributed toward the venular regions (Fig. 4-4). Branching from the A-V capillaries are the "true" capillaries, which are intricately joined to form complex networks lying between adjacent thoroughfare channels. The "true" capillaries have no smooth muscle except for muscular cuffs (precapillary sphincters) at their points of origin from the A-V capillaries. Capillaries from the vascular network rejoin the A-V capillaries near the venular end, but there are no smooth muscle sphincters at these junctions. If all the precapillary sphincters serving a capillary bed closed simultaneously, blood would not flow through these channels. However, at any one instant, some precapillary sphincters are open and others are closed. At intervals of one-half to three minutes some sphincters

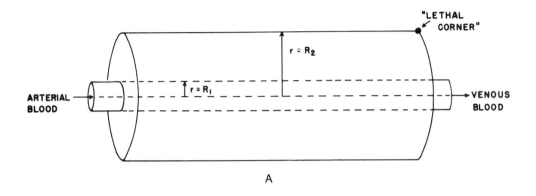

A

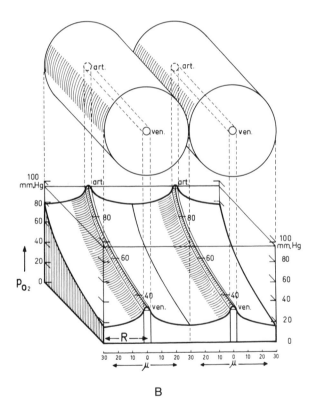

B

FIGURE 4-2   CONCENTRATION GRADIENTS NEAR CAPILLARIES

A, Each capillary delivers oxygen to a roughly cylindrical volume of surrounding space by means of diffusion along concentration gradients.

B, The concentrations of oxygen along two parallel capillaries are displayed in three dimensions to show the progressive reduction in oxygen pressure during flow from arteriole to venule and at the periphery of the cylindrical zones. (From Thews.[5])

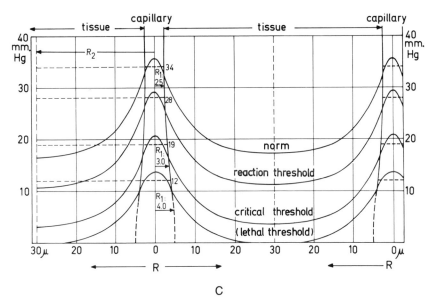

FIGURE 4-2 *Continued.*

C, The concentration of oxygen around capillaries under conditions of progressively greater hypoxia (see text). (From Thews.[5])

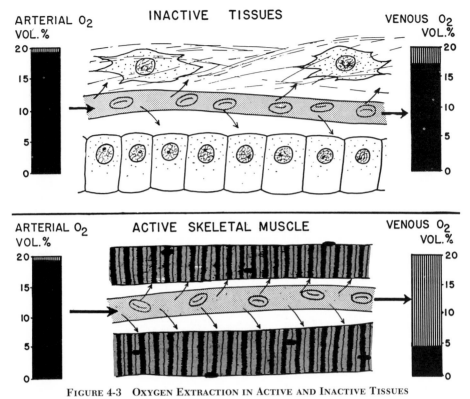

FIGURE 4-3   OXYGEN EXTRACTION IN ACTIVE AND INACTIVE TISSUES

The quantity of oxygen extracted from the blood during its flow through capillaries is determined by the relationship between the rate of oxygen utilization and the blood flow.

A, Slight oxygen extraction and small arteriovenous oxygen differences occur in tissues with relatively small oxygen requirements and active blood flow, e.g., skin.

B, Tissues which release energy at rapid rates, e.g., contracting muscle, extract a major portion of the oxygen from the blood.

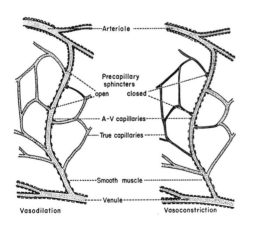

FIGURE 4-4   VASOMOTION IN A CAPILLARY NETWORK

Capillary networks, in some tissues at least, consist of arteriovenous capillaries (thoroughfare channels) and "true" capillaries. The blood flow through the different portions of the capillary bed is affected by contraction and relaxation of smooth muscle in the arterioles, A-V capillaries and precapillary sphincters. Phasic changes in the caliber in these regions produce cyclic alterations in the amount and distribution of blood flow through the various true capillaries (vasomotion).

close and others open. The caliber of the A-V channels also fluctuates asynchronously.

Dilatation and constriction of the A-V capillaries and the different combinations of dilated precapillary sphincters produce a continuously changing pattern of flow through the capillary networks. In a particular segment of the capillary bed, the blood may flow rapidly through one channel for a period of time, then cease to flow or even flow in the opposite direction, depending on which sphincters are open. The phasic changes in the caliber of the arterioles, A-V capillaries and precapillary sphincters have been termed "vasomotion" (Fig. 4-4). The rate of blood flow through the individual channels is an expression of a gradient in capillary pressure. Blood flow is rapid when capillary pressure in the arteriolar end of an A-V capillary is high in relation to venular pressure. When flow ceases, the pressure throughout the capillary approximates that in the venules.

The functional significance of vasomotion is being intensively investigated. It is apparent that this aspect of vascular control has important implications for normal function. For example, phasic vasomotor activity is expressed in periodic changes in the volume of the finger and in fluctuations in the arterial blood pressure. The existence of vasomotion implies a more precise regulation of capillary blood flow in response to local tissue demands than could result if control were exerted only by the arterioles. At the same time, descriptions of capillary blood pressure become more complicated because the pressure levels and gradients are continuously changing. However, certain generalizations can be made. If the pressure in the venules remains constant, vasomotion would affect only the pressure

gradients from arterioles to venules. When the arterioles, A-V capillaries and precapillary sphincters are dilated, the pressure gradients along the channels are steep and blood flow is rapid. When the caliber of these channels is reduced by constriction, more potential energy is lost as friction before the blood reaches the capillaries. The pressure at the arteriolar end of the capillaries is thus lowered, the pressure gradients become shallow or are eliminated and blood flow diminishes or ceases. Total blood flow through a tissue is increased by prolonging the intervals of vasodilatation and reducing the periods of vasoconstriction. The organization of capillaries illustrated in Figure 4-4 is believed to occur in those tissues which have widely varying levels of activity. Vasomotion, as a characteristic pattern of peripheral circulatory control, has been observed in a number of tissues, including rat mesentery, bat wing, subcutaneous connective tissues and canine and human hearts.

Capillary Morphology in Various Tissues. The functional requirements and environmental conditions of capillaries are not the same in different tissues. Contracting skeletal muscles, as compared to connective tissues or glands, have grossly different requirements for blood flow through their capillary networks (see Fig. 4-3). Similar diversity is readily demonstrated in the structural relationships of the capillary tubes as well. The capillaries in skeletal muscle, myocardium and skin consist of endothelial cells joined firmly at their edges with no evidence of pores or fenestrations (Fig. 4-5A, B). Pericapillary cells enclose the capillary but the investment seems incomplete, and perivascular spaces are not generally observed in fixed specimens on either light or electron microscopy.

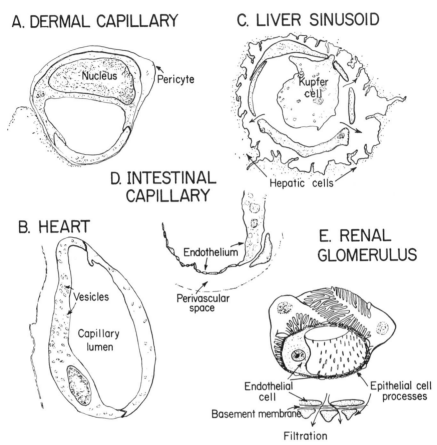

A. DERMAL CAPILLARY

C. LIVER SINUSOID

D. INTESTINAL CAPILLARY

B. HEART

E. RENAL GLOMERULUS

FIGURE 4-5 VARIATIONS IN CAPILLARY STRUCTURE

Schematic diagrams of electron micrographs indicate the extent to which capillaries display different characteristics in various tissues.

A, Dermal capillaries appear to be formed by endothelial cells joined at their edges without visible spaces between. Such capillaries may be enveloped by pericytes.

B, Capillaries in the heart also consist of continuous membranes of endothelial cells. Capillary endothelial cells characteristically contain large numbers of vesicles which have been implicated by some investigators in active transport of substances across the capillary membrane (Bennett et al.[8]).

C, Liver sinusoids are discontinuous membranes with large spaces between cells through which cellular elements can pass freely.

D, Intestinal capillaries may exhibit very thin regions in endothelial cells which may not be a continuous barrier between the capillary lumen and perivascular space (after Bennett et al.[8]).

E, The renal glomerulus is a complex structure composed of endothelial cells, basement membrane and epithelial cells through which filtration occurs (after Yamada[7]).

Openings or fenestrations between the processes of endothelial cells are found in several tissues such as liver sinusoids (Figs. 4-5C) or intestinal capillaries (Fig. 4-5D). The capillaries in the renal glomerulus are extremely complex as illustrated in a composite drawing by Yamada.[7] Bennett, Luft and Hampton[8] proposed a rather complicated classification of various types of capillaries based on the basement membranes, porosity or perforations and pericapillary investment:

Type:

A With complete continuous basement membrane

B Without complete continuous basement membrane

1 Without fenestrations or pores

2 With *intra*cellular fenestrations or perforations

3 With *inter*cellular fenestrations or perforations

α Without a complete pericapillary cellular investment interposed between parenchymal cells and the capillary

β With a complete capillary cellular investment interposed between parenchymal cells and capillary

Majno[9] presented a comprehensive description of the ultrastructure of capillaries, including a pictorial classification based on the continuity of the main filtration barrier: the endothelial sheet (Fig. 4-6). On this basis three main types are designated: continuous, fenestrated and discontinuous. For each of these categories, the endothelial cells may be high or low (thin). The low variety of continuous endo-

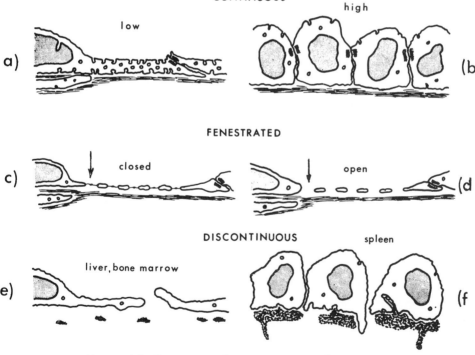

FIGURE 4-6 FUNCTIONAL CLASSIFICATION OF CAPILLARIES

The capillaries in various tissues have widely different architecture which can be distinguished in terms of the degree and type of fenestration in the endothelial cells and the height or thickness of the endothelial cells. (From Majno, G.[9]).

thelium (Fig. 4-6A) is found in striated muscle, myocardium, central nervous system, smooth muscle of digestive and reproductive systems and subcutaneous and adipose tissues.

Postcapillary venules of lymph nodes and thymus had high endothelial cells (Fig. 4-6B). Endothelial cells with intracellular fenestrae may be closed in endocrine glands, choroid plexus, ciliary body and intestinal villi (Fig. 4-6C). In the renal glomeruli, the fenestrae appear to be open (Fig. 4-6D). Sinusoids of liver, bone marrow and spleen have gross intercellular gaps as shown in Figures 4-6E and F. Clearly, the barrier to bulk flow, filtration and diffusion offered by endothelial cells must be very different in capillaries as varied in structure as those illustrated in Figures 4-5 and 4-6. The differences in function of various tissues and organs are also clearly represented by differences in blood flow and oxygen extraction.

NORMAL OXYGEN DISTRIBUTION

In most tissues other than skeletal muscles and myocardium, adjustments of blood flow in relation to oxygen consumption or metabolic activity would be inappropriate. For example, the oxygen consumption in skin is quite trivial and yet extremely large amounts of blood may flow through this organ to support its function of dissipating heat. Similarly, the amount of blood flowing through the kidney is very large in relation to its metabolic activity. Thus, only a small fraction of the oxygen presented to the kidney substance is taken up and the blood leaving the kidney does not differ greatly from arterial blood.

To illustrate these points, the quantity of blood flowing each minute through several organs is plotted on the abscissa in Figure 4-7. The quantity of oxygen presented to the tissues in the arterial blood was 19 cc. per 100 cc. of blood (ordinate in Fig. 4-7). Thus, the area of each rectangular figure represents the quantity of oxygen presented to each organ each minute. The stippled area represents the quantity of oxygen in the venous blood leaving the organ, and the remaining area (vertical lines) indicates the amount of oxygen extracted by the tissue. Note the very small quantity of oxygen extracted from blood in the kidney. Myocardium extracts about 70 per cent or more of the oxygen presented to it. Resting skeletal muscle utilizes only about one third of the oxygen in the blood it receives, but contracting skeletal muscle extracts about three fourths of the oxygen from the blood. Thus, the difference between the oxygen contents of arterial and venous blood (A-V oxygen difference) varies widely from tissue to tissue. The average A-V oxygen difference at rest, based on mixed venous blood, ranges around 4 to 6 cc. per 100 cc. of blood.

RESISTANCE TO BLOOD FLOW

The blood pumped by the heart is distributed to the various tissues according to their functions. The rate at which the blood flows through the vascular channels is dependent upon the energy lost in the form of friction. Little pressure energy is dissipated in the long arterial conduits (Fig. 1-7), but the pressure gradient becomes steeper as the blood flows through the smaller and smaller branches toward the periphery. Thus, a substantial fraction of the pressure head available in the aorta is dissipated as the blood flows through the terminal arteries, arterioles and capillaries. The amount of pressure dissipated is regulated by

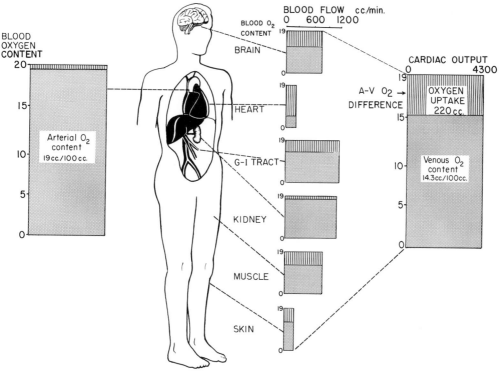

FIGURE 4-7   THE ARTERIOVENOUS OXYGEN DIFFERENCES IN VARIOUS TISSUES

The blood flow through some tissues is voluminous in relation to the oxygen requirements (kidney and skin). In contrast, the myocardium extracts most of the oxygen from the blood. The arteriovenous oxygen differences represent the relationship between blood flow and oxygen utilization in various tissues.

variations in the caliber of the vascular channels. The extent to which the vessels change their diameters for this type of regulation becomes progressively greater and more significant toward the peripheral ramifications of the arterial tree. The wall of the aorta contains a substantial quantity of elastic tissue (about 40 per cent by weight). The proportion of elastic tissue diminishes and the proportion of smooth muscle is greater in the more peripheral arterial branches (Fig. 4-8).

The pressure within the lumen of the blood vessels must be supported by tension in their walls in accordance with the law of Laplace $(P = T/r)$; so that the greater the radius of the tube,

the greater the wall tension required to support a given internal pressure (see Fig. 1-11). The tension supported by various components of the vascular wall has been analyzed by Burton.[10] The tensile strength of the elastic tissue in the aorta is capable of supporting three times the normal aortic pressure, providing a good margin of safety. The force required to break the collagenous tissue in the aorta is so great that in most experiments the clamps holding the tissue slip before breakage occurs. The caliber of the vascular channels is adjusted by changing tension exerted by smooth muscle (see Fig. 4-8), which can maintain tension for a long time with a very small expenditure of energy.[10]

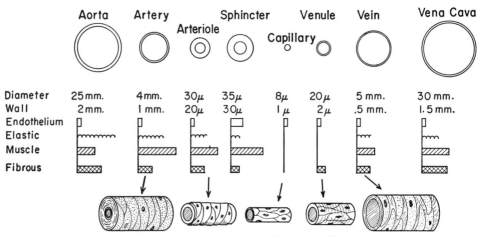

FIGURE 4-8   COMPONENTS OF VASCULAR WALLS

The relative amount of elastic tissue and fibrous tissues is largest in the aorta and least in small branches of the arterial tree. Smaller vessels have more prominent smooth muscle in the media. Capillaries consist only of endothelial tubes. The walls of the veins are much like the arterial walls but are thinner in relation to their caliber.

Critical Closing Pressure. By virtue of Laplace's law, active tension exerted by smooth muscle in the wall of a cylindrical tube may produce a fundamental instability. Suppose that when the wall tension is precisely balanced against the pressure in a blood vessel $(P = T/r)$ the tension exerted by the smooth muscle is slightly increased. The radius of the vessel decreases slightly, and the tension required to maintain the pressure is further reduced so that the radius continues to shrink. If this occurred, the caliber would progressively diminish until the lumen of the vessel closed. Thus, if smooth muscle predominates in the wall, as in arterioles, precapillary sphincters and arteriovenous shunts, the vessels would tend to be either fully open or fully closed. Burton proposed the concept of a *critical closing pressure* at which the lumina of such small vessels would close because the wall tension was being supported predominantly by smooth muscle. According to this con-

cept, the sites of controlled resistance in the terminal vascular networks should be either wide open or closed. Microscopic examination fails to confirm this prediction completely since graded variations in the caliber of vessels and sphincters can be observed. However, the control of capillary flow distribution clearly involves changing patterns of closure of the vascular sphincters.

The concept of critical closing pressure neglects the influence of the thickness of the vascular walls. In vessels with walls which are thick in relation to the radius, $P = T\delta/r$, where P is the pressure, T is the tension in the wall, δ is the thickness of the wall and r is the radius of the tube. With constriction of the vessel, the wall becomes thicker. Internal stresses develop in the wall as the lumen is progressively constricted until extremely great tension must be developed to obliterate the lumen completely.

Mechanisms of Vascular Constriction. The lumina of larger arteries can be reduced but are not completely obliterated by contraction of the smooth muscle in the walls. Reduction in the caliber of such arteries involves severe deformation of the smooth muscle cells, the internal elastic membrane and the endothelial cells. The forces required to completely occlude the lumen can be simulated by encircling a piece of gum rubber tubing with a strong ligature or string and pulling on its two ends in an attempt to close the lumen. The smallest terminal arteries, arterioles and precapillary sphincters can be completely constricted by contraction of the layers of smooth muscle. In the transition from the normal dilated state to maximal constriction, the wall components of small arteries and arterioles are greatly distorted. Van Citters et al.[11] studied serial histological sections of mesenteric arteries (about 1 mm. O.D.) in which a localized constriction was produced by local application of a drop of epinephrin. Quick freezing preserved the normal relationships disclosing a wall thickness only about 1/30 of the radius in the normal dilated state (Fig. 4-9). Sections obtained in the maximally constricted regions showed the lumen reduced to about 25 per cent of the total diameter, with a wall-to-lumen ratio of about 1:2. The endothelial cells were rounded and perched on the folds of a highly convoluted internal elastic membrane. The smooth muscle cells were severely distorted and the nuclei rounded. Similar histological changes were subsequently reported by Hayes.[12] Measurements of various components of the walls in contracted small arteries and arterioles were examined as potential objective criteria for the degree of vasoconstriction by Stromberg et al.[13]

Complete occlusion of the lumen of small arteries was not observed in the studies just described. In contrast, the terminal branches or arterioles may become completely obstructed by smooth muscle contraction and deformation of the rounded endothelial cells[14] which serve as a plastic plug as illustrated by three examples on the right of Figure 4-9.

BASIC REQUIREMENTS FOR CARDIOVASCULAR CONTROL

The tissues and organs served by the vascular system have widely varying functions and ranges of activity. If the changing requirements of tissues for blood flow had no priority or coordinating mechanism, the circulatory responses might easily become chaotic and break down, e.g., during running on a hot day after a full meal. At the risk of oversimplification, the fundamental requirements for cardiovascular regulation can be described in terms of uncomplicated hydraulic systems.

A common form of such systems consists of a large tank supported at sufficient height to give a head of pressure. In such a system, the pump can be set to operate at constant speed, variations in demand being accommodated at the expense of the reserve volume in the tank. However, this type of system could not easily be adapted to man or animals because a large quantity of blood would have to be carried around above the head. Portability can be achieved only if the capacious storage tank is replaced by a small pressure tank. In this case, however, an increase in outflow from the system must be rapidly and precisely compensated by adjusting the output of the pump.

Consider a model circulation consisting of a pump, a compression chamber and several variable orifices (Fig. 4-10). By adjustments in stroke vol-

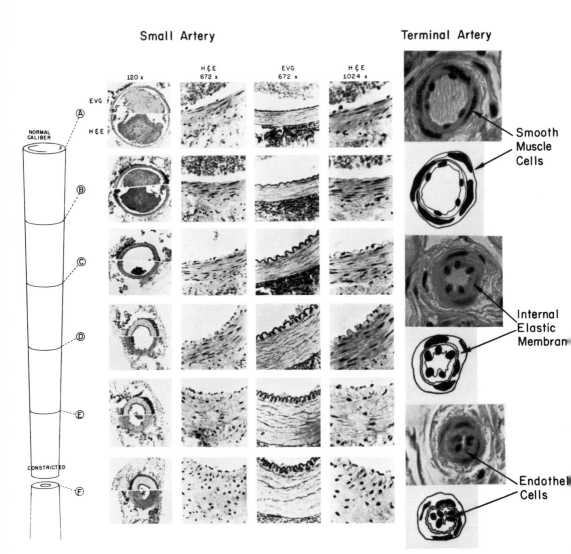

FIGURE 4-9   ARCHITECTURAL CHANGES DURING VASOCONSTRICTION

Left, The wall of a small artery (about 1 mm. outside diameter) is very thin in the dilated state (upper figure) and the components are stretched out circumferentially. As the artery constricts, the wall thickens and the components become rounded and deformed. Such vessels do not become occluded at maximal constriction. (From Van Citters, Wagner and Rushmer.[11])

Right, Terminal branches may become occluded by the endothelial cells, which have become rounded, tending to serve as a plastic plug. (From Ruch and Patton, *Physiology and Biophysics,* 19th Ed., W. B. Saunders Co., 1965.)

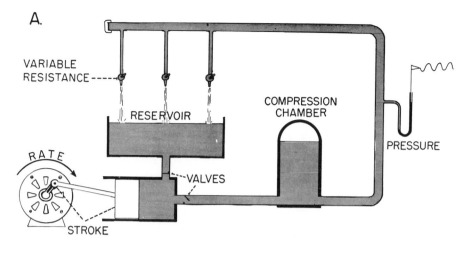

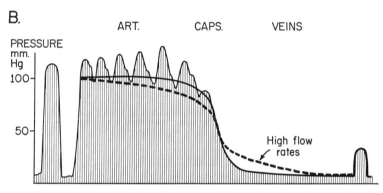

FIGURE 4-10   PRESSURE GRADIENTS

A, The principles of cardiovascular control can be illustrated by a simple hydraulic model. In this system, the pressure head is determined primarily by the relation between the resistance to outflow and the pump output (stroke volume × heart rate). To maintain the pressure at a constant level, any change in outflow resistance must be promptly compensated by an adjustment in the pump output. The pressure head, outflow resistance and pump output are so intimately related that none can be altered without effect on the others.

B, The pressure gradient along the arteries and veins is very shallow under resting conditions. However, if the blood flow is greatly acelerated, the pressure gradient in the terminal arteries and veins becomes steeper, diminishing the pressure gradient along the small vessels (arterioles, capillaries and venules). The magnitude of the change is exaggerated in the figure.

ume, stroke frequency and total outflow resistance, the mean pressure in the system can be maintained at constant levels for indefinite periods of time. If the stroke frequency and outflow resistance are properly set, the pressure in the system never drops to zero between strokes. Once such an equilibrium is established, alterations in any one of the three variables will be immediately reflected in changes in pressure within the system. To maintain a constant pressure, any alteration in one variable must be simultaneously balanced by adjustments in the others so that inflow always equals outflow. For example, if the stroke frequency is increased and the outflow resistance is not changed, the stroke volume must be reduced until pump output is restored to previous levels. Similarly, opening one outflow orifice more widely would produce a fall in pressure unless the resistance to outflow from other valves was increased or the pump output was rapidly augmented by an increase in either stroke volume or stroke frequency. In this system, maintenance of a constant mean pressure automatically provides a precise balance between inflow and outflow. This schematic model illustrates the fundamental principle by which the cardiac output is continuously adjusted to compensate for changes in peripheral resistance. The mean arterial blood pressure tends to stay within a relatively narrow range both at rest and during activity. To the extent that the requirements of the tissues for blood flow are reflected by their changes in peripheral resistance, cardiac output is continuously adjusted to equal the total blood flow in all the tissues.

The quantity of blood flowing through a set of vessels per unit of time is determined by two factors: (1) the pressure gradient from the arteries to the veins and (2) the resistance of the vascular bed as influenced by constriction in the smaller and terminal branches. The mechanisms by which the systemic arterial blood pressure is maintained within a reasonable range despite wide fluctuations in the distribution and total quantity of blood flowing through the peripheral tissues are described in Chapter 5. In the following discussion of the mechanisms of vascular control, the arterial pressure head will be considered to be relatively fixed.

Pressure Gradients at High Flow Rates. Despite the gradual reduction in the caliber of the long arterial trunks, the pressure drop along them is very slight (2 to 4 mm. Hg from the axillary to the radial arteries) at rest in a cool environment. As a result, flow along the arteries is normally slow (Fig. 4-10B). However, peripheral vasodilation in the extremities of man during reactive hyperemia may accelerate the flow rates as much as ten times. Under such conditions, the pressure drop between the brachial and radial arteries increases from 5 mm. Hg to 25 mm. Hg.[15] The rate of pressure drop along the terminal branches of the arterial system also steepens so that the pressure at the arterioles is markedly depressed. The increased pressure required to propel the increased flow along the veins also results in a high pressure head at the venules because central venous pressure cannot be greatly depressed. Thus, in the presence of high flow rates through a segment of the vascular tree, the arterial and venous pressure gradients are steepened and the pressure drop across the arterioles and capillary networks is reduced far below the normal resting conditions. Under these conditions, the resistance to flow through the larger arterial and venous conduits assumes major importance in the dissipation of pressure energy during flow.

MECHANISMS OF VASCULAR REGULATION

The quantity of blood flowing through various vascular beds and its distribution among the myriad vascular channels depend primarily upon smooth muscle contraction at the sites of controlled resistance. Histologic examination of vascular smooth muscle fails to reveal structural differences from one vessel to another. Yet the functional disparity between the vessels of different organs is so great that a single substance may produce constriction in one organ and dilation in another.

The Role of the Nervous System.
In a hydraulic system like that in
Figure 4-10 there must be sensitive
and responsive controls to quickly
adapt to abrupt changes in levels of
activity of the various tissues without
precipitous or soaring changes in arterial blood pressure. The involvement of the nervous system in such
control is a matter of everyday experience. Individuals with impairment of
the sympathetic nervous system are
subject to fainting merely on assuming
the erect position. Obvious flushing or
pallor of the skin can develop rapidly
in response to emotions (embarrassment or fear) as well as by changes in
environmental temperature. The functional role of neural control of the vascular system is to adjust the cardiac
output and the distribution of this total
flow to meet the varying needs of
tissues, maintain systemic arterial
pressure and still preserve the essential functions of the heart, brain and
other vital tissues. The specifications
for such a system have been presented
in an engaging and imaginative summary by Burton.[16] To preserve the vital
functions, the neural controls are generally powerful enough to override
hormonal mechanisms.[17] These vascular adjustments are effected involun-
tarily by the sympathetic nervous system. Contrary to previous concepts,
the sympathetic nervous system rarely
discharges en masse but rather displays well developed functional differentiation.[18] The discharge of sympathetic nerves to blood vessels of skin,
kidney or viscera is a constantly changing pattern accompanying changes in
type and level of functional activity.
Renkin and Rosell[19] present evidence
supporting the view that arterioles and
precapillary sphincters are controlled
separately, contributing to the shifting
patterns of flow in capillary networks
like those illustrated in Figure 4-4.

According to Lutz and Fulton,[20]
however, some vascular smooth muscle has dual innervation (constrictor
and dilator), only vasoconstrictor or
vasodilator nerves serve some vascular smooth muscle and a third class
of muscle cells apparently does not receive any innervation. Vascular
smooth muscle without a nerve supply
reacts to both epinephrine and acetylcholine (the transmitter substances for
the sympathetic and parasympathetic
nervous systems, respectively), and
vessels highly sensitive to acetylcholine may have no demonstrable
cholinergic innervation. Some vascular beds respond to changes in the
carbon dioxide tension in arterial
blood; others dilate in response to
unidentified metabolites. Thus, concise descriptions of peripheral vascular
control are impossible because the system is very complex and because not
nearly enough is known about it. For
the present discussion, some of the
more important controls will be considered in terms of neural, hormonal,
chemical and physical mechanisms.
Then, the factors which appear to be
prominent in the control of certain
key organs will be discussed.

Sympathetic Vasomotor System.
Neural control over the peripheral vascular system is dominated by the sympathetic division of the autonomic
nervous system. Nerve cell bodies
lying in the intermediolateral cell
column of the thoracic division of the
spinal cord give off axons that pass out
the ventral root and synapse either in
the ganglia of the sympathetic chain or
in accessory ganglia. The postgan-
glionic axons follow the segmental
nerves to the peripheral vessels or
pass directly to perivascular plexuses
through which the fibers pass to the
periphery. The terminal branches of
the sympathetic constrictor fibers pass
to vascular smooth muscle and appar-

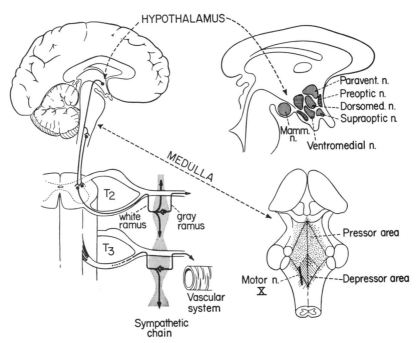

FIGURE 4-11   CENTRAL CONTROL OF SYMPATHETIC VASOCONSTRICTION

Sympathetic constrictor nerves, distributed to peripheral vascular system, originate from the intermediolateral cell column of the thoracic cord. Impulses descend from the medullary region and the hypothalamus to modulate the sympathetic nerve discharge. The hypothalamus plays an important role in autonomic control of many different visceral functions. Changes in systemic arterial pressure can be readily produced by stimulation of the "pressor" and "depressor" areas in the medulla. However, these medullary areas may actually represent pathways from higher levels down to the spinal cord, rather than "vasomotor centers."

ently release transmitter substances which induce contraction or relaxation of the smooth muscle components in the walls.

The collections of nerve cell bodies in the intermediolateral column serve as spinal vasomotor centers, receiving impulses over afferent fibers entering the spinal cord from various structures and also receiving regulatory impulses descending from higher neural structures (Fig. 4-11). Immediately after cervical spinal section in man the blood pressure tends to be poorly sustained.[21] Since the spinal lesion has interrupted descending pathways but has neither injured the cells at the thoracic level nor interfered with their afferent input, this

condition indicates that volleys of impulses descending the spinal cord normally modulate the discharges of the spinal vasomotor centers. Sometime later such patients regain vascular reactivity. This reactivity is a function of the spinal centers and is reflex in nature. For example, when the spinal cord is bombarded by impulses aroused by experimental distention of the bladder, the systemic arterial pressure may rise to 300 mm. Hg or more.[25]

MEDULLARY CENTERS. Electrical stimulation of some areas in the medulla oblongata produces prompt elevation in blood pressure (pressor areas), and stimulation of other medullary areas causes a sharp reduction in blood pressure (depressor areas; Fig. 4-11). These regions are generally termed the vasoconstrictor and vasodilator "center," respectively. These so-called centers are not strictly localized but are diffuse networks of interconnected neuron groups. The nature of the interaction between the pressor and depressor zones is not known, and they are continuously influenced by impulses from many sources such as pressoreceptors, chemoreceptors, somatic afferent sources and the higher levels of the nervous system (see later discussion). These medullary centers of cardiovascular regulation appear to be essential to normal control of systemic arterial pressure (see Chapter 5).

DIENCEPHALIC CENTERS. The region of the hypothalamus contains control centers integrating reactions which involve the vascular system. These reactions include temperature regulation, water balance, thirst and hunger and cardiovascular responses to exertion. Electrical stimulation of discrete hypothalamic and subthalamic sites produces profound changes in the heart rate, ventricular contractility and arterial pressure and also dilation of blood vessels in skeletal muscle by means of the familiar sympathetic cholinergic vasodilator fibers (see later discussion). Supplementing such functional evidence of central nervous system control is a growing body of anatomical evidence of neural pathways descending from the diencephalon to the midbrain and spinal cord.[22]

Impinging on the hypothalamic centers are nerve impulses from many parts of the brain, including the motor and premotor cortex, the frontal cortex, the orbital cortex, the temporal lobe, the amygdala, the insula and the cingulate gyrus.[23, 24] In general, if electrical stimulation of an area in the brain consistently yields behavior responses, cardiovascular responses are also induced. Conversely, if electrical stimulation of a cerebral area does not induce cardiovascular responses, it rarely evokes behavioral changes.

SYMPATHETIC CONSTRICTOR NERVES. The sympathetic constrictor fibers exert their most profound effects on the blood vessels of skeletal muscle, the skin and the splanchnic bed (see Figs. 4-13 and 4-14). The sympathetic constrictor nerve fibers apparently exert their action on smooth muscle at the so-called alpha (α) receptor sites at which l-epinephrine and norepinephrine also act (Fig. 4-12A). The blood vessels of skeletal muscles are served by both adrenergic constrictor fibers and cholinergic dilator fibers. The constrictor fibers to the skin are involved in conservation of heat, and the direct vascular connections between the small arteries and small veins (arteriovenous anastomoses) in the skin are directly controlled by the hypothalamic heat loss center. Through these channels large volumes of blood pass directly from the terminal arteries into the voluminous venous plexuses for heat dissipation. The arteriovenous anastomoses are completely dominated by the constrictor fibers, dilating maximally when the constrictor nerves are cut. In other areas, severance of the constrictor fibers leaves the blood vessels with considerable constrictor "tone" (i.e., they are partially constricted).

SYMPATHETIC VASODILATOR SYSTEM. Stimulation of the sympathetic chain in the lumbar region of cats or dogs may cause initial dilation followed by constriction in the vascular beds within skeletal muscle. When the constriction was eliminated by adrenergic blocking drugs, pure vasodilation was obtained.[23] The vasodilator response was restricted to skeletal muscle and was potentiated by eserine

A. GENERAL VASOMOTOR CONTROL MECHANISMS

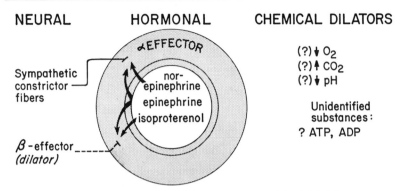

B. SPECIAL VASOMOTOR MECHANISMS

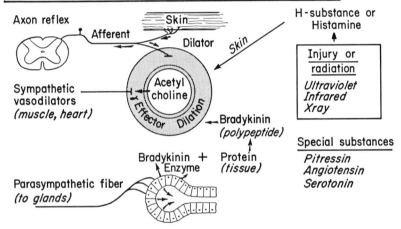

FIGURE 4-12   VASOMOTOR CONTROL

A, Vasoconstriction or vasodilation can be produced in various tissues by means of many neural, hormonal and chemical mechanisms. Sympathetic fibers and circulating norepinephrine and *l*-epinephrine are widely believed to act at specific sites (α effectors). The β effectors are not innervated. The chemical dilators are proposed mechanisms for explaining vasodilation following temporary occlusion of blood supply to a vascular bed (reactive hyperemia).

B, The special vasomotor mechanisms are found prominently in the skin although the sympathetic vasodilators are found in skeletal muscle and heart and the postulated bradykinin mechanism affects glands. No definite role in normal vascular regulation has been assigned to the special constrictor substances, vasopressin (Pitressin), angiotensin and serotonin.

and eliminated by atropine.[23] A substance like acetylcholine was found in the effluent perfusate from such muscles.[24] These observations form the basis for the concept of a sympathetic cholinergic vasodilator system (Fig. 4-12*B*). It is believed that this system originates in the motor cortex and that impulses descend from there to the hypothalamus, pass through the medullary centers and leave the spinal cord with the sympathetic nerves to induce vasodilation of the blood vessels in skeletal muscles. When the sympathetic constrictor fibers to the skeletal muscle are blocked or inactivated, the blood vessels dilate somewhat but continue to display considerable basal tone (partial constriction). Upon stimulation of the sympathetic cholinergic vasodilator system the blood flow may become five or six times greater. The evidence for active neurogenic vasodilation in muscle and skin of man has been reviewed by Greenfield.[25] Species variability has been clearly shown by Uvnäs[26] in that cholinergic vasodilator nerves have been demonstrated in dog, cat, mongoose, fox and jackal but appear to be absent in lemur, old world monkey, rabbit, badger and polecat. There may be basic differences in vasomotor mechanisms in these different animals.

Axon Reflex. Stimulation of the peripheral ends of severed dorsal roots (afferent fibers) produces vasodilation in skin vessels. This response was formerly ascribed to activity of motor fibers issuing from the spinal cord against the stream of the sensory fibers that normally enter the cord by this route. A preferred explanation for this phenomenon is the hypothetical axon reflex. According to this concept, sensory nerve fibers in the skin may have collateral fibers distributed to adjacent blood vessels (Fig. 4-12B). Impulses generated from the sensory endings may pass directly to the dilator termination in the blood vessel as well as to the spinal cord. Such a mechanism has been invoked to explain the dilatory effects of certain irritants and mechanical stimulation of the skin.

Parasympathetic Dilator Mechanism. Stimulation of the parasympathetic nerves supplying certain glands (e.g., salivary glands) induces a profuse secretion and an intense vasodilation. Existence of parasympathetic vasodilators was postulated to explain the hyperemia. Hilton and Lewis[27] presented evidence that the glandular cells, activated by the parasympathetic fibers, release an enzyme (bradykinin) into the interstitial spaces. There this enzyme acts on tissue proteins to split off a polypeptide which diffuses to vessels in the vicinity, and produces vasodilation (see Fig. 4-12B). Bradykinin was apparently recoverable from the glandular excretion, and, after saline was perfused under the skin during profuse sweating, a substance like bradykinin was recovered in the perfusate.[28] Thus, the bradykinin mechanisms may be involved in the vasodilation of the skin which accompanies profuse sweating. It is tempting to postulate that the same type of mechanism is involved in the vasodilation which accompanies other visceral activity induced by parasympathetic activity (e.g., that in the gastrointestinal tract). Bradykinin injected into arteries produces marked vasodilation in man, being among the most active on a molar basis. The observation that carboxypeptidase B, which blocks bradykinin dilatation, failed to influence exercise hyperemia or cholinergic sympathetic vasodilation serves as a note of caution in ascribing a role for kinins in these responses.[30]

Hormonal Mechanisms. Impulses arriving at the terminals of the autonomic nervous system exert their influence on the effectors by release of transmitter substances. In the parasympathetic nervous system, this transmitter is acetylcholine, a rather potent vasodilator substance in some vascular beds. Through Euler's investigations,[31] the transmitter substance for sympathetic constrictor fibers has been identified as norepinephrine, which is found in high concentration in sympathetic nerves and in tissues with an intact sympathetic innervation. This substance differs from *l*-epinephrine, which is excreted primarily from chromaffin cells in the adrenal medulla and from other chromaffin cells scattered in different parts of the body, particularly in the heart. In man, norepinephrine produces vasoconstriction in those vascular beds where it produces any response at all. In contrast, *l*-epinephrine also has a vasodilator action in skeletal muscle, and perhaps in the heart, and a powerful effect on myocardial performance.

THE CONCEPT OF VASCULAR RECEPTORS. Catechol amines exert either of two effects on the vascular beds in skeletal muscle — vasoconstriction or vasodilation. Norepinephrine is a powerful vasconstrictor, but *l*-epinephrine can have either a dilator or a constrictor action, depending upon the circumstances. Ahlquist[32] was therefore led to propose that two distinct types of receptors, or binding sites — α and β receptors — are involved at the smooth muscle. (Since the term "receptor" might be misconstrued to mean the sensory or afferent receptors of reflex activity, the word "effector" has been substituted for "receptor" in Figure 4-12.)

It is thought that norepinephrine acts only on the α receptors and that these receptors excite the constrictor mechanism. *l*-epinephrine is also believed to have the same effect when acting on α receptors. A substance called kinekard of unknown composition has been extracted from blood plasma and has been shown to produce vasoconstriction and is believed to act on adrenergic receptors.[33] If these receptors are blocked by an appropriate drug (azapetine; Ilidar), then injected *l*-epinephrine produces vasodilation by its action on the receptors. The β receptor is blocked by very large doses of adrenergic blocking agents and is believed to be without innervation. The β receptors are believed to be confined to the blood vessels in skeletal muscle and perhaps in myocardium. Gamma (γ) receptors are believed responsible for the cholinergic vasodilation initiated by the sympathetic vasodilator in skeletal muscle.

The pharmacology of vascular smooth muscle, including the concept of receptors, has been reviewed by Green and Kepchar.[34] Although existence of these receptors, or effectors, has excited much interest among physiologists, it seems doubtful that the circulating catechol amines are very important in the normal peripheral vascular control. On the other hand, the action of norepinephrine as the transmitter substance for the sympathetic constrictor nerves is undoubtedly important in the control of certain vascular beds.

ACETYLCHOLINE. The transmitter substance issuing from the parasympathetic nerve endings is quite definitely acetylcholine. If the proposed bradykinin mechanism withstands the tests of time and critical evaluation, direct action of acetylcholine in vascular smooth muscle as a normal control mechanism need be postulated only for the sympathetic cholinergic vasodilator fibers which serve skeletal muscle and perhaps the coronary vessels. Intravenously administered acetylcholine produces vasodilation in various vascular beds, but this effect is probably not a significant facet of normal peripheral vascular control. The cholinesterase levels in the blood are so high that circulating acetylcholine is rapidly destroyed. Thus, very large doses must be administered intravenously to produce vascular effects.

Chemical Dilators. It is common experience that, if the blood supply to a limb is obstructed for a few minutes and then released, the skin supplied by these vessels flushes a vivid red.

Such vasodilation induced by temporary occlusion of the blood supply is termed *reactive hyperemia*. Roy and Brown[35] studied these vascular reactions and concluded that it "seems to us to throw much light on the manner in which the local circulation is carried on under normal conditions. It shows us that there is a local mechanism independent of the centres in the medulla and spinal cord by which the degree of dilation of the vessels is varied in accordance with the requirements of the tissues." This was in 1879; the same views are widely held today, and we are still unable to identify the substance, substances or other mechanisms which actually induce the vascular dilation in reactive hyperemia or during increases in the metabolic activity of the tissues. Lewis[36] described a series of astute observations and subscribed to the view that the vasodilator substance is a normal metabolite.

UNIDENTIFIED VASODILATOR SUBSTANCES. The effects of obstructed blood flow or increased metabolism which are perhaps the most obvious include: diminished oxygen tension in the tissues, increased carbon dioxide and lowered pH due to accumulation of acid metabolic products. As a matter of fact, perfusion with arterial blood of diminished oxygen content may produce vasodilation in some organs, particularly the heart, skeletal muscles, skin and, to a lesser extent, the gastrointestinal tract. If the low oxygen were the immediate cause of the vasodilation, however, the blood flow should return to control levels by the time the oxygen debt is repaid. Evidence has been presented that the oxygen debt is overpaid in both skin[37] and muscle,[38] and the excess blood flow may vary from 50 to 200 per cent of that necessary to repay the calculated oxygen debt.[39] Furthermore the

increased flow may persist after the venous oxygen content has returned to normal or even attained supernormal values. On the contrary, Hymen[40] found an exact quantitative repayment of effective blood flow debt indicating control by some unidentified vasodilator substance. The identity of such substances is clouded by evidence that potassium, ATP and lactic acid injected into arteries may have a marked effect but produce little change when injected locally by intramuscular injection.[41] Mellander *et al.*[42] showed that locally induced hyperosmolarity was associated with vasodilation in muscle.

At the present time reactive hyperemia is attributed to vasodilator metabolite(s) accumulating during hypoxia, but the cause is not histamine. In short, the vascular reaction must be attributed to *unidentified vasodilator substance(s)*.[34] To provide such a hypothetical substance with an attractive name might gain some measure of reassurance but will certainly not accelerate progress toward its identification. In fact, the label "unidentified vasodilator substance" is used in Figures 4-12 and 4-13 as a signpost directing attention to an important unsolved problem.

ADENYLIC ACID DERIVATIVES. Adenosine triphosphate (ATP) is an important source of energy for metabolism. During the release of energy, this substance is converted into adenosine diphosphate (ADP). If ADP were a strong vasodilator, it might qualify as a mechanism for adjusting the blood flow in accordance with metabolic demands. Considerable evidence has been compiled to demonstrate that ATP, ADP, adenosine monophosphate and even adenosine have vasodilator effect.[43] They all probably act on the same inhibitory sites to permit vasodilation, but ATP and

ADP are more powerful than the others. Although these substances deserve further study, there is no evidence that they are released from cells so that they might act on the vascular smooth muscle. One difficulty in such studies is that the vascular beds are so exquisitely sensitive to these substances that the concentrations necessary for vasodilation are less than can be detected with current methods.

VASOPRESSIN (PITRESSIN). The neurohypophysis excretes a polypeptide, vasopressin, which has a fairly strong vasoconstrictor action in coronary vessels. This substance does not appear to react at the effector (receptor) sites involved by epinephrine, serotonin or histamine. The close spatial and functional relations between the hypothalamic centers and the neurohypophysis certainly suggest that release of vasopressin might contribute to vascular control, but no specific action of this mechanism has ever been demonstrated. Vasopressin is composed of eight amino acids, a characteristic shared by two other substances which induce smooth muscle contraction: oxytocin, which induces contraction of the uterus, and angiotensin.

ANGIOTENSIN. Under some circumstances the kidney releases a protein, renin, that acts on a blood protein (renin substrate) to produce angiotensin I, which is composed of ten amino acids. This decapeptide does not affect the caliber of blood vessels, but under the influence of converting enzyme it loses two amino acids to form angiotensin II, which has potent vasoconstrictor qualities (see Fig. 5-19). The synthesis of these substances is a most notable achievement by Page and his collaborators.[44] This mechanism was explored in a search for the cause of systemic arterial hypertension and has been proposed as one

of the mechanisms for normal peripheral vascular control which go awry in patients who developed hypertension. Since the cellular sources of renin are not known, the mechanism or mechanisms by which its production is accelerated or depressed are completely obscure. The sensing element which monitors the concentration of angiotensin I or II or renin in blood has not been discovered, and it thus seems premature to assign this mechanism a role in normal peripheral vascular control. This subject will receive more attention in Chapter 5.

SEROTONIN. The serum of clotted blood causes contraction of blood vessels. Since the substance responsible for this reaction could easily complicate research on hypertension, Page and his colleagues[45] investigated the problem and isolated a substance called serotonin or, more exactly, 5-hydroxytryptamine. When injected intravenously this substance has a very complex action on the pulmonary circulation,[46] which otherwise is quite unresponsive (Figs. 4-13 and 4-16). Serotonin also is a vasodilator in peripheral beds, notably the coronary vessels; however, under normal conditions it is confined within platelets and mast cells, and release into the blood stream has not been demonstrated. Thus, its role in normal vascular control remains doubtful.

H-SUBSTANCE AND HISTAMINE. Mechanical stimulation of the skin (e.g., by firm stroking) produces a sequence of vascular changes including local vasoconstriction, a surrounding vasodilation or flare and, finally, local swelling or edema. Lewis[36] attributed this "triple response" to the release of "H-substance" from the injured tissue. This substance is generally identified as histamine, which can be derived from histidine by splitting off carbon dioxide. Experimentally, histamine causes vasodilation in the terminal capillary beds but constriction of the larger arterial branches. Histamine-like substances are generally considered to be present during vascular responses to tissue injury caused by such forms of radiation as ultraviolet light (sunburn), infrared (thermal burns) and roentgen rays and by mechanical stress and trauma. However, this substance is not apparently involved in normal control.

MYOGENIC RESPONSES. In 1902 Bayliss[47] reported experiments which indicated that "the muscular coat of the arteries reacts, like smooth muscle in other situations, to a stretching force by contraction" independent of the nervous system. More recently Folkow[48] and others have investigated this concept that elevated internal pressure produces vasoconstriction in denervated vascular beds. The evidence of this type of reaction is quite universally indirect. Without any questioning of these observations it seems illogical, as McDonald and Taylor have pointed out, to emphasize this mechanism as the physiologically dominant one since it would appear to act as a positive feed-back loop and so to be completely unstable. "Thus, a rise in blood pressure would cause a vasoconstriction which would cause further rise in pressure."[49] If smooth muscle is indeed capable of a myogenic response, then it must act in conjunction with, and be governed by, built-in sensing and control systems.

VASCULAR CONTROL IN SPECIFIC TISSUES

The anatomic arrangement and environmental conditions of arteries, arterioles and sphincters vary from one vascular bed to another, but the smooth muscle cells which invest these vessels and induce changes in their caliber look the same in all vascular beds. Nevertheless, the vascular smooth muscle in different tissues responds in widely different ways under the influence of the mechanisms illustrated in Figure 4-12. Under these conditions, control of the vascular system cannot be considered in general terms. The characteristics of the vascular responses peculiar to each major tissue or organ must be detailed individually. In the following discussion, the organs of the body will be discussed roughly in the order of increasing reactivity or diversity of mechanisms inducing vasomotor responses. Green and Kepchar's[34] excellent review is a valuable reference to supplement the following discussion.

Brain. The cerebral vasculature is probably the most resistant to vasomotor influences to be found in the body. According to Kety,[50] the cerebral blood flow of healthy young men is about 54 ml. per 100 gm. of brain tissue per minute and the respiratory quotient is approximately unity, indicating that carbohydrate is the prime source of energy. The energy requirement of the brain is about 20 watts, compared to the thousands of watts required by electronic computors.

It is well established that autonomic nerves supply the cerebral vessels. This innervation may influence the cerebral blood flow in lower animals, but there is little evidence of its effectiveness in man. After reviewing a great many potential factors, Sokoloff[51] concluded, "an overall view of the action of drugs on the cerebral circulation is the great resistance of the cerebral blood flow to change" (Fig. 4-13). Increased carbon dioxide tension has the most potent effects on cerebral vessels, but it rarely elevates cerebral flow as much as twofold. Reduced oxygen tension in the arterial blood has also been reported to dilate cerebral vessels.[52]

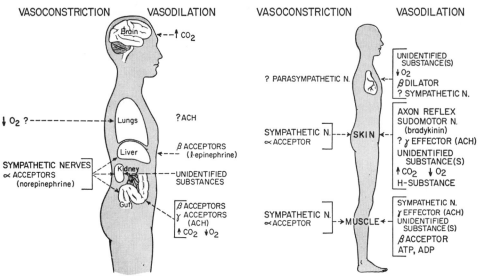

FIGURE 4-13   VASOMOTOR MECHANISMS IN VARIOUS TISSUES

Vascular beds in some tissues are very unresponsive to all normal vasomotor mechanisms; e.g., cerebral vessels are slightly affected by CO_2 and pulmonary vessels by O_2 content. The splanchnic vascular bed is quite reactive and responds to many different controlling mechanisms. The vascular reactivity of the coronary vessels is difficult to determine because most of the mechanisms affect cardiac function as well. The vessels of skin and muscle respond to a very large number of different control mechanisms and are extremely reactive.

Reflecting the constancy of the overall cerebral metabolism, the total cerebral blood flow is remarkably constant. However, the blood flow is not uniform throughout the brain substance, varying from 0.14 ml. per gram in spinal white matter to 1.8 mg. per gram in the inferior colliculus.[53] Primary sensory areas subserving visual, auditory and somatosensory functions receive significantly higher blood flows than do other cortical areas. Under thiopental anesthesia, the differences in blood flow through sensory areas disappear.

Lungs. The pulmonary circulation appears to be almost as unresponsive as the cerebral to normal controlling mechanisms (Fig. 4-13). The pulmonary vascular bed is an extremely low resistance system (Chapter 1), and its resistance readily becomes even less. Thus the amount of blood flow-

ing through this system can increase two or three times with very little increase in the pressure gradient from the pulmonary artery to the left atrium. Because definitive demonstration of any active vasomotor change induced by neural, hormonal or chemical agents has proved very difficult, the reduction in resistance as flow increases has been ascribed to passive distention of the vascular bed. At higher pulmonary blood flow rates, however, the pressure gradient increases in direct proportion to the flow rate as though the vascular bed had reached a maximum cross-sectional area and was behaving more like a system of rigid tubes.[54]

Hypoxia apparently induces some vasoconstriction, which would tend to shunt blood from collapsed or inactive lung parenchyma toward regions where gases could be interchanged.

Fairly large concentrations of acetylcholine infused directly into the pulmonary artery produce a slight and questionable fall in pulmonary arterial pressure.[54] There is, however, no evidence that either hypoxia or acetylcholine is normally a regulator of pulmonary vessels.

The evidence on the action of vasodilator drugs on pulmonary vessels is inconclusive. They are constricted by serotonin and under these conditions respond with vasodilation to acetylcholine, histamine and adenosine triphosphate.[55] The functional significance of this observation remains obscure. Some evidence for a parasympathetic innervation of the lung activated by stimulation of the carotid chemoreceptors has been presented by Daly and Daly,[56] but such a mechanism would play little or no role in normal control.

It thus seems safe to consider the pulmonary vascular bed as one that does not share in peripheral vasomotor alterations. This attitude appears entirely logical since all of the cardiac output flows through the lungs. There is no obvious need for a means of changing the distribution of blood flow from one part of the lungs to another under normal conditions, because all parts serve the same function.

Liver. The liver, like the lung, is a low-pressure system served by two vascular systems. A major portion (about four fifths) of the blood flowing through the liver arrives by way of the portal vein under low pressure after having passed through the capillaries in the gastrointestinal tract upstream. The remainder enters under the systemic arterial pressure head by way of the hepatic artery. Both stimulation of sympathetic nerves and norepinephrine apparently produce some constriction of both the hepatic and portal arterial systems, but the effects are

relatively mild. Since epinephrine, isoproterenol and acetylcholine have little or no effect on either vascular system, neither β nor γ effectors are believed to exist here. Reactive hyperemia does not follow temporary occlusion of the blood flow. Thus, the liver is a system that is quite unresponsive to the available control systems.

Spleen. Stimulation of the splenic nerve greatly increases the vascular resistance and activates the mechanism by which the cells concentrated in the spleen are dumped into the active circulation. The changes in resistance apparently are mediated by norepinephrine; the emptying mechanism by *l*-epinephrine. Dilation follows administration of extremely small concentrations of cholinergic substances, although existence of a parasympathetic innervation has not been demonstrated.

Kidney. The splanchnic sympathetic nerves exert a vasoconstrictor effect on the renal vessels. Norepinephrine and *l*-epinephrine act on effectors to produce constriction. Temporary occlusion of renal blood flow results in reactive hyperemia induced by unidentified dilator substances. Above a certain critical pressure (i.e., 70 mm. Hg) the blood flow through the kidney tends to remain quite constant in spite of progressively elevated arterial perfusion pressure. This has been termed *autoregulation* and may result from elevation of perivascular pressures in step with increases in perfusion pressure, so that flow remains relatively constant.

Gastrointestinal Tract. The splanchnic nerves are profusely distributed to the vessels of the splanchnic bed and are believed to play an important role in the maintenance of systemic arterial blood pressure. These nerves apparently act through α effectors so that administration of nor-epinephrine induces similar effects on this bed. Prolonged stimulation of intestinal vasoconstrictor fibers induces a pattern termed "autoregulatory escape," an initial constriction followed by an escape of resistance vessels from the nervous influences within 1 to 2 minutes while the perfused capillary exchange area remains reduced.[58] Significant dilation follows injection of isoproterenol, indicating the presence of β effectors. Mild dilation from administration of acetylcholine suggests the presence of γ effectors. However, according to presently available information, the autonomic nerves act on the α effectors but not on the β effectors. Since such levels are beyond the physiologic range, the resulting dilation has very limited significance.

Heart. The terminal coronary vessels penetrate the walls of the heart. There they are compressed by the contracting myocardium, particularly within the wall of the left ventricle (see Chapter 9). During ventricular systole, the outflow from the coronary veins is accelerated and the inflow through the coronary arteries is impeded. However, the pumping action of ventricular systole apparently does not facilitate blood flow. Sudden arrest of the heart immediately increases both the arterial inflow and the venous outflow, indicating that ventricular contraction impedes flow through the coronary vessels.[59] More vigorous contraction of the myocardium, induced by catechol amines or sympathetic stimulation, tends to increase simultaneously the work load on the myocardium and the impedence to coronary flow. A close relation between the cardiac effort, the myocardial oxygen consumption and the coronary flow has been repeatedly reported. Gregg[59] pointed out that

most of the oxygen is normally removed from the coronary blood so that the oxygen content of coronary sinus (venous) blood cannot be reduced very much. Therefore increased oxygen delivery must be achieved primarily by increased coronary flow.

It seems likely that low oxygen tension or low oxygen content in the blood produces coronary dilation, but this dilation could reflect the effects of unidentified vasodilator substances since the coronary vessels exhibit reactive hyperemia. Carbon dioxide and altered pH apparently have no effect. According to Green and Kepchar,[34] the only agents which consistently cause constriction of the coronary arterioles are vasopressin and angiotensin. Many drugs appear to produce coronary dilation but have no known functional significance in normal control. (see also Chapter 9.)

Skeletal Muscle. The blood vessels supplying skeletal muscles generally are now believed to have double sympathetic innervation. The sympathetic constrictor fibers activate typical α receptors and, apparently, participate in the generalized sympathetic discharges which tend to support systemic arterial blood pressure. When this sympathetic constrictor mechanism is eliminated, the blood vessels of muscle maintain a substantial degree of vasoconstriction. Sympathetic vasodilator fibers act through cholinergic γ receptors, which can produce maximal dilation and can be readily blocked by atropine. The sympathetic vasodilator system is confined to skeletal muscle and is apparently dissociated from the control of the blood pressure regulatory system of the medullary vasomotor areas. Instead, the nerve impulses which ultimately reach the sympathetic vasodilator nerve endings have been traced from the motor cortex of the cerebrum near the cruciate sulcus to the supraoptic part of the hypothalamus, to the collicular area and through the medullary regions, apparently bypassing the medullary cardioregulator centers, to impinge rather directly on the sympathetic outflow in the spinal cord.[60]

Thus there are four postulated mechanisms by which vasodilation in skeletal muscle may be achieved: (1) inhibition of the sympathetic constrictor mechanism (twofold to threefold increase), (2) activation of the sympathetic vasodilator system (fivefold to sixfold increase), (3) the β effectors and (4) unidentified vasodilator substances present immediately after exercise (sixfold to tenfold increase). The β effectors are not innervated but are activated by circulating l-epinephrine or injected isoproterenol (Fig. 4-12). The function of this mechanism in normal body economy has not been established.

The skeletal muscles are prone to develop extremely intense reactive hyperemia following temporary occlusion of their blood supply. This state is attributed to unidentified metabolic vasodilator substances.

Extremely small quantities of adenosine triphosphate (ATP) produce profound vasodilation in skeletal muscle. A similar degree of vasodilation can be produced by adenosine diphosphate (ADP). In fact, these substances are such potent dilators that the effective doses for the skeletal vessels defy chemical detection. Although ATP and ADP are fine potential candidates for the position of "unidentified vasodilator substances," their role has not been conclusively demonstrated.

The contraction of skeletal muscle impedes blood flow just as ventricular contraction does (see previous discussion). Thus, the blood flow through an extremity is greater immediately after the cessation of exercise than during the exertion itself. The compression of blood vessels by contracting muscle can actively pump venous blood against a very high resistance (see Fig. 7-8).

Skin. The skin has the most complex assortment of available control mechanisms (Fig. 4-13) and contains a vascular bed which is very accessible for study by physiologists and clinicians. The result is an imposing, almost overwhelming mass of literature that defies precise description.

The predominant neural control is exercised by the sympathetic vasoconstrictor nerves; the mediator is probably norepinephrine. In contrast with vessels in muscle, skin vessels dilate maximally when the sympathetic constrictor influence on them is eliminated. Consequently, the full range of cutaneous flow can be achieved by release of constrictor tone. No sympathetic or parasympathetic vasodilator fibers directly affecting cutaneous vessels have been described. Injection of acetylcholine induces a slight dilation of these vessels which suggests the presence of γ effectors that are not innervated. Stimulation of the peripheral ends of several dorsal roots produces vasodilation which can best be explained in terms of an axon reflex (see Fig. 4-12B). The normal course of impulses in such a mechanism is from sensory nerve endings in the skin to collaterals which directly impinge on blood vessels. Recent evidence suggests that the parasympathetic supply to the sweat glands (sudomotor) triggers the release of an enzyme (bradykinin enzyme) that acts on tissue proteins to form bradykinin which diffuses to adjacent blood vessels and induces a vasodilation of the deep and superficial vascular plexuses. (Fig. 4-12).

The skin exhibits severe reactive

hyperemia following temporary occlusion to blood supply. Thus, it can be postulated that unidentified vasodilator substances participate in the control of the skin vessels. A vasomotor role of low oxygen or elevated carbon dioxide has not been established.

Local warming of the skin produces a vasodilation which is believed to result from release of constrictor tone through central reflexes rather than from a direct action of the heat on the blood vessels. These reflexes probably involve the hypothalamic temperature regulating centers, acting through sympathetic vasoconstrictor nerves. Excessive cold applied to the skin may produce a brief vasodilation which may be independent of the nerve supply.

Finally, flushing of the skin from embarrassment or emotional stimuli represents vascular changes induced from higher levels of the nervous system.

EFFECTS OF CONTROL MECHANISMS ON FLOW DISTRIBUTION

When ultrasonic flowmeters are installed on arteries or veins, the instantaneous flow through these regions can be continuously registered during the spontaneous activity of healthy dogs and during reactions experimentally induced in the presence or absence of anesthesia.[61]

Flow Distribution During Spontaneous Activity. The instantaneous flow through the superior mesenteric or hepatic artery, the renal artery and the terminal abdominal aorta of intact dogs was continuously recorded while the animals were engaged in various activities, including: reacting to a startling event, standing erect with the head up (60 degrees), standing with the head down (50 degrees), sit-ting, drinking water, entering a treadmill and exercising at 3 m.p.h. on a 12 per cent grade (Fig. 4–14). As the changes in the wave form of the instantaneous flow do not indicate the changes in volume flow per unit time, the flow records have been integrated with an analogue computer so that the flow during intervals of 2.5 seconds is accumulated. In this manner the influences of both changes in wave form and changes in heart rate are taken into account, and the height of the resulting deflection is an accurate measure of volume flow during a particular period. The contribution of each stroke can be identified from the distance separating pairs of darker spots representing diastole on the integrated flow line.

Each of the preceding spontaneous actions was associated with obvious deflections in the records of instantaneous flow. The integrated flow per unit of time through the superior mesenteric and renal arteries, however, remained remarkably constant, although slight changes accompanied the startle reaction and standing erect with the head up. In all seven dogs studied, volume flow was remarkably constant in the renal artery and in the superior mesenteric or hepatic artery during virtually all forms of spontaneous activity which were studied. On the other hand, the integrated flow as well as the instantaneous flow in the terminal abdominal aorta was very responsive to most forms of activity. During exercise the forward flow of blood through the hindquarters exceeded zero throughout the cardiac cycles, a condition indicating both a considerably reduced peripheral resistance and a greatly increased blood flow. The mean pressure in the abdominal aorta was quite constant except when standing erect with the head up. The heart

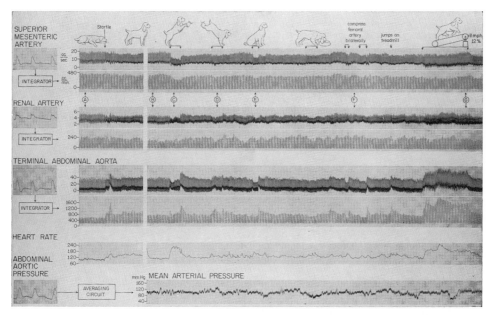

FIGURE 4-14   FLOW DISTRIBUTION DURING SPONTANEOUS ACTIVITY

Instantaneous and integrated flow through the superior mesenteric artery, renal artery and terminal abdominal aorta as recorded simultaneously and continuously in an intact dog during a series of cardiovascular adjustments to spontaneous activity including startle reaction, standing erect with head up, head down, eating, constriction of femoral arteries bilaterally, entering treadmill and exercise. Note that blood flow per unit of time (integrated) through the superior mesenteric and renal arteries changes very little during most responses except standing with head up. Flow to the hindquarters increased greatly during treadmill exercise.

rate increased notably during the startle reaction, standing erect and exercise.

Effects of Diencephalic Stimulation. Stimulation of selected sites in the diencephalon produced a wide variety of flow patterns in dogs under chloralose anesthesia. Changes in flow distribution reminiscent of those during exercise consistently resulted from stimulation in the region of the H_2 fields of Forel; stimulation of this region was already known to cause changes in cardiac function comparable to the changes accompanying exercise.[62] In the studies of blood flow, repeated stimulation as the electrode was advanced at 1 mm. increments toward this area produced the changes illustrated in Figure 4–15. No significant alterations followed stimulation

at the first two points selected. After the electrode was advanced only 1 mm., the superior mesenteric and renal flows definitely decreased and the flow through the terminal aorta increased. Stimulation after the electrode was moved 1 mm. farther produced an even greater response, but, as the electrode was advanced still farther, the response lessened. The influence of diencephalic stimulation on the blood flow through these arteries and the promptness of the response indicate that their nerve supplies were intact. Thus, the relative slightness of the changes in superior mesenteric and renal flow during spontaneous activity probably cannot be attributed to damage of essential innervation during application of the flow sections.

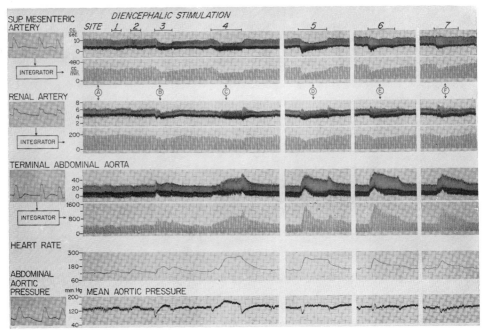

FIGURE 4-15   EFFECTS OF DIENCEPHALIC STIMULATION ON FLOW DISTRIBUTION

A series of stimuli was applied as the electrode was advanced in 1 mm. increments to and through the H_2 fields of Forel. The changes in flow distribution resemble those observed during spontaneous exercise by the same animal. Stimulation in this diencephalic region simultaneously produces these changes in flow distribution, changes in cardiac rate and function resembling the exercise response (see Fig. 7-4), increased respiratory ventilation and, on some occasions, running movements.

SUMMARY

The basic principles of peripheral vascular control are generally considered in terms of mechanisms by which the blood flow through various tissues are adjusted in relation to metabolism and the oxygen requirement. Actually, many tissues have functional requirements for blood flow which are unrelated to the oxygen consumption (e.g., kidney, skin, liver, and perhaps the gastrointestinal tract; Fig. 4–16). In fact, the principal tissues that require blood flow related to their metabolic rates (oxygen uptake) are the striated muscles: myocardium and skeletal muscles. After temporary occlusion of the blood supply to these tissues they exhibit a most powerful reactive hyperemia apparently caused by unidentified metabolic vasodilator substances.

The blood flow, oxygen extraction and vasomotor control are quite different in the various vascular beds. The neural control mechanisms are clearly important in the regulation of blood flow through many tissues, but not all. Neural controls are based principally on the sympathetic constrictor system, which continuously maintains varying degrees of constriction within the vascular beds. In addition there is a sympathetic vasodilator system, which is restricted to skeletal muscle (and, perhaps, the heart). Vasodilation is attributed currently to parasympathetic activation of certain structures, notably glands, with resulting formation of bradykinin by an enzyme released from the gland into the interstitial

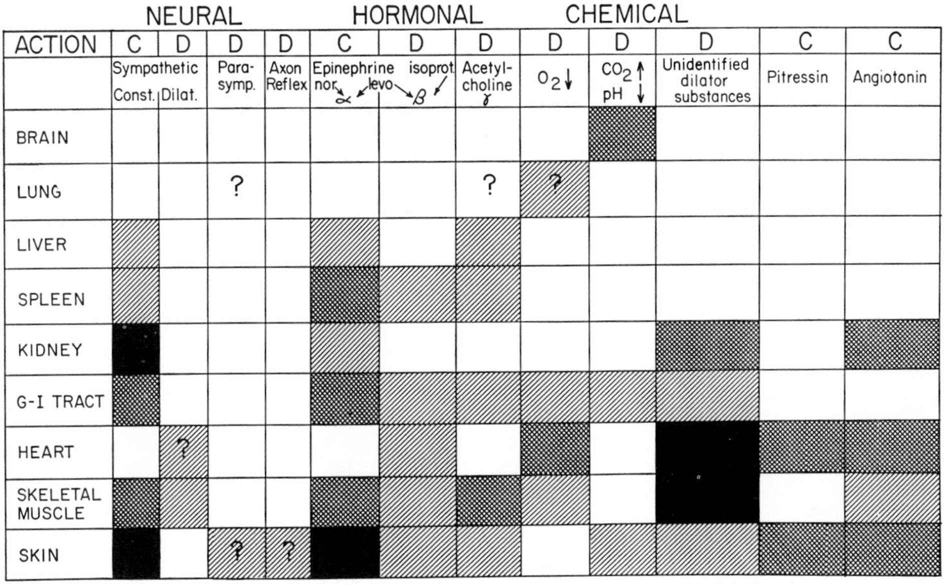

ACTION	NEURAL				HORMONAL			CHEMICAL				
	C	D	D	D	C	D	D	D	D	D	C	C
	Sympathetic Const.	Sympathetic Dilat.	Para-symp.	Axon Reflex	Epinephrine nor α, levo β	isoprot	Acetyl-choline γ	O_2 ↓	CO_2 ↑ pH ↓	Unidentified dilator substances	Pitressin	Angiotonin
BRAIN												
LUNG			?				?	?				
LIVER												
SPLEEN												
KIDNEY												
G-I TRACT												
HEART		?										
SKELETAL MUSCLE												
SKIN			?	?								

FIGURE 4-16   VASCULAR REACTIVITY IN VARIOUS ORGANS

The responsiveness of the various vascular beds illustrated in Figure 4-13 is here indicated schematically by the density of the shading under each of the neural, hormonal and chemical factors. The action of the mechanisms is indicated by C for constriction and D for dilation. The question marks indicate that the response is controversial. Note that both the diversity of the response and the intensity of the response tend to be much greater in the gastrointestinal tract, heart, skeletal muscle and skin than in the brain, lung, liver and spleen.

tissues. Circulating autonomic hormones, l-epinephrine, norepinephrine and acetylcholine have powerful vasomotor activity when injected, but their role in normal peripheral vascular control remains questionable. The vasodilator substances, which seem to accumulate when tissues metabolize in an environment containing inadequate oxygen, have not been definitely identified and represent an important challenge in this field.

The vascular reactivity in various organs is strikingly different (Fig. 4-16). For example, the cerebral circulation is little affected by neural or hormonal substances and is mildly dilated by increased carbon dioxide tension. Control of the pulmonary circulation is difficult to demonstrate experimentally. The coronary vessels dilate readily in response to metabolic vasodilator substances but are otherwise quite nonreactive so far as can be determined experimentally. In contrast, the splanchnic bed, kidney, liver and spleen are fairly responsive to a variety of mechanisms, and skeletal muscles and the skin are influenced by a bewildering number of factors.

REFERENCES

1. ZWEIFACH, B. W. The microcirculation of the blood. Sci. Amer., 200:54–60, 1959.
2. ROMANUL, F. C. A. Distribution of capillaries in relation to oxidative metabolism of skeletal muscle fibres. Nature, 201:307–308, 1964.
3. MYERS, W. W., and HONIG, C. R. Number and distribution of capillaries as determinants of myocardial oxygen tension. Amer. J. Physiol., 207:653–660, 1964.
4. SCHMIDT-NIELSEN, K., and PENNYCUIK, P. Capillary density in mammals in relation to body size and oxygen consumption. Amer. J. Physiol., 200:746–750, 1961.

5. THEWS, G. Gaseous diffusion in the lungs and tissues. Chapter 20 in *Physical Bases of Circulatory Transport: regulation and exchange*. E. B. Reeve and A. C. Guyton, Eds. Philadelphia, W. B. Saunders Co., 1967.

6. ZWEIFACH, B. W., and KOSSMANN, C. E. Micromanipulation of small blood vessels in the mouse. *Amer. J. Physiol.*, 120:23–35, 1937.

7. YAMADA, E. The fine structure of the renal glomerulus of the mouse. *J. Biophys. Biochem. Cytol.*, 1:551–556, 1955.

8. BENNET, H. S., LUFT, J. H., and HAMPTOM, J. C. Morphological classification of vertebrate blood capillaries. *Amer. J. Physiol.*, 196:381–390, 1959.

9. MAJNO, G. Ultrastructure of the vascular membrane. In *Handbook of Physiology, Section II Circulation*, Vol. 3. William Hamilton, Ed. Bethesda, Amer. Physiol. Soc., 1965.

10. BURTON, A. C. Physical principles of circulatory phenomena; the physical equilibria of the heart and blood vessels. In *Handbook of Physiology, Section II Circulation*, Vol. I. William Hamilton, Ed. Bethesda, Amer. Physiol. Soc., 1962.

11. VAN CITTERS, R. L. WAGNER, B. M., and RUSHMER, R. F. Architectural changes in the walls of small arteries during vasoconstriction. *Circulat. Res.*, 10:668–675, 1962.

12. HAYES, J. R. Histological changes in constricted arteries and arterioles. *J. Anat.*, 101:343–349, 1967.

13. STROMBERG, D. An index for quantitative measurement of vasoconstriction in histologic sections of blood vessels. *Vascular Surg.*, 3:68–80, 1960.

14. VAN CITTERS, R. L. Occlusion of lumina in small arteries during vasoconstriction. *Circulat. Res.*, 18:199–204, 1966.

15. WALLACE, J. M., and STEAD, E. A. Fall in pressure in radial artery during reactive hyperemia. *Circulat. Res.*, 7:876–879, 1959.

16. BURTON, A. C. Why have a circulation? In *Physiology and Biophysics of Circulation*. Year Book Medical Publishers, Inc., 1965.

17. FOLKOW, B. Range of control of the cardiovascular system by the central nervous system. *Physiol. Rev.*, 40 (Suppl. 4):93–99, 1960.

18. FOLKOW, B., JOHANNSON, B., and LÖFVING, B. Aspects of functional differentiation of the sympatho-adrenergic control of the cardiovascular system. In *Medicina Experimentalis*, R. Domenjoz and S. Karger, Eds. Basel, New York. (*Med. Exp.* 4:321–328, 1961.)

19. RENKIN, E. U., and ROSELL, S. Independent sympathetic vasoconstrictor innervation of arterioles and precapillary sphincters. *Acta physiol. scand.* 54:381–384, 1962.

20. LUTZ, B. R., and FULTON, G. P. Smooth muscle and blood flow in small blood vessels. Pp. 13–23 in *Factors Regulating Blood Flow*, G. P. Fulton and B. Zweifach, Eds. Washington, Amer. Physiol. Soc., 1958.

21. WHITTERIDGE, D. Cardiovascular reflexes initiated from afferent sites other than the cardiovascular system itself. *Physiol. Rev.*, 40 (Suppl. 4): 198–200, 1960.

22. SMITH, O. A. Anatomy of central neural pathways mediating cardiovascular functions. In *Nervous Control of the Heart*, W. C. Randall, Ed. Baltimore, The Williams and Wilkins Co., 1965.

23. FOLKOW, B. Nervous control of blood vessels. *Physiol. Rev.*, 35:629–663, 1955.

24. ERICI, I., FOLKOW, B, and UVNÄS, B. Sympathetic vasodilator nerves to the tongue of the cat. *Acta physiol. scand.*, 25:1–9, 1952.

25. GREENFIELD, A. D. M. Survey of evidence for active neurogenic vasodilatation in man. *Fed. Proc.*, 25:1607–1610, 1966.

26. UVNÄS, B. Cholinergic vasodilator nerves. *Fed. Proc.*, 25:1618–1622, 1966.

27. HILTON, S. M., and LEWIS, G. P. The relationship between glandular activity, bradykinin formation and functional vasodilatation in the submandibular salivary gland. *J. Physiol.*, 134:471–483, 1956.

28. FOX, R. H., and HILTON, S. M. Sweat gland activity, bradykinin formation and vasodilation in human forearm skin. *J. Physiol.*, 137:43p–44p, 1957.

29. FOX, R. H., GOLDSMITH, R., KIDD, D. J., and LEWIS, G. P. Bradykinin as a vasodilator in man. *J. Physiol.*, 157:589–602, 1961.

30. WEBSTER, M. E., SKINNER, N. S., JR., POWELL, W. J. Role of the kinins in vasodilation of skeletal muscle in the dog. *Amer. J. Physiol.*, 212:553–558, 1967.

31. VON EULER, U. S. *Noradrenaline.* Springfield, Ill., C. C Thomas, 1956, 382 pp.

32. AHLQUIST, R. P. Adrenergic drugs. Pp. 378–407 in *Pharmacology in Medicine*, Vol. 2, V. A. Drill, Ed. New York, McGraw-Hill, 1958.

33. DOREVITCH, N., NAYLER, W. G., LOWE, T. E. The action on isolated smooth muscle of kinekard, a cardioactive fraction isolated from human plasma. *J. Pharmacol. Exptl. Therap.* 155:367–375, 1967.

34. GREEN, H. D., and KEPCHAR, J. H. Control of peripheral resistance in major systemic vascular beds. *Physiol. Rev.*, 39:617–686, 1959.

35. ROY, C. S., and BROWN, J. G. The blood pressure and its variations in the arterioles, capillaries and small veins. *J. Physiol.*, 2:323–359, 1879–1880.

36. LEWIS, THOMAS. *The Blood Vessels of the Human Skin and Their Responses.* London, Shaw & Sons Ltd., 1927, 322 pp.

37. PATEL, D. J., and BURTON, A. C. Reactive hyperemia in the human finger. *Circulat. Res.*, 4:710–712, 1956.

38. YONCE, L. R., and HAMILTON, W. F. Oxygen consumption in skeletal muscle during reactive hyperemia. *Amer. J. Physiol.*, 197: 190–192, 1959.

39. KORNER, P. I. Circulatory adaptations in hypoxia. *Physiol. Rev.*, 39:687–730, 1959.

40. HYMAN, C., PALDINO, R. L., and ZIMMERMAN, E. Local regulation of effective blood flow in muscle. *Circulat. Res.*, 12: 179–181, 1963.

41. CROSS, R. B., GIMLETTE, T. M. D. The effect of intramuscular injections of K, ATP and lactic acid on muscle blood flow estimated by ^{133}Xe clearance from the point of injection. *J. Physiol.*, 189:43p, 1967.

42. MELLANDER, S., JOHANSSON, B., GRAY, S., JONSSON, O., LUNVALL, J., and LJUNG, B. The effects of hyperosmolarity on intact and isolated vascular smooth muscle; possible role in exercise hyperemia. *Angiologica*, 4:310–322, 1967.

43. FOLKOW, B. The vasodilator action of adenosine triphosphate. *Acta physiol. scand.*, 17:311–316, 1949.

44. PAGE, I. H., McCUBBIN, J. W., SCHWARZ, H., and BUMPUS, F. M. Pharmacologic aspects of synthetic angiotonin. *Circulat. Res.*, 5:552–555, 1957.

45. PAGE, I. H. Serotonin (5-hydroxytryptamine): the last four years. *Physiol. Rev.*, 38:277–335, 1958.

46. ROSE, J. C., and LAZARO, E. J. Pulmonary vascular responses to serotonin and effects of certain serotonin antagonists. *Circulat. Res.*, 6:282–293, 1958.

47. BAYLISS, W. M. On the local reactions of the arterial wall to changes of internal pressure. *J. Physiol.*, 28:200–231, 1902.

48. FOLKOW, B. Description of the Myogenic Hypothesis. *Circulat. Res.*, Supplement 1, Vols. 14 and 15:1279–1287, 1964.

49. McDONALD, D. A., and TAYLOR, M. G. The hydrodynamics of the arterial circulation. *Progr. Biophys. Biophys. Chem.*, 9:105–173, 1959.

50. KETY, S. S. The physiology of the cerebral circulation in man. Pp. 324–340 in *Circulation*, J. McMichael, Ed. Oxford, Blackwell Scientific Publications, 1958.

51. SOKOLOFF, L. The action of drugs on the cerebral circulation. *Pharmacol. Rev.*, 11: 1–85, 1959.

52. LASSEN, N. A. Cerebral blood flow and oxygen consumption in man. *Physiol. Rev.*, 39:183–238, 1959.

53. SOKOLOFF, L. Factors regulating the total and regional circulation of the brain. Pp. 79–88 in *Factors Regulating Blood Flow*, G. P. Fulton and B. Zweifach, Eds. Washington, Amer. Physiol. Soc., 1958.

54. COURNAND, A. Control of the pulmonary circulation in normal man. Pp. 219–237 in *Circulation*, J. McMichael, Ed. Oxford, Blackwell Scientific Publications, 1958.

55. RUDOLPH, A. M., KURLAND, M. D., AULD, P. A. M., and PAUL, M. H. Effects of vasodilator drugs on normal and serotonin-constricted pulmonary vessels of the dog. *Amer. J. Physiol.*, 197:617–623, 1959.

56. DALY, I. DE B., and DALY, M. DE B. The effects of stimulation of the carotid body chemoreceptors on pulmonary vascular resistance in the dog. *J. Physiol.*, 137:436–446, 1957.

57. FOLKOW, B., and LANGSTON, J. The interrelationship of some factors influencing renal blood flow autoregulation. *Acta physiol. scand.*, 61:165–176, 1964.

58. WALLENTIN, I. Studies on intestinal circulation. *Acta physiol. scand.*, 69 (supplementum 279):1–38, 1966.

59. GREGG, D. W. Regulation of the collateral and coronary circulation of the heart. Pp. 163–186 in *Circulation*, J. McMichael, Ed. Oxford, Blackwell Scientific Publications, 1958.

60. LINDGREN, P., and UVNÄS, B. Vasoconstrictor inhibition and vasodilator activation — two functionally separate vasodilator mechanisms in the skeletal muscles. *Acta physiol. scand.*, 33:108–119, 1955.

61. RUSHMER, R. F., FRANKLIN, D. L., VAN CITTERS, R. L., and SMITH, O. A., JR. Changes in peripheral blood flow distribution in healthy dogs. *Circulat. Res.*, 9:675–687, 1961.

62. SMITH, O. A., JR., RUSHMER, R. F., and LASHER, E. P. Similarity of cardiovascular responses to exercise and to diencephalic stimulation. *Amer. J. Physiol.*, 198:1139–1142, 1960.

CHAPTER 5

SYSTEMIC ARTERIAL PRESSURE

The distribution of blood flow through the various peripheral vascular beds is controlled primarily by changes in caliber at the sites of resistance in the vessels leading to the capillary networks (Chapter 4). This form of flow control depends upon the maintenance at all times of an adequate pressure head within the systemic arterial system (Fig. 4–10).

FACTORS DETERMINING MEAN SYSTEMIC ARTERIAL PRESSURE

The high pressures maintained within the systemic arteries constitute a pressure reservoir to supply the driving force propelling blood through the complex networks of narrow channels in the microcirculation. This hydrostatic head of pressure is normally in the range of 120/80 mm. Hg and must not fall below some critical level (i.e., 60/40 mm. Hg) lest perfusion of the brain be insufficient to maintain consciousness or to maintain functional integrity of rapidly metabolizing tissues such as the heart and kidney. The control of the arterial pressure is a complex problem because it can be

altered by a very large number of factors as illustrated schematically in Figure 5–1.

The systemic arterial pressure is ultimately determined by the relationship between the cardiac output and the total peripheral resistance. An uncompensated reduction in either can lead to reduced pressure in the arterial system. The cardiac output is, in turn, determined by the product of the heart rate and the stroke volume. Since the left ventricle does not always fill completely during diastole nor empty completely during systole, the stroke volume must be regarded as the difference between the diastolic and systolic ventricular volumes.

Numerous factors influence the stroke volume, as indicated schematically in Figure 5–1. Among the influences on diastolic ventricular volume are the effective ventricular filling pressure and the resistance of the ventricular walls to distention (distensibility). The ventricular filling pressure depends upon the total volume of blood in the cardiovascular system and the distribution of this blood as it is affected by the venous capacity in various channels and

148

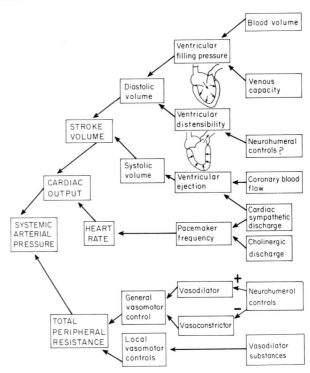

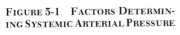

FIGURE 5-1 FACTORS DETERMIN-
ING SYSTEMIC ARTERIAL PRESSURE

The many interacting factors which determine the level of the systemic arterial pressure present a wide variety of alternative mechanisms for control. Note that each branch point represents a potential site of control or compensation for any perturbation of the system (see text).

reservoirs. The distensibility, or compliance of the ventricular walls, is not a simple elastic relation between length and tension but changes during the sequence of filling and is affected by the rate of filling. The sympathetic discharge to the ventricular myocardium affects the rate and degree of systolic ejection. The energy released by the contracting myocardium to expel the blood must be replenished continuously by processes dependent upon the continued flow of blood through the coronary arteries.

Control over heart rate can be readily traced to the balance of sympathetic and parasympathetic discharges into the region of the pacemaker. This balance is affected by a very wide variety of neural pathways. Reflexes initiated by distortion receptors in the carotid sinus and aortic arch are generally recognized as mechanisms for producing tachycardia in response to lowered systemic arterial pressure. Spontaneous variations in heart rate apparently stem from diverse central mechanisms acting through the autonomic system as final common pathways. For example, visual images, sounds, cold, pain and cerebration can all affect heart rate. Our knowledge of these mechanisms is woefully inadequate.

General control over the peripheral resistance is exerted by the autonomic nervous system and circulating hormones, which are both predominantly constrictor in nature, except in skeletal muscles and glands. In addition, local accumulation of various chemicals (carbon dioxide, acids, adenosine triphosphate, adenosine disphosphate and histamine) have a predominantly vasodilator action.

Systemic arterial pressure could theoretically be reduced by an appropriate and uncompensated alteration in any of the controlling factors, as illustrated in Figure 5–1. It is obvious, however, that the analysis could be readily extended further to include factors controlling the total blood volume, those affecting the venous capacity, the causes of changes in coronary blood flow and so on. Even an oversimplified scheme like that in Figure 5–1 inevitably leads to the conclusion that many mechanisms are potentially capable of causing a depression of systemic arterial pressure. With but a moderate stretching of the imagination, a clinical cause of arterial hypotension was listed for virtually every mechanism indicated in Figure 5–1. Thus, either blood loss (hemorrhage) or reduced plasma volume (deshydremia) could lead to reduced blood pressure, reduced diastolic volume, diminished stroke volume, smaller cardiac output and lower systemic arterial pressure. Similarly, venodilatation could reduce ventricular filling pressure by changing the distribution of blood and lowering central venous pressure and so on down the list.

COMPENSATORY MECHANISMS

When factors that influence the systemic arterial pressure are represented schematically like the branchings of a tree, each fork in the arborization constitutes an opportunity for a functional compensation. For example, a reduction in cardiac output can be offset by a corresponding increase in total peripheral resistance, so that the systemic arterial pressure remains unchanged. Similarly, a reduction in total peripheral resistance can be completely compensated for by a corresponding increase in cardiac output (e.g., during exercise). A reduction in ventricular stroke volume can be balanced by an increase in heart rate, so that cardiac output is unchanged. A

local vasodilatation can be compensated by a generalized vasoconstriction. If the ventricular diastolic volume is diminished, the stroke volume can be maintained by more complete systolic ejection. A reduction in the sympathetic discharge to the cardiac pacemaker can be balanced by a correspondingly effective reduction in the parasympathetic discharge to prevent a change in heart rate. The ventricular filling pressure is established by the relationship between total blood volume and the capacity of the cardiovascular system, with particular reference to the venous system. A reduction in total blood volume can theoretically be compensated for by a constriction of the venous capacity, maintaining the central venous pressure unchanged. Thus, any change in arterial pressure signifies an alteration in some mechanism(s) in Figure 5–1 which was not fully compensated for by other mechanisms.

A monitoring system which senses systemic arterial pressure and induces appropriate cardiovascular compensations to maintain this pressure within a relatively narrow range will automatically adjust the balance between inflow and outflow so that the total flow through capillary networks does not exceed the capacity of the pump.

The requirements of a pressure-regulating system are indicated schematically in Figure 5–2. By adjustment of the pump motor and the resistance valves, the pressure head can be set at a predetermined level. Pressure-sensing elements which continuously monitor this pressure can act upon a black-box control system. In such a system, wider opening of one resistance valve increases the outflow from the high pressure side, dropping the pressure head. This lowers the output from the pressure transducers which in turn acts on the control sys-

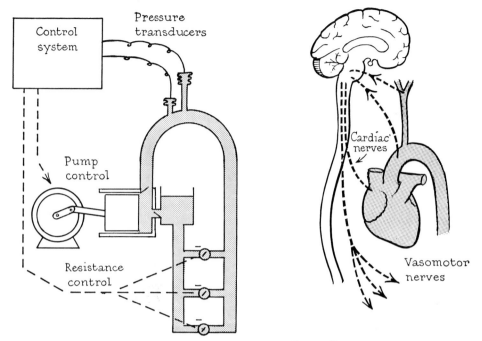

FIGURE 5-2   CONTROL OF ARTERIAL BLOOD PRESSURE

The pressure head in a simple hydraulic system could be controlled by means of pressure-sensing elements transmitting signals proportional to pressure through leads to a black-box integrating system which appropriately adjusts the pump output and valve settings in response to any deviation from some preset level. The corresponding elements for the control of arterial blood pressure include carotid sinus and aortic arch pressoreceptors feeding into the nervous system which provides integration of nerve impulses to the pump and peripheral vascular system.

tem to close other resistance valves, speed up the pump, or do both. In other words, the pressure level is set, the pressure-sensing elements detect a shift in pressure from this level as an error signal, and proper corrective adjustments to return the pressure to the "normal" level are instituted.

The systemic arterial pressure is apparently controlled essentially in this manner. There are, however, some complications. First, the process by which the "normal range" of systemic arterial pressure is originally set at a mean of about 90 mm. Hg is not obvious. Second, to detect an error, the pressure-sensing elements must continuously register actual pressure above atmospheric pressure even

though they are stretch receptors located in flexible walls apparently capable of varied distensibility. The pressure-sensing mechanism must integrate a fluctuating arterial pressure and induce responses which are related to changes in mean pressure rather than to changes in either the systolic or the diastolic pressure.

ARTERIAL PRESSURE PULSES

The principal function of the arterial system is to accept the repetitive spurts of blood injected by the heart and to convert this intermittent inflow into a relatively steady outflow through the peripheral resistance ves-

A. DISTORTION OF THE ARTERIAL PULSE WAVE ALONG THE AORTA

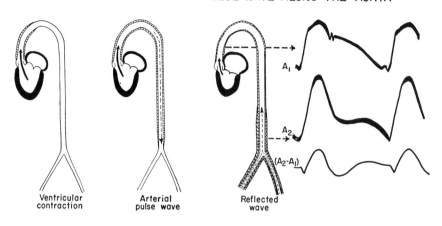

Ventricular   Arterial   Reflected
contraction   pulse wave   wave

B. THE VELOCITY OF BLOOD FLOW AND ARTERIAL PULSE IN THE AORTA

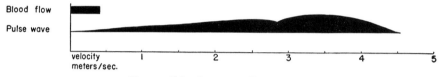

Blood flow

Pulse wave

velocity
meters/sec.

FIGURE 5-3   ARTERIAL PRESSURE PULSE

A, The arterial pressure pulse is a wave of pressure which passes rapidly along the arterial system. Blood suddenly ejected into the ascending aorta at the beginning of systole has insufficient energy to overcome all the inertia of the long columns of blood in the arteries. Therefore, blood tends to pile up and distend the ascending aorta, causing a sudden local increase in pressure. Blood is then forced into the next portion of the aorta, extending the region of distention and initiating a pulse of pressure which travels rapidly along the arteries toward the periphery. These waves of pressure, reflected by peripheral structures, travel back toward the heart and become superimposed on the advancing pulse wave. This produces a higher peak of systolic pressure, a slurring of the incisura and a lower diastolic pressure in the femoral artery. If the peripheral arterial pulse wave is subtracted from the pulse recorded at the arch of the aorta, the resulting wave form $(A_2 - A_1)$ suggests a natural frequency of the peripheral arterial system.

B, The pulse wave velocity (4 to 5 m. per second) is much faster than the velocity of blood flow (less than 0.5 m. per second). The pulse wave velocity is determined by the elasticity (compliance) of the arterial walls.

sels into the capillary networks. The geometry of the vascular bed and the visco-elastic properties of the arterial walls play important roles in conveying of blood down the long arterial channels with a minimal loss of pressure head but with a damping of the violent pressure fluctuations in the peripheral vessels.

At the onset of ventricular ejection, blood flows into the aorta faster than it leaves through the arterioles. The inertia of the long columns of blood in the arteries opposes acceleration. Blood ejected by the left ventricle

accumulates in the first portion of the aorta (Fig. 5–3A), increasing the tension in the walls of this region. The increased pressure and wall tension in the root of the aorta force blood into the adjacent segment of aorta which, in turn, is stretched and develops increased tension. In this way, a pulse of pressure moves rapidly down the aorta at a velocity which is determined by the elasticity of the walls and the pressure of the blood (Fig. 5–3B).

During the latter part of systole ventricular ejection slows, and the pressure in the root of the aorta falls.

Ventricular pressure drops rapidly to a level below the arterial pressure, and the aortic valves close.

SYSTOLIC PRESSURE

The peak systolic pressure in the central aorta is determined largely by the left ventricular stroke volume, the peak rate of ejection and the distensibility of the aortic walls. For example, the slow ejection of a small stroke volume into an easily distensible aorta produces a small elevation in systolic pressure. A rapid ejection of a large volume into a rigid aorta produces a large rise in systolic pressure, as does a normal stroke volume injected at normal velocity into a rigid atherosclerotic artery. The greatly accelerated ventricular ejection associated with sympathetic stimulation also produces greatly increased systolic pressure in the aorta (see Fig. 3–17).

DIASTOLIC PRESSURE

After ventricular systole is completed, the aortic valves are closed by a retrograde surge of blood, represented on the pressure pulse by the dicrotic notch (see Fig. 5–4). After the aortic valves snap shut, the arterial pressure gradually falls as blood flows out through the myriad of peripheral vascular networks. The rate at which the diastolic pressure falls is determined by the pressure at the end of the systolic interval, the rate of outflow through the peripheral resistances and the diastolic interval. If the next systole were delayed for 3 or 4 seconds, the arterial pressure would continue to fall, asymptotically approaching a level of about 10 mm. Hg. The minimal diastolic pressure is determined primarily by the total peripheral resistance and by the heart rate (Fig. 5–4). The pulse pressure (the maximum systolic minus the minimum diastolic pressure) is increased by the factors that increase systolic pressure and reduce diastolic pressure.

DISTORTION OF THE ARTERIAL PULSE DURING TRANSMISSION

The form of the arterial pressure pulse changes as it passes down the arterial tree (Figs. 5–3 and 5–4). The systolic wave becomes considerably higher, is more sharply peaked and falls abruptly; the gradual decline in central diastolic pressure becomes replaced by several damped oscillations. These changes in the form of the pulse have been variously attributed to (a) pressure waves reflected from the periphery[1] or from abdominal aortic branches,[2] (b) a damping transmission line,[3] (c) the resonant frequency and damping coefficient of the arterial walls[4] and (d) highly damped steady-state oscillations. Although the exact cause has not been completely determined, it is clear that the pulse pressure becomes progressively greater as the pulse traverses the major branches of the arterial tree, so that the systolic pressure peak in the femoral or brachial arteries reaches values as much as 15 to 20 mm. Hg higher than those in the central aorta.

It is important to recognize that an increase in systolic pressure, with an increase in both pulse pressure and mean pressure, can occur without a change in peripheral resistance by three different mechanisms: (a) increased stroke volume, (b) increased ejection rate and (c) reduced arterial distensibility. These factors can be exaggerated by the distortion of the pressure pulse during its transmission to the site of measurement at the brachial artery.

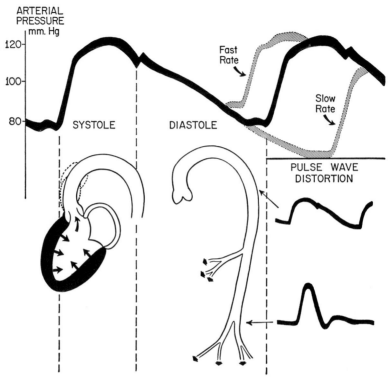

FIGURE 5-4   FACTORS AFFECTING SYSTOLIC AND DIASTOLIC ARTERIAL PRESSURE

The systolic pressure is determined primarily by the rate and volume of ventricular ejection in relation to the arterial distensibility. The diastolic pressure is determined by the rate of diastolic pressure drop (related to peripheral resistance) and the heart rate as it affects the duration of diastole. The pulse wave is distorted by damping and reflections as it travels along the arterial trunks such that the peak systolic pressure is higher and the diastolic pressure is flatter but the mean arterial pressure is only slightly less than at the arch of the aorta.

I. MEASUREMENT OF ARTERIAL PRESSURE

Measuring arterial blood pressure involves determining both the systolic and the diastolic pressure. These two pressure levels actually represent the excursions of the arterial pressure pulse at the point of measurement.

SPHYGMOMANOMETRY

Since the pulse waves rapidly spread through the arterial system and are modified to varying degrees, the arterial pressure at any instant varies throughout the arterial tree. Determinations of arterial pressure generally represent the maximal and minimal pressure of the pulse wave at the point of measurement.

The most accurate records of arterial pressure pulses are obtained through intra-arterial needles connected to suitable pressure recordings systems (see later). To reproduce the wave as it appears in the artery, the

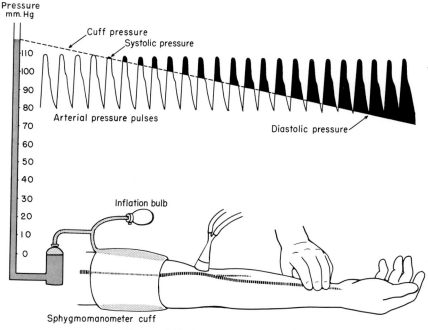

FIGURE 5-5 SPHYGMOMANOMETRY

When the pressure within the sphygmomanometer cuff is increased above arterial blood pressure, the arteries under the cuff are occluded and no pulse can be palpated at the wrist. As the cuff pressure is gradually released, the systolic peaks of pressure finally exceed cuff pressure and blood spurts into the arteries below the cuff, producing palpable pulses at the wrist. The sudden acceleration of blood below the cuff produces vibrations which are audible through a stethoscope. The pressure in the mercury manometer at the time the pulse is heard or felt indicates systolic pressure. As cuff pressure is further diminished, the sounds increase in intensity and then rather suddenly become muffled at the level of diastolic pressure where the arteries remain open throughout the entire pulse wave. At still lower pressures, the sounds disappear completely when laminar flow is re-established.

recording paper would have to move at the velocity at which the pulse travels past the needle (Fig. 5–3B). Since this is impractical, the records are generally obtained on paper moving relatively slowly, and the pulse waves are compressed in time (Fig. 5–5).

The arterial blood pressure is generally measured with a sphygmomanometer consisting of an inelastic cuff containing an inflatable rubber bag. The rubber bag is connected by rubber tubing to a rubber bulb and to a device which continuously records the pressure within the cuff (e.g., a mercury manometer, Fig. 5–5). When the cuff is snugly applied to the arm, inflation of the rubber bag compresses the tissues under the cuff. If the rubber bag is inflated to a pressure which exceeds the peak of the arterial pulse wave, the artery is continuously collapsed and no pulse wave can be palpated in the artery peripheral to the occlusion. If the pressure in the cuff is gradually reduced, a point will be reached at which the peak of the pulse wave slightly exceeds the pressure in the surrounding tissues and in the rubber bag (Fig. 5–5). At that level, the pulse becomes palpable and the pressure indicated on the mercury manometer is a measure of the peak of the arterial pulse or systolic pressure.

The spurt of blood flowing through the artery under the cuff rapidly accelerates the column of blood in the peripheral arterial tree, producing turbulence and distinctive sounds (Korotkoff sounds) which can be heard through a stethoscope applied over the artery just below the cuff. As the pressure in the cuff is reduced further, the difference between systolic pressure and cuff pressure progressively widens and the artery is open during a greater proportion of the time. In general, the quantity of blood surging under the cuff is similarly increased, and the sounds heard through the stethoscope tend to become louder. When the pressure in the cuff falls below the minimal pressure of the arterial pulse wave, the artery remains open continuously and the emitted sounds become muffled because the blood flows continuously and the degree of acceleration of the blood by the pulse wave is suddenly reduced. At still lower cuff pressures, the sounds disappear altogether as laminar flow is re-established.

Origins of Korotkoff Sounds.

In his original publication, Korotkoff[6] described two distinct types of sounds heard over the brachial artery as the pressure was reduced in a pressure cuff above the elbow. The first "short tones" appear with passage of part of the pulse wave under the cuff. With further fall in the pressure, the "systolic compression murmurs" are heard, which pass again into "tones (second)." An experimental analysis of the mechanisms of production of these sounds[7] indicated that the first "short tones" or tapping sounds were due to acceleration transients produced by abrupt arterial wall distension as a jet of blood surged under the cuff into the distal artery. The "compression sound" appeared to stem from the turbulent jet distal to the compressed arterial segment. Criteria for measurement of arterial pressure appear to be largely dependent upon the appearance of the acceleration transient (systolic pressure) and its disappearance to produce the characteristic muffling (diastolic pressure).

Sources of Error in Measuring Arterial Pressure.

Significant errors in arterial blood pressure readings result from improper selection or application of sphygmomanometer cuffs.[8, 9] The pressure which exists in the rubber bag is transmitted to the greatest depth at the center of the cuff. If the cuff is sufficiently wide and is properly adjusted, the pressure indicated by the manometer extends to the tissues immediately surrounding the artery (Fig. 5–6A). However, if the limb is too thick in relation to the width of the cuff, the pressure around the artery may be significantly less than that recorded from the rubber bag (Fig. 5–6B). Under these conditions, the cuff pressure required to collapse the artery must exceed the pressure which exists in the artery at that point. Thus, the systolic (and diastolic) pressure readings will be too high. If the cuff is loosely applied (Fig. 5–6C) so that the rubber bag must be partially inflated before it exerts pressure on the tissues, the area of contact is seriously reduced, corresponding to a very narrow cuff.

The Auscultatory Gap.

In some patients, the sounds emitted from the artery below the cuff disappear over a fairly large range in pressure between the systolic and diastolic pressures. The cause of this auscultatory gap is not known. If the cuff pressure is increased only to levels within the range of the auscultatory gap, the pressure at the lower end of this silent range may be mistaken for a normal systolic pressure when, in fact, the true systolic pressure is excessively high. Since the pulse wave persists in the

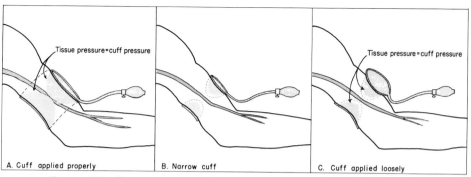

FIGURE 5-6   TRANSMISSION OF CUFF PRESSURES TO TISSUES OF THE ARM

A, When a sphygmomanometer cuff of sufficient width in relation to the diameter of the arm is properly applied, the tissue pressure around deep arteries under the cuff equals cuff pressure. However, pressure under the edge of the cuff does not penetrate as deeply as that under the center of the cuff.

B, A cuff which is too narrow in relation to the diameter of the limb does not transmit its pressure to the center of the limb. Under these conditions, the cuff pressure must greatly exceed arterial pressure to produce complete occlusion of the artery, and erroneously high systolic and diastolic pressures will be read from the mercury manometer.

C, If a cuff of sufficient width is applied too loosely, it becomes rounded before exerting pressure on the tissues and produces the same sort of error as a narrow cuff.

range of the auscultatory gap, this source of error can be eliminated by routinely checking systolic pressure by both the auscultatory and the palpatory methods (Fig. 5–5).

Mean Arterial Blood Pressure. Since the arterial blood pressure fluctuates during each cardiac cycle, the mean arterial pressure is often used in clinical and experimental reports. The arithmetic average of the systolic and diastolic pressures would be an accurate indication of the mean arterial perfusion pressure if the arterial pressure pulse were a true sine wave (see Fig. 5–7). However, the arterial pulse wave in no way resembles a sine wave and the arithmetic average of systolic and diastolic pressures is not an accurate expression of the mean pressure. The true mean arterial pressure can be determined by damping out the pulses or by integrating the arterial pulse wave on accurate records of the pressure pulse. Vertical lines are dropped from corres-

ponding points on arterial pulse waves to the zero pressure line. The arterial pressure pulses then correspond to a serrated upper border of a rectangular area. If the area enclosed by these lines, measured by means of a planimeter, is divided by the length of the horizontal base line (Fig. 5–7, line *L*), the quotient represents the vertical distance above the zero line (Fig. 5–7, line *H*) at which the mean arterial pressure lies. By this method the mean arterial pressure is usually about one third of the way between diastolic and systolic pressures but varies with the configuration of the arterial pulse wave.

CONTINUOUS RECORDING OF ARTERIAL BLOOD PRESSURE

Measurement of arterial blood pressures has long played an important role in cardiovascular research. Recent developments in cardiac catheterization and the pulse-contour method of

DETERMINATION OF MEAN ARTERIAL PRESSURE

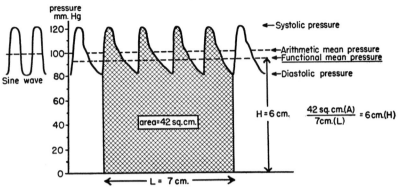

FIGURE 5-7 MEAN ARTERIAL PRESSURE

If the systolic pressure is 120 mm. Hg and the diastolic pressure 80 mm. Hg, the arithmetic mean pressure is 100 mm. Hg. If the arterial pulse wave were symmetrical (a sine wave), this value would represent the average perfusion pressure. However, the interval during which the arterial pressure is less than 100 mm. Hg is longer than that during which it is elevated above this level, so the functional mean pressure is less than 100 mm. Hg. The functional mean pressure is determined by dividing the area of the shaded region (area = 42 sq. cm.) by the horizontal dimension (L = 7 cm.) to determine the height of a rectangle having the same area (H = 6 cm.). The functional mean pressure tends to be higher than diastolic pressure by about one-third the pulse pressure, but this estimate does not apply to pulse waves having different contours, e.g., with changes in heart rate.

computing cardiac output have created widespread interest in accurately recording both pulmonary and systemic arterial pressures. Pressure transducers, suitable for recording the rapidly fluctuating arterial and intraventricular pressures, have certain essential requirements which should be understood by anyone who either uses them or wishes to appraise the multitude of clinical reports involving such equipment.

A mercury manometer is inadequate for recording pressures which fluctuate widely and rapidly, especially when the extremes of pressure are significant. The inertia of the fluid and the resistance to its flow into the manometer keep the fluid level from following the rapid changes in pressure. If a mercury manometer is connected directly to an artery through a hypodermic needle, the mercury column oscillates slightly above and below the mean pressure. The manometer obviously does not indicate the magnitude of either the systolic or the diastolic pressure. The same problem arises in measuring the widely fluctuating pressures in the ventricular cavities. Thus, more complicated apparatus is required to measure arterial and ventricular pressures accurately.

Rapidly fluctuating pressures can be accurately recorded only by apparatus with an adequate frequency response. The frequency response is a measure of the rate at which a recording system responds to a sudden change in pressure. The factors which determine the responsiveness of a pressure-sensitive device can best be described in terms of simple mechanical systems.

Mechanical Pressure Transducers. A common pressure transducer consists of a tambour with a rubber membrane coupled to a writing lever. If the rubber membrane is quite flaccid, very slight pressures will stretch the membrane and displace the writing lever

MECHANICAL RECORDERS

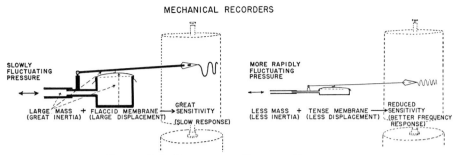

FIGURE 5-8 MECHANICAL PRESSURE RECORDERS

Pressure recording ordinarily involves the displacement of some type of elastic membrane. To displace the membrane, fluid must move into the recording capsule. The inertia of the fluid, the membrane and the recording mechanisms tends to resist displacement. When the moving mass is large and the membrane is flaccid, the recording system may be very sensitive to slowly fluctuating pressures, but will not respond to rapid changes in pressure. Reducing the moving mass and utilizing stiff membranes diminish sensitivity but improve the frequency response.

(Fig. 5–8). In response to an increased pressure, a considerable quantity of fluid must pass along the tubing and enter the tambour to produce a corresponding displacement of the membrane and writing lever. The inertia of the fluid and lever opposes a rapid response to a change in pressure, and the rubber membrane provides a relatively weak force to restore the fluid and lever to their original positions when the pressure is reduced. Clearly, such a system could not respond rapidly enough to follow the fluctuating arterial pressure. The natural frequency of a pressure transducer can be visualized in terms of a mass suspended on a spring. The smaller the mass and the stiffer the spring, the faster the oscillations which occur after a displacement from the rest position. When the mass of the fluid and of the lever is large in relation to the tension of the membrane, the oscillations are slow. If the rubber membrane is very tense, the frequency response is increased, but the sensitivity (deflection per unit of pressure) is correspondingly reduced. A more complete

description of different mechanical pressure transducers was presented by Green.[10]

Electrical Pressure Transducers. In this electronic age it is not surprising that slight movements of stiff membranes should be used to affect currents or voltages which can be amplified by electronic amplifiers. Various types of electronic pressure transducers are available in which movements of membranes produce changes in (*a*) resistance, (*b*) capacitance or (*c*) inductance (Fig. 5–9A, B, C). In each case, stiff membranes with small fluid displacement and relatively high frequency response can be used because the output signals can be amplified enough to activate recording galvanometers of various types.

No ideal pressure recording system exists. For any particular application the transducer, amplifier and recorder must be matched to obtain optimal performance. This process invariably involves compromise of sensitivity, convenience, stability or frequency response. The nature and significance of frequency response is

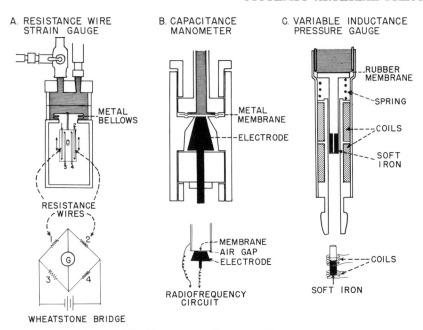

A. RESISTANCE WIRE STRAIN GAUGE

B. CAPACITANCE MANOMETER

C. VARIABLE INDUCTANCE PRESSURE GAUGE

FIGURE 5–9   ELECTRICAL PRESSURE TRANSDUCERS

A, The unbonded resistance wire strain gauge (Statham gauge) consists of a metal bellows which is compressed by increased pressure within the chamber. Downward displacement of the bellows is transmitted to a metal slide supported by four sets of strain-sensitive wires wound under tension and connected to form a Wheatstone bridge. Displacement of the metal slide stretches two sets of wires and relaxes the other two. These changes in resistance imbalance the bridge in proportion to the applied pressure. The resulting voltage output from the bridge is amplified and recorded by various means.

B, The electrical capacitance diaphragm manometer is a condensor formed by an electrode (black) separated from a stiff metal membrane by a carefully adjusted air gap. Displacement of the membrane changes the thickness of the air gap. This results in a change in capacitance which is recorded by a radio frequency circuit. (From Lilly.[11])

C, Variations in magnetic flux in two coils of wire can be produced by movements of an iron slug positioned within the coils. In a differential transformer pressure transducer, the iron slug is fastened to the center of an elastic membrane so that changes in pressure produce changes in magnetic flux. (From Gauer and Gienapp, *Science*, 1950, 112:404.)

widely misunderstood even by some individuals routinely engaged in physiologic recording.

The Frequency Response of Recording Systems. It is generally agreed that a high fidelity reproduction of a wave form can be recorded by a system which has a uniform response to the tenth harmonic of its fundamental frequency. With a heart rate of 240 beats per minute, the pulse frequency is 4 per second and the tenth harmonic of this frequency is 40 c.p.s. Such a high frequency response is deemed necessary if the most rapid changes in pressure during the pulse are to be faithfully recorded.

Although it is possible to determine the frequency response characteristics of the transducer, amplifier and galvanometer individually, it is more important to test the dynamic response of the entire system assembled for use. When the transducer is connected to a fluid-filled catheter or through tubing to a hypodermic needle, the frequency response of the gauge becomes greatly reduced. The fluid in the system represents a mass which must move with changes in pressure, and its inertia markedly reduces the frequency response of the gauge. When the diaphragm is displaced by an increased pressure, its elasticity must overcome the inertia of the entire mass of fluid within the connecting tubes. The mass of fluid can be reduced by using tubing of small caliber, but only at the price of increasing the frictional resistance to movement of fluid. Thus, some of the pressure energy is dissipated as friction in fluid within narrow tubes. Increasing the frictional resistance of a system is a form of "damping." Careful matching of the frequency response of the system with an optimal degree of damping can greatly improve the response characteristics (Fig. 5–10). Damping is attained by reducing the caliber of the catheter or tube, by locally constricting the tubing with a clamp or by inserting a short section of tube with appropriate caliber.

Virtually identical arterial and ventricular pulse contours have been obtained with damped systems having uniform response to 5, 30, and 50 c.p.s.[12] The frequency response and the degree of damping of any system should be routinely established by methods indicated in Figure 5–10. Such a procedure eliminates inaccurate records caused by temporary malfunction of the system. For example, a small bubble remaining in the tubing or gauge after it is filled with fluid reduces the frequency response of the system to very low levels because air is much more elastic than the diaphragm. Additional details regarding this most important topic may be found in an excellent discussion by Fry.[13]

Artifacts from the Movement of Cardiac Catheters. Pressures from within the heart and great vessels are frequently measured through long catheters. Owing to movements of the heart, the tip of the catheter may oscillate in time with the cardiac cycle. Such movements produce artifacts which are superimposed upon the pressure pulses and often attain amplitudes equivalent to 10 mm. Hg. These motion artifacts are much more prominent when recorded with high frequency systems and are largely eliminated by using an optimally damped system responding uniformly to 5 c.p.s.[14]

The systolic and diastolic values for arterial pressure can be obtained with reasonable accuracy by a system with low frequency response, but the very rapid changes in pressure are generally slurred. With increasing interest in the dynamic properties of ventricular ejection (see Figs. 3–17 and 3–18), the rates of change of pressure as indicated by the slopes are assuming great importance. For example, Shaper et al.[15] emphasized that the maximum rate of change of left ventricular pressure in a normal resting dog varies between about 2000 and 6000 mm. Hg/sec. and under the influence of epinephrine, the upslope can reach values as high as 15,000 mm. Hg/sec. The rates of changes of pressure and flow as judged by the slopes of high fidelity records are destined to become extremely important in evaluating the dynamic performance of the ventricular myocardium in health and disease. For such purposes, recording systems must have extremely high frequency responses with proper damping and with minimal artifacts. These results can best be achieved using miniature pressure transducers located at the very tip of a cardiac catheter. These are commercially available and their clinical application will become more widespread as their cost becomes more moderate with volume production.

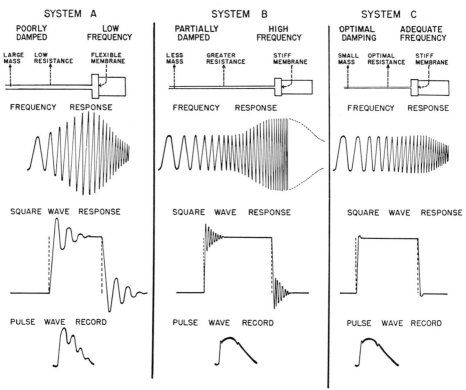

FIGURE 5-10   THE DYNAMIC RESPONSE CHARACTERISTICS OF PRESSURE RECORDING SYSTEMS

The response characteristics of a recording system should be carefully established and rechecked frequently.

System A has a large mass of fluid in a large caliber tube and a flexible membrane. Thus, the system is very sensitive to changes in pressure but is poorly damped. If fluctuating pressures of constant amplitude and progressively increasing frequency are applied to the end of the tube, the output from the system increases with higher frequencies up to the natural frequency of the system and then declines. The characteristics of the system can be more easily checked by suddenly raising or abruptly lowering the pressure (a square wave of pressure). In this particular system, the recorded deflection was considerably delayed in reaching the new pressure level (slow rise time). The deflection had considerable overshoot and oscillations persisted at the natural frequency of the system for a considerable time (poor damping). This system would be entirely unreliable for recording arterial pressure pulses.

System B has a stiff membrane and partial damping. Pressure waves of equal amplitude produced a response of uniform height over a considerable range of frequency. However, the deflections became exaggerated near the natural frequency of the system. In response to a square wave, the rise time was very short and the oscillations at the natural frequency of the system died down rather promptly. This system would be adequate for recording pressure pulses unless certain portions of the pulse had frequencies near the natural frequency of the system. The square wave response should be determined just before using such a system because a single small air bubble in the catheter or the gauge may so reduce the response characteristics that system B acts like system A.

In system C the membrane is more flexible than that in system B, but system C has been critically damped. In other words, the output from the system is uniform throughout a wide range of frequencies. A square wave of pressure produced a rapid response and a very slight overshoot, but no sustained oscillations. A critically damped system accurately reproduces arterial pressure pulses even though its uniform frequency response is limited to 20 or even 10 c.p.s. (From records presented by Lambert, E. H., and Jones, R. E.: *Proc. Staff Meet. Mayo Clin.*, 23:487–493, 1948.)

II. CONTROL OF SYSTEMIC ARTERIAL PRESSURE

A stabilizing mechanism must exert an overall regulation of systemic arterial pressure to prevent circulatory collapse when several major areas of the body simultaneously require increased blood flow. For example, running at full speed on a hot day after a full meal would theoretically require increased blood flow through active skeletal muscles, the skin and the gastrointestinal tract. If all these vascular beds suddenly dilated, the arterial blood pressure would drop precipitously and blood flow through vital organs (heart and brain) would be jeopardized.

medial surface where the sinus nerve arises. In this part of the media, the smooth muscle is almost completely replaced by elastic fibers and the adventitia is fairly dense. The sensory endings in the wall of the sinus have multiple branchings like a vine (Fig. 5-11). Impulses are set off at the very fine terminations, apparently by any type of distortion. The thinning of the media seen in the carotid sinus is believed to occur at other places where such distortion receptors lie, including

ARTERIAL STRETCH RECEPTORS (PRESSORECEPTORS)

The role of receptors in the walls of cardiovascular structures in the regulation of the circulation and respiration has been studied by many investigators,[16-20] whose work has been fully reviewed by Heymans and Neil.[21] The aortic depressor nerve was discovered by Cyon and Ludwig in 1866. Since then, a great deal of information has been gathered regarding the function of neural elements in the reflex regulation of the cardiovascular system.

CAROTID SINUS

At the bifurcation of the common carotid artery into the internal and external branches there is a local dilation of the very first portion of the internal carotid artery called the carotid sinus. It has a much thinner wall than other arteries of the same size because the smooth muscle in its media is relatively sparse, particularly on the ventro-

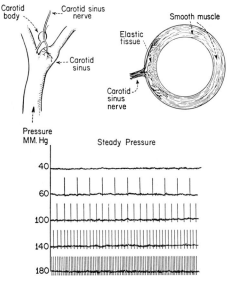

FIGURE 5-11   CAROTID SINUS STRETCH RECEPTORS

Nerve endings sensitive to stretch or distortion are located in the wall of a localized expansion at the origin of the internal carotid artery. At this site the walls contain an unusually large amount of elastic tissue and the smooth muscle of the media is somewhat deficient. Such an arrangement is particularly suited to the monitoring of pressure by these receptors, which discharge at greater and greater frequencies in response to increasing steady pressures, maintained artifically. (After Heymans and Neil.[21])

sites along the common carotid arteries, the aortic arch and the brachiocephalic artery.[21] Although these nerve endings are sensitive to any form of distortion of the wall in which they lie, they serve as pressure-sensitive elements since they are located in elastic segments of walls supporting high and fluctuating internal pressure. To be effective in regulation the receptors should monitor "absolute" arterial pressure. However, their sensitivity could theoretically be influenced by changes in the distensibility of the walls resulting from smooth muscle contraction or stiffening of the walls with aging.

Bronk and Stella[17] recorded the action potentials in single afferent nerve fibers from stretch receptors located in isolated and perfused carotid sinus. Within the sensitivity range of a receptor, an increase in distending pressure was associated with an increase in the frequency at which the receptor discharged impulses. One receptor may increase its discharge rate from zero to maximum frequency when the pressure ranges from 30 to 200 mm. Hg, and others may function within different ranges of pressure. The overlap of sensitivity between fiber groups assures responses from very low to very high pressures. If the isolated carotid sinus is distended with a steady pressure, the discharge frequency is also steady over a long period. In other words, the stretch receptors do not exhibit fatigue or adaptation. If the carotid sinus is distended by a fluctuating pressure, bursts of impulses occur during a rapid rise of pressure. Similar bursts of impulses appear during the abrupt increase in arterial pressure (Figs. 5–12 and 5–13). Thus, the discharge rate of the receptors is increased not only by the pressure in the artery but also by the rate of rise of pressure. The nerve

fibers from the stretch receptor endings in the carotid sinus travel by way of the glossopharyngeal (IXth) nerve and those from the aortic arch pass by way of the vagus (Xth) nerve to the "cardiovascular regulatory centers" in the medulla (see Fig. 3–4).

Pressoreceptor Reflexes. An increase in arterial pressure increases the rate of discharge from the stretch receptors. These impulses impinge upon the medullary centers to slow the heart by stimulating the motor nucleus of the vagus and inhibiting the "cardioaccelerator center," which acts through the cardiac sympathetic nerves. The increased sympathetic discharge also enhances atrial and ventricular contractility. At the same time, the medullary "vasoconstrictor center" is inhibited, so that the total peripheral resistance is reduced. Of all the potential mechanisms for changing peripheral resistance, the excitation or inhibition of the sympathetic vasoconstrictor outflow is the only one which has a demonstrated role in the control of arterial pressure.

Although the distortion receptors actually respond to stretch, the words "pressoreceptor" and "baroreceptor" are usually used to describe the reflexes induced by activation of these fibers. To avoid confusion, these terms will be employed in the following discussion with the reservation that they may eventually prove to be somewhat misleading.

Theoretically, the cardiovascular system can respond to an elevation in blood pressure with a reduction in heart rate, a reduction in stroke volume or a reduction in total peripheral resistance. In general, the vasomotor effects have been assigned the predominant role, and the protection of the arterial pressure level during hemorrhage has also been ascribed primarily to increased peripheral resist-

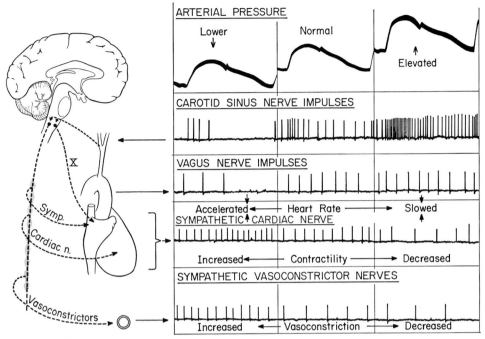

FIGURE 5-12   CAROTID SINUS REFLEXES

Single stretch receptors in the carotid sinus discharge at frequencies dependent upon the arterial pressure. When the arterial pressure is lower, the pressoreceptor impulse frequency diminishes, the vagus nerve impulses diminish and sympathetic cardiac nerve impulses increase (accelerating the heart) and the sympathetic vasoconstrictor fibers become more active and increase peripheral resistance. The net effect is to raise the blood pressure. If the arterial pressure rises above the normal set value, the impulse frequency increases on carotid sinus nerves, reducing the sympathetic discharge and increasing the vagal discharge. Slowing of heart rate and peripheral vasodilation restore the blood pressure to normal again.

ance. The growing tendency, however, is to recognize the importance of both cardiac output and peripheral resistance in such reactions. For example, Carlsten et al.[22] reported that direct stimulation of the carotid sinus nerve in man produced reflex bradycardia, peripheral dilation in the forearm and reduced pulse pressure — ascribed to reduced stroke volume. On the other hand, no baroreceptor effect on the pulmonary vascular system could be demonstrated.[23] This finding is consistent with the impression that the pulmonary vasculature is highly non-reactive to neural or humoral control mechanisms and does not participate in general systemic vascular responses (see Chapter 4).

The pressoreceptor mechanism illustrated in Figures 5–2, 5–12 and 5–13, acting alone, would appear to provide a simple and straightforward explanation for the maintenance of systemic arterial blood pressure within a very narrow range. Actually, the arterial pressoreceptors constitute only one of many different sources of potent influences on cardiovascular responses. Thus, the regulation of systemic arterial pressure must involve the net result of many interacting mechanisms.

Chemoreceptors. The carotid

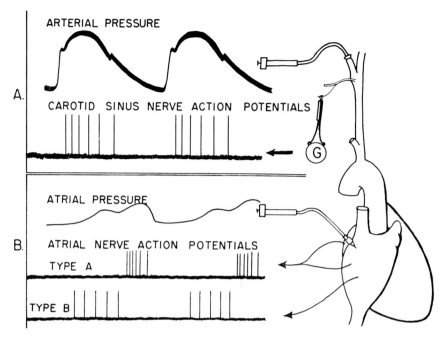

FIGURE 5-13   STRETCH RECEPTORS IN THE ATRIA AND CAROTID ARTERY

A, Individual stretch receptors in the carotid sinus discharge impulses at a frequency dependent primarily upon the arterial pressure (after Bronk and Stella[17]).

B, Stretch receptors from the atria have been divided into two groups: type A, which discharge during atrial systole, and type B, which discharge during atrial diastole (after Paintal[27]).

body, lying near the carotid bifurcation, is a reddish glomus structure which is profusely supplied with nerves and has one of the most active blood supplies in the body (equivalent to 2000 cc. per 100 gm. of carotid body tissue). The carotid bodies are stimulated by reduced oxygen, increased carbon dioxide and lowered pH in the arterial blood perfusing them. Conditions which stimulate the chemoreceptors lead to elevated systemic arterial pressure. These chemoreceptors are strongly stimulated by experimental occlusion of the carotid sinus, a fact which complicates studies of pressoreceptor mechanisms. Other chemoreceptors of similar nature are found near the aortic arch. Since the oxygen content and pH of arterial blood are diminished and its carbon dioxide content is increased only when the cardio-

vascular-pulmonary system is overtaxed or incompetent, such chemoreceptors probably have no function during normal conditions of rest. It may also be that they become involved in responses to activity only under extreme conditions.

STRETCH RECEPTORS AT VARIOUS SITES

In various experiments the results have suggested the presence of stretch receptors at many sites in the cardiovascular system including the descending thoracic aorta, abdominal vessels, cerebral vessels, lungs, atria and even the ventricular walls.[16, 24] Most of these receptors have not been implicated in the control of blood pressure. Thus, bradycardia reportedly follows distention of the left ventricular wall.[25] Rapid infusion of fluids into the systemic veins was once widely believed to be a mechanism for inducing tachycardia in association with increased venous return (Bainbridge reflex). Receptors suitable for such a response have not been found, and the original observations have not been consistently confirmed. In fact, acceleration, deceleration or no change in heart rate has recently been reported to result from intravenous infusions into isolated hearts, denervated hearts or hearts in intact animals.[26] In contrast, profound bradycardia and fainting responses, resembling the reactions induced by pressure applied to the carotid sinus in persons with hypersensitive carotid receptors, can be produced by mechanical stimulation of peripheral arteries and veins. Stretch receptors in the left atrium have been postulated as contributors to the control of blood volume. Paintal[27] has described the discharges from vagal afferent nerve fibers which fired during atrial contraction (A fibers) or during atrial filling (B fibers), as illustrated in Figure 5–13. A role for these impulses in hemodynamic regulation has not been demonstrated.

The complexity of the neural reflex mechanisms which may significantly affect the systemic arterial pressure under different conditions is illustrated in Figure 5–14. Included are the fibers from pressoreceptors and chemoreceptors, atrial afferent fibers and visceral afferents from the various organs within the abdomen and from the blood vessels throughout the body. Virtually all of these reflex actions induce lowered blood pressure and slow the heart rate. In contrast, application of cold or painful stimuli to the skin produce elevated blood pressure and tachycardia. Pathways from the higher centers of the nervous system also produce powerful vascular adaptations, associated with rage, embarrassment, fainting, and so forth. Practically all of these pathways descend through the medulla and reach the vascular system and the heart by way of the sympathetic outflow (Fig. 5–14B) plus the vagal distribution to the heart.

SUMMARY

A large number of factors and mechanisms *influence* the systemic arterial blood pressure. All the factors which affect cardiac function in terms of the heart rate, stroke volume and rate of ejection also affect the pulse pressure and, to some extent, the mean pressure. In general, the peak amplitude of the rise in systolic pressure is a manifestation of the rate and amount of systolic ejection by the left ventricle. In addition, the systemic arterial pressure is influenced by the peripheral resistance produced by all the neural, hormonal and chemical mechanisms discussed in Chapter 4. Finally, the wide variety of visceral and somatic afferent impulses converging on the medulla may significantly alter the level of the blood pressure.

Although all of these mechanisms are potentially capable of changing the blood pressure, none of them could be regarded as regulating it. Regulation of the blood pressure must involve a sensing mechanism (arterial pressoreceptors), an integrating mechanism (medullary or higher centers) and an effector mechanism (autonomic outflow), so that a deviation in arterial pressure is automatically compensated. So far as we know, only the pressoreceptor reflexes qualify as a regulatory mechanism. Such a mechanism is inherently static, tending to cause a re-

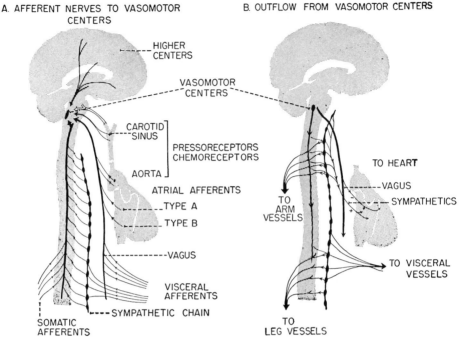

A. AFFERENT NERVES TO VASOMOTOR CENTERS

B. OUTFLOW FROM VASOMOTOR CENTERS

FIGURE 5-14   NEURAL MECHANISMS FOR PERIPHERAL VASCULAR CONTROL

A, The vasomotor centers in the medulla receive afferent impulses originating from many different areas in the body, including the higher centers of the nervous system, pressoreceptors from the heart and great vessels, afferent nerves from the viscera and somatic pain afferents.

B, Impulses discharged from the vasomotor centers descend the spinal cord and influence cell bodies in the intermediolateral cell column which in turn initiate sympathetic nerve impulses conducted to the blood vessels in all parts of the body.

turn to a particular level. Other factors (e.g., pain, cold, emotion) tend to produce a deviation of the blood pressure and are not known to have the sensing mechanisms required for stabilization. Whenever any of these factors causes a significant change in systemic arterial pressure, that factor must have been able to override, suppress or modify the pressoreceptor mechanism. The many mechanisms which can produce a deviation of the systemic arterial pressure from its baseline condition are unquestionably responsible for the great variation in blood pressure noted when it is repeatedly measured in one person. On the other hand, the potency of the pressoreceptor mechanism is displayed in the fact that, among most normal individuals, the blood pressure remains within a fairly circumscribed range with a fairly constant mean value. The causes of sustained variations in systemic arterial pressure should be considered from this point of view.

III. MECHANISMS OF ARTERIAL HYPOTENSION AND SHOCK

The control mechanisms which normally maintain systemic arterial pressure within a relatively narrow range despite wide variations in activity are necessarily complex. Insight into the many facets of arterial pressure regulation is provided by Figure 5–1. A failure of regulation producing low blood pressure is an important clinical problem.[28, 29] The branching representation of factors determining arterial pressure can also be employed to indicate various mechanisms which cause it to fall to abnormally low levels (right-hand column in Fig. 5–15).

The "primary" mechanisms can

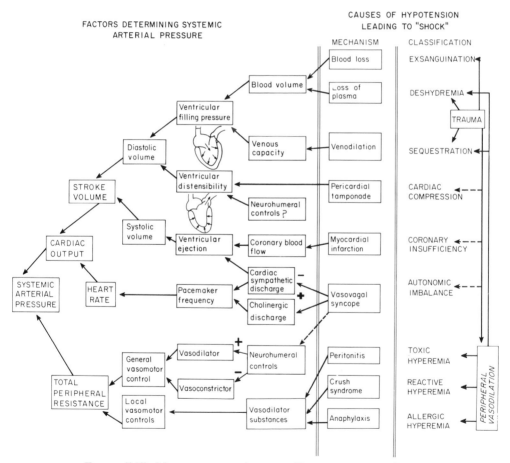

FIGURE 5-15   MECHANISMS OF ARTERIAL HYPOTENSION AND SHOCK

The various factors which determine systemic arterial pressure can be utilized as a framework for classifying causes of diminished blood pressure (hypotension) leading to a state called "shock." The mechanisms listed in the right hand column operate through the mechanisms listed to perturb the blood pressure equilibrium. Compensatory adjustments could occur theoretically at each branch point, indicating the complexity of responses even when only a single stimulus or disturbance initiated the lowered blood pressure.

affect the systemic arterial pressure only by undergoing changes that are not, or cannot be, balanced by the net effect of all the compensatory mechanisms in the chain extending from right to left in Figure 5–15. Viewed in this light, a change in any item listed under "causes of hypotension" can theoretically call forth either additive or compensatory effects among virtually all interacting factors in the chart. This does not, however, preclude identification of the initiating factors primarily responsible for the lowered blood pressure. If primary mechanisms of the sort illustrated in Figure 5–1 can ultimately be identified with specific clinical forms of shock, then an essential step in solving this complex problem can be taken by providing a group of tentative definitions of discrete forms of hypotension and shock. The classification of "shock" suggested on the right side of Figure 5–15 is intended to be only a first approximation as a basis for defining clinical disturbances of various origins.

EXSANGUINATION

The average human adult can lose somewhat more than 500 ml. of blood without significant cardiovascular disturbance, as judged by widespread experience at blood banks. If exsanguination is of such magnitude that the neural and hormonal controls fail to compensate fully, then the systemic arterial blood pressure will fall. Simple loss of blood accompanied by low blood pressure is insufficient evidence, however, to delineate exsanguination hypotension, because many people faint merely from the sight of blood. Effective criteria for the presence of exsanguination hypotension should include evidence for each step

in the functional chain of events leading from blood loss to systemic arterial hypotension in Figure 5–15. In addition, evidence for appropriate compensatory reactions should be demonstrable. Thus, a functional definition of exsanguination hypotension should include specified diminution in blood volume, ventricular filling pressure, diastolic volume, stroke volume and cardiac output. Evidence for compensatory peripheral vasoconstriction, tachycardia and increased systolic ejection (smaller end-systolic volume) would indicate that appropriate compensatory mechanisms were active.

Patients and experimental animals can survive for many hours with a mean systemic arterial pressure of 40 to 50 mm. Hg and quickly respond to restoration of the blood volume without ill effects. The term "exsanguination hypotension" should be reserved for the previously described pattern in which the blood pressure is stabilized at a low level (i.e., below a mean value of 60 mm. Hg). If the compensatory reactions begin to fail and the systemic arterial pressure is not sustained even after full restoration of the blood volume, the term "decompensating exsanguination hypotension" would appear appropriate (see *Vicious Circles in Terminal Circulatory Collapse*).

If the problem were really this simple, further research on the subject would not be needed. There is no assurance whatever that the functional definition of "exsanguination hypotension" indicated in Figure 5–15 is the correct or final one, but it is a more explicit and unique designation than is commonly employed. Some of the physiologic and semantic problems that appear during various forms of hypotension are described later.

DESHYDREMIA

The loss of large quantities of body fluids (i.e., due to cholera, burns, Addison's disease, water depletion and so forth) leads to a reduced plasma volume. Systemic arterial hypotension can also result from losses of plasma fluid into the tissues.[30] Deshydremic hypotension, characterized by increased blood viscosity and hematocrit level due to concentration of the blood cells and blood elements, theoretically can be distinguished from exsanguination hypotension with hemodilution by body fluids absorbed from the tissue spaces.

SEQUESTRATION

Nearly three fourths of the total blood volume is normally contained within the venules, venous channels and venous reservoirs. If the capacity of some large portion of the venous system suddenly increased, a substantial part of the total blood volume could be sequestered, producing effects corresponding to external blood loss. (The term sequestration is used here to denote a net increase in the quantity of blood contained within vascular channels through which forward flow may or may not persist.) For example, when a man stands, a substantial quantity of blood is displaced into his legs from the heart, lungs and upper portion of his body. During prolonged quiet standing (e.g., on parade ground) further accumulation of blood in the dependent vessels predisposes to a drop in systemic arterial pressure sufficient to cause fainting. However, sequestration of blood probably assumes far greater importance in the production of shock-like states by trauma, peritonitis or the crush syndrome (Fig. 5–15). In these conditions, sequestration probably occurs in capillaries and venules as well as in the veins and reservoirs. Lacking suitable methods of determining the amount of blood contained in various regions of the body, information concerning the incidence, significance and quantitative contribution of this mechanism is woefully inadequate.

TRAUMA

"Trauma" is a nonspecific term, and the effects of injury are so widespread and diverse that no single functional mechanism could reasonably be labeled as an initiating cause of the resulting hypotension. If blood escapes from the vascular system into the tissues or outside the body, the blood volume is diminished. Damage to capillaries may lead to loss of plasma into the tissues. Vascular distention and hyperemia in injured parts lead to sequestration of blood. In addition, hemopericardium can produce ventricular compression in some instances. Autonomic controls to heart and peripheral vessels may be disturbed by massive discharge in somatic and visceral afferent nerves. Finally, vasodilatation in the injured tissues should tend to reduce peripheral resistance. These mechanisms could contribute in various degrees to systemic arterial hypotension following injury.

CARDIAC COMPRESSION

Rapid collection of blood or fluid within the pericardial sac can be viewed as interfering with ventricular distention and preventing normal ventricular diastolic filling. Theoretically, extracardiac compression diminishes the diastolic and systolic ventricular volumes, reduces the stroke volume and lowers the cardiac output in spite of tachycardia. Systemic arterial hypotension develops when the drop in cardiac output is not adequately compensated by increased total peripheral resistance. Although pericardial tamponade may exert its effects through the same final pathway as exsanguination and sequestration, the distinction can be readily made. The total blood volume is essentially normal, and the central venous pressure should be elevated in the presence of extracardiac compression.

CORONARY INSUFFICIENCY

Acute myocardial infarction may produce severe or fatal systemic arterial hypotension by mechanisms indicated in Figure 5–15. Acute interference with the blood supply to a substantial area of the myocardium reduces ventricular ejection and the stroke volume. The infarcted myocardium not only fails to contribute to ejection, but actually expands during systole so that the effectiveness of the remaining myocardium is reduced. Under these conditions the cardiac output could be reduced in spite of increased ventricular volume and tachycardia. A full blown clinical picture of shock may then appear as compensatory mechanisms are activated in response to diminished systemic arterial blood pressure.

AUTONOMIC IMBALANCES

The sympathetic division of the autonomic nervous system directly affects the stroke volume by acting on the myocardium, affects the heart rate by acting on the pacemaker and affects the total peripheral resistance by acting on the peripheral vessels. Severe depression of arterial pressure resulting from autonomic imbalance is characterized by bradycardia and regional vasodilatation (e.g., in skeletal muscle), as though the normal baroreceptor reflexes were depressed or overridden.

The well-known syncopal reactions to carotid sinus pressure, intense visceral afferent pain or unpleasant sights exhibit transient bradycardia with peripheral vasodilatation in muscle beds. Transient autonomic imbalance frequently produces brief loss of consciousness but rarely leads to prolonged hypotension or the typical symptoms of shock. Severe disturbances of the central nervous system (e.g., head injury) may produce a shock-like state characterized by prolonged systemic arterial hypotension. The exact mechanism involved is not clear, but the importance of depression of the central nervous system in the terminal events of various kinds of shock is discussed later.

PERIPHERAL VASODILATATION

A reduction in the total peripheral resistance could be the primary mechanism producing hypotension in a number of clinical conditions. For example, peritonitis, crush injury and anaphylaxis are all characterized by extreme vasodilatation. The expected compensatory reaction to vasodilatation in one portion of the vascular system would be an appropriate increase in cardiac output, as in exercise, and vasoconstriction in other vascular areas. Severe arterial hypotension produced solely by net peripheral vasodilatation would signify that the level of cardiac output was insufficient to balance the vasodilatation. In other words, these clinical conditions should be accompained by extreme tachycardia and increased cardiac output. Sustained reduction in arterial pressure from lowered total peripheral resistance indicates either massive vasodilatation, limited compensatory vasoconstriction, or interference with a full increase in cardiac output.

VARIATIONS IN THE COURSE AND TERMINATION OF HYPOTENSION

Theoretically, effective elimination of the factor or factors that initiated the systemic arterial hypotension should be promptly followed by a return of the blood pressure to normal levels and restoration of good health. For example, exsanguination can produce an arterial hypotension lasting many hours and can be followed by a prompt return of the blood pressure to normal by restoration of the shed blood. Experience has shown, however, that most types of hypotension may be of sufficient degree and duration that deterioration and death may occur even after the apparent initiating factors are removed. Thus the condition of patients or animals suffering from protracted exsanguination hypotension may improve only transiently following restoration of the blood volume. The blood pressure returns to normal briefly and then gradually falls despite all efforts to maintain blood volume, peripheral resistance and cardiac output. This condition has been called "irreversible" shock, but should probably be considered as a group of separate entities. Just as there are many different factors capable of initiating hypotension and shock, so there are many different terminal mechanisms or pathways leading to death. An experimental example will illustrate this concept. In a healthy alert dog the mean arterial pressure was reduced to 45 mm. Hg by allowing blood to flow from the femoral artery into a reservoir slowly at first and then more rapidly (Fig. 5–16). After 2 hours about 300 ml. of blood had spontaneously returned into the dog at the same low arterial pressure. This autoinfusion was a signal of beginning cardiovas-

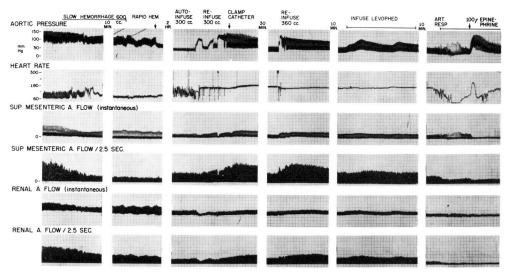

FIGURE 5-16 EFFECTS OF EXSANGUINATION

Continuous measurements of aortic pressure, heart rate and splanchnic blood flow in an intact, unanesthetized dog illustrate the effects of exsanguination (see Fig. 5–15) during a two hour period. During the period following "autoinfusion," the dog was on the brink of death from three different causes: (a) progressive fall in arterial pressure, despite restoration of blood volume, (b) respiratory arrest and (c) severe bradycardia. This example illustrates that circulatory collapse can occur from many mechanisms as suggested in Figure 5–15.

cular deterioration. An additional 300 ml. of blood was forceiably reinfused, and the femoral catheter was clamped at the time indicated by the abrupt widening of the arterial pulse pressure. The arterial pressure fell progressively for 30 minutes, when the last (360 ml.) of the shed blood was reinfused. The decline persisted, but the pressure was transiently raised by the infusion of levarterenol (Levophed), without which the animal would have died from the progressive fall in pressure. Abruptly respiration ceased, but death of the animal was prevented by artificial respiration. After ventilation had been restored, the heart rate suddenly slowed, and death would surely have ensued from bradycardia had not the arterial pressure been rapidly elevated by a heroic dose of epinephrine.

The sequence of events illustrated in Figure 5–16 is representative of the common observation that the terminal patterns and final causes of death are quite variable. Prompt remedial action postponed death from one mechanism only to be followed by a different threat. In effect the animal was on the brink of death from three different causes in rapid succession: (a) progressive fall in arterial pressure in spite of restoration of blood volume and vasopressor agents, (b) respiratory arrest and (c) severe bradycardia.

Respiratory arrest might result from severe cerebral depression as indicated by other manifestations of impaired function of the brain. The animals generally remained responsive and alert until they began to exhibit autoinfusion and other signs of circulatory deterioration. Then they became unresponsive, appeared to lose consciousness and frequently exhibited depressed or absent corneal and pupillary reflexes. Severe bradycardia was a fairly common terminal event.

DEPRESSION OF CENTRAL NERVOUS SYSTEM IN TERMINAL STATES

Subnormal responsiveness or unconsciousness with sluggish reflexes has been regularly manifest when animals began to display autoreinfusion, abrupt bradycardia or respiratory arrest. In two dogs fully equipped with instruments, electrodes were chronically implanted at sites in the diencephalon where stimulation produced exorbitantly elevated heart rate and blood pressure. In these two dogs, the diencephalic sites were stimulated repeatedly during exsanguination hypotension produced in the standard manner. When autoinfusion and depression of reflexes developed, the same stimulus strength produced greatly attenuated cardiovascular response. In one of these animals, systemic arterial pressure was restored by levarterenol; the animal then lifted his head and looked around. The corneal reflex again became active and stimulation of the diencephalon again produced a response as large as during the control period. These observations were interpreted as indicating that depression of the central nervous system may be important during the terminal stages of shock, confirming the views of Ossipov[31] and Kovách and Takács.[32] The observed depression could actually occur anywhere along the relatively direct pathway from the point of stimulation to the effectors.

VICIOUS CIRCLES IN TERMINAL CIRCULATORY COLLAPSE

A reduction in blood flow through virtually all tissues is a natural result of a greatly lowered systemic arterial pressure (Fig. 5–17A). The reduced arterial pressure correspondingly di-

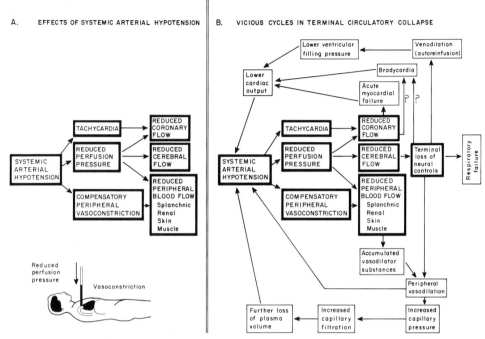

FIGURE 5-17 SYSTEMIC ARTERIAL HYPOTENSION WITH VICIOUS CYCLES

A, Some functional effects of compensation to systemic arterial hypotension include reduced coronary and cerebral blood flow as well as reduced peripheral blood flow through important visceral organs.

B, Severe and prolonged hypotension can induce vicious cycles which tend to further depress cardiac output or to induce vasodilation rendering the hypotension progressively more intractable.

minishes the arteriovenous perfusion gradient. Lower perfusion pressure tends to slow up vascular flow in every tissue, in some more than in others. The cerebral blood flow would be diminished by this mechanism primarily. In addition, a compensatory response to hypotension is a generalized vasoconstriction induced by baroreceptor reflexes. Thus, flow through the splanchnic bed, kidney, muscles and skin may be greatly curtailed. A compensatory tachycardia might also contribute to a reduction in coronary flow. No tissue would be fully spared from a diminution of blood flow.

The blood supply to the central nervous system should be adversely affected by a reduction in arterial pressure because the cerebral circulation is not very responsive to diminished blood flow. Cerebral vasodilatation is difficult to produce experimentally by neural, hormonal or chemical means except for moderate effects from increased carbon dioxide content of the blood. Thus, the cerebral blood flow is generally regarded as dependent primarily upon the perfusion pressure. A pronounced reduction in mean arterial pressure should therefore produce a corresponding reduction in cerebral blood flow (Fig. 5–17).

Respiratory arrest might result from cumulative effects of inadequate cerebral blood flow producing failure of the respiratory control centers (Fig. 5–17). On the other hand, the autoreinfusion may represent a release of the venoconstrictor tone that had caused compensatory shrinkage of venous channels and reservoirs. The relaxation of these channels could increase the capacity of the venous system and thus further diminish ventricular filling pressure and cardiac output. Abrupt appearance of bradycardia (Fig. 5–16) might signal serious autonomic imbalance from depression of the nervous system. The combined effect of lowered perfusion pressure and tachycardia could lead to acute myocardial failure with a further drop in cardiac output and lower arterial pressure.

Loss of neural controls could be expressed as a release of compensatory vasoconstriction. The resulting reduction in peripheral resistance would directly diminish arterial pressure without a further reduction in cardiac output. The compensatory constriction in peripheral vessels could be sufficiently severe and prolonged to curtail drastically flow through many vascular beds. Chemical vasodilators could accumulate and finally reach levels high enough to overcome the constrictor tone by a mechanism resembling reactive hyperemia.

The cardiovascular control could deteriorate by mechanisms like those illustrated in Figure 5–17 despite efforts at combating them. Determination of the pathways of circulatory collapse would depend upon appropriate measurements on patients in these final stages of shock. Although the difficulties involved in collecting such data are extremely severe, they must be circumvented before rational methods of therapy can be based on a full understanding of appropriate physiologic mechanisms.

SUMMARY

The first step in analyzing any clinical problem must be the identifica-

tion and precise definition of the entity. An adequate definition must be based on accurate and quantitative description in terms of crucial variables. Since many of the essential variables can be measured or estimated on patients, shock can be approached in a series of logical steps for each type:

1. A discrete clinical condition currently classified under the term "shock" could be identified.

2. A specific and unique name and definition of this condition could be derived by direct and quantitative measurements of variables such as those represented in Figure 5–15.

3. The initiating factors would become apparent from these measurements.

4. The compensatory reactions that are inadequate should be distinguished from responses that are inappropriate.

5. With this knowledge at hand, a suitable model of the circulatory disturbance could be evolved and validated by quantitative measurements in experimental analysis.

6. Appropriate therapy of the defined condition could then be based on knowledge of the nature of the basic disturbance. Obviously, treatment that would effectively correct the fundamental defect from extravasation or anaphylaxis might be dangerous if applied to a patient with myocardial infarction.

7. The terminal events in fatal shock-like states can be regarded as a group of potential vicious circles that may have no obvious connection with the original cause of the systemic arterial hypotension. Effective therapy during the final stages of circulatory deterioration requires a great deal more knowledge regarding the various mechanisms of circulatory collapse than we now possess.

IV. CAUSES OF HIGH BLOOD PRESSURE (HYPERTENSION)

The cardiovascular system is equipped with a simple pressure regulating mechanism of the sort illustrated in Figure 5–2. Theoretically, such a system should ensure prompt compensation for any change in blood pressure. Such extreme stability of the systemic arterial pressure is achieved consistently in animals and men under surgical anesthesia. Under these conditions, the systemic arterial pressure remains remarkably constant over extended periods of time unless the level of anesthesia changes or external influences are introduced. The same situation is achieved in decerebrate animals, indicating that an important source of fluctuation in systemic arterial pressure stems from overriding or "resetting" of the regulating system by higher levels of the nervous system.

In normal human subjects, systemic arterial pressure diminishes more than 20 mm. Hg during sleep, reaching a minimum at 3:00 or 4:00 A.M.[33] The "basal" blood pressure has been defined as the arterial pressure present when all physical, emotional and metabolic activities are reduced to a physiologic minimum. This state is rarely achieved, so the "basal" blood pressure has been approximated with measurements made before the subject arises from a good night's sleep. This, too, is difficult to accomplish routinely, so many investigators collect their data on patients who have reclined quietly in a comfortable, soothing environment for at least 30 minutes, ten to twelve hours after the previous meal. Even under these conditions a single determination of systemic arterial pressure is almost meaningless because of fluctuations, so that average values from repeated measurements must be used. The emotional reaction to the act of recording the blood pressure can be alleviated by measuring blood pressure repeatedly for half an hour.[34] The difficulties involved in obtaining reproducible "basal" blood pressure values have been stressed to indicate how much caution must be used in interpreting the "casual" blood pressure recorded routinely in a physician's examining room or in a hospital.

VARIABILITY IN SYSTEMIC ARTERIAL PRESSURE

In addition to emotions, expressed or repressed, a great many factors affect the systemic arterial pressure. A complete list is beyond the scope of this book, so a few examples will have to suffice.

1. Technical Errors. The values obtained by sphygmomanometry may be in error for a number of reasons including the width of the cuff, the method of applying it, the position of the arm in relation to heart level, the rate of pressure release and the subjective nature of the end points (see Fig. 5–6).

2. Posture. Assumption of the erect posture usually produces a transient reduction in systolic pressure and a more sustained increase in diastolic pressure, with a reduction in pulse pressure (see Chapter 7).

3. Exercise. Physical exertion generally induces an increase in both systolic and pulse pressures. These increases may persist for varying periods after the termination of the exertion (see also Chapter 8).

4. Eating. Ingestion of a large

meal is usually followed by a significant increase in systolic pressure.

5. Diurnal Variation. From early morning until dinner time, the blood pressure tends to rise progressively by about 15 to 20 mm. Hg.

6. Temperature. In warm weather the blood pressure tends to diminish somewhat.

7. Race. Chinese, Filipinos, Puerto Ricans, East Africans, Indians, Arabs and aboriginal Australians seem to have lower blood pressure than do North American or Western European peoples.

8. Weight. The blood pressure tends to increase with greater body weight. The incidence of patients with "high" blood pressure is greater among groups that are overweight.

9. Sex. The blood pressure is lower among women under 40 years of age and higher in women over 50 years of age than in men in the corresponding age groups.

10. Age. Both systolic and diastolic arterial pressures increase with age, so that different standards must be established for the various age groups (see Figure 5–18).

Additional discussion of these factors appears in the excellent texts by Master et al.,[33] Smirk,[34] Pickering[35] and Page.[36]

HOW HIGH IS HIGH?

The "normal" arterial blood pressure is commonly said to be 120/80 mm. Hg. This statement is clearly meaningless from a practical point of view if one considers all the causes of variability listed previously and described in the first part of this chapter (see also Chapter 4). The commonly accepted upper limit for normal blood pressure, 140/90 mm. Hg, has been established largely by life insurance companies during the past four decades. Actually, single values for the upper limits of systolic and diastolic pressure are unacceptable because they fail to take into account the sources of variability.

The problem of physiologic variability is most effectively approached by statistical methods, based on frequency distribution. Master and his colleagues[33] proposed new and broader limits for the range of normal blood pressure after studying 15,706 persons in 11 industrial plants. A frequency distribution curve of diastolic and systolic pressures was established for each five-year group of men and women. A sample frequency distribution for men 40 to 44 years old is shown in Figure 5–18A. The mean value for systolic pressure was 130 mm. Hg. The normal range was arbitrarily set to include 40 per cent of the subjects above and 40 per cent of the subjects below the mean. By definition, 80 per cent of the population was considered "normal." The borderline range included the next 7.5 per cent of all observations, and the remaining values (2.5 per cent) above the borderline were regarded as "abnormally high blood pressure." Note that this partitioning arbitrarily defines "high blood pressure" as the values found in the top 2.5 per cent of each group in Figure 5–18. The ranges of "normal," "borderline" and "abnormal" for men are presented in Figure 5–18; the ranges for women are quite similar.

The progressive rise in mean values and borderline ranges in the older age groups is interpreted as a tendency for blood pressure to increase with age. However, some individuals may have little or no increase in systemic arterial pressure with advancing age, and others may develop high pressures more rapidly than indicated by these figures. Pick-

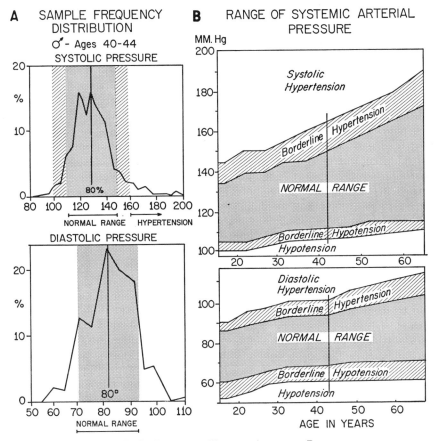

FIGURE 5-18   RANGE OF NORMAL ARTERIAL PRESSURE

   A, In males age 40 to 44, the normal arterial blood pressure is generally described in terms of range of values which will include a major portion of normal subjects (80 per cent in this graph). The "normal systolic pressure range" extends from 110 to 150 mm. Hg. Abnormal blood pressure is defined as extending above and below some borderline range.

   B, Assembling the frequency distributions for various age groups demonstrates a distinct tendency for broadening of the normal systolic and diastolic pressure ranges and a tendency for higher pressures in older people. This fact must be considered in defining "high blood pressure" or hypertension.

ering[35] directed attention to the fact that the individuals with high blood pressure represent only the upper end of the frequency distribution curves and not a separate group or population. He also presented observations indicating that when high blood pressure had existed for a long time, it is not necessarily completely reversed when the original causative lesion is removed. This led him to query whether hypertension tends to produce persistent changes in vascular walls.

   Since the mean systemic arterial pressure increases with age in a sample population, the number of people with blood pressures over some arbitrary level (e.g., 140/90 mm. Hg) is very great indeed. In many persons the blood pressure fluctuates more widely and tends to rise more rapidly than in the general population. In a small percentage of these people, elevation of blood pressure is obviously or suggestively associated with a recognizable disease state. However, in a vast majority of them the development of "hypertension" cannot be explained at present. In this last large category the elevated blood pressure is called "primary" or "essential" hypertension, signifying that it seems to arise without a distinctive or recognizable cause.

HYPERTENSION ASSOCIATED WITH SPECIFIC DISEASE PROCESSES

Elevated systemic arterial pressure is not a disease state; it is one sign (among many) which is common to a variety of physiologic and pathologic conditions. From the vast pool of individuals displaying this sign, a few patients may be identified in whom the elevated arterial pressure is the direct result of a specific cause and can be alleviated by removal of that cause (Fig. 5–19). A rare form of tumor consisting of chromaffin cells like those in the adrenal medulla (pheochromocytoma) provides an exceptionally good example.

ADRENAL GLAND DYSFUNCTION

Pheochromocytoma. Chromaffin cells in the adrenal medulla and elsewhere in the body normally secrete norepinephrine and *l*-epinephrine. When chromaffin cells multiply to produce a tumor or adenoma, these catechol amines are released periodically into the circulating blood to produce bouts of severe symptoms consisting of mounting hypertension, palpitation, headaches, anxiety and tremor, nausea, vomiting, blanching and coldness of the skin—in short, the signs and

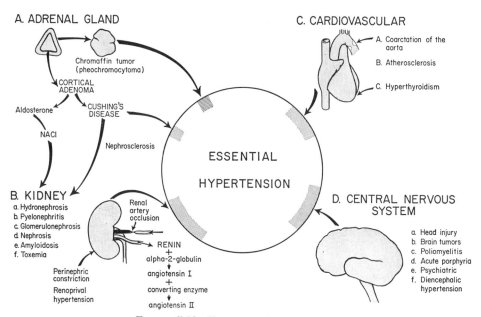

FIGURE 5-19   ESSENTIAL HYPERTENSION

Elevation of the systemic arterial pressure is a common feature in many different disease processes involving the adrenal glands, kidneys, brain and cardiovascular system (see text). Of the very large population with elevated systemic arterial pressure, only a small proportion have these specific disease processes. The very large remainder are defined as having "essential hypertension" which means that its cause is undetermined.

symptoms of a massive release of sympathetic transmitter substances. The blood pressure is elevated intermittently and tends to return toward normal in the intervals between attacks. These attacks may last for minutes or days and induce severe exhaustion. In some patients the blood pressure fluctuates widely but remains persistently elevated. The signs, symptoms, duration, course, diagnostic tests and treatment are discussed in detail elsewhere[34-36] and will not be considered here. Suffice to say that complete removal of the chromaffin tumor abolishes the symptomatic attacks. In some patients in whom the attacks have been eliminated by surgery, the systemic arterial pressure remains elevated for reasons which are not at all clear. The persistence of elevated blood pressure after elimination of its cause leads to the concept that hypertension begets hypertension (see later).

Adrenal Cortical Tumors. Changes in the blood pressure are consistently observed in patients with diseases affecting the adrenal cortex. For example, hypertension occurs in about 85 per cent of patients with Cushing's syndrome—an adrenogenital syndrome resulting from excessive secretion of adrenocortical hormones and consisting of sexual precocity, hemaphroditism, virilism of females or feminization in males and obesity. The elevated blood pressure is the most important cardiovascular manifestation of the disease. The incidence of hypertension is also high in patients with cortical adenomata but without the other signs of Cushing's syndrome.[34] At present it is impossible to identify the abnormality in cortical steroid metabolism which is responsible for the hypertension. Administration of desoxycorticosterone acetate (DOCA) produces hypertension in rats; the hypertensive effect of this hormone is accentuated by the administration of salt.[37] The same results can be achieved in human subjects. As might be expected, diminished function of the adrenal cortex (Addison's disease) is characterized by diminished systemic arterial pressure.

The potentiating effect of sodium chloride administered along with adrenal cortical hormones suggests a role for aldosterone in the induction of hypertension. Aldosterone, one of the steroid hormones normally excreted by the adrenal cortex, acts on the kidney tubules to induce retention of sodium and accelerated excretion of potassium. A few patients with primary aldosteronism resulting from tumors of the adrenal cortex have been described, and in most of them the systemic arterial pressure was above normal levels. Moser and Goldman[38] summarized a sequence following the narrowing of a main renal artery producing decreased perfusion pressure in the affected kidney and a release of renin from specialized cells within the afferent glomerular arteriole (juxtaglomerular apparatus). Renin acts on a protein substrate to produce angiotensin I which is converted into angiotensin II by an activator or converting enzyme. Angiotensin II stimulates the adrenal cortex to elaborate aldosterone which in turn causes retention of sodium and water, adding to the increase in blood pressure by a volume effect. This postulate is mentioned to indicate the degree of complexity one may encounter in such a biological control system as blood pressure regulation.

The precise mechanism by which salt excess might be linked to the development of systolic hypertension remains obscure. No single hypothesis satisfactorily explains the many conflicting observations. For example, in rats fed very large quantities of sodium chloride there is an elevation of blood pressure which correlates well with the percentage of sodium chloride in the diet.[39] Furthermore, the pathologic changes seen in rats with severe salt-induced high blood pressure resembled those observed in human patients with malignant hypertension, and the life expectancy of the animals was materially reduced. However, administration of potassium chloride along with the excess sodium chloride ameliorated the hypertension and pathologic changes, extending the life expectancy. Whereas most patients with excessive production of aldosterone exhibit elevated systemic arterial pressure, those who experience intermittent aldosteronism associated with periodic paralysis are no more susceptible to hypertension than the population at large. To confound the problem even more, hypertension can also be induced by administration of the cortical hormones which influence metabolism of glucose rather than salt, and this effect may actually be enhanced if the salt intake is reduced. Skelton[40] demonstrated that hypertension can be induced in the presence of hypofunction of the adrenal gland. For example, if one adrenal gland is excised and the medulla and most of the cortex is removed from the other, hypertension is more readily induced during the regeneration of the cortical tissue than when the regenerating gland is removed.

The kidney obviously plays an important role in the action of mineralocorticoids and in the retention or elimination of electrolytes. Thus, it is not possible to dissociate the adrenal cortical effects from kidney function. Furthermore, administration of excessive amounts of such cortical hormones leads to widespread lesions in arterial walls within the kidney (nephrosclerosis) and pathologic degeneration of renal substance. Such changes are also prominent in Cushing's disease. Attention has therefore been directed to participation of the kidneys in provoking elevated systemic arterial pressure.

KIDNEY DISEASES

More than 100 years ago Richard Bright recognized a relation between protein in the urine and pathologic changes in the kidney with hypertrophy of the left ventricle attributable to changes in the "quality" or composition of the blood which led to constriction of the small vessels. This remains a fair description of increased peripheral resistance associated with altered kidney function.

The systemic arterial pressure is elevated during a wide variety of kidney diseases—in fact nearly all. A few of these disorders are indicated in Figure 5–19.

Interference with the arterial blood supply to the kidney or external compression of the renal parenchyma may be associated with elevated systemic arterial pressure. For example, the systemic arterial pressure may increase in patients with unilateral obstruction of the renal artery or its branches. Such lesions are commonly caused by encroachment upon the arterial lumen by local mural thickening (atherosclerosis) or by local constriction of the vessel. In a majority of such patients, successful elimination of the obstruction or excision of the affected kidney is curative. Such recovery provides strong evidence that the kidney itself is involved in the production of this form of hypertension. The number of patients with these disorders is relatively small, but they represent the counterpart in man of the experimental hypertension which Goldblatt produced years ago by graded constriction of the renal arteries of animals. It is now generally agreed that any mechanism which interferes with the blood supply to the renal parenchyma may be expected to cause elevation of systemic arterial pressure.

The renal pressor mechanism is believed to be activated by many different forms of kidney disease, most of which can be presumed to disturb renal blood flow by one means or another. Included among these disorders are hydronephrosis, pyelonephritis, glomerulonephritis, nephrosis, amyloidosis and toxemia of pregnancy. For example, obstruction of the ureter (e.g., by kidney stones) leads to expansion of the pelvis and compression of the kidney parenchyma. Pyelonephritis is stated to produce obliteration and destruction of the medium-sized renal arteries; atherosclerotic occlusion of the renal arteries may or may not be complicated by pyelonephritis. Glomerulonephritis, an inflammatory reaction in the kidney usually following streptococcal infections, causes obstruction of glomerular capillaries.

By a different mechanism, excision of both kidneys leads to a severe increase in systemic blood pressure. This increase is best demonstrated when the survival of experimental animals is being supported by means of artificial kidneys. This form of hypertension ("renoprival" hypertension) is distinctly different from that produced by the renin mechanism and is probably more closely related to the electrolyte metabolism normally involving both the kidneys and the adrenal cortical hormones. Such hypertension may be encountered in terminal states of renal disease.

CARDIOVASCULAR HYPERTENSION

Systemic arterial pressure may rise as a result of changes within the cardiovascular system itself. The cardiovascular disorders causing elevated blood pressure are exemplified by coarctation of the aorta, generalized atherosclerosis of the systemic arteries and periarteritis nodosa (Fig. 5–19).

Near the site of the ductus arteriosus a constriction of the thoracic aorta occasionally occurs as a developmental defect. This local constriction reduces the lumen of the aorta to a very small channel and greatly impedes the flow of blood from the arch to the descending thoracic aorta. Collateral channels develop around this obstruction, but blood pressure is usually far above normal in the systemic arteries arising above the constriction. In the past, this hypertension in the upper part of the body was attributed to interference with the blood supply to the kidneys, as indicated in the preceding section. However, an occasional patient develops such an obstruction below the renal arteries and still displays hypertension.[34] Moreover, the diastolic pressure in the lower extremities may be higher than normal. Surgical correction of the aortic constriction is followed by a prompt fall of blood pressure, which returns to normal over a few days.

DISEASES OF THE CENTRAL NERVOUS SYSTEM

Elevated blood pressure is associated with diverse pathologic and functional disturbances of the central nervous system such as head injury, brain tumors, selective destruction of brain tissue as in rare cases of poliomyelitis, acute porphyria, psychiatric disturbances, cardiovascular hyperreaction and disturbances of the pressoreceptor mechanism (Fig. 5–19). This list by itself indicates that hypertension can result from damage to selected portions of the central nervous system or from overactivity of other regions. To illustrate these conditions, a few will be described briefly.

Increased Intracranial Pressure. Head injuries or strategically placed brain tumors may lead to a rise in the pressure of the cerebrospinal fluid surrounding the central nervous system. Under these conditions, the systemic arterial pressure tends to increase as the cerebrospinal fluid pressure rises. This consequence is commonly attributed to compression of the brain stem in the medullary regions which contain centers of cardiovascular regulation.[34]

Destructive Lesions. Some patients with acute poliomyelitis involving the brain stem (bulbar paralysis) develop severe hypertension; the lesions lie in the medial portion of the medullary reticular substance. In general, the hypertension is transient.

Occasionally severe mental disturbances are combined with neural lesions resulting from peripheral neuritis and ascending myelitis. Examination of the urine discloses excessive excretion of porphyrin as a result of abnormal pigment metabolism. Such patients are prone to display disturbances of autonomic function (vomiting, constipation, cramping abdominal pain) as well as hypertension with tachycardia. The hypertension appears and subsides in relation to the psychoneurotic behavior.

Psychiatric Disturbances. Widespread recognition of the fact that excitement and other psychologic factors may greatly influence the level of systemic arterial pressure has led many investigators to examine the incidence of hypertension among patients with neuroses or psychoses. The results are not clear-cut because conflicting evidence has been obtained by different approaches. However, the consensus of current opinion is a conservative or doubtful attitude toward this mechanism as a dominant cause of chronic hypertension.

Diencephalic Syndrome. A labile form of hypertension associated with blotchy flushing of the face and upper chest, cold pale extremities, tachycardia and hyperperistalsis may be induced by embarrassment and excitement in young and middle-aged women. This group of symptoms and signs has been termed the "diencephalic syndrome" because it can be brought on by diffuse stimulation of the human diencephalon.

Patients with hypertension related to disturbances of the nervous system frequently display tachycardia and increased cardiac output. In patients with diseases of the adrenal glands, kidneys or cardiovascular system, on the other hand, the hypertension is generally the result of increased peripheral resistance with little or no increase in heart rate or cardiac output. This distinction should be kept in mind when attempting to assign a cause to hypertension of unknown origin.

Surprisingly enough, the wide variety of causes of elevated systemic arterial pressure discussed are responsible for a very small proportion of the cases of abnormally high blood pressure. The remainder represents patients with "primary" or "essential" hypertension (Fig. 5–19).

ESSENTIAL HYPERTENSION

The causes of sustained hypertension can be identified in only about 5 to 10 per cent of such patients; the remaining 90 to 95 per cent are generally classified as having "essential" or "primary" hypertension (see Fig. 5–19). A more realistic term would be "hypertension of undetermined origin."

THE NATURE OF ESSENTIAL HYPERTENSION

Essential hypertension is a term applied to high blood pressure which cannot be attributed to a specific lesion. Since blood pressure rises progressively with age—faster in some individuals than in others—the patients with essential hypertension are those at the high end of the frequency distribution curves for each age. Inheritance, environment and sex may affect the rate at which the blood pressure rises. In general, the higher the blood pressure, the shorter the life expectancy. Headache and vertigo are common complaints of such patients and cerebral vascular accidents (strokes) are frequent complications. The elevated systemic arterial pressure leads to left ventricular hypertrophy. Since vascular disease may interfere with coronary blood supply, congestive heart failure occurs frequently in later stages.

In most patients with benign hypertension, the blood pressure fluctuates more widely than normal, but rises progressively and slowly over many years. In a small percentage of such patients, the hypertension becomes "malignant" or rapidly progressing. Characteristic vascular changes in the retina of the eye (hypertensive neuroretinopathy) appear early in this phase of the disease, and kidney function often becomes rapidly impaired. Patients with malignant hypertension have a very limited life expectancy, usually succumbing with-

in a few months but occasionally surviving one or two years. Left ventricular failure or cerebral vascular accidents may cause death before renal failure becomes fully developed.

CAUSES OF ESSENTIAL HYPERTENSION

The problem of establishing the cause of "essential" hypertension is comparable to attempting to determine the origin of fever in a group of patients after all known causes have been specifically eliminated. A great deal of effort has been expended in attempts to determine which of the mechanisms illustrated in Figure 5–19 might be responsible for such hypertension. The search for renal hypertension without renal disease, adrenal hypertension without adrenal dysfunction, vasomotor hypertension without central nervous system abnormality and cardiovascular hypertension without cardiovascular lesions has provided much controversy and semantic confusion but has shed little light on the subject at hand.

Exclusion of Standard Mechanisms. During the early stages of essential hypertension none of the hypertensive mechanisms illustrated in Figure 5–19 can be shown to be operative. Electrolyte metabolism and excretion are entirely within normal limits. Renal blood flow and function are normal, and the extent of atherosclerotic lesions is not greater than that among patients with normal blood pressure. The presence of neural lesions cannot be demonstrated.

Although there is considerable evidence that angiotensin may be involved in certain spontaneous and experimental hypertensive states, it seems doubtful that this mechanism is the common exciting cause of "essential" hypertension for several reasons. During the early phases of moderate hypertension in younger persons, the kidneys appear to be entirely normal functionally and anatomically. Dogs with moderate hypertension from unilateral renal ischemia may have no evident renal vascular disease in the other kidney. Abnormal amounts of renin have not been found consistently in human patients with primary hypertension. Finally, patients with congestive heart failure may have easily demonstrable increases in the amount of renin in the plasma without having hypertension. Thus it is difficult to believe renin in *undetectable* concentrations in the plasma of hypertensive patients is the cause of their high blood pressure. One of the most confusing elements in the puzzle stems from evidence that hypertension is self-perpetuating.

Hypertension Begets Hypertension. Since patients with "essential" hypertension exhibit no identifiable cause of it, the therapy of it has been largely directed toward reduction of the blood pressure by various means. Without casting doubt on the wisdom or success of this approach, one should recognize that the implied basis of this therapy is that elevated systemic arterial pressure acts in some manner to produce even greater increases in this pressure. It is true that the elevation of the systemic pressure produced by several experimental procedures may persist after the exciting cause has been removed. One explanation of this phenomenon depends upon the pronounced tendency toward development of degenerative lesions in the walls of the renal blood vessels. According to one view, this "nephrosclerosis" impedes blood flow through the renal parenchyma, exciting the renin mechanism so that the amount of circulating angiotensin II increases and produces generalized vasocon-

striction. Theoretically, then, elevated systemic arterial pressure from any cause would become self-sustaining though the development of nephrosclerosis and the original cause might disappear, effectively confounding investigators. Experimental hypertension induced by neural mechanisms (section of the carotid sinus nerves or chronic stimulation of sympathetic nerves) is not generally associated with renal lesions, nor is this type of hypertension self-perpetuating. Another mechanism for self-sustaining hypertension could be related to resetting of the pressoreceptor mechanism.

Reseting the Pressoreceptor Mechanism. Kubicek et al.[41] produced arterial hypertension which was sustained over several weeks (up to 38 days) by continuous electrical stimulation of the splanchnic nerves. Within 20 hours of sustained stimulation the systemic arterial pressure rose significantly; but the pulse rate was normal, indicating that the pressoreceptor mechanism was no longer attempting to compensate. As soon as the stimulation was interrupted, the blood pressure began to fall toward the control level and the heart rate accelerated. In other words, the pressoreceptor mechanism had been reset to the new higher level and was acting to oppose the fall of pressure. This resetting could occur at the cardiovascular control centers in the central nervous system or at the peripheral receptors in the carotid sinus.

Interestingly enough, McCubbin et al.[42] demonstrated that the frequency at which carotid sinus stretch receptors discharged in response to a given pressure was clearly lower in chronically hypertensive dogs than in normal animals (Fig. 5–20). In other words, the peripheral pressoreceptors themselves apparently can adapt to a sus-

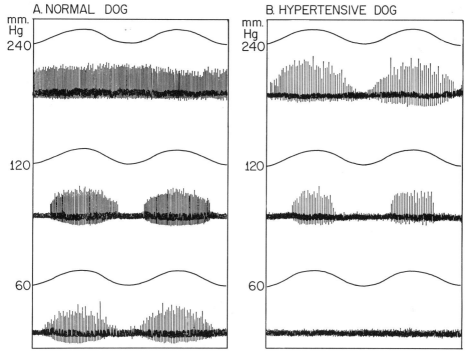

FIGURE 5-20   CAROTID SINUS SENSITIVITY IN HYPERTENSIVE DOGS

The frequency of discharge of carotid sinus stretch receptors was recorded during induced pressure fluctuations at various mean pressure levels in normal control dogs and in dogs with chronic renal hypertension. The carotid sinus discharge frequency at the same pressure levels was much lower in the hypertensive dogs suggesting reduced sensitivity of the pressure monitoring system. (After McCubbin, Green and Page.[42])

tained increase in arterial pressure, with only a slight lag. The adapted pressoreceptor mechanism would act to sustain the pressure at the higher level to which it had been reset rather than to compensate toward "normal." Adaptation of the integrating centers in the nervous system might also occur. The concept of resetting of the pressoreceptor mechanism is not a wholly satisfactory explanation of the sustained elevation of systemic arterial pressure because the blood pressure does tend to return to normal levels over longer periods of time when the stimulus to neurogenic hypertension is removed. A more sustained depression of carotid sinus pressoreceptor activity would result from pathologic

changes in the walls of the vessels that would restrict their distensibility.

Atherosclerosis of the Carotid Sinus. The carotid sinus region is a site of predilection for atherosclerosis.[43] This has been recognized since Burns first described the condition in 1811. Pathologic thickening and even calcification may occur here when other portions of the arterial tree are relatively unaffected. Such changes may begin at relatively early ages (as young as 19 years). If the wall of the carotid sinus is stiffened by this process, the amount of stretch in the wall for a particular pressure range would be reduced, curtailing the stretch on the distortion receptors in the wall. Under these conditions, the nerves might still be quite responsive to external compression and yet display greatly reduced discharge frequency from changes in internal pressure.

Generalized Vasoconstriction. Theoretically, the mean arterial blood pressure would be doubled if half of the vascular channels were completely closed or if the circumference of all the resistance vessels were reduced by only about 20 per cent. Generalized reduction in circumference is more effective than a decrease in the number of *channels* open because the pressure gradient and resistance to flow are related to the reciprocal of the radius to the fourth power $(1/r^4)$ in accordance with Poiseuille's law (see Fig. 1–6). In blood vessels with appreciably thick walls, the reduction in external circumference would be even less and would most certainly be imperceptable without the most meticulous quantitative measurements. Several mechanisms might be involved in a generalized vasoconstriction sufficient to induce hypertension.

The administration of norepinephrine or nitroglycerin produces a greater response in hypertensive patients but its duration is the same as in normal subjects. This observation led Conway[44] to conclude that the increased reactivity might result from structural changes in the arterial wall. Furthermore, some of the increased resistance in hypertensives was not overcome by nitrite, indicating that the vessels could not dilate as greatly as could those in normal subjects. Gaskell[45] found that abnormally high vascular tone persisted in the vessels of the finger after digital nerve block in patients with persistent hypertension. This tone was attributed to an "abnormal force" exerted by the vascular smooth muscle not under the immediate control of the nervous system.

Hypertrophy in the medial layers of the arterial walls is a prominent feature in the resistance vessels of patients with hypertension. Such hypertrophy might result from repetitive or continuous exposure to elevated internal pressure or from intermittent increases in sympathetic constrictor nerve activity. Folkow *et al.*[46] postulated that thickening of the arterial walls would reduce the vascular lumen and also significantly increase the degree of vascular constriction induced by a specific degree of smooth muscle shortening. They demonstrated that the resistance through "maximally" distended forearm vessels was higher in hypertensive than in normal subjects. Furthermore, a 30 per cent shortening of the smooth muscle could theoretically increase the resistance as much as two times.

VASCULAR SWELLING. Tobian and Binion[47] found an increased concentration of water and sodium in the renal artery and psoas muscle in humans with hypertension and in the aortic walls of hypertensive rats. Swelling of the arteriolar walls was regarded as a potential cause of increased peripheral resistance since a 13 per cent swelling of the arteriolar wall was computed to increase flow resistance by 54 per cent. A retention of salt and water might represent a change in the electrolyte metabolism in such patients, and low-salt diets might then alleviate hypertension by reducing the fluid content of the vascular walls. Edema of the vascular walls would be roughly equivalent to medial hypertrophy.

UNIDENTIFIED VASOCONSTRICTOR SUBSTANCES. Finally, vasoconstrictor substances yet to be identified might be primarily responsible for the production of essential hypertension. Such substances should have more or less equal effects on such vascular beds as those in the brain and skin and the splanchnic bed, with a slightly more intense effect on renal vessels and a slightly less intense effect on vessels of the skeletal musculature.

SUMMARY

Elevated systemic arterial pressure is a clinical sign which is common to a wide variety of disease states. The many potential mechanisms for the production of sustained high blood pressure are generally grouped into four main classes: endocrine (primarily adrenal glands), renal, cardiovascular and neural. Several specific diseases in each category are characteristically associated with elevated systemic arterial pressure. All these causal mechanisms combined will account for only about 5 to 10 per cent of all patients with high arterial blood pressure. The remaining 90 to 95 per cent of these patients have "essential" hypertension or elevated arterial pressure of unknown origin. Among these patients, the blood pressure rises at different rates. In a small percentage, the blood pressure rises abruptly ("malignant hypertension"); death usually supervenes within a year from severe heart failure, advanced kidney disease or cerebral vascular accident.

The cause of essential and malignant hypertension is not known. Attempts to explain this condition in terms of recognized mechanisms which elevate the blood pressure have been unsuccessful. The distribution of blood flow in the presence of this hypertension is very nearly normal even though the total peripheral resistance is increased. This distribution means that the degree of increased resistance must be more or less equal in all major vascular beds. None of the vasomotor control mechanisms discussed in Chapter 4 produces such widespread, uniform constrictor responses. It thus seems reasonable to seek other mechanisms affecting the various vascular beds which might be responsible for a progressive increase in blood pressure.

First, the presence of elevated arterial blood pressure apparently tends to be self-perpetuating in that it tends to persist after the initiating cause is removed. This persistence may be due to the development of sclerotic vascular lesions in the renal vessels (nephrosclerosis) in the presence of systemic hypertension. Furthermore, the pressoreceptor mechanisms can be shown to be reset to higher levels when the blood pressure is elevated for even a few hours. Thus, the neural control mechanisms may actually tend to sustain a hypertension rather than to induce compensatory reactions to restore the pressure to the control levels. The carotid sinus area is exceptionally susceptible to the development of atherosclerosis. The stiffening of the walls would tend to reduce the sensitivity of the stretch receptors in them, and reflexly induce vasoconstriction in the peripheral vascular system.

Generalized vasoconstriction in the various vascular beds might result from structural changes in the resistance vessels. For example, the smooth muscle in the media apparently hypertrophies in these vessels. If this condition develops in response to repeated vasoconstrictor impulses or to repeated episodes of transient elevation of systemic arterial pressure, a sustained increase in peripheral resistance will occur. Also, the same degree of shortening of the smooth muscle will produce greater constriction of the vessels owing to the greater thicknesses of their walls. Edema of the vascular walls due to increased concentrations of sodium and water in them has been demonstrated in hypertensive patients. This edema would have the same functional effect as hypertrophy of the smooth muscles in the media. Finally, currently unidentified vasoconstrictor substances may be discovered and may turn out to be the primary cause of the progressive rise in systemic arterial pressure observed in this large group of patients.

REFERENCES

1. HAMILTON, W. F., and DOW, P. An experimental study of the standing waves in the pulse propagated through the aorta. *Amer. J. Physiol.*, 125:48–59, 1939.

2. ALEXANDER, R. S. The genesis of the aortic standing wave. *Circulat. Res.*, 1:145–151, 1953.

3. PETERSON, L. H., and GERST, P. H. Significance of reflected waves within the arterial system. *Fed. Proc.*, 15:144–145, 1956.

4. WARNER, H. R. A study of the mechanism of pressure wave distortion by arterial walls using an electrical analog. *Circulat. Res.*, 5:79–84, 1957.

5. ATTINGER, E. O. Pulsatile blood flow. *Proc. of International Symposium on Pulsatile Blood Flow*, April 11-13, 1963. New York, Blakiston Division. McGraw-Hill Book Company, 1964.

6. KOROTKOFF, N. S. A contribution to the problem of methods for the determination of blood pressure. Pp. 126–133 in *Classics in Arterial Hypertension*, A. Rushin, Ed., Springfield, Charles C Thomas, 1956.

7. McCUTCHEON, E. P., and RUSHMER, R. F. Korotkoff Sounds. *Circulat. Res.*, 20:149–160, 1967.

8. THOMSON, A. E., and DOUPE, J. Causes of error in auscultatory blood pressure measurements. *Rev. Canad. Biol.*, 8:337, 1949.

9. WENDKOS, M. H., and ROSSMAN, P. L. The normal blood pressure in the lower extremity. *Amer. Heart J.*, 26:623–630, 1943.

10. GREEN, H. D. Circulatory system: methods. Pp. 208–222 in *Medical Physics*, O. Glasser, Ed. Chicago, Year Book Publishers, 1950.

11. LILLY, J. C. The electrical capacitance diaphragm manometer. *Rev. Sci. Instrum.*, 13:34–37, 1942.

12. ELLIS, E. J., GAUER, O. H., and WOOD, E. H. An intracardiac manometer: its evaluation and application. *Circulation*, 3:390–398, 1951.

13. FRY, D. L. Physiologic recording by modern instruments with particular reference to pressure recording. *Physiol. Rev.* 40:752–788, 1960.

14. WOOD, E. H., LEUSEN, I. R., WARNER, H. R., and WRIGHT, J. L. Measurement of pressures in man by cardiac catheters. *Circulat. Rev.*, 2:294–303, 1954.

15. SCHAPER, W. K. A., LEWI, P., and JAGENEAU, A. H. M. The determinants of the rate of change of the left ventricular pressure (dp/dt). *Archiv für Kreislaufforschung.* 46:27–41, 1965.

16. HEYMANS, C., DELAUNOIS, A. L., and VAN DEN HEUVEL-HEYMANS, G. Tension and distensibility of carotid sinus wall, pressoceptors and blood pressure regulation. *Circulat. Res.*, 1:3–7, 1953.

17. BRONK, D. W., and STELLA, G. The response to steady pressures of single end organs in the isolated carotid sinus. *Amer. J. Physiol.*, 110:708–714, 1935.

18. LANDGREN, S. On the excitation mechanism of the carotid baroceptors. *Acta physiol. scand.*, 26:1–34, 1952.

19. LANDGREN, S., NEIL, E., and ZOTTERMAN, Y. The response of the carotid baroceptors to the local administration of drugs. *Acta phsyiol. scand.*, 25:24–37, 1952.

20. LEUSEN, I., DEMEESTER, G., and BOUCKAERT, J. J. La regulation de la pression arterielle apres hemorragie. *Acta cardiol.*, 11:556–566, 1956.

21. HEYMANS, C., and NEIL, E. *Reflexogenic Areas of the Cardiovascular System*. Boston, Little, Brown & Co., 1958, 271 pp.

22. CARLSTEN, A., FOLKOW, B., GRIMBY, G., HEMBERGER, C. A., and THULESIUS, O. Cardiovascular effects of direct stimulation of the carotid sinus nerve in man. *Acta physiol. scand.*, 44:138–145, 1958.

23. DALY, I. DEB., and DALY, M. DEB. Observations on the changes in resistance of the pulmonary vascular bed in response to stimulation of the carotid sinus baroreceptors in the dog. *J. Physiol.*, 137:427–435, 1957.

24. AVIADO, D. M., JR., and SCHMIDT, C. F. Reflexes from stretch receptors in blood vessels, heart and lungs. *Physiol. Rev.*, 35:247–300, 1955.

25. AVIADO, D. M., JR., and SCHMIDT, C. F. Cardiovascular and respiratory reflexes from the left side of the heart. *Amer. J. Physiol.*, 196:726–730, 1959.

26. PATHAK, C. L. Alternative mechanism of cardiac acceleration in Bainbridge's infusion experiments. *Amer. J. Physiol.*, 197:441–444, 1959.

27. PAINTAL, A. S. The conduction velocities of respiratory and cardiovascular afferent fibres in the vagus nerve. *J. Physiol.*, 121:341–359, 1953.

28. RUSHMER, R. F., VanCITTERS, R. L., and

FRANKLIN, D. Definition and classification of shock. In *Shock: Pathogenesis and Therapy, An International Symposium.* Berlin, Springer Verlag, 1962.

29. RUSHMER, R. F. Shock: a semantic enigma. *Circulation,* 26:445–459, 1962.

30. CLARKSON, B., THOMPSON, D., HORWITH, M., and LUCKEY, E. H. Cyclical edema and shock due to increased capillary permeability. *Amer. J. Med.,* 29:193–216, 1960.

31. OSSIPOV, B. K. On the pathogenetic therapy of shock. In *Shock: Pathogenesis and Therapy: An International Symposium.* Berlin, Springer Verlag, 1962.

32. KOVÁCH, A. G. B., and TAKÁCS, L. Responsiveness of the vegetative nervous system in shock. *Acta Physiol., Acad. Sci., Hung.,* 3:91–101, 1952.

33. MASTER, A. M., GARFIELD, C. L., and WALTERS, M. B. *Normal Blood Pressure and Hypertension.* Philadelphia, Lea & Febiger, 1952, 144 pp.

34. SMIRK, F. H. *High Arterial Pressure.* Oxford, Blackwell Scientific Publications, 1957.

35. PICKERING, G. W. *The Nature of Essential Hypertension.* London, J. and A. Churchill Ltd., 1961.

36. PAGE, I. H. Hypertension, an important disease of regulation. *Advances in Chemistry Series,* 45:50–66, 1964.

37. MILLS, L. C. Clinical observations on the general effects of steroids and the adrenal cortex on blood pressure and relationship to hypertension. Pp. 232–242 in *Hypertension: The First Hahnemann Symposium on Hypertensive Disease.* J. Moyer, Ed. Philadelphia, W. B. Saunders Co., 1959.

38. MOSER, M., and GOLDMAN, A. *Hypertensive Vascular Disease: Diagnosis and Treatment.* Philadelphia, J. B. Lippincott Co., 1967.

39. MENEELY, G. M. The effect of salt and other electrolytes in hypertension. Pp. 250–261 in *Hypertension: The First Hahnemann Symposium on Hypertensive Disease.* J. Moyer, Ed. Philadelphia, W. B. Saunders Co., 1959.

40. SKELTON, F. R. A study of the natural history of adrenal-regeneration hypertension. *Circulat. Res.,* 7:107–117, 1959.

41. KUBICEK, W. G., KOTTKE, F. J., LAKER, D. J., and VISSCHER, M. B. Adaptation in the pressor-receptor reflex mechanisms in experimental neurogenic hypertension. *Amer. J. Physiol.,* 175:380–382, 1953.

42. MCCUBBIN, J. W., GREEN, J. H., and PAGE, I. H. Baroceptor function in chronic renal hypertension. *Circulat. Res.,* 4:205–210, 1956.

43. ADAMS, W. E. *The Comparative Morphology of the Carotid Body and Carotid Sinus.* Springfield, Ill., Charles C Thomas, 1958, 272 pp.

44. CONWAY, J. Vascular reactivity in experimental hypertension measured after hexamethonium. *Circulation,* 17:807–810, 1958.

45. GASKELL, P., and DOISY, A. Persistence of abnormally high vascular tone in vessels of the fingers after digital nerve block in patients with chronic high blood pressure. *Circulat. Res.,* 7:1006–1010, 1959.

46. FOLKOW, B., GRIMBY, G., and THULESIUS, O. Adaptive structural changes of the vascular walls in hypertension and their relation to the control of the peripheral resistance. *Acta physiol. scand.,* 44:255–272, 1958.

47. TOBIAN, L., JR., and BINION, J. T. Tissue cations and water in arterial hypertension. *Circulation,* 5:754–758, 1952.

CHAPTER 6

EFFECTS OF POSTURE

I. CIRCULATORY RESPONSE TO ARISING

The cardiovascular system is generally studied in supine subjects or animals. Circulatory dynamics are most stable while the individual is lying down because many of the arteries and veins are horizontally oriented at or near heart level. When one stands upright, many of the arteries and veins are oriented vertically and large hydrostatic pressures are produced by the long, uninterrupted columns of blood. The arterial, capillary and venous pressures are markedly elevated in the dependent extremities, and the circulatory system must promptly make appropriate compensatory adaptation.[1,2] If these compensatory mechanisms are insufficient or retarded, orthostatic hypotension results. Fainting reactions are frequently produced in erect subjects by stimuli that would have virtually no effect on the supine individual. Recognition that much of man's effective existence is spent in the erect position makes it appropriate to consider the cardiovascular adjustments required in this position.

MEASUREMENT OF VENOUS PRESSURES

A vertical column of fluid in a manometer and an accurate ruler are the only tools needed for measuring steady pressures. It is well to remember that even the most intricate pressure measuring devices require calibration by such simple pressure indicators. Thus, the fluid manometer is the basic instrument for pressure recording.

PERIPHERAL VENOUS PRESSURE

The venous pressure can be measured by a needle connected through a three-way stopcock to a vertical manometer. From the syringe, sterile saline is expressed into the manometer to a level above the expected venous pressure (Fig. 6–1A). The valve on the stopcock is then turned so the vertical tube becomes continuous with the needle. The saline runs into the vein until the vertical height of the column of saline is in equilibrium with the venous pressure at the point of the needle.

Alternatively, the phlebomanometer of Burch and Winsor[3] is well suited to measurement of pressure in both large and small peripheral veins (Fig. 6–1B). In this apparatus, a small needle is fastened to a capillary tube which is connected by a rubber tube

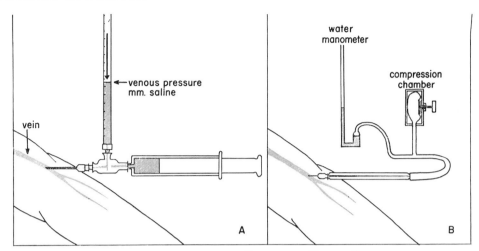

FIGURE 6-1   MEASUREMENT OF PERIPHERAL VENOUS PRESSURE

A, Venous pressure can be measured by a simple vertical manometer filled with saline and connected to a needle which has been thrust into a vein. The fluid column in the vertical tube descends until its pressure is in equilibrium with venous pressure at the point of measurement.

B, The phlebomanometer of Burch and Winsor[3] consists of a small hypodermic needle fastened to a glass capillary partially filled with sterile fluid. The remainder of the system except the water manometer is filled with air. The manometer registers the pressure in the system as adjusted by twisting the screw on the compression chamber until the fluid in the glass capillary is stationary. The pressure in the water manometer then indicates venous pressure when corrected for capillary and hydrostatic pressures in the needle and observation tubing.

to a small air chamber, the capacity of which can be adjusted to elevate the pressure in the system. A water manometer indicates the air pressure within the tubes. Sterile saline is drawn into the capillary tube until the meniscus lies at a reference line. When the needle is inserted into a vein, the meniscus will move farther along the capillary tube if the venous pressure exceeds the pressure within the phlebomanometer. By elevation of the pressure in the system, the meniscus can be brought to a standstill at the reference line when the pressure in the manometer equals the venous pressure. A correction (about 20 mm. H_2O) must be made for the capillarity of the needle and observation tube. A more compact version of this instrument has been described by Sodeman.[4] The advent of sensitive electronic pressure monitoring systems has greatly increased the ease and continuity of venous pressure measurement. A variety of pressure transducers is now available commercially and permit continuous recording of pressures from veins, large and small, from virtually all parts of the body. The nature and performance characteristics of such gauges have been described in some detail by Fry[5] and by Frank.[6] Techniques of venous catheterization have been described in detail by Thompson and McIntosh.[7]

The Significance of Venous Pressure. The veins originate at the capillaries and terminate at the heart. Thus, venous pressure has important bearing on the function of both the capillaries and the heart. The pressure in the smallest peripheral veins is a basis for deducing the minimal pressure in the capillaries of the region, since the capillary pressure must exceed venous pressure. The effective pressure in the large intrathoracic veins reflects the diastolic filling pressure of the ventricles.

Right atrial pressure ranges just above or below atmospheric pressure but the pressure in extrathoracic veins is 2 to 5 cm. H_2O higher. A rather sudden drop in pressure often occurs as the veins penetrate the thoracic walls, where the extravascular pressure becomes subatmospheric. Branches of the superior vena cava in normal erect subjects are collapsed from the point of entrance into the thorax to a level a few centimeters above the right atrium. The sudden drop in pressure indicates local constriction at or near the point at which the veins pass through the thoracic musculature. In any case, the venous pressure in the arms does not normally reflect right ventricular diastolic pressure. However, if central venous pressure rises, e.g., in congestive failure, the difference between intrathoracic and extrathoracic venous pressure disappears, and the brachial venous pressure becomes a fairly reliable indicator of central venous pressure.

The Phlebostatic Level. To obtain comparable values in different individuals or in a series of measurements, the venous pressure is frequently measured at the level of the right atrium. For this purpose, Burch and Winsor[3] described a reference line (the phlebostatic axis) which passes transversely through the thorax midway between the anterior and posterior surfaces of the trunk at the level of the fourth interspace at the sternum (Fig. 6–2A). The phlebostatic level is a horizontal plane at the level of the phlebostatic axis. Venous pressures anywhere in the body can be meas-

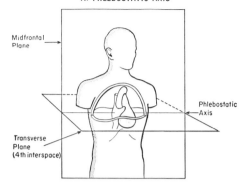

A. PHLEBOSTATIC AXIS

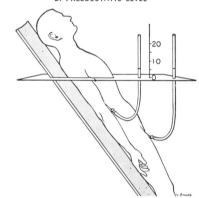

B. PHLEBOSTATIC LEVEL

FIGURE 6-2   BASELINE FOR CENTRAL VENOUS PRESSURE

A, The phlebostatic axis is defined as the line of junction between two planes: a midfrontal plane and a plane at right angles passing through the junction of the fourth rib with the sternum. The phlebostatic axis passes through or near the mid-portion of the right atrial chamber.

B, The phlebostatic level is used as the zero reference for venous pressures measured in different locations with the body in various positions. The phlebostatic level is a horizontal plane passing through the phlebostatic axis.

ured as the vertical height of a fluid column above this plane (Fig. 6–2B).

EXTRAVASCULAR PRESSURES

Water manometers are generally employed for measuring tissue pressures in various sites. For example, pressures in the skin, subcutaneous

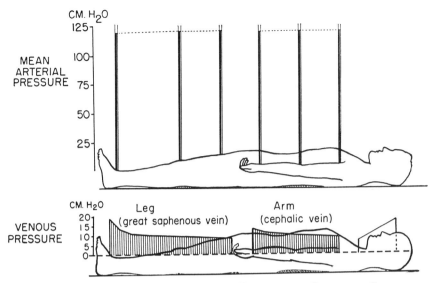

FIGURE 6-3   MEAN ARTERIAL AND VENOUS PRESSURES IN RECLINING SUBJECTS

A, The mean arterial pressure diminishes but slightly from the arch of the aorta to the arterial branches, e.g., the radial. This pressure gradient is responsible for the flow of blood through the system.

B, The peripheral venous pressure also has a very gradual diminution in pressure from the periphery toward the heart. In the smaller venous branches the pressure gradient is considerably steeper. (After Ochsner et al.[8])

tissue and muscle have generally been recorded with apparatus resembling the phlebomanometer (Fig. 6–1B). Cerebrospinal fluid pressure is usually measured with simple vertical manometers of the type illustrated in Figure 6–1A.

VASCULAR PRESSURES IN RECLINING SUBJECTS

When the long axis of the body is horizontal, the long columns of blood are at or near heart level. The mean pressure throughout the entire systemic arterial tree is fairly uniform except for the slight pressure gradients incident to the frictional energy loss during flow through these tubes (Fig. 6–3). The mean arterial pressure diminishes only a few millimeters of mercury during flow of the blood from the aorta to arterial branches the size of the radial artery at the wrist.

In the same way, the venous pressure declines only slightly between the smallest venous branches in the extremities and the large central venous channels. The pressure in peripheral veins of various calibers was measured at various points over the body surface by Ochsner et al.[8]; their data are schematically illustrated in Figure 6–3B. Note that the pressure in the smallest peripheral veins averaged about 17 mm. Hg in the lower extremity and that capillary pressure must exceed the pressures in the corresponding veins.

PRESSURES PRODUCED BY HYDROSTATIC COLUMNS

The pressure in a rigid tube containing a continuous column of stationary fluid is determined by the ver-

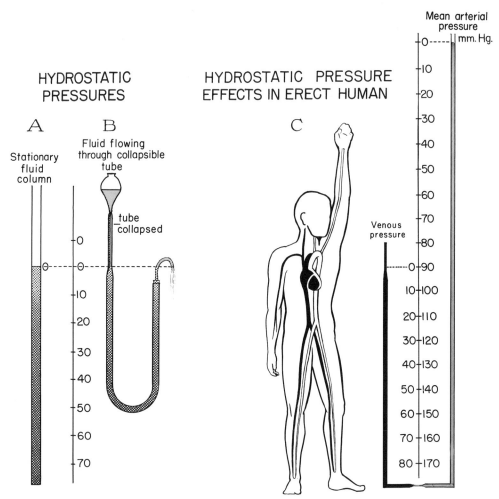

FIGURE 6-4   THE NATURE AND SIGNIFICANCE OF HYDROSTATIC PRESSURES

A, The pressure in a column of fluid is dependent upon its specific gravity and the vertical distance from the point of measurement to the meniscus.

B, A collapsible tube is distended only so long as the internal pressure exceeds the external pressure. These two pressures are exactly equal in the portion of the tube which is collapsed.

C, In the erect position, the arterial and venous pressures are both increased by some 85 mm. Hg at the ankle. With the arm held above the head, the arterial pressure at the wrist is about 40 mm. Hg and the effective venous pressure is zero down to a level just above the heart.

tical distance from the point of measurement to the top of the fluid (Fig. 6–4). At lower levels within the tube, the pressure in the fluid progressively increases owing to the action of gravity on the column of fluid above each point of measurement. Strictly speaking, the meniscus of the fluid represents an interface between the fluid

medium and the atmosphere, so the total pressure equals the hydrostatic pressure in the fluid column plus the ambient atmospheric pressure. In the present discussion the hydrostatic pressure will be considered in relation to the specific gravity of the fluid and the vertical distance from the point of measurement to the level at which fluid pressure equals the pressure immediately outside the tube.

The venous system consists of a series of collapsible tubes, so there is no interface between the venous blood and the external environment of the vein. If at any point along the vein, the pressure within it equals the external tissue pressure, the vessel collapses at that level. If a thin-walled tube containing no air is arranged as indicated in Figure 6–4B, the fluid from the reservoir will flow through the tube in response to a pressure gradient. The tube collapses at a level just above that of the outflow tube. Below this level, the internal pressure exceeds the external pressure, and the tube is distended by hydrostatic pressures which increase progressively toward the lower portion of the system. Above the zero level, the pressure within the collapsed tube is equal to the external pressure. Technically, a free-falling body has no weight because all the potential energy is converted into kinetic energy (movement) or lost as friction (heat). Thus, even though there is fluid flowing through the collapsed portion of the tube, the lateral pressure exactly equals the external pressure. If a normal man assumes a semi-reclining position with his head and trunk oriented about 30 to 45 degrees from the horizontal plane, the lower portion of the jugular vein is distended, but at some point along its course the vein becomes collapsed because venous pressure equals tissue pressure. This represents the level of zero effective venous pressure.

When a normal man is standing, the level of zero effective venous pressure is within the thorax (Fig. 6–4C). If there is a continuous column of blood extending from the foot to heart level, the pressure in an ankle vein should be about 85 mm. Hg (125 cm. H_2O). It has been demonstrated ex-perimentally that this is approximately true so long as the subject remains relaxed and motionless. Similarly, if the mean arterial blood pressure at heart level is 90 mm. Hg the arterial blood pressure at the ankle should be increased by a corresponding amount, i.e., to about 175 mm. Hg, neglecting the slight frictional losses during flow indicated in Figure 6–3. Since the arterial and venous pressures in dependent extremities are increased to the same extent by hydrostatic pressure, the energy lost during circulation through dependent parts is no greater than that lost when the same vascular bed is at heart level. The pressure differences between arteries and veins at the ankle are essentially the same as those at heart level. The frictional energy loss along a tube is not increased when it is formed into a U tube. For example, the pressure head is the same for tubes A and B in Figure 6–5 and the flow from each tube is essentially identical. Forming a tube into a dependent loop does not increase the amount of energy required to propel fluid through the tube. Thus, the erect position does not require an increased energy output by the heart, but capillary pressure increases tremendously in the dependent parts of the body.

CEREBRAL CIRCULATION

Whenever a man is erect, the pressure within the skull drops well below atmospheric pressure while the pressure in the lower spinal canal is well above this value. It has long been recognized that cerebrospinal fluid protects the cerebrospinal vascular bed. The cerebrospinal fluid pressure and the cerebral venous pressure vary together because these fluids are confined within a relatively rigid chamber

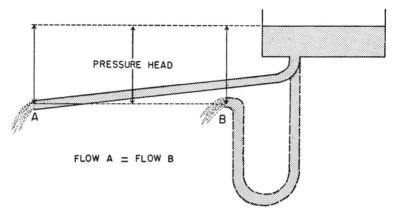

FIGURE 6-5   THE EFFECTS OF DEPENDENCY ON THE FLOW OF FLUID

This simple model illustrates the point that assuming the erect position per se places no additional burden upon the heart. Since the frictional energy loss is essentially the same, the same energy release (pressure head) provides equal flow from A and B.

(Fig. 6–6). The intravenous and extravenous pressure must be precisely equal at all levels of the cerebrospinal cavity regardless of its position or orientation.

Since the hydrostatic columns in the arteries, capillaries and veins are precisely balanced by equal changes in extravascular hydrostatic pressure,[9] the cerebrospinal circulation exhibits a stability not exceeded in any other tissue of the body. The pressure gradient from the arteries to the veins is precisely equal across all capillary beds. The only mechanism for altering flow through any part of the enclosed circulation is by means of local vasoconstriction or vasodilation. However, the cerebral circulation is remarkably unresponsive to the usual neural, humoral or chemical mechanisms (see Chapter 4). The blood flow through the cerebrospinal vessels is extremely constant, a condition compatible with the more or less uniform oxygen requirements of the central nervous system. The effective capillary pressure is also very similar at all levels within the cerebrospinal canal, and the fluid balance postulated by

Starling (see Fig. 1–15) is probably in effect in all capillary networks. Net filtration probably does not occur in cerebral capillaries other than those of the choroid plexus, which has the specialized function of producing cerebrospinal fluid. In fact, many substances in the blood are greatly impeded in their movement into the cerebrospinal fluid, a fact ascribed to the so-called "blood-brain barrier."

The circulatory pattern and extravascular support within the eye are quite analogous to those of the cerebrospinal cavity. The ciliary body is a structure specialized to produce capillary filtrate (aqueous humour). A similar kind of external support of the vascular beds probably obtains within the medullary cavity of bones.

COUNTER PRESSURES IN PERIPHERAL CIRCULATION

It is obvious that a capillary pressure exceeding a pressure of 85 mm. Hg in an ankle vein must also greatly exceed the maximum colloid osmotic pressure of the plasma proteins (about 30 mm. Hg). If the effective capillary

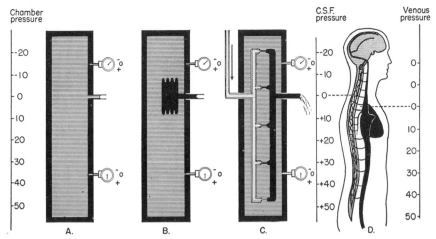

FIGURE 6-6   THE RELATION OF CEREBROSPINAL FLUID PRESSURE TO VENOUS PRESSURE

In a rigid container filled with fluid, the pressure at the level of the horizontal tube equals atmospheric pressure. Below this level the pressure progressively increases owing to the hydrostatic column of fluid. Above the reference level, the pressure progressively diminishes below atmospheric pressure. This situation is unaltered by the presence of a distensible barrier between the contents of the chamber and the outlet tube. If fluid flows into the chamber through rigid tubes and out through collapsible tubes, the pressure within the collapsible tubes is precisely equal to the pressure outside the tube at any level within the rigid system. By the same token, the venous pressure determines the cerebrospinal fluid pressure within the cerebrospinal cavity.

pressure throughout the vascular networks of a region significantly exceeds the maximal colloid osmotic pressure, fluid will filter from all parts of the capillary system, resorption will be impossible and accumulation of fluid in the tissue spaces (edema) can result. It is important to consider the extent to which this kind of situation is alleviated in various regions of the body by such mechanisms as (*a*) the balancing of intravascular pressures by extravascular or tissue pressure, (*b*) the reduction of the hydrostatic columns in veins by "pumping" action and (*c*) the return of unabsorbed capillary filtrate to the circulation by way of the lymphatic system.

INTRAMUSCULAR TISSUE PRESSURE

In reclining subjects the intramuscular pressure ranges from 2 to 5 cm.

H_2O in muscles with loose fascial investment,[10] e.g., biceps brachii and gastrocnemius. Slightly higher values have been obtained from anterior tibial and soleus muscles, which are invested with a tight fascial sheath. After the subject has been tilted into the erect position, intramuscular pressures rise abruptly a few centimeters of water and then gradually increase to values of 20 or 30 cm. H_2O in muscles with tight fascial covering. Maximal pressures developed during voluntary muscular contraction are rarely reported to be over 50 cm. H_2O, although the venous pressure in the legs exceeds this amount. In muscles without tight fascial sheaths the increase in pressure is relatively slight during maximal voluntary contraction. For example, pressure in the rectus femoris could not be raised above 20 cm. H_2O by maximal effort.[10] Although the recorded values for intramuscular

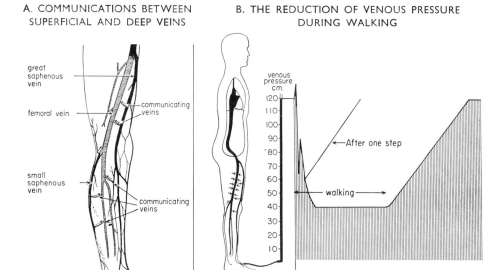

A. COMMUNICATIONS BETWEEN   B. THE REDUCTION OF VENOUS PRESSURE
   SUPERFICIAL AND DEEP VEINS   DURING WALKING

FIGURE 6-7   PUMPING ACTION OF MUSCLES DURING WALKING

A, Venous blood may ascend the leg along both deep and superficial channels, which are in communication at many points. To reduce the venous pressure at the ankle, each vertical column of blood draining the area must be interrupted at some point in the leg.

B, After taking one step the venous pressure in a dorsal vein of the foot is markedly reduced and then gradually ascends to the control level; repetitive steps keep the venous pressure depressed (after Pollack and Wood[13]).

pressure are surprisingly low, muscular contraction has important cardiovascular significance. A relationship between low intramuscular pressure and syncope has been demonstrated by Mayerson and Burch.[11] Even more impressive is the fact that voluntary muscular contraction can apparently force blood under a cuff inflated to levels of 90 mm. Hg.[12] By some unknown means, contraction of skeletal muscle in the legs is sufficient to compress the veins of the legs even when their internal pressure is very high. This is the basis of a muscular pumping mechanism by which the venous pressure in dependent extremities may be significantly lowered during ordinary walking or shifting of position.

Muscular Pumping Mechanisms. The veins of the extremities are equipped with many valves located at strategic positions along their course. So long as blood flows continuously throughout the peripheral venous system, the valves along all the venous channels are open and the columns of blood are not interrupted at any point. Under these conditions, the pressure in the veins at the dorsum of the foot is equal to that in a vertical column of blood extending from the point of measurement to heart level (Fig. 6-4). If the subject takes one step (Fig. 6-7), the venous pressure at the ankle drops to a level equivalent to that in a column of fluid extending to the knee and then gradually returns to the previous level at a rate determined by the volume flow of blood through the limb.[13] There are alternate pathways by which blood from the foot may ascend the leg. If any single uninterrupted column of blood from ankle to heart persisted after the step, the venous pressure at the dorsum of the foot would not be altered. Thus, muscular contraction must produce complete or partial emptying of both the deep and superficial veins within the leg or thigh. As the muscles relax, columns of blood are supported by closed intravenous valves. According to Höjensgard and Stürup,[14] the pressure in the deep and superficial leg veins may be reduced simultaneously during walking. The superficial veins must empty into the deep veins of the thigh so that all the veins above the knee are decompressed. This could be accomplished by complete emptying of veins or by segmenting the columns of blood so that each valve in the thigh is closed and supports a column of blood which does not extend to the valve above. As blood flows through the capillaries into the veins, the partially collapsed deep and superficial veins gradually refill, elevating the pressure at the dorsum of the foot back to the initial levels. Repetitive movements of the lower extremities, as in walking, maintain the venous pressures at the lower level (Fig. 6–7) if each successive step occurs before the venous columns in the thighs are refilled.

This muscular pumping mechanism has important functional connotations: (a) It drastically lowers the venous and capillary pressures, reducing the effective capillary filtration pressures. (b) It reduces the volume of blood contained within the veins of the leg and to this extent these veins act as a reservoir which releases stored blood during muscular exercise (see later). (c) It momentarily acceler-

ates the return of venous blood from the legs at the onset of walking or running. After the pumping mechanism is established, the rate of venous return again depends upon the rate of blood flow through the capillaries into the veins. When venous blood flows upward from the leg into the abdomen, the pressure in the veins of the thigh must exceed the pressure in the abdominal portion of the inferior vena cava, which has no valves. In general, the veins within the abdomen are filled with uninterrupted columns of blood under a pressure equivalent to that of a vertical column extending slightly above heart level. A critical analysis of the pumping mechanisms in the leg by Stegall[15] disclosed that muscle contraction of the legs can contribute significantly to the propulsion of the blood during running. The abdominal pressure was found to be elevated by about 22 mm. Hg during exertion, apparently to splint the trunk and pelvis. The contracting leg muscles must elevate venous pressure sufficiently to overcome elevated abdominal pressure and propel blood upward against hydrostatic pressure to the heart. Measured by ultrasonic Doppler flow detector, blood was accelerated in both the deep and superficial veins during contraction of the leg muscles (Fig. 6–8A). Measurements of venous pressures by catheters from the right atrium down the vena cava to the ankle revealed an increase in venous pressure above the popliteal veins and a decrease in venous pressure at the ankle (Fig. 6–8B). The power developed by the leg muscles in pumping blood upward to the heart was computed utilizing data on muscle blood flow from the literature and the pressure drops indicated in Figure 6–8B. The surprising result was an estimate that at least 30 per cent of the

CALF MUSCLE PUMP

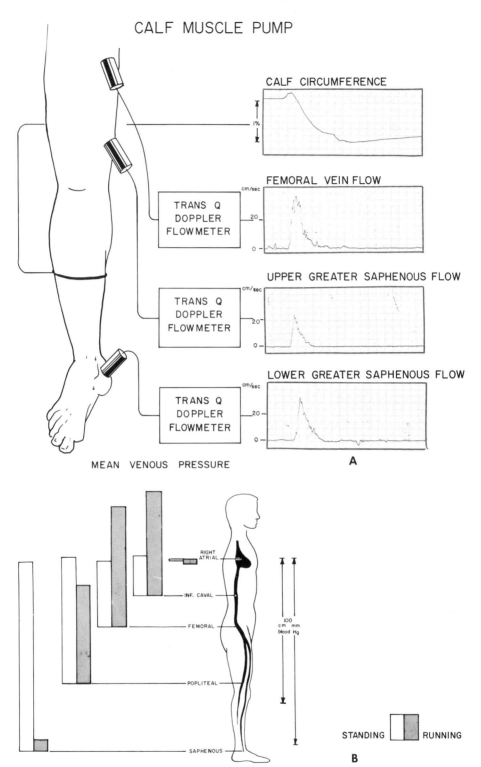

FIGURE 6-8 MUSCULAR PUMPING MECHANISMS

A, Upper calf circumference and venous flow velocity with a brief ankle flexion. Paper speed 25 mm./sec.

B, Mean venous pressures at rest and during running in one subject. The figure is scaled as shown. The bottom of each bar represents atmospheric pressure at the level shown; bar height is proportional to the mean pressure obtained during running. (From *Circulat. Res.* 19:182.)

202

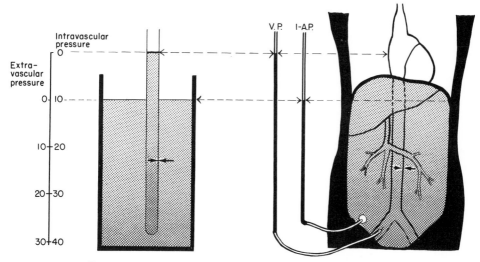

FIGURE 6-9   TRANSMURAL PRESSURES OF ABDOMINAL VEINS

If a collapsible tube is filled with fluid and suspended in a tank of water, the walls must support only the difference in pressure between the inside and the outside. In the case illustrated, the walls of the tube support no more than 10 cm. H_2O pressure at any level in the tube. The abdomen contains movable organs with a specific gravity similar to that of blood. For this reason the transmural pressure of intra-abdominal veins is less than 10 cm. H_2O at any level in the abdominal cavity.

total systemic circulatory work during running must be done by pumping action of the musculature in the legs.

INTRA-ABDOMINAL PRESSURE

The abdominal cavity is filled with organs having a specific gravity approximating that of blood. The hydrostatic pressure of a vertical column of abdominal organs is similar (Fig. 6–9) to that which would be produced if the abdomen were filled with fluid.[16] At rest the venous pressure apparently exceeds the intra-abdominal pressure by only 5 to 10 cm. H_2O at any level within the abdomen in either the supine or the erect position. However, the diaphragm and the abdominal walls may simultaneously exert tension during deep inspiration or straining, so that the overall intra-abdominal pressure exceeds venous pressure in

the thorax and compresses the abdominal veins. Blood is forced onward into the veins of the thorax because retrograde flow out of the abdominal cavity is prevented by closure of venous valves. Since the diaphragm can exert no force in the upward direction, intrathoracic pressure never exceeds intra-abdominal pressure.

INTRATHORACIC PRESSURE

The collapsed volume of the lungs is much smaller than the capacity of the thoracic cage. Since the lungs are stretched or distended to fill their allotted space, the elastic tissue is under stretch even at the end of a forced expiration. This elastic tension of the pulmonary tissue is expressed as a subatmospheric intrathoracic pressure which exerts a distending force on the structures within the chest. An elastic tube filled with fluid is further distended if the tube is confined within a chamber containing a subatmospheric pressure. The level of zero transmural pressure occurs at the point where the internal fluid pressure is balanced by the extravascular pressure. The central venous pressure measured with a catheter ranges slightly above or slightly below the atmospheric pressure. The transmural pressure of the veins and atria, however, is greater than the recorded values because of the subatmospheric pressure in the thorax. If the negative intrathoracic pressure is applied to the top of an external fluid column connected to an intrathoracic vein (Fig. 6–10), the top of the fluid column is elevated by the "suction" of the subatmospheric intrathoracic pressure. The "effective" venous pressure within the chest is indicated by such a manometer. The distending influence of the subatmospheric intrathoracic pressure tends to increase the transmural pressures throughout the thoracic cavity. It augments the central

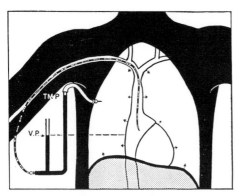

FIGURE 6-10   TRANSMURAL PRESSURE IN THE
THORAX

The central venous pressure recorded with a catheter approximates atmospheric pressure. The transmural pressure of the intrathoracic vessels is actually represented by the combined effects of intrathoracic and intravascular pressures. The intrathoracic pressure exerts a distending influence on vasculature within the thorax.

venous pressure in distending the large veins and the heart, reducing, to this extent, the lower end of the pressure gradient from the periphery to the right ventricle.

The intrathoracic pressure fluctuates during normal respiratory activity, averaging about −5.4 cm. H_2O (−4 mm. Hg) at the end of a normal expiration. Inspiration further distends the lungs, lowering the pressure to about −10.8 cm. H_2O (−8 mm. Hg). Increased respiratory excursions produce correspondingly greater fluctuations in the intrathoracic pressure. Changes in intrathoracic and intra-abdominal pressure associated with diaphragmatic movements provide a pumping mechanism that facilitates transfer of blood into the thorax.

THE ABDOMINOTHORACIC PUMPING MECHANISM

During inspiration, the contracting diaphragm descends and the intrathoracic pressure is lowered by increased stretch of the inflated lungs. Simultaneously, the abdominal organs are displaced downward and forward; this displacement tends to stretch the anterior abdominal wall and increases the overall intra-abdominal pressure. Thus, during inspiration, the gradient in pressure between the abdomen and the thorax is increased and the flow of blood into the thoracic veins is accelerated (Fig. 6–11). In addition, the shortening of the inferior vena cava reduces its capacity, contributing to the blood flow into the thorax.[17] The increased intra-abdominal pressure temporarily impedes flow from the periphery into the abdomen; flow is accelerated after the intra-abdominal pressure is lowered during the subsequent expiratory movement.

Exhalation releases tension within the inflated lungs, and the intrathoracic

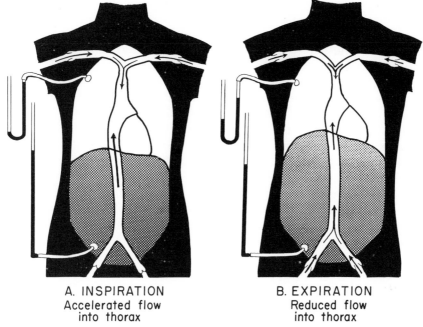

A. INSPIRATION
Accelerated flow into thorax

B. EXPIRATION
Reduced flow into thorax

FIGURE 6-11   ABDOMINOTHORACIC PUMP

A, During inspiration, reduced intrathoracic pressure coupled with increased intra-abdominal pressure accelerates the flow of blood from the abdominal veins into the thorax.

B, During expiration, flow into the thorax is retarded by simultaneous increase in intrathoracic pressure and reduction in intra-abdominal pressure.

pressure rises toward atmospheric pressure. Intra-abdominal pressure is reduced as the diaphragm relaxes and ascends. The inferior vena cava becomes elongated and accommodates more blood.[17] Thus, blood flow from abdomen to thorax is accelerated during inspiration and slowed during expiration. If expiration is continued beyond the normal range by active contraction of the abdominal muscles, the diaphragm is stretched as it is elevated beyond the position of rest so that intra-abdominal pressure is increased more than intrathoracic pressure rises. Since the diaphragm applies force only toward the abdominal cavity, and elastic tension in the lungs is continuously present, intra-abdominal pressure always exceeds intrathoracic pressure. By this mechanism, a favor-able pressure gradient from abdomen to thorax is always maintained under normal conditions.

CONTROL OF CENTRAL VENOUS PRESSURE

The pressure in the intrathoracic portions of the superior and inferior venae cavae is of great importance because the transmural pressure in these veins represents the distending pressure of the heart. A positive effective filling pressure must be maintained in these veins at all times regardless of the position of the body, the magnitude of the blood volume, the redistribution of blood in dilated capillary beds or the accumulation of blood in distended dependent veins. Otherwise, filling of the heart would be deficient during the diastolic intervals. On the other hand, excessive pressure in these veins would raise the gradient in pressure in both the venous and the lymphatic systems, which would promote accumulation of fluid in the tissues. The maintenance of central venous pressure between these two critical levels requires that the venous system compensate for variations in total blood volume and changes in its distribution. The right ventricular pressure during diastole represents the minimal pressure in the systemic venous system, since it is the point of outflow from the entire system. At rest in the horizontal position, the right ventricular pressure varies between +2 and −2 mm. Hg during diastole. Angiocardiographic studies[18] have revealed that, in the supine position, both the superior and inferior venae cavae are distended with blood. In the erect position, the inferior vena cava is distended, but the superior vena cava is partially collapsed just above the level of the right atrium. The point of collapse of the veins represents the level at which the effective venous pressure (intravascular pressure minus extravascular pressure) is essentially zero. If the pressure in the inferior vena cava fell until the point of collapse was just below the right atrium, the effective filling pressure of the right ventricle would be zero. Thus, a decrease in venous pressure of only a few centimeters of water in the right atrium would represent a serious impairment of right ventricular filling. This contingency is prevented by continuous and precise adjustments in the venous reservoir system to maintain the central venous pressure at levels only slightly above that of the right atrium regardless of the body's position.

The mechanism which controls the central venous pressure is best de-scribed by a schematic diagram (Fig. 6–12). Consider a distensible tube filled with water until there is a slight positive internal pressure when it is horizontal. In the vertical position, the fluid level in the tube would descend because the hydrostatic pressure would produce greater distention of the dependent portions. The fluid level could be restored to the previous height only by compression of some portion of the tube (Fig. 6–12). Exactly the same considerations apply whether the fluid is stationary or is flowing through the tube (see Fig. 6–4). The central venous pressure is only slightly above atmospheric pressure in normal reclining subjects. When the individual assumes a vertical position, the hydrostatic pressures produce a distention of the dependent veins which may accumulate relatively large quantities of blood (more than 500 cc.). Unless some portions of the venous vascular bed were compressed, effective central venous pressure would probably fall below that of the heart. A major portion of this blood may come from the lungs. However, external compression of veins by skeletal muscles in the legs, and probably by contraction of large venous channels and other venous reservoirs, restores the central venous pressure so that it is just above the pressure in the right atrium. The exact mechanisms controlling this important adjustment have not yet been elucidated.

The probability that central venous pressure is precisely controlled was strengthened by exposing animals to positive and negative radial acceleration on a large centrifuge.[9] Under forces as great as five times the force of gravity (5 g) the pressures in "dependent regions" became very high, but the level at which venous pressure remained essentially unchanged was at or near heart level whether these

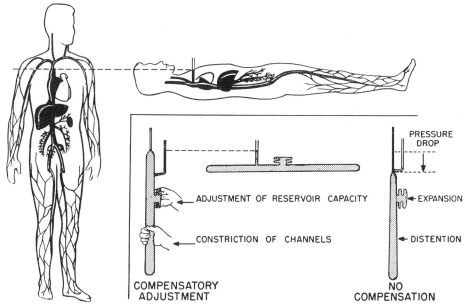

FIGURE 6-12   MAINTENANCE OF CENTRAL VENOUS PRESSURE

The veins in various regions of the body tend to be distended to about the same degree when a subject is recumbent. In the erect position the hydrostatic columns of blood produce distention of the vessels below the heart and collapse of veins above the heart. Since most of the venous reservoir capacity is below heart level, the central venous pressure theoretically could fall below heart level unless compensatory adjustments were promptly instituted. These compensatory mechanisms are illustrated schematically as a constriction of venous channels and regulation of reservoir capacity.

forces were directed toward the head or toward the lower parts of the body. Since the capacity of the veins below the diaphragm greatly exceeds that of those above the diaphragm, the large hydrostatic pressures would tend to cause massive accumulations of blood in dependent regions when the forces acted from head to feet. Control of central venous pressure must certainly involve regulation of the capacity of the venous reservoirs.

THE EFFECTS OF POSTURE ON VENTRICULAR SIZE

In earlier times the ventricular chambers were thought to be nearly empty at the end of each systole. This impression probably stemmed from observation of hearts exposed by thoracotomy, which induces marked shrinkage of the heart (see Fig. 3–9). Measurements under more normal conditions consistently indicate that relatively large volumes of blood remain within the ventricular chambers at the end of a normal ventricular systole. In fact, the ventricles apparently eject only about half of the end diastolic volume.[19, 20] In normal human subjects and in patients with heart disease resting quietly in the supine position the heart functions at or near its maximum dimensions.[21, 22] In resting recumbent dogs, the left ventricle tends to attain near maximum dimensions as recorded by gauges of diameter, length and circumference.

The rapid increase in the left ventricular diameter of a dog during a

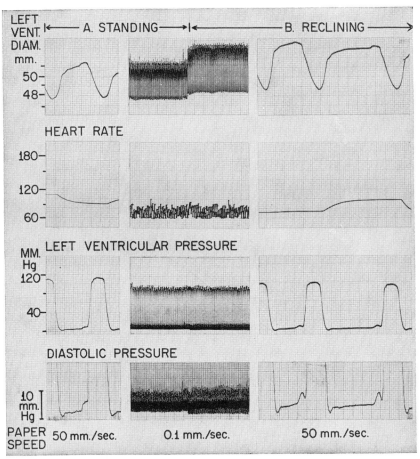

FIGURE 6-13 EFFECTS OF RECLINING ON VENTRICULAR FUNCTION

The changes in left ventricular diameter, heart rate and ventricular pressures as a healthy dog, standing with his trunk horizontal, spontaneously reclines. Note that the diastolic distention increased in spite of a slight drop in mean atrial pressure. The increased stroke deflections in the diameter record indicate an increase in stroke volume which has been amply confirmed by aortic flowmeters. These changes are in accordance with the Frank-Starling mechanism.

change from the standing (with trunk horizontal) to the reclining position is illustrated in Figure 6–13. The transition from sitting (or standing) to the recumbent position was accompanied by a progressive increase in diastolic dimensions over a series of cardiac cycles in which the stroke deflection increased and the systolic pressure was elevated (Fig. 6–14A, B). Thus, the increase in diastolic size was accompanied by an increase in energy release, in accordance with the Frank-Starling mechanism.[22] The diastolic diameter expanded to a maximum as evidenced by the fact that it reached a plateau early in diastole and atrial contraction produced little or no additional distention.

After the dog was anesthetized and thoracotomized, the heart was observed as it distended to its "maximum" dimensions when the animal succumbed to asphyxia. The diastolic

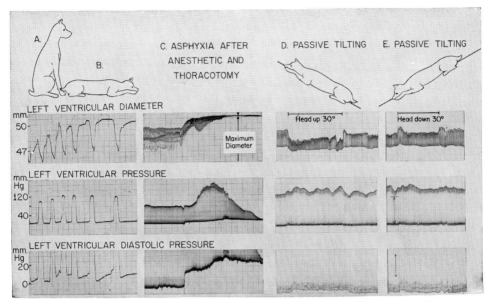

FIGURE 6-14 MAXIMAL DIASTOLIC DISTENTION DURING RECUMBENCY

A, As indicated in Figure 6-13, the left ventricular diameter promptly increases during the next few cycles after a dog assumes the reclining position.

B, After anesthesia, thoracotomy and asphyxia, the left ventricle distended under direct vision. The ventricular diameter after this extreme distention was essentially the same as in the recumbent position in *A,* indicating that under these conditions left ventricular distention may be "maximal" for that ventricle.

C, Changes in ventricular diameter with changes in posture are not due to the effort because they occur during passive tilting with the head up but to a much lesser extent with the head down.

diameter recorded during the distention produced by asphyxia was essentially the same as that recorded previously while the dog was relaxed (Fig. 6–14*B*).

The reduction in ventricular size was not due to the exertion involved in standing since both the diastolic diameter and the stroke deflection were reduced when the head was passively tilted up 30 degrees (Fig. 6–14*C*). However, vertical orientation of the trunk per se is not an essential factor in the reduction in heart size and stroke volume because the trunk is horizontal during both reclining and standing in the dog. Furthermore, the heart size promptly diminishes to about the same extent if the animal merely lifts his head in response to an unexpected noise. In other words, the cardiac chambers function at or near their maximum dimensions in the relaxed recumbent dog and their size is promptly reduced in all other circumstances observed.

A reduction in stroke volume on arising has been consistently observed in normal human subjects;[23] the average heart rate is slightly accelerated, but the net effect is a diminution in cardiac output. The same observation was made on intact dogs in which aortic flow was measured continuously by means of an indwelling ultrasonic flowmeter.[24] A reduction in cardiac output when the erect position is assumed indicates that the total flow through the peripheral circulation has been curtailed, presumably by vasoconstriction in some peripheral vascular bed.

THE CONCEPT OF VENOUS RETURN

The stroke volume of the heart-lung preparation was generally increased by elevating the venous reservoir. This experimental technique formed the basis for the concept that a prominent factor in the initiation of increased cardiac output was an increase in "venous return" in many cardiovascular responses. A precise definition for the term "venous return" is difficult to derive since it has been employed in many different ways so that it has, at one time or another, included increased volume flow into the ventricles, increased velocity of flow in the central veins, increased central venous pressure, increased filling pressure in the ventricles and so forth. However, there might be general agreement that stroke volume and cardiac output are increased by greater venous return when the central venous pressure, the volume flow into the ventricles, the diastolic ventricular volume, the stroke volume and the cardiac output are all increased. On the basis of these criteria, the increase in stroke volume and cardiac output occurring when an erect man or dog lies down is a most clear-cut example of the results of an increased venous return. Similarly, the reduced stroke volume and cardiac output accompanying standing could be described in terms of reduced venous return. An exaggerated form of this response is seen when positive radial acceleration with centrifugal forces of three to five times the force of gravity (3 to 5 g) are applied. Under these conditions, the ventricles become progressively smaller until they appear to empty maximally during each systole. Evi-

dence of changes in venous return in the initiation of circulatory responses cannot be easily recognized in other spontaneous circulatory adjustments by normal animals or man.

THE EFFECTS OF STANDING ON PERIPHERAL FLOW DISTRIBUTION

When a normal person arises from the recumbent to the erect position, less blood flows through the splanchnic bed and the dependent extremities (Fig. 6–15). For example, the estimated blood flow through the liver decreased on the average from 1713 cc. to 1070 cc. per minute in a group of human subjects.[25] The blood flow through the hand promptly diminishes and then rises somewhat to reach a mean level just below that recorded in the reclining subject. The blood flow through the legs decreases significantly, and the oxygen content of femoral venous blood is reduced, indicating that a much greater proportion of the oxygen reserve is utilized. A most pronounced reduction in flow through renal and superior mesenteric arteries occurred when the dogs in Figure 4–14 stood on their hind legs with the trunk held erect. According to recent evidence, the arteriovenous oxygen difference in blood passing through the leg increases about two-fold without a demonstrable increase in oxygen consumption, and oxygen extraction is augmented by this amount even if the leg bears no weight.

Teleologic explanations for vaso-constriction in the dependent leg are not difficult to imagine. In the erect position, the long columns of blood elevate the pressure in both the arteries and veins of the legs. An increase in the internal pressure within the arteries, arterioles, capillaries and

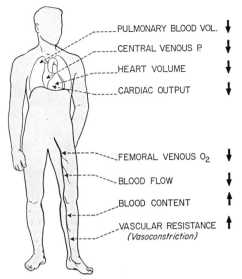

FIGURE 6-15 SOME EFFECTS OF ARISING

Changes in blood distribution and blood flow when a man stands are summarized schematically. Blood content diminishes in the lungs and heart and increases in the legs. Blood flow through the legs and cardiac output both diminish. The oxygen extraction from the blood flowing through the legs is necessarily more complete.

venules by 50 to 90 mm. Hg would tend to produce distention of all these vessels, producing a passive vasodilation throughout these vascular beds unless this tendency were opposed by active vasoconstriction. Vasoconstriction might also serve to diminish the rate at which fluid filters through the dependent capillary beds. If an erect subject moves his legs, as in walking, venous pressure in the lower legs drops to much lower levels owing to the pumping action of the muscles (Fig. 6–7). Under these conditions, the pressure gradient from the arteries to the veins may suddenly increase from about 90 mm. Hg to about 140 mm. Hg. This increase would cause considerably augmented flow through the dependent vascular beds. The consequent accelerated outflow from the

arterial system, coupled with the reduced stroke volume (Figs. 6–13 and 6–14), might produce a precipitous fall in systemic arterial blood pressure unless a peripheral vasoconstriction were promptly induced. The principal sign of a severe reduction in systemic arterial pressure attendant upon standing is a loss of consciousness.

THE TIME SEQUENCE OF POSTURAL RESPONSES

The directional changes illustrated in Figure 6–15 fail to convey the need for very prompt circulatory compensation to avoid precipitous fall in systemic arterial pressure. The vertical orientation greatly increases the hydrostatic pressure in dependent blood vessels which should cause distention and a lowered peripheral resistance at the same time that cardiac output is reduced. The central blood volume and heart volumes are diminishing, and the cardiac output is reduced by some 20 to 30 per cent. Diminished cardiac output accompanying reduced peripheral resistance should result in sharply falling arterial pressure unless reflex vasoconstriction occurs at the same time. In normal individuals actual measurements of systemic arterial pressure reveal no significant change even at the very onset of passive tilting from horizontal to erect positions on a tilt table where muscular pumping action of the legs is minimal or absent. To study the time relations of the integrated response to passive tilt to 60 degrees, Stegall and I recorded the overall reactions in a group of six normal subjects as illustrated in Figure 6–16. The course of changes in venous pressure and volume in the extremities (Fig. 6–16A) demonstrates a prompt but slight reduction in arm volume (10 to 30 ml.) and a sustained drop in

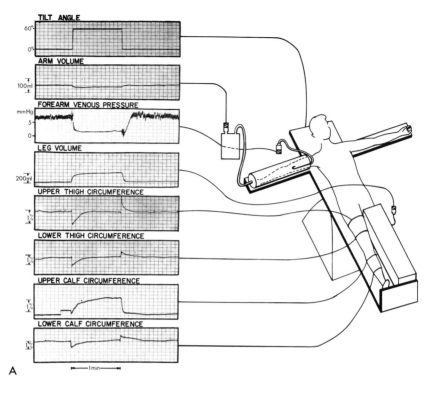

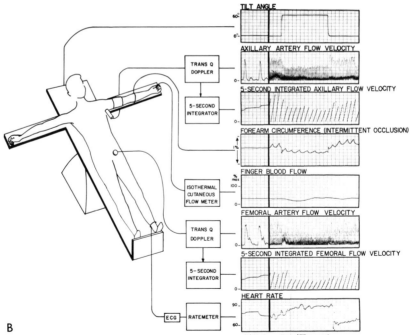

Figure 6-16 CHANGES IN VENOUS PRESSURE AND VOLUME AND BLOOD FLOW DURING PASSIVE TILT

A, Changes in venous pressure, arm and leg volumes and leg circumference at four levels during a passive tilt upright to 60 degrees. The initial downward spike in the circumference records represents easily visible sagging of tissues; the swelling of the leg follows the artifact.

B, Changes in axillary and femoral flow velocity recorded by ultrasonic Doppler flow sensors, forearm circumference changes with intermittent venous occlusion, finger blood flow and heart rate during passive tilting to 60 degrees like that illustrated in part A.

212

forearm venous pressure while the leg volume (by plethysmography) increased very rapidly by some 200 ml. in 10 to 15 seconds and another 50 ml. at the end of a minute. The circumference of the leg at four levels displayed an initial artifact due to visible sagging of tissues on all records. The increase in circumference due to swelling began immediately after the artifact. The upper calf showed the greatest change in circumference. Computations from the circumference gauges indicated that about 130 ml. accumulated in the thigh and some 80 ml. in the calf, accounting for 80 to 90 per cent of the swelling observed by plethysmography. The remaining 10 to 20 per cent must have gone to the foot. On return to the horizontal position, the blood rapidly leaves the legs, reaching pretilt levels within 15 to 20 seconds. The blood pressure recorded by sphygmomanometer repeatedly remained within a few mm. Hg of the pretilt values throughout.

The changes in blood flow during tilting are presented in Figure 6–16B. The instantaneous flow velocity in the axillary and femoral arteries (recorded by ultrasonic Doppler flow sensor) diminished very promptly, and the integrated flow velocity (related to volume flow per 5 seconds) also fell by one-third or one-half within about 10 to 15 seconds, indicating extremely prompt vasoconstriction in both arm and leg. The reduction in blood flow was confirmed by venous occlusion plethysmography using a circumference gauge, showing a reduction in estimated flow from 4.4 to 2.2 m./min./100 ml. of forearm. An isothermal skin blood flow sensor on the finger also showed an initial reduction in apparent blood flow during the first part of the tilt. The heart rate rose gradually after upright tilting from about 75 to about 90 beats/min. On the return to

horizontal, the heart rate dropped abruptly to a level below the control within one or two beats.

The net result of the changes observed in Figure 6–16A and B represents evidence of extremely rapid and effective compensation for the downward displacement of blood by a prompt vasoconstriction and reduction in peripheral blood flow to maintain arterial pressure very near the control levels. Under a wide variety of conditions, the compensatory vasoconstriction is either delayed or insufficient in amount, the arterial pressure falls and the individual experiences giddiness or fainting. This is the fundamental functional disturbance of the so-called orthostatic hypotension discussed in Part II of this chapter.

SUMMARY

In the standing adult of average height, the arterial and venous pressures recorded at the ankle are both as much as 85 mm. Hg higher than the pressures in the reclining subject. The pressure difference between the arteries and veins remains unchanged. The cardiac output has been reported to be diminished when the subjects are relaxed in the upright position rather than when they are supine. The major circulatory change produced by the hydrostatic columns is an increase in the capillary pressure in the dependent extremities and displacement of blood into dependent extremities.

Changes in the position of the body have no functional effect on the vasculature within the cerebrospinal cavity and the eye, and probably not on those in bone, because the extravascular pressure precisely balances the venous pressure.

Contraction of the leg muscles during walking brings into play the so-called "muscular pumping action" which has three effects: (*a*) At the beginning of muscular contraction, blood is displaced from the veins of the legs owing to external compression. (*b*) The pressure in the veins and capillaries in the lower extremities tends to be maintained at lower levels during active walking. (*c*) The arteriovenous pressure difference is increased so that blood flow through the capillaries into the veins would be increased if the state of arteriolar constriction remained unchanged. The quantity of blood flowing through the veins depends upon the rate of flow through the capillaries.

The external pressure provided by the hydrostatic column of abdominal organs tends to balance the hydrostatic pressures in the veins of the abdomen. By this mechanism, the vast splanchnic venous bed is largely protected from being distended by the increased venous pressures developed in the erect position. The subatmospheric pressure within the thorax provides a favorable pressure gradient from abdomen to thorax. Contraction of the diaphragm can act only to increase intra-abdominal pressure and reduce intrathoracic pressure.

The effective or transmural pressure in the thoracic veins, atria and ventricles is greater than that recorded externally because the subatmospheric pressure acts as a distending force. The filling pressure of the right ventricle is normally maintained at very low and constant levels by adjustments in the capacity of the venous reservoir system to compensate for variations in the distribution of blood and in the total blood volume.

II. POSTURAL HYPOTENSION

Diminished systemic arterial pressure, often accompanied by dizziness, sweating, visual disturbances and even loss of consciousness, is occasionally produced by sudden assumption of the erect posture after an individual has been relaxed while seated or lying down. The principal effects of arising from the recumbent to the standing position result from the hydrostatic pressures of vertically oriented columns of blood. The arterial and venous pressures increase in the dependent regions of the body. In regions above the heart, the veins collapse and the venous pressure becomes approximately equal to the surrounding tissue pressure. The arterial pressure in these regions diminishes by an amount equivalent to the height of the column of blood above the level of the heart. The cerebral circulation, however, is protected against the effects of the reduction in arterial pressure because the gravitational influences on hydrostatic columns affect equally the intravascular and extravascular pressures within the rigid cerebrospinal canal. During standing the arterial pressure at the base of the skull[15] (about 30 cm. above the heart) is about 25 mm. Hg less than the arterial pressure at heart level. The pressure of the cerebrospinal fluid within the skull is also about 25 mm. Hg less than the systemic venous pressure at heart level (i.e., is approximately 25 mm. Hg below atmospheric pressure). Since the arterial, capillary, venous and extravascular pressures within the skull are all reduced by the same amount (25 mm. Hg), the perfusion pressure from the arteries to the veins is not reduced when the erect position is assumed.

The cerebral blood flow is affected by a reduction in the systemic arterial pressure that acts to reduce the perfusion pressure, i.e., the pressure gradient from the cerebral arteries to the veins.

The cerebral circulation is unresponsive to virtually all mechanisms normally exerting control over peripheral blood flow. Lacking effective compensatory mechanisms, the cerebral perfusion diminishes with any significant drop in systemic arterial pressure.

SYNCOPE (FAINTING)

Fainting is characterized by an abrupt fall in blood pressure, bradycardia, pallor, dizziness, dimming or loss of vision and unconsciousness.[12, 26] These changes may be induced by many and varied conditions including emotional reactions (e.g., the sight of blood), standing quietly for long periods, hemorrhage and pain—particularly the diffuse, poorly localized pain carried by visceral afferent fibers.[26] Fainting reactions can be elicited experimentally by passively tilting the subject into the erect position during withdrawal of blood by venesection or trapping of blood in the legs with cuffs, after administration of various dilator drugs or during application of painful stimuli.

Because fainting most commonly develops in erect individuals and is promptly alleviated by falling or lying down, many investigators once attributed it to reduced cardiac output resulting from a combination of the bradycardia with pooling of blood in the dependent veins. Since then, evidence obtained in a variety of ways suggests that such a combination is not necessarily concurrent with fainting. Prevention of the bradycardia with atropine does not affect the fall in blood pressure. By means of cardiac catheterization, a reduction in both right atrial pressure and cardiac output was observed after passive tilting and during venesection while the arterial blood pressure was well maintained. At the abrupt onset of the fainting reaction the blood pressure drops precipitously to lower levels (i.e., 60/40) with no drop in cardiac output.

Barcroft[12] accidentally discovered that during fainting reactions the blood flow through skeletal muscle increases greatly owing to both release of vasoconstrictor tone and activation of vasodilator fibers serving skeletal muscles. He compared the blood flows in the forearms of subjects with and without sympathetic nerve block during induced fainting reactions and found a flow through the innervated muscles exceeding that through the denervated muscles. These observations led to the concept of sympathetic vasodilator fibers serving skeletal muscles. Although the blood flow through the liver diminishes abruptly at the onset of a fainting reaction, the concurrent fall in blood pressure is disproportionately great. This observation suggests the occurrence of some vasodilation in the splanchnic bed as well as in the skeletal muscle.[26] Resistance to blood flow through the kidney may also be reduced. The loss of consciousness is apparently caused by diminished cerebral blood flow, as evidenced by a marked reduction in the amount of venous blood flowing from the brain.

HYPERSENSITIVE CAROTID SINUS

External pressure on the carotid sinus may activate the pressoreceptor reflex which normally compensates for an abrupt rise in systemic arterial blood pressure. The heart rate slows, and the peripheral vessels dilate as though to correct an increased arterial pressure. Thus, the systemic arterial pressure is abruptly but inappropriately reduced, and the individual experiences lightheadedness or even unconsciousness.

In 1933 Weiss and Baker[27] described 15 patients complaining of dizziness and fainting apparently related to unusual sensitivity of the carotid sinus mechanism. Some of these patients developed cardiac standstill for 2 to 12 seconds when pressure was exerted on their necks by tight collars, during shaving or even by the turning of their heads in a particular manner. Digital pressure over the sinus region readily produced the attacks. In six of these patients there was a definite aneurysmal dilation of one or both carotid sinuses, and in three a small tumor pressed on the sinus. In the remaining six patients no gross lesion was noted.

Four main types of syncope can be produced by compression of the carotid sinus: (a) transient cardiac standstill, (b) precipitous fall in blood pressure with slowing of the heart rate, (c) precipitous fall in blood pressure without bradycardia and (d) cerebral syncope now regarded as a form of epilepsy rather than as cardiovascular collapse.

Circulatory collapse accompanied by a precipitous fall in blood pressure, bradycardia, profuse sweating and pallor can be induced in many erect normal subjects by mechanical stimulation of the brachial arterial wall with a hypodermic needle.[28] Stimulation of visceral afferent fibers in general and pain fibers in particular produces depressor responses in most normal subjects and frequently produces syncopal reactions. The vasodilation in peripheral vascular beds during syncopal reactions or in response to hyperactive carotid sinus reflexes represents an inappropriate response in the circulatory system which has accommodated to the erect position.

Systemic arterial pressure is most apt to drop during a sudden transition from lying down to standing up. The normal response to this change is a prompt vasoconstriction in the dependent parts, accompanied by a reduction in stroke volume and cardiac output. If the peripheral vasoconstriction is not prompt enough or not great enough, the individual is likely to faint. Thus, patients who have been bedridden for days or weeks may suffer from dizziness or faintness the first few times they stand. This is commonly attributed to a reduced sympathetic constrictor "tone" or to "sluggish" sympathetic responses. A person is much more prone to exhibit a transient drop in systemic arterial pressure on arising if his blood pressure is chronically low.

SYSTEMIC ARTERIAL HYPOTENSION

In any large group of normal individuals the values for systemic arterial pressure conform to the frequency distribution shown in Figure 5–18. Among people with blood pressures below the "normal range" are many who experience transient dizziness, loss of vision or even occasional unconsciousness if they stand up too abruptly, particularly first thing in the morning. These symptoms can be alleviated by arising more gradually or by sleeping on a bed tilted slightly with the head elevated. Such individuals are also prone to develop these symptoms on arising suddenly after kneeling, squatting or stooping. These people have "orthostatic hypotension" primarily because their sympathic constrictor activity is always limited and the response to arising is too slow or too slight. For example, Stead and Ebert[29] reported that the blood vessels of the hands did not constrict normally during a fall in blood pressure when such subjects were in an upright position. The heart rate remained unchanged or increased moderately. The signs and symptoms developed when the systolic pressure was 50 mm. Hg or less. The absence of normal vasoconstriction in response to a fall in arterial pressure was indicated by the following observations: (a) the diastolic pressure dropped markedly when the subject stood up, (b) the blood flow in the hand was higher than that in normal subjects for a given decrease in arterial pressure and (c) trapping blood in the extremities produced a greater reduction in arterial pressure in these patients than normal subjects. Thus, the reflex vasoconstriction which normally accompanies standing does not occur in patients with postural hypotension.

The same sort of symptoms are experienced following surgical excision of the sympathetic chains as a treatment for severe arterial hypertension.

POSTURAL HYPOTENSION FOLLOWING SYMPATHECTOMY

If postural hypotension and syncope result from an inadequate sympathetic constrictor response, elimination of the sympathetic outflow should produce a similar reaction which is more severe. Cutting of the sympathetic fibers running to various organs releases the vasoconstrictor "tone" and increases the blood flow through most tissues except the brain and kidney. (The effects of sympathectomy on the coronary circulation are equivocal for reasons described in Chapter 9.) Since the sympathetic constrictor mechanism is dominant in the maintenance of systemic arterial pressure, elimination of this system produces a prompt and severe reduction in arterial blood pressure. However, the increased peripheral blood flow produced by the diminished peripheral resistance does not persist even if the entire sympathetic chains are removed bilaterally. In experimental animals, the peripheral resistance begins to rise again within one or two days and attains preoperative levels within a week or two. This restoration of the blood pressure is an expression of the increased reactivity of the peripheral vessels to catechol amines and other vasoconstrictor substances. This so-called denervation sensitivity has not been satisfactorily explained. Since the arterial blood pressure returns to preoperative levels even after extirpation of the adrenal medullae, the exact mechanism for the return of vascular tone remains a most perplexing problem.

Sympathectomy as a treatment for hypertension has been less than satisfactory because the arterial blood pressure returns to approximately the preoperative levels in about 80 per cent of patients within two years. Immediately after sympathectomy, all patients suffer from hypotension on arising. This orthostatic hypotension persists in very severe form for days or weeks but gradually subsides spontaneously in most instances. Within a few months these patients are able to function quite normally without their sympathetic outflow. In recent years, sympathetic blocking agents have become available for therapy of hypertension. These drugs act to reduce the

Table 6-1.   TYPES OF POSTURAL HYPOTENSION

Primarily an Inadequate Cardiac Output Carotid sinus syndrome—cardiac or vagal inhibitory type Adams-Stokes syndrome Ventricular asystole Ventricular fibrillation Paroxysmal tachycardias Cardiac tamponade Valvular heart disease (aortic and mitral stenosis) Ball-valve thrombus and pedunculated myxoma of heart Myocardial injury Infection (diphtheria, rheumatic fever) Acute coronary insufficiency Infarction (cardiogenic shock) Massive pulmonary embolism Post-tussive syncope (Valsalva maneuver) Pregnancy: Decubitus position with large gravid uterus **Primarily an Inadequate Peripheral Resistance** Neurogenic disturbances Mediated through the autonomic nervous system Chronic orthostatic hypotension Surgical splanchnicotomy Debilitating infections (atypical pneumonia) Mediated through the vasomotor centers Direct Brain tumor Cerebral vascular disease Indirect Vasodepressor syncope Carotid sinus syndrome—peripheral vasodilator type	Primary pulmonary hypertension Hypotensive drugs (modified after Wilkins) Sympatholytic or adrenergic blocking agents Ganglionic blockers, e.g., tetraethylammonium and hexamethonium Centrally acting, e.g., dihydrogenated ergot alkaloids, *l*-hydrazinophthalazine Peripherally acting, e.g., Dibenamine Vasodilator agents, e.g., nitrites (peripheral), veratrum (central neurogenic) Agents with modes of action as yet uncertain, e.g., thiocyanates, pyrogens Acute fulminating infections Allergic reactions **Primarily an Inadequate Effective Blood Volume** Hemorrhagic and traumatic shock Venesection Venous congestion of extremities Large varicosities and angiomas of lower extremities Postexertional hypotension **Mechanisms Mixed or Not Completely Understood** Adrenal cortical insufficiency, crisis Diabetic coma Low salt syndrome Anoxia Anemia Congenital heart disease, right-to-left shunt

systemic arterial pressure by blocking the sympathetic outflow. Like surgical sympathectomy they may induce postural hypotension.

SUMMARY

These few examples illustrate the manner in which physiologic mechanisms for the control of systemic arterial pressure may become involved in circulatory collapse. Obviously, reduction in blood pressure could result from combinations of those factors which reduce the heart rate, stroke volume and cardiac output, reduce peripheral resistance or retard or diminish the vasoconstriction which is a normal component of the cardiovascular response to arising. Judson[30] has based a more comprehensive discussion of these mechanisms on the classification presented in Table 6-1.

REFERENCES

1. HELLEBRANDT, F. A., and FRANSEEN, E. B. Physiological study of the vertical stance of man. *Physiol. Rev.*, 23:220-255, 1943.
2. MAYERSON, H. S. Effect of gravity on the

blood pressure of the dog. *Amer. J. Physiol.*, 135:411–418, 1942.

3. BURCH, G. E., and WINSOR, T. The phlebomanometer. A new apparatus for direct measurement of venous pressure in large and small veins. *J.A.M.A.*, 123:91–92, 1943.

4. SODEMAN, W. A. Direct venous pressure determinations by use of a new instrument. *Amer. Heart J.*, 43:687–690, 1952.

5. FRY, E. L. Physiologic recording by modern instruments with particular reference to pressure recording. *Physiol. Rev.*, 40:753–788, 1960.

6. FRANK, E. K. Physiologic pressure transducer. In *Methods in Medical Research*, Vol. 11, R. F. Rushmer, Ed. Chicago, Year Book Medical Publishers, Inc., 1966.

7. THOMPSON, H. K., JR., and McINTOSH, H. D. Cannulation and catheterization procedures. In *Methods in Medical Research*, Vol. 11, R. F. Rushmer, Ed. Chicago, Year Book Medical Publishers, Inc., 1966.

8. OCHSNER, A., JR., COLP, R., JR., and BURCH, G. E. Normal blood pressure in the superficial venous system of man at rest in the supine position. *Circulation*, 3:674–680, 1951.

9. RUSHMER, R. F., BECKMAN, E. L., and LEE, D. Protection of the cerebral circulation by the cerebrospinal fluid under the influence of radial acceleration. *Amer. J. Physiol.*, 151:355–365, 1947.

10. WELLS, H. S., YOUMANS, J. B., and MILLER, D. G., JR. Tissue pressure (intracutaneous, subcutaneous and intramuscular) as related to venous pressure, capillary filtration, and other factors. *J. Clin. Invest.*, 17:489–499, 1938.

11. MAYERSON, H. S., and BURCH, G. E. Relationships of tissue (subcutaneous and intramuscular) and venous pressures to syncope induced in man by gravity. *Amer. J. Physiol.*, 128:258–269, 1940.

12. BARCROFT, H., and SWAN, H. J. C. *Sympathetic Control of Human Blood Vessels*. London, Edward Arnold, 1953.

13. POLLACK, A. A., and WOOD, E. H. Venous pressure in the saphenous vein at the ankle in man during exercise and changes in posture. *J. Appl. Physiol.*, 1:649–662, 1949.

14. HÖJENSGARD, I. C., and STÜRUP, H. Static and dynamic pressures in superficial and deep veins of the lower extremity in man. *Acta physiol. scand.*, 27:49–67, 1952.

15. STEGALL, H. F. Muscle pumping in the dependent leg. *Circulat. Res.*, 19:180–190, 1966.

16. RUSHMER, R. F. The nature of intraperitoneal and intrarectal pressures. *Amer. J. Physiol.*, 147:242–249, 1946.

17. FREMONT-SMITH, F. The role of elongation and contraction of the inferior vena cava, coincident with respiration, in the return of blood to the heart: report of an observation on men. *J. Mt. Sinai Hosp.*, 9:432–434, 1942.

18. DUOMARCO, J. L., RIMINI, R., and SAPRIZA, J. P. Attempted evaluation of venous pressure by angiocardiography. *Rev. argent. cardiol.*, 17:15–28, 1950.

19. HOLT, J. P. Estimation of the residual volume of the ventricle of the dog's heart by two indicator dilution technics. *Circulat. Res.*, 4:187–195, 1956.

20. SJÖSTRAND, T. Regulatory mechanisms relating to blood volume. *Minnesota Med.*, 37:10–15, 1954.

21. MUSSHOFF, V. K., and REINDELL, H. Zur Röntgenuntersuchung des Herzens in horizontaler und vertikaler Körperstellung. Der Einfluss der Körperstellung auf das Herzvolumen. [Radiographic examination of the heart in erect and lying position. The influence of the body's position on heart volume.] *Deutsch. med. Wchnschr.*, 81:1001–1008, 1956.

22. RUSHMER, R. F. Postural effects on the baselines of ventricular performance. *Circulation*, 20:897–905, 1959.

23. WEISSLER, A. M., LEONARD, J. J., and WARREN, J. W. Effects of posture and atropine on the cardiac output. *J. Clin. Invest.*, 36:1656–1662, 1957.

24. FRANKLIN, D. L., ELLIS, R. M., and RUSHMER, R. F. Aortic blood flow in dogs during treadmill exercise. *J. Appl. Physiol.*, 14:809–812, 1959.

25. CULBERTSON, J. W., WILKINS, R. W., INGELFINGER, F. J., and BRADLEY, S. E. The effect of the upright posture upon hepatic blood flow in normotensive and hypertensive patients. *J. Clin. Invest.*, 30:305–311, 1951.

26. EDHOLM, O. G. Physiological changes during fainting. Pp. 256–270 in *Visceral Circulation, a Ciba Foundation Symposium*. G. E. W. Wolstenholme, Ed. London, J. & A. Churchill Ltd., 1952.

27. WEISS, S., and BAKER, J. P. The carotid sinus reflex in health and disease: its role in the causation of fainting and convulsions. *Medicine*, 12:297–354, 1933.

28. RUSHMER, R. F. Circulatory collapse following mechanical stimulation of arteries. *Amer. J. Physiol.*, 141:722–729, 1944.

29. STEAD, E. A., and EBERT, R. Postural hypotension; a disease of the sympathetic nervous system. *Arch. Int. Med.*, 67:546–562, 1941.

30. JUDSON, W. E. Hypotension; physiologic mechanisms and treatment. *Med. Clin. North Amer.*, 37:1313–1339, 1953.

CHAPTER 7

CARDIOVASCULAR RESPONSES DURING EXERTION

In everyday life, the adjustments in blood flow accompanying increased activity of tissues or organs impose little stress on the capacity of the cardiovascular system. Digestion of food, formation of urine, secretion of enzymes or synthesis of substances in the liver or glands requires little or no increase in cardiac output above its resting level. Heat dissipation by the skin may involve increased blood flow and slightly augmented cardiac output. In contrast, exercise taxes the ability of the cardiovascular system to convey blood to the peripheral vessels and is the principal normal activity to do so. In man, dog and horse, the cardiac output during exertion is directly related to oxygen consumption.[1] The oxygen consumption of a resting man is about 250 cc. per minute, but during sustained exercise a maximum rate of oxygen consumption of 5350 cc. per minute has been recorded, an increase of 21 fold.[2] This represents a sustained increase in energy release from 0.12 horsepower to 2.6 horsepower. Ekblom and Hermansen[3] reported extremely high values in selected athletes attaining cardiac output up to 42 l./min. with stroke volume of 212 ml. at maximum. In the 10 seconds required to

run 100 yards, the athlete consumes oxygen at a rate of about 30 liters per minute, equivalent to 14.4 horspower. During this brief period, however, he burns only about 0.5 liter, so that his oxygen debt is about 5 liters. The rate of energy expenditure increases about 120 times as a man goes from rest to maximum exertion. Fenn[2] computed the actual work done while sprinting as corresponding to 3.95 horsepower of actual external work; the efficiency was thus about 21.5 per cent. Based on these observations, the increased oxygen utilization by exercising muscle must be achieved by (1) increased cardiac output, (2) redistribution of blood flow from inactive to active tissues, (3) increased oxygen extraction from the blood and (4) oxygen debt.

INCREASED OXYGEN UTILIZATION DURING EXERTION

The oxygen consumption of the body is normally increased by significant amounts only during muscular exertion. The magnitude of the increased oxygen requirement is closely related to the quantity of external work which is involved in the exertion. The

220

changes in oxygen consumption from a condition of rest in the supine position to the erect position is so slight that cardiac output need not increase and stroke volume generally decreases considerably (see Chapter 6). Leisurely walking on level ground increases oxygen requirements slightly, but this can be readily accommodated by stroke volume at levels approximating those in the supine position. This effect is discussed in more detail in subsequent sections of this chapter. Moderate exercise can be well sustained by normal individuals utilizing the kinds of control mechanisms described in previous chapters. For any particular individual, maximum exercise which can be sustained for several minutes calls into play an integrated series of mechanisms illustrated in Table 7–1.

Oxygen delivery is increased by a combination of increased total blood flow through the tissues and more complete oxygen extraction from each increment of blood flowing through the tissues. Oxygen extraction is represented by the difference in oxygen content of arterial and venous blood. The oxygen content of arterial blood is normally in the range of 200 cc./liter of blood. The oxygen content in venous blood from all the various tissues averages about 150 cc./liter of

blood. During exercise, the oxygen content of arterial blood is well-sustained, but the oxygen content of venous blood drops to much lower levels in most tissues. In resting muscle and other tissues which do not participate in the increased metabolic requirements, the oxygen uptake is about the same, but the blood flow is generally reduced to some degree by selective vasoconstriction. The resulting redistribution of blood flow shunts blood generally away from relatively inactive tissues (e.g., splanchnic bed, kidneys) and toward the actively metabolizing muscle, but the magnitude of this shift appears to be variable, depending upon the severity of the exertion and on species differences. For example, exercising dogs exhibit little or no reduction in splanchnic or renal blood flow while humans appear to utilize this mechanism to a much greater extent as discussed in subsequent sections.

The increased cardiac output can be achieved by accelerated heart rate, larger stroke volume or a combination of the two. The changes in autonomic discharge to the heart which would result in tachycardia also induce sympathetic effects on the myocardium producing more rapid tension development and fiber shortening. The effects of increased sympathetic discharge to the ventricles was discussed in detail in Chapter 3 (see Figs. 3–17 and 3–18). Another mechanism which could contribute to increased stroke volume is the Frank-Starling mechanism which proscribes increased energy release in elongated myocardial fibers. If the ventricular myocardium were stretched by greater diastolic distention during exertion, increased energy release during systole would be expected. The relative roles of the sympathetic discharge and the Frank-Starling mechanism has been subject

Table 7–1. *MECHANISMS FOR INCREASED OXYGEN UTILIZATION DURING EXERTION*

Stroke volume	Heart rate	
Cardiac output	A-V oxygen difference	
	Oxygen delivery	Oxygen debt
	Oxygen utilization	

to protracted controversy, in large measure because of differences in control conditions, in experimental procedures, severity of exercise, species differences, types of measurements, and interpretation of the same or similar data. This complex and controversial argument cannot be fully resolved, but we can at least avoid augmentation of disagreement by dealing with the exercise response where it can be most comprehensively described: in dogs with chronically implanted devices for continuously measuring changes in pressures, cardiac dimensions and blood flow. Some sources of variability in canine responses are apparent. The role of the central nervous system in initiating cardiovascular responses in exercise has been demonstrated experimentally, contributing greatly to the variability in observed responses. Finally, recognizable differences between cardiovascular adaptation to exercise in man and dogs will be summarized.

LEFT VENTRICULAR RESPONSE TO EXERTION IN HEALTHY DOGS

Recently, the traditional concepts of cardiac control during exertion have been evaluated by means of new techniques for continuous analysis of left ventricular performance in healthy dogs.[4, 5] Changes in the diameter of the left ventricle and the effective pressure in it were recorded directly, and additional variables were derived by electronic analogue computers as indicated in Figure 7–1.

Comprehensive descriptions of cardiac responses during exercise can be gleaned from continuous and simultaneous recording of the critical physical variables of the type illustrated in Figure 2–23. In dogs, fully recovered from the surgical implantation of re-cording devices for intraventricular pressure, ventricular outflow and dimensions (ventricular diameter or circumference) can be recorded continuously. Using analogue computers, other essential variables can be derived to provide a remarkably complete picture of the sequential changes in ventricular performance reclining, at rest, standing and during treadmill exercise (Fig. 7–1).

The simultaneous records in Figure 7–1 begin with the dog reclining quietly and then display a sequence of responses of the dog when hearing a loud noise, standing, doing treadmill exercise at 3 m.p.h. on a 12 per cent grade, standing, reclining, repeating exercise, reclining, and so forth. Note the startle response to the loud noise which produced a sharp peak in all the records except the ventricular diameter (top record) and the duration of systole (bottom record). A similar overshoot appeared in most of the records at the beginning of exercise, a pattern characteristic of a dog's initial or early experience with treadmill exercise. The initial overshoot is considerably smaller on the second exercise and after two or three more trials, most if not all the variables would promptly rise to a plateau and remain there during the remainder of the exercise without initial overshoot. This phenomenon has been confirmed in careful studies by Ninomiya and Wilson.[6] They found that the initial overshoot had a response time (63.2 per cent) for all cardiac variables of about 9 seconds. The magnitude of the overshoot was largely dependent upon the number of previous exercise periods, diminishing rapidly with repeated trials. The plateau levels established during more nearly steady state were dependent upon the magnitude of the work loads. The initial response of the inexperienced dogs were clearly re-

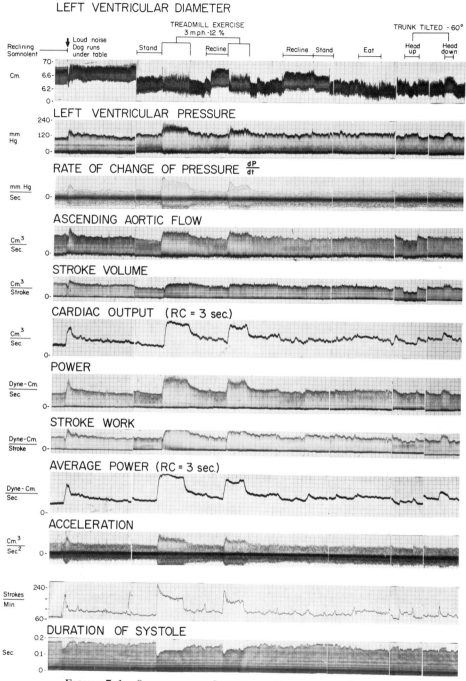

FIGURE 7–1. SPONTANEOUS CHANGES IN VENTRICULAR FUNCTION

The function of the left ventricle, monitored by the techniques illustrated in Figure 2–22, displays marked changes in all significant variables during both postural adaptations and exertion on a treadmill.

lated to the startle response when the treadmill belt started moving without advance warning. It indicates the major contribution of the central nervous system to variability in exercise responses in dogs and probably in man as well.

The magnitude and direction of changes in stroke volume during sustained exercise in dogs remains somewhat equivocal. For example, Wang, Marshall and Shepherd[7] found little or no change in stroke volume at wide ranges of exercise, often less than 5 per cent and the highest reaching 19 per cent. Smulyan *et al.*[8] reported a reduction in stroke volume at the onset of exertion with a modest increase in stroke volume developing when the heart rate diminished after the initial overshoot. Variability in the responses reported in different animals and by different investigators complicates the problem of providing a "generally accepted" pattern of response.

From more than 200 records of the responses of more than 30 dogs to a standard exercise (running on a treadmill at 3 m.p.h. on a 5 per cent grade), a "typical" ventricular reaction to moderate exertion can be summarized as follows:

1. *Heart rate.* Tachycardia appears promptly, without a lag, and is well sustained throughout the period of exercise.

2. *The left ventricular diameter* tends to change only slightly if the animal is standing at the onset of exertion. Systolic ejection may increase slightly and, on occasion, the diastolic distention may also increase somewhat. In general, the stroke deflections are either unchanged or slightly increased (see also Figs. 7–10 and 7–11).

3. *The left ventricular systolic pressure* is elevated in practically all records.

4. *The left ventricular diastolic pressure* is somewhat variable; the most common changes include a lower pressure during the early rapid filling phase and a higher end diastolic pressure (apparently due to more vigorous atrial contraction) with little change in mean atrial pressure. In some instances the diastolic pressures are definitely reduced.

5. *The instantaneous aortic flow rate* increases, particularly in the early part of systole.

6. *The stroke volume* (integrated instantaneous aortic flow) is unchanged or slightly increased in dogs. In Figure 7–1, the stroke volume increased about as much as was observed in any of the animals studied. In most animals, the stroke volume was increased slightly or not at all at this moderate level of exercise. In dogs exhibiting marked tachycardia, the stroke volume was sometimes reduced during moderate exertion.

7. The peak "power" (rate of doing work) of the ventricle is increased, representing the combined effects of high peak flow and ventricular pressure.

8. *The "stroke work"* increases slightly in dogs, reflecting the increased ventricular systolic pressure combined with the same or slightly augmented stroke volume. The increase in stroke work is undoubtedly greater in man than in the dog. The accumulated stroke "work" ("work" per stroke times heart rate) is definitely greater.

9. *The rate of change of pressure* (dP/dt) is much more rapid during both the rise in systolic pressure and the fall in pressure at the end of systole.

Thus, the principal changes in ventricular performance in dogs during exercise involved a combination of an accelerated heart rate and more dynamic ventricular contraction of the sort produced by increased sympathetic stimulation to the myocardium (see Figs. 3–17 and 3–18). Significant differences between the exercise responses in dogs and in man are described in a subsequent section of this chapter.

Variability in Exercise Responses. Comparison of two successive exercise responses in the same dog and single responses from two other dogs demonstrates fairly similar fundamental patterns, although the details differ. Significant differences in the diastolic diameter, the amplitude of the stroke deflection and the systolic and diastolic pressures are observed. Physiologic variability is a common feature of biologic systems, stemming from individual differences in structure, function, previous state of training and other characteristics. The responses of different animals tend to be more divergent than the responses of the same animal to different bouts of exercise. Successive exercise periods tend to reduce the variability and to produce more stereotyped responses.

The differences in repeated exercise reactions by the same animal can usually be reduced. On a subsequent day, the first exercise may again be associated with an overshoot. Thus, learning or conditioning may play a role in the nature and magnitude of the cardiac responses to exercise.

Some dogs have become so accustomed to the laboratory and so well trained that they will exercise freely on the treadmill for as long as desired without any restraint. When a trained dog is standing quietly on the treadmill, showing him the switch that activates the treadmill may induce a response much like the typical exercise response without any external evidence of muscular movement or tensing (Fig. 7–2). The variability in the ventricular responses of different ani-

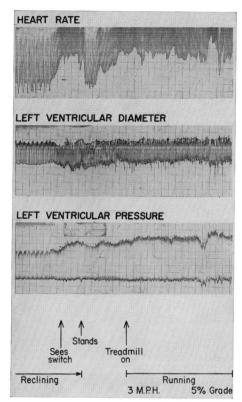

FIGURE 7–2. RESPONSE TO IMPENDING EXERCISE

A dog with extensive experience running on the treadmill was shown the electric switch that activates the treadmill, producing a left ventricular response very similar in kind and magnitude to the subsequent adaptation to running on the treadmill. This example is somewhat more dramatic than is generally seen.

mals, coupled with such evidence of control by higher levels of the nervous system, indicates the interaction of multiple mechanisms. Thus it seems futile to attempt to describe or explain the exercise response in terms of any simple generalization. These observations have required a critical evaluation of a long standing concept that cardiac compensation to exercise characteristically includes marked increase in stroke volume by virtue of the Frank-Starling mechanism.

POSTULATED RESPONSE TO EXERTION BASED ON THE FRANK-STARLING MECHANISM

For many years, the mechanisms for increasing peripheral vascular flow and cardiac output were discussed in terms of increased "venous return" and Starling's law of the heart. In these traditional formulations, the increased cardiac output resulted from two parallel sequences originating with the onset of skeletal muscle contraction (Fig. 7–3).

According to this postulation the cardiac response to exercise should follow the pattern presented schemati-

cally in Figure 7–3B. A brief time after exertion begins, the diastolic pressure in the ventricles should increase.[9] The diastolic, systolic and stroke volumes should all increase and remain elevated during the exercise. The systemic arterial pressure should fall, exciting the pressoreceptor mechanisms to induce tachycardia and peripheral vasoconstriction which restore the blood pressure to normal. This hypothetical sequence of events was generally believed to occur until serious deviations from it were seen during direct measurements on human subjects and intact animals.[10]

In this traditional view five mech-

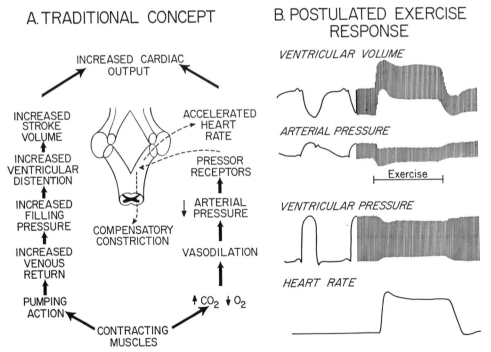

FIGURE 7–3.   VENTRICULAR RESPONSE TO EXERCISE (TRADITIONAL CONCEPTS)

A, Schematic representation of the ventricular response, envisioned in terms of the Frank-Starling mechanism. According to this hypothesis, stroke volume would be increased by greater diastolic and systolic distention of the ventricles, reduced systemic arterial pressure, increased ventricular diastolic pressure and tachycardia.

B, The sequence of events postulated to explain the increased stroke volume by increased "venous return" and tachycardia in response to diminished systemic arterial pressure through the pressoreceptor mechanisms.

anisms were assigned prominent roles in promoting increased cardiac output during exercise: (*a*) a drop in arterial blood pressure, (*b*) cardio-acceleration induced reflexly by pressoreceptors, (*c*) an increase in "venous return," (*d*) elevated central venous pressure and (*e* increased diastolic ventricular volume leading to increased stroke volume.

Arterial blood pressure (systolic) is characteristically elevated during exercise with mean pressure remaining relatively unchanged. If a drop in arterial pressure occurs at all, it is so transient at the beginning of exertion that it cannot be consistently demonstrated in man or experimental animals.

Tachycardia often occurs in anticipation of exertion, before muscular contractions begin. During exercise, the elevated arterial blood pressure should slow the heart. What sustains the accelerated heart rate during exertion? Furthermore, cardio-acceleration per se does not increase cardiac output. With constant "venous return" the cardiac output cannot be increased by tachycardia.

"Venous return" is a term which is widely used but rarely defined. It appears to stem from experiments with heart-lung preparations in which an ample venous reservoir of blood could be artificially maintained. The intact circulation, in contrast, is a closed system. A sustained increase in volume flow through the entire circuit has been correspondingly increased. Some authors have used the expression *increased venous return* as though it implied an elevated central venous pressure or increased filling pressure of the ventricles.

Increased ventricular filling pressure. Although an increase in peripheral venous pressure during exercise has been repeatedly demonstrated,

evidence of changes in central venous pressure has been somewhat equivocal.

Changes in ventricular volume. Although the traditional concepts of cardiovascular control appear to call for an increase in diastolic volume whenever the stroke volume is increased, there is considerable evidence that the heart often becomes smaller during exertion.[11, 12]

Critical Evaluation of These Traditional Concepts. The traditional concepts of cardiac adaption to exercise were based for many years on the Frank-Starling mechanism, calling for an increase in central venous pressure, increased ventricular distention and greater stroke volume resulting from increased "venous return" and greater diastolic extension of the myocardium. A drop in systemic arterial pressure was predicted to result from reduced peripheral resistance from net vasodilation as illustrated schematically in Figure 7–3. These concepts stemmed directly from certain experiments with anesthetized animals. The development of techniques for continuous analysis of cardiac function during spontaneous exercise has made it possible to re-evaluate the role of these hypothetical mechanisms by directly comparing the response to treadmill exercise with the responses to the classic experimental procedures in the same dog on the same day.[4]

Increased venous return to the heart clearly corresponds to an elevation of the venous reservoir in the heart-lung preparation (Fig. 3–11). Similar effects are commonly expected to follow intravenous infusion of blood or other fluids. Increasing "venous return" (by rapid or slow infusion of blood, by compression of the abdomen with pneumatic cuffs or by tilting dogs into the head-down position) failed to produce cardiac responses bearing any obvious relation to the normal exercise responses even when the central venous pressure was greatly elevated.[4] Studies on human subjects have demonstrated that increased cardiac output does not result when central venous pressure has been elevated by intravenous infusion of blood. Infusion of fluids containing no blood cells may be followed by an increase in cardiac output to compensate for the relative anemia produced by the dilution of the blood.[13, 14] Thus, there is little positive evidence that an increase in "venous return," in the most common usage of the term, is essential for initiation of an increase in cardiac output when exercise begins.

Reduced peripheral resistance was simulated experimentally by rapidly pumping blood from a femoral artery into a femoral vein exposed under local anesthesia. The systemic arterial pressure declined and this reduction was accompanied by tachycardia. However, the overall response did not resemble the normal exercise response.

Naturally occurring catechol amines, l-epinephrine and norepinephrine, were infused intravenously in doses calculated to be within the physiologic range. In virtually all experiments on dogs, these substances in physiological doses produced bradycardia along with elevation of the systemic arterial pressure. Under these conditions the normal ventricular exercise response cannot be reproduced unless tachycardia is induced artificially. When the right atrium was stimulated with an artificial pacemaker during infusion of catechol amines, normal exercise responses were simulated with a fair degree of precision.

Stimulation of sympathetic nerves distributed to the heart from the stellate ganglia profoundly affected both the heart rate and the dynamic ventric-

ular performance as defined in Chapter 3 (see Figs. 3–17 and 3–18). Prompt and sustained tachycardia can be produced by relatively weak stimulation. The ventricular contraction was much more vigorous, as indicated by a more rapid rise in ventricular pressure, a more rapid ejection, a higher peak pressure, a more rapid fall in pressure and a shorter systole. Stimulation of the same sympathetic fibers through electrodes implanted in a healthy dog produced changes in ventricular performance of the same general type as those commonly observed during spontaneous exercise.[15]

Stimulation in the central nervous system was next undertaken to locate sites from which impulses could reach the heart through the autonomic pathways. Since the hypothalamic region is generally recognized as the locus of important integrating mechanisms governing autonomic activity, the diencephalon was explored by means of stimulating electrodes.[16-18] The success of the search for sites of electrical stimulation which would produce cardiac responses similar to the natural exercise responses is indicated in Figure 7–4.

After a typical treadmill exercise response was recorded, the dog was anesthetized with chloralose and an electrode was positioned in the subthalamus (H_2 fields of Forel). Stimulation there produced changes in cardiac function of the proper type, and the similarity of responses to unipolar and bipolar stimulation indicated that the electrode tip was directly in or very near the source of the nerve impulses producing this change. The electrode shaft was cemented to the skull, and the animal was permitted to recover. Three days later the same locus was stimulated through the implanted electrode while the unanesthetized dog stood quietly. The

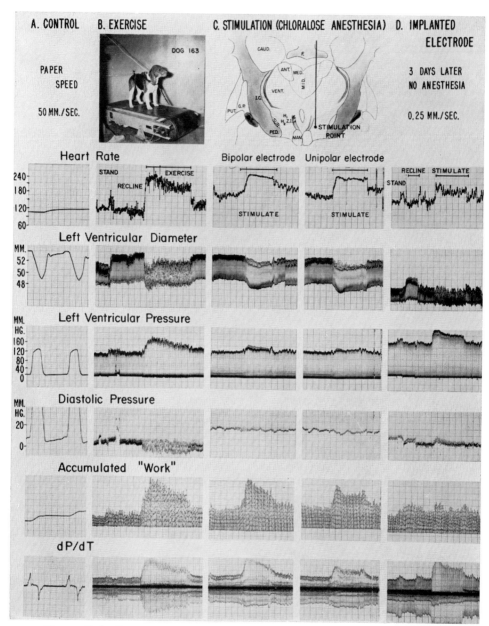

FIGURE 7–4.   EXERCISE RESPONSE SIMULATED BY DIENCEPHALIC STIMULATION

A, Control records at fast paper speed (50 mm./sec.).

B, Left ventricular response to exercise on a treadmill at 3 m.p.h. on a 5 per cent grade.

C, On the same day, unipolar and bipolar stimulation in the H_2 fields of Forel under chloralose anesthesia produced changes of the same general type as were recorded during exercise. The electrode was implanted at that site.

D, Three days later, without any anesthesia, stimulation using the implanted electrode reproduced the original left ventricular response to exercise with considerable precision. The principal difference was in the ventricular diastolic pressure change.

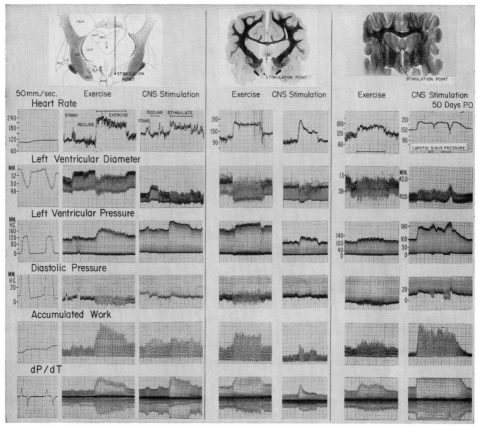

FIGURE 7–5.   COMPARISON OF RESPONSES TO EXERCISE AND DIENCEPHALIC STIMULATION

Diencephalic stimulation in the region of the H_2 fields of Forel and in the periventricular gray matter produces changes in left ventricular function comparable to those produced by spontaneous exercise.

response to stimulation reproduced nearly all details of the exercise response with considerable precision (Fig. 7–4B). The same kind of cardiac responses can be elicited routinely by stimulation of the H_2 fields of Forel or the periventricular gray matter, as evidenced by records from three different dogs (Fig. 7–5).

When the animal is under chloralose anesthesia, electrical stimulation of these areas often results in increased ventilation and distinct running movements as well as the cardiovascular response. Syncurine completely abolished the limb and respiratory movements but did not affect the magnitude of the cardiac response. If the electrode was moved a very short distance up or down, cardiac responses without running movements or running movements without cardiac responses could be elicited. Unfortunately, the activated neural structures are never exactly the same during electrical stimulation and normal activity. For this reason, the role of these diencephalic sites in normal function cannot be assessed with confidence by stimulation alone. Additional evidence obtained by selective destruction of such areas is also necessary.

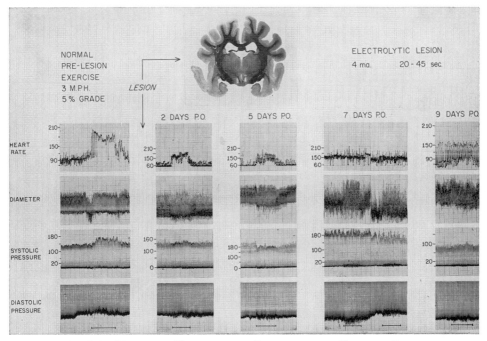

FIGURE 7–6. EFFECT OF DIENCEPHALIC LESIONS ON THE EXERCISE RESPONSE

The response to the standard treadmill exercise was recorded. Small bilaterally symmetrical lesions were placed in the H$_2$ fields of Forel. Two days later the systolic ventricular pressure rise during exercise was slightly reduced. After five days, the systolic ventricular pressure fell during exercise. Seven days after the lesions, the heart rate did not accelerate. After nine days, the animal performed the standard exercise without any significant changes in the recorded variables. The explanation for this sequence is not obvious, but it suggests that, before the lesions, these discretely localized sites may have played a significant role in the normal response to exercise.

Diencephalic lesions of a very small size were made bilaterally in regions which produced powerful cardiac responses. In one animal with such lesions the ventricular response to exertion decreased progressively during successive treadmill exercises (Fig. 7–6). By the seventh day after the lesions were made, the animal's ventricular performance did not change significantly when he exercised. Obviously, he could run only a short time. He then stopped and let the treadmill slide beneath him. During the period after the diencephalon was damaged, the animal displayed other signs of autonomic disturbance including vomiting, diarrhea, reduced food intake and easy fatigability. In spite of these complications it seems evident that the bilateral lesions destroyed pathways or collections of nerve cells important to normal cardiovascular regulation.

In summary, the changes in ventricular performance during exercise in dogs can be characterized by increased heart rate, increased ejection velocity and acceleration of blood leaving the ventricles, shorter systolic interval with little or no increase in stroke volume (Fig. 7–7). The differences between the recorded exercise responses in dogs and the traditional postulates are illustrated in Figure 3–14.

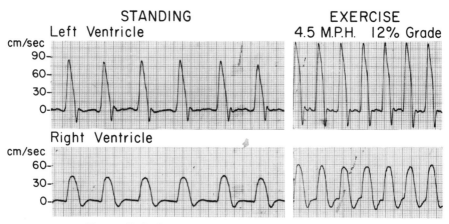

FIGURE 7–7. VENTRICULAR OUTFLOW WITH EXERCISE

The instantaneous outflow velocity of blood from the right and left ventricles displays steeper upslope to a higher peak velocity during exertion. This signifies greater outflow acceleration of blood. The duration of ejection is reduced so that the stroke volume (area under each stroke deflection) may not be increased to any significant degree.

REDISTRIBUTION OF BLOOD FLOW DURING EXERTION

Contracting skeletal muscles need a greatly increased blood flow, which can be supplied by an increase in cardiac output. The load on the heart can be reduced somewhat by diversion of some flow from relatively inactive tissue to the active muscle. For example, about one fourth of the total cardiac output at rest flows through the kidney, a quantity far greater than necessary to meet that organ's oxygen requirement. A significant proportion of the renal blood flow could be diverted to serve active muscles at the expense of a reduction in the oxygen content of renal venous blood. If this mechanism is operable, the cells in the renal parenchyma must function in an environment of reduced oxygen tension to achieve the greater oxygen extraction. Curtailment of renal blood flow during exercise not only is a very reasonable concept but is supported by evidence from normal human subjects. For example, Bucht *et al.*[19]

catheterized the renal veins and measured renal clearances to determine the blood flow during mild and moderately severe exercise. When the work was slight, the renal blood flow was unchanged but the cardiac output was somewhat augmented. During more strenuous work the renal blood flow decreased by 20 per cent and the cardiac output was almost doubled.

The blood flow through the splanchnic bed and liver might also be curtailed during exertion. During supine exercise the hepatic blood flow, measured indirectly, was about 400 ml. per minute below a mean resting level of approximately 1500 ml. per minute.[20] The extent to which differences in posture would affect these observations is not known (see later discussion). The blood flow in the arm diminishes 50 per cent in the early minutes of exercise, primarily because circulation through the skin decreases;[21] this reduced flow does not persist throughout the exertion. According to Scheinberg *et al.*,[22] cerebral blood flow increased in subjects walking on a treadmill.

The distribution of blood flow during exercise most commonly has been studied in human subjects by means of indirect methods applied to one portion of the circulation at a time. Installation of ultrasonic flowmeters at several sites in the canine circulation makes possible continuous, simultaneous monitoring of several patterns of flow at rest, during exercise and under other conditions. When a dog ran on the treadmill, the flow through the lower abdominal aorta to the hindquarters increased promptly and was sustained throughout the exercise (Fig. 7–8). The instantaneous flow velocity and the integrated flow (flow per stroke) rose, and there were more strokes per minute. In contrast, the blood flow through the renal artery was essentially unchanged, not only in the example presented in Figure 7–8 but also, consistently, in a series of exercise responses by six dogs. The flow through the hepatic artery to the liver and stomach was substantially

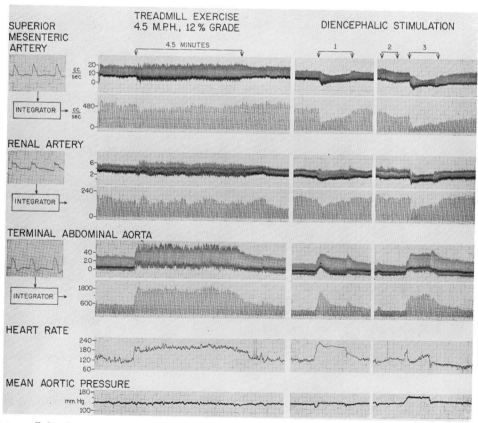

FIGURE 7–8. BLOOD FLOW DISTRIBUTION DURING EXERTION AND DIENCEPHALIC STIMULATION

During exercise, the flow through the superior mesenteric and renal arteries may change transiently, but the integrated flow is essentially unchanged, while the flow to the hindquarters is greatly increased. A similar change in flow distribution can be induced by stimulation in the same regions that produced the pronounced changes in cardiac function illustrated in Figure 7–5.

reduced, as was the flow through the hepatic portal vein; these observations suggest that the splanchnic flow diminished. The blood flow through the common carotid artery was generally greater than at rest. Since flow through the internal carotid could not be distinguished from that through the external, the flow through soft tissues of the head might have increased without a change in the cerebral vascular bed.

The hypothesis that blood flow to the visceral organs would be reduced during exertion was not confirmed by these experiments. Van Citters and Franklin[23] utilized telemetry to record the blood flow velocity to kidneys and gut in husky dogs pulling sled and driver during cross country races. Although the flow in terminal aorta increased by 9 to 12 fold and coronary flow increased 5 to 6 fold, the mesenteric and renal flows were unchanged during this violent and prolonged exercise.

Electrical stimulation of selected sites in the diencephalon consistently influenced flow distribution directionally as exercise did (Fig. 7–8B). These sites were at or near those which induced corresponding changes in cardiac function, hyperpnea and running movements (see previous discussion). Thus, complete patterns of somatic and visceral adaptation (e.g., exercise) can be induced by selective diencephalic stimulation. It should be emphasized, however, that the motor and visceral components can appear individually after stimulation of slightly different diencephalic loci, so that the motor activity is not the cause of the changes in visceral function. Abrahams and Hilton[24] reported that stimulation of certain hypothalamic sites produced muscle vasodilation in anesthetized cats and defense reactions in conscious cats — pupillary

dilation, hissing, snarling, massive pilo-erection and running about the cage.

Uvnäs[25] noted that, although the vasodilator mechanism induces additional blood flow through muscle, the clearance of radioactive materials from the muscle is somewhat retarded and its oxygen consumption decreases. These observations were interpreted as evidence that the sympathetic vasodilator system tends to open arteriovenous shunts (or arteriovenous capillaries) and to reduce flow through true capillaries. Such a mechanism would at least deliver more blood to the muscles. It could then be distributed to the true capillaries by an opening of the precapillary sphincters during exercise (i.e., opening induced by local metabolic products).

BLOOD FLOW IN MUSCLES DURING EXERTION

At the beginning of exercise the flow of blood through the contracting muscles increases greatly to maintain and restore the supply of energy that is being released as work and wasted as heat. Barcroft and Dornhorst[26] presented evidence that contraction of skeletal muscles actually hinders the flow of blood through them; thus, the vasodilation must be great enough to permit very large flows in the intervals between contractions.

The widely accepted concept that vasodilation in active muscle results directly from the diminution of oxygen tension, decline of pH and accumulation of carbon dioxide and other metabolites appears to be logical and to be evidenced by the extreme vasodilation occurring after temporary obstruction of the arterial supply to an extremity (reactive hyperemia). As mentioned in Chapter 4, the evidence that a lowered oxygen level or an elevated carbon dioxide level is normally an important regulator of blood flow to muscles and certain other tissues is tenuous and indirect. The blood flow through the human calf immediately after exercise does not consistently reflect the severity of the preceding exertion[27] and remains elevated after the oxygen debt has been repaid and the heart rate has returned to normal. Then, too, the venous blood from the legs may contain more oxygen during recovery from either exercise or temporary arterial occlusion than during rest.

Most concepts of the intimate nature of the control exercised by metabolites, hormones or neural mechanisms over the peripheral vasculature are based on very indirect evidence and remain extremely controversial.[28] Evidence can be marshalled to support any one of several widely divergent views, and the solution to the dilemma does not appear close at hand. The specific chemical(s) which produce local vasodilation in active muscle have not been identified with certainty. Kjellmer[29] presented evidence that potassium ions released from within muscle cells during exercise can reach concentrations high enough to account for a major portion of vascular dilation during exertion. Intra-arterially injected potassium appears to simulate vascular responses observed during exercise. It is generally agreed that the sympathetic nerves serving vessels in skeletal muscle are predominantly constrictors. If the constrictor portion of this action is blocked, a vasodilation is elicited by stimulating sympathetic trunks which has been ascribed to a specialized sympathetic vasodilator system (see also Chapter 4).

Sympathetic Vasodilator Fibers to Skeletal Muscle. Nerve fibers are assigned to the sympathetic system on purely anatomic grounds. Although the vast majority of these fibers release a transmitter substance closely resembling norepinephrine, exceptions exist. For example, the fibers innervating the sweat glands of the skin are anatomically sympathetic, but they release acetylcholine as a transmitter substance and thus may be blocked by atropine. In recent years an eminent group of Swedish investigators has presented a great deal of experimental evidence[30-32] which suggests that some sympathetic fibers distributed to skeletal muscles (and possibly to the heart) release acetylcholine as a transmitter substance to induce vasodilation.

The use of the term "vasodilator" in this connection deserves additional consideration. After all accessible sympathetic fibers to the extremities are cut, the smooth muscle in vessels serving skeletal muscle retains a fairly high degree of tone, evidenced by the fact that the blood flow increases five- or six-fold when acetylcholine is administered. This effect is blocked by atropine. Activation of the sympathetic vasodilator fibers can also increase the blood flow above the level sustained under "basal tone." This effect can also be blocked by atropine administered in doses too small to affect the vasodilation caused by inhibition of vasoconstrictor tone. Such dual innervation of vessels in skeletal muscle is generally interpreted as mediating two forms of vascular reaction, the vasoconstrictor activity serving in the control of systemic arterial pressure and the vasodilator activity serving to accelerate muscle blood flow promptly at the onset of muscular exertion.[31]

The pathway of the sympathetic vasodilator system has been traced from the motor cortex[32] to the supra-optic area in the hypothalamus, through the medulla and thence down to spinal levels. Quite naturally, it has been suggested that impulses from higher neural levels traverse these connections to elicit vasodilation in skeletal muscles, "in circumstances when a sudden increase in blood flow in the skeletal muscles is needed in order to create optimal conditions for muscular effort."[33]

POSTURAL EFFECTS ON THE EXERCISE RESPONSE

Over some five years the changes in the ventricular dimensions of healthy dogs were measured hundreds of times by different techniques during various spontaneous adjustments. When the animal had stood quietly on the treadmill during the control period, exercise at 3 m.p.h. on a 5 per cent grade was accompanied by only slight changes in the ventricular dimensions. The diastolic dimensions might increase slightly in some instances and not at all in others. The systolic dimensions might decrease slightly, but, in general, the systolic deflections were not significantly augmented during the moderate exercise employed. The

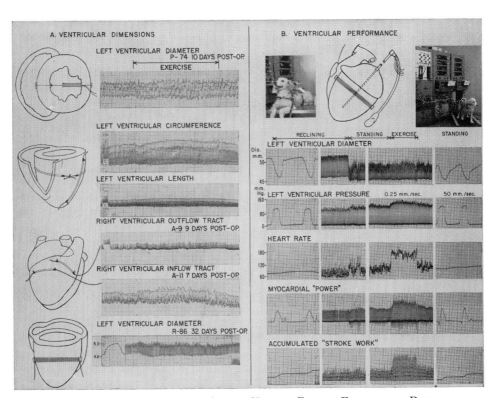

FIGURE 7–9.   CONSTANCY OF STROKE VOLUME DURING EXERTION IN DOGS

A, Direct recordings of changing internal left ventricular diameter, external left ventricular circumference and length, various dimensions of the right ventricular wall and the external left ventricular diameter consistently demonstrated little or no shift in baseline or increase in the amplitude of the deflections. This observation indicates that the total ventricular volume and stroke volume remain essentially unchanged in dogs during moderate exercise from a standing control.

B, When a recumbent dog stands up, the diastolic and systolic dimensions abruptly diminish and the stroke deflections become much smaller (see also 6–13 and 6–14). These changes in ventricular dimensions are much greater than were typically recorded during exertion.

examples in Figure 7–9A represent about the greatest changes in the stroke deflections of the left and right ventricles recorded by each of three different techniques. These observations suggested that the stroke volume did not increase materially when the standing animal began to run. This conclusion was confirmed by measuring the aortic flow directly with the ultrasonic flowmeter. On the other hand, if the dog was reclining quietly during the control period, the diastolic and systolic ventricular dimensions

and the stroke deflections all diminished significantly when he began to exercise (Fig. 7–9B). Clearly the cardiac output was augmented in either case primarily by an increase in heart rate rather than by greater stroke volume.

Tachycardia alone does not effectively increase cardiac output. This fact is shown clearly by the left ventricular response to cardio-acceleration induced by an artificial pacemaker (Fig. 7–10). Stimulating electrodes were implanted in the region of

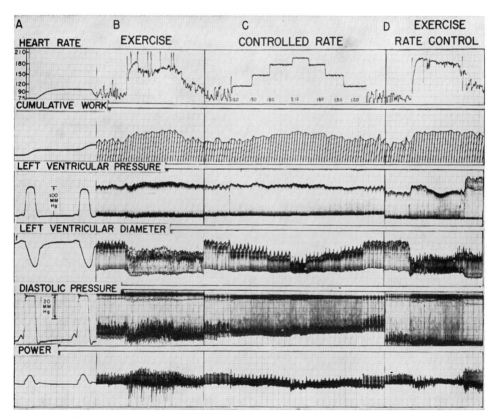

FIGURE 7–10. RELATION OF TACHYCARDIA TO STROKE DEFLECTIONS

A, B, The principal change in left ventricular function during spontaneous exercise is a pronounced acceleration of the heart with little increase in stroke deflections (see also Fig. 7–9).

C, Stepwise increase in heart rate induced by an artificial pacemaker in the same alert dog produced a progressive decline in diastolic and systolic dimensions and stroke deflections.

D, The changes in heart rate during exercise were precisely reproduced from a tape recording activating the artificial pacemaker, and the stroke deflections were greatly diminished as compared with the normal exercise response.

the sino-atrial node during an aseptic operation in which recording devices were also attached to the heart. After recovery the animal was exercised on the treadmill (Fig. 7–10B). The left ventricular dimensions decreased as the animal stood up and began to run. The stroke deflections were now slightly larger than those after exertion, during a standing control period. Stimulation through the electrodes near the sino-atrial node was then begun to increase the heart rate in a stepwise fashion (Fig. 7–10C). This artificial tachycardia was accompanied by a progressive reduction in the diastolic and systolic dimensions and the stroke deflections. Similarly, an artificially induced tachycardia reproducing the rates recorded during exercise resulted in a markedly reduced stroke deflection (Fig. 7–10D). Thus, an

artificial tachycardia does not produce the normal increase in cardiac output because the stroke volume is decreased. The normal exercise response involves no change or a slight increase in the stroke volume.

The nature of the cardiac response to exertion depends to a considerable extent on the state of the animals during the control period. For example, if a dog is lying quietly on the treadmill during a control period and then stands and begins to exercise abruptly, systolic and diastolic left ventricular diameters diminish along with stroke deflections (Fig. 7–11B). On the other hand, if the animal is standing quietly on the treadmill during the control period, the left ventricular diameter is not greatly altered when the exercise begins (Fig. 7–11D).

To summarize, the cardiovascular

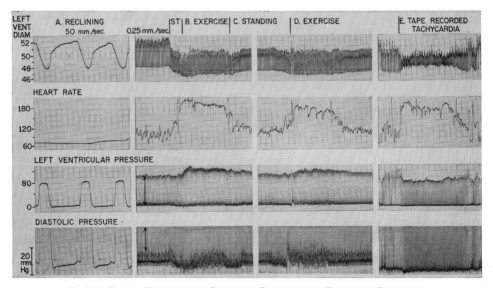

FIGURE 7–11. EFFECTS OF CONTROL POSTURE ON EXERCISE RESPONSE

A, In reclining dogs, the left ventricular diameter is approximately maximal and the stroke deflections are large.

B, If the animal stands and immediately begins to exercise, the ventricular dimensions and stroke deflections appear to diminish promptly in relation to the exercise.

C, D, Exercise begun from a standing control demonstrates that the ventricular dimensions and stroke deflections are not greatly affected by the exercise.

E, Artificial tachycardia produced greatly reduced stroke deflections.

response to physical exertion in dogs can be characterized as follows. If the dog is reclining during the control period, his heart rate will range around 70 beats per minute and his diastolic ventricular dimensions and stroke volume are at or near their maximal levels. When the dog stands, diastolic and systolic dimensions are abruptly reduced and the stroke volume diminishes by as much as 30 per cent. (See also Chapter 6.) Exercise of moderate degree is accompanied by a substantial increase in heart rate and little or no change in stroke volume (generally less than 10 per cent according to Wang, Marshall and Shepherd[34]). Strenuous exercise produces greater tachycardia and wider variability in stroke volume in either intact or sympathectomized dogs.[35] However, dogs without cardiac nerves revealed less tachycardia and larger stroke volumes, particularly during mild exercise.[36] With cardiac nerves intact, the cardiac output is increased primarily by increased heart rate, with stroke volume generally maintained or slightly increased, depending upon the magnitude of the tachycardia, particularly at the onset of exertion. In our experiments, the stroke volume during exertion failed to reach the recumbent values even during the maximum exertion we could induce the animals to sustain.

The blood flow is greatly augmented through arteries serving actively contracting muscles (e.g., terminal aorta). In contrast with traditional concepts, the visceral blood flow (e.g., to kidneys and gastrointestinal tract) was well maintained; indeed it did not diminish even during extremely severe exertion by husky sled dogs pulling heavy loads over long distance.[23] The redistribution of blood away from inactive or visceral tissues was not displayed by these studies as compensation to exertion in dogs.

EXERTIONAL RESPONSES IN MAN

The cardiovascular adaptation to exercise in dogs has been described quantitatively and comprehensively by continuous recordings capable of rapid responses to abrupt changes. Available information regarding cardiovascular adaptations in man are neither so comprehensive nor so dynamic. However, the data at hand suggest many points of similarity between human and canine exercise responses.

The constancy of the stroke volume which had been so consistently observed in the animal experiments (Figs. 7–9 and 7–11) led to a survey of the literature to determine how the stroke volume behaves during exercise by human subjects.[38] In eight different studies, summarized in Figure 7–12, the stroke volume changed only slightly over a wide range of exercise levels, graded for severity on the basis of oxygen consumption. This apparent failure of stroke volume to increase progressively as the work load increased was not consistent with observations by certain investigators, notably Mitchell, Sproule and Chapman.[39] In a personal communication Chapman pointed out that this discrepancy might be partly explained by the fact that the stroke volume during exercise is very little higher than that in the recumbent position. It seems quite possible that the stroke volume in the relaxed recumbent subject is at or near the maximal level ordinarily reached during heavy work. When the individual stands up, his stroke volume, and his heart volume, consistently diminish.[40] Beginning at this smaller baseline, the stroke volume in-

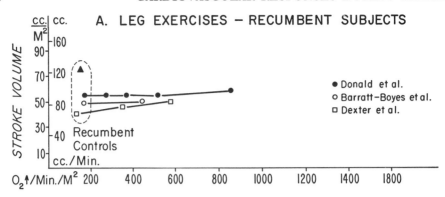

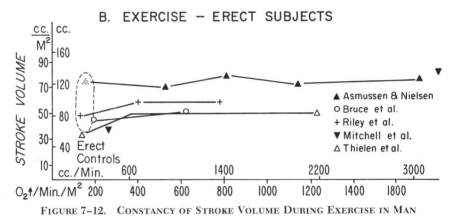

FIGURE 7–12.   CONSTANCY OF STROKE VOLUME DURING EXERCISE IN MAN

A, Human subjects exercising in the recumbent position exhibit little increase in stroke volume over a fairly wide range of exercise as judged by the oxygen consumption.

B, Normal human subjects in the erect position have smaller stroke volumes during the control period, and at the onset of exercise the stroke volume increases to a higher level where it tends to remain over a wide range of oxygen consumption. At the extreme levels of exercise, a further increase in stroke volume is observed (see Fig. 15–2).

creases promptly with even slight exertion, but does not necessarily increase progressively as the external work becomes more intense. Chapman has, however, presented evidence that there is an additional increase in stroke volume under conditions of maximal exertion.[41]

In summary, relaxed men typically appear to have a slow heart rate, large ventricular dimensions and large stroke volume (at or near maximum). Exercise in the supine position produces little or no increase in stroke volume even when the exertion is severe. Athletes tend to have slower heart rates, larger blood volumes,

higher ventricular filling pressures, larger ventricular dimensions and larger stroke volume than sedentary individuals equally relaxed and recumbent. Athletes also tend to respond to supine exercise primarily by tachycardia with little or no increase in stroke volume.[42]

On assuming the erect position, the heart rate increases somewhat and stroke volume declines precipitously by some 30 to 40 per cent.[42] Wang and Shepard[43] demonstrated that even the mildest exercise (alternately lifting the feet two inches off the floor) was sufficient to restore stroke volume to approximately the recumbent control values. Increasing exertion up to rather extreme levels produced only slight increases in stroke volume above either mild exercise or recumbent control levels.

Distribution of blood flow in man. Evidence for a shift of blood flow from inactive or visceral tissues to actively contracting muscle during exercise remains controversial. For example, Brod[44] reported no pronounced change in blood flow to kidney or splanchnic bed with light work. Greater reduction in kidney flow could be much more readily produced by neural mechanisms (such as the suggestion of heavy work, disagreeable situations, mental arithmetic), more or less as startle reactions produce profound renal vasoconstriction in dogs. In contrast, Rowell *et al.*[45] found that hepatic blood flow (estimated using indocyanin green) was reduced by 50 to 70 per cent during prolonged treadmill exercise requiring 48 to 70 per cent of maximum oxygen uptake. With more severe exertion, estimated hepatic blood flow was diminished by as much as 80 per cent or more.

Conditions Under Which Stroke Volume Increases. According to Yandell Henderson,[46] "The athlete's heart is supernormal." Many other investigators have also observed this tendency,[47] although Freedman *et al.*[48] could find no differences attributable to training in the way a trained and an untrained athlete meet the tissues' demands for oxygen. In any event, there seems little doubt that, during exertion, the heart rate accelerates less and the stroke volume is higher in trained athletes than in average subjects. Warner *et al.*[49] demonstrated that, if tachycardia is prevented by artificial control of the heart rate, the cardiac output increases normally during exertion through an increase in stroke volume.

Patients with chronically high cardiac output (resulting from anemia, thyrotoxicosis or an arteriovenous fistula) also tend to have a normal heart rate and an increased stroke volume at rest and to utilize increased stroke volume rather than cardioacceleration during exertion.[50] The cardiac responses of such patients resemble those of trained athletes.

Normal persons who stand during the control period will generally exhibit an increase in stroke volume at the onset of exertion, be it severe or mild. There is little evidence that stroke volume increases progressively with more strenuous work in average normal subjects. Subjects whose apprehensions induce tachycardia and reduced stroke volume during the control period will tend to display greater increases in stroke volume than relaxed subjects will.

SUMMARY

Traditional concepts of the cardiac response during exertion, based primarily on the Frank-Starling mechanism, have been evaluated for human subjects and intact dogs and found wanting. The patterns of ventricular response to exercise could not be duplicated by many different standard experimental methods including increased "venous return," reduced peripheral resistance, intravenous administration of natural autonomic hormones or by artificial tachycardia. Electrical stimulation of specific areas in the diencephalon reproduced ventricular responses similar to those occurring during exercise both with and without anesthesia. Lesions in the regions which produced these responses have been shown to produce profound changes in the responses to treadmill exercise. In both dogs and man, the stroke volume does not necessarily increase with increased severity of exertion as judged by oxygen consumption. The stroke volume is characteristically smaller during standing control measurements than in the recumbent position. During exercise in the erect position, the stroke volume may increase above the values measured during standing control but rarely exceeds the recumbent controls to any great extent. The stroke volume does not necessarily increase from very mild to quite severe exercise in human subjects. A further increase in stroke volume may occur at maximal levels of exertion.

REFERENCES

1. BARGER, A. C., RICHARDS, V., METCALFE, J., and GUNTHER, B. Regulation of the circulation during exercise. *Amer. J. Physiol.*, 184:613–623, 1956.
2. FENN, W. O. Acute and sustained high energy output. Pp. 8–17 in *Symposium on Stress* (16–18 March, 1953). Washington, D. C., Army Medical Service Graduate School, 1953.
3. EKBLOM, B., and HERMANSEN, L. Cardiac output in athletes. *J. Appl. Physiol.*, 25: 619–625, 1968.
4. RUSHMER, R. F., SMITH, O. A., JR., and FRANKLIN, D. Mechanisms of cardiac control in exercise. *Circulat. Res.*, 7:602–627, 1959.
5. FRANKLIN, D. L., VAN CITTERS, R. L., and RUSHMER, R. F. Left ventricular function described in physical terms. *Circulat. Res.*, 11:702–711, 1962.
6. NINOMIYA, I., and WILSON, M. F. Cardiac adaptation at the transition phases of exercise in unanesthetized dogs. *J. Appl. Physiol.*, 21:953–958, 1966.
7. WANG, Y., MARSHALL, R. J., and SHEPHERD, J. T. Stroke volume in the dog during graded exercise. *Circulat. Res.*, 8:558–563, 1960.
8. SMULYAN, H., CUDDY, R. P., VINCENT, W. A., KASHEMSANT, U., and EICH, R. H. Initial hemodynamic responses to mild exercise in trained dogs. *J. Appl. Physiol.*, 20:437–442, 1965.
9. RUSHMER, R. F. Anatomy and physiology of ventricular function. *Physiol. Rev.*, 36: 400–425, 1956.
10. RUSHMER, R. F., and SMITH, O. A., JR. Cardiac control. *Physiol. Rev.*, 39:41–68, 1959.
11. LILJESTRAND, G., LYSHOLM, E., and NYLIN, G. The immediate effect of muscular work on the stroke and heart volume in man. *Scand. Arch. Physiol.*, 80:265–282, 1938.
12. SJÖSTRAND, T. Regulatory mechanisms relating to blood volume. *Minnesota Med.*, 37:10–15, 1954.
13. SUNAHARA, F. A., HATCHER, J. D., BECK, L., and GOWDEY, C. W. Cardiovascular responses in dogs to intravenous infusions of whole blood, plasma, and plasma followed by packed erythrocytes. *Canad. J. Biochem.*, 33:349–360, 1955.
14. FOWLER, N. O., FRANCH, R. H., and BLOOM, W. L. Hemodynamic effects of anemia with and without plasma volume expansion. *Circulat. Res.*, 4:319–324, 1956.
15. ANZOLA, J., and RUSHMER, R. F. Cardiac responses to sympathetic stimulation. *Circulat. Res.*, 4:302–307, 1956.
16. SMITH, O. A., JR., RUSHMER, R. F., and LASHER, E. P. Similarity of cardiovascular responses to exercise and to diencephalic stimulation. *Amer. J. Physiol.*, 198:1139–1142, 1960.
17. RUSHMER, R. F., SMITH, O. A., JR., and LASHER, E. P. Neural mechanisms of cardiac control during exertion. *Physiol. Rev.*, 40(Suppl. 4): 27–34, 1960.
18. SMITH, O. A., JR., JABBUR, S. J., RUSHMER, R. F., and LASHER, E. P. Role of hypothalamic structures in cardiac control. *Physiol. Rev.*, 40 (Suppl. 4):136–145, 1960.
19. BUCHT, H., EK, J., ELIASCH, H., HOLMGREN, A., JOSEPHSON, B., and WERKÖ, L. The effect of exercise in the recumbent position on the renal circulation and sodium excretion in normal individuals. *Acta physiol. scand.*, 28:95–100, 1953.
20. BISHOP, J. M., DONALD, K. W., TAYLOR, S. H., and WORMALD, P. N. Changes in arterial-hepatic venous oxygen content difference during and after supine leg exercise. *J. Physiol.*, 137:309–317, 1957.
21. BISHOP, J. M., DONALD, K. W., TAYLOR, S. H., and WORMALD, P. N. The blood flow in the human arm during supine leg exercise. *J. Physiol.*, 137:294–308, 1957.
22. SCHEINBERG, P., BLACKBURN, L. I., RICH, M., and SASLAW, M. Effects of vigorous physical exercise on cerebral circulation and metabolism. *Amer. J. Med.*, 16:549–554, 1954.
23. VAN CITTERS, R. L., and FRANKLIN, D. L. Cardiovascular responses in Alaska sled dogs during exercise. *Circulat. Res.*, 24: 33–42, 1969.
24. ABRAHAMS, V. C., and HILTON, S. M. Active muscle vasodilatation and its relation to the "flight and fight reactions" in the conscious animal. *J. Physiol.*, 140:16P–17P, 1958.
25. UVNÄS, B. Sympathetic vasodilator system and blood flow. *Physiol. Rev.*, 40 (Suppl. 4):69–80, 1960.

26. BARCROFT, H., and DORNHORST, A. C. The blood flow through the human calf during rhythmic exercise. *J. Physiol.*, 109:402–411, 1949.

27. HALLIDAY, J. A. Blood flow in the human calf after walking. *J. Physiol.*, 149:17P, 1959.

28. FOLKOW, B. Nervous control of the blood vessels. *Physiol. Rev.*, 35:629–663, 1955.

29. KJELLMER, I. The effect of exercise on the vascular level of skeletal muscle. *Acta physiol. scand.*, 62:18–30, 1964.

30. UVNÄS, B. Sympathetic vasodilatory outflow. *Physiol. Rev.*, 34:608–618, 1954.

31. LINDGREN, P., and UVNÄS, B. Vasoconstrictor inhibition and vasodilator activation—two functionally separate vasodilator mechanisms in the skeletal muscles. *Acta physiol. scand.*, 33:108–119, 1955.

32. ELIASSON, S., LINDGREN, P., and UVNÄS, B. Representation in the hypothalamus and the motor cortex in the dog of the sympathetic vasodilator outflow to the skeletal muscles. *Acta physiol. scand.*, 27:18–37, 1952.

33. ELIASSON, S., FOLKOW, B., LINDGREN, P., and UVNÄS, B. Activation of sympathetic vasodilator nerves to the skeletal muscles in the cat by hypothalamic stimulation. *Acta physiol. scand.*, 23:333–351, 1951.

34. WANG, Y., MARSHALL, R. J., and SHEPHERD, J. T. Stroke volume in the dog during graded exercise. *Circulat. Res.*, 8:558–567, 1960.

35. ASHKAR, E., and HAMILTON, W. F. Cardiovascular response to graded exercise in the sympathectomized-vagotomized dog. *Amer. J. Physiol.*, 204:291–296, 1963.

36. DONALD, D. E., and SHEPHERD, J. T. Response to exercise in dogs with cardiac derevation. *Amer. J. Physiol.*, 205:393–400, 1963.

37. FRANKLIN, D. L., ELLIS, R. M., and RUSHMER, R. F. Aortic blood flow in dogs during treadmill exercise. *J. Appl. Physiol.*, 14:809–812, 1959.

38. RUSHMER, R. F. Constancy of stroke volume in ventricular responses to exertion. *Amer. J. Physiol.*, 196:745–750, 1959.

39. MITCHELL, J. H., SPROULE, B. J., and CHAPMAN, C. B. The physiological meaning of the maximal oxygen intake test. *J. Clin. Invest.*, 37:538–547, 1958.

40. LINDERHOLM, H., and STRANDELL, T. Heart volume in the prone and erect positions in certain heart cases. *Acta med. scand.*, 162:247–261, 1958.

41. FISHER, J. M., CHAPMAN, C. B., and SPROULE, B. J. Effect of exercise on stroke volume in human subjects. *Clin. Res.*, 8:73, 1960.

42. BEVEGARD, S., HOLMGREN, A., and JONSSON, B. Circulatory studies in well trained athletes at rest and during heavy exercise with special response to stroke volume and the influence of body position. *Acta physiol. scand.*, 57:26–50, 1963.

43. WANG, Y., MARSHALL, R. J., and SHEPHERD, J. T. The effect of changes in posture and of graded exercise on stroke volume in men. *J. Clin. Invest.*, 39:1051–1061, 1960.

44. BROD, J. Haemodynamic changes in the body during severe muscular exercise and preparation for exercise under physiological and pathological conditions. *Proc. 5th National Cong. Czechoslovak Physiol. Soc.*, June 13, 1961.

45. ROWELL, L. B., KRANING, K. K., EVANS, T. O., KENNEDY, J. W., BLACKMON, J. R., and KUSUMI, F. Splanchnic removal of lactate and pyruvate during prolonged exercise in man. *J. Appl. Physiol.*, 21:1773–1783, 1966.

46. HENDERSON, Y., HAGGARD, H. W., and DOLLEY, F. S. The efficiency of the heart, and the significance of rapid and slow pulse rates. *Amer. J. Physiol.*, 82:512–524, 1927.

47. MUSSHOFF, K. VON, REINDELL, H., and KLEPZIG, H. Stroke volume, arteriovenous difference, cardiac output and physical working capacity and their relationship to heart volume. *Acta cardiol.*, 14:427–452, 1959.

48. FREEDMAN, M. E., SNIDER, G. L., BROSTOFF, P., KIMELBLOT, S., and KATZ, L. N. Effects of training on response of cardiac output to muscular exercise in athletes. *J. Appl. Physiol.*, 8:37–47, 1955.

49. WARNER, H. R., and TORONTO, A. F. Regulation of cardiac output through stroke volume. *Circulat. Res.*, 8:549–552, 1960.

50. BISHOP, J. M., DONALD, K. W., and WADE, O. L. Circulatory dynamics at rest and on exercise in the hyperkinetic states. *Clin. Sci.*, 14:329–360, 1955.

CHAPTER 8

DETECTION OF PERIPHERAL VASCULAR DISEASE

By D. E. Strandness, Jr.

Peripheral vascular diseases usually encompass those entities which occur in vessels that lie outside the confines of the thoracic and cranial cavities. Vessels of both macroscopic and microscopic size are altered in ways which interfere with either delivery of blood to the tissues or return of blood to the heart. The entire field is too extensive for complete coverage in this chapter which is devoted to methods of detecting and evaluating diseases of the macroscopic arteries and veins. The discussion will be limited to the two major occlusive diseases, namely atherosclerosis and thrombophlebitis.

ATHEROSCLEROSIS

Atherosclerosis is a progressive disorder which begins with the deposition of lipid material in the intima which gradually increases in size and extent of involvement. In its earliest stages the arterial plaque does little to interfere with the delivery of blood but ultimately reduces the arterial cross-sectional area and distorts the

244

constituents of the vessel wall.[1] In its fully developed form there are often seen (1) surface ulceration, (2) fragmentation of the elastic fibers, (3) hemorrhage into the plaque, (4) calcium deposition in the plaque, (5) thinning of the media and (6) adventitial fibrosis. Since the process so commonly obstructs the vessel, the label most frequently applied to its involvement of the large and medium-sized arteries is arteriosclerosis obliterans.

DIAGNOSIS

With few exceptions the presence of arteriosclerosis obliterans is discovered only when the disease has reached a sufficiently advanced stage to interfere with the delivery of a normal amount of blood flow either at rest or during exercise. A correct diagnosis requires the proper association of the symptoms and signs with the location of the disease. This is important because the disease tends to occur preferentially in areas at or near branch points or bifurcations. In the upper extremity the origin of the subclavian artery is most frequently involved, but the arm vessels distally are rarely occluded. Symptoms secondary to the subclavian artery obstruction itself are uncommon but may occur in combination with the flow reversal that occurs down the ipsilateral vertebral artery, the so-called subclavian steal syndrome.[2]

In the lower extremity, symptoms commonly develop secondary to the arterial occlusion and are characteristic enough to make the diagnosis of arteriosclerosis obliterans relatively easy. For convenience the clinical picture can be subdivided into symptoms with exercise and symptoms at rest.

SYMPTOMS WITH EXERCISE

If the forearm muscles are vigorously contracted while the arterial inflow is arrested by an inflated cuff, intense pain develops within a very few minutes. When arterial narrowing or occlusion develops to the point of interfering with the delivery of a normal volume flow of blood to the exercising muscle, similar pain develops which promptly disappears with rest. This symptom complex is referred to as intermittent claudication. The location of the muscle pain is important since it provides information concerning the most proximal level of arterial occlusion. Pain in the calf muscles can occur with disease of the arterial supply proximal to the level of the popliteal artery. If the claudication involves the thigh muscles as well, the obstruction is proximal to the origin of the profunda femoris artery. Disease of the common iliac artery or distal aorta may result in buttock claudication due to interference with the arterial inflow to the hypogastric arteries. If the terminal aorta is occluded, impotence

may be a complaint in addition to the symptoms in the lower limb.

It must be emphasized that it is not uncommon for calf claudication to be the sole symptom even though the arterial inflow to more proximal muscle groups is also compromised. The basis for this is obvious when one considers the nature of the collateral blood supply that bypasses areas of obstruction. These critical channels are generally intermuscular in location and tend to supply the more proximal muscle groups first, thus tending to divert blood destined for the calf muscles. Therefore, it is not unusual for patients with terminal aortic or common iliac artery occlusion to complain of calf claudication alone.

SYMPTOMS AT REST

While the location of atherosclerotic obstructions responsible for claudication is segmental in distribution, the extent of the involvement is usually different when symptoms are present at rest. Because of the excellent available collateral blood supply normally present for most single segment occlusions, ischemic pain at rest, ulceration or gangrene signifies extensive involvement of the arteries serving the region. The disease process most commonly involves multiple levels of the arterial inflow. A single occlusion will rarely produce ischemia at rest unless it occurs in a very critical location blocking both the exit and reentry collateral arteries.

The development of symptoms at rest or frank tissue necrosis is an ominous sign indicating that early amputation is likely unless direct arterial surgery can effectively increase arterial inflow to the limb. This is in contrast to intermittent claudication which does not carry the same serious outlook for limb survival.

PHYSICAL FINDINGS

On inspecting the limb with arterial obstruction, a wide spectrum of signs may be present which extend from a normal appearing extremity to the limb with gangrene. The normal appearing limb simply indicates that the nutritional blood supply is sufficient to maintain integrity of the skin, hair and nail growth.

Arterial occlusion can usually be confirmed by palpation and auscultation. Pulses are normally palpable at the common femoral artery, popliteal and posterior tibial and dorsalis pedis arteries. With complete arterial obstruction, the pulses distal to the site of involvement are not palpable. If the artery is only partially narrowed, audible sounds may be noted at the site of the stenosis and for a variable distance downstream. These abnormal sounds (called bruits) are presumably secondary to vibrations of the arterial wall distal to sites of narrowing (see chapter on *Heart Murmurs*). Auscultation should always be performed in the examination of the arteries and carried out from the level of the abdominal aorta to the popliteal artery.

ARTERIOGRAPHY

Once the diagnosis of arteriosclerosis obliterans has been made by history and physical examination, a decision must be made as to the necessity for further studies and therapy. The common practice today is to follow the clinical evaluation by some type of arteriographic procedure which will outline the exact location of the disease, its extent and the state of the existing collateral circulation[3] (Fig. 8–1). The method by which the arteriograms are performed is dependent upon the most proximal level of the occlusive disease. Aortography is employed when there is suspected aorto-iliac disease. Femoral arteriography is most useful for evaluating

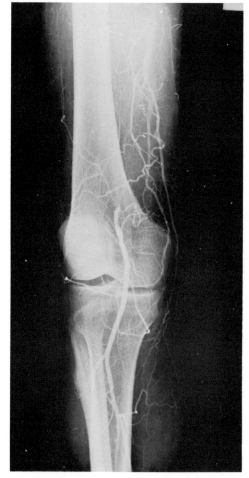

FIGURE 8–1   FEMORAL ARTERIOGRAM

This femoral arteriogram shows the type of information that must be available when direct arterial surgery is contemplated. This data includes: (1) location of occlusion, (2) size and location of collateral arteries, (3) caliber of the vessels at the proposed site of operation and (4) the patency of those arteries which will be used as "run-off" vessels.

those vessels distal to the inguinal ligament. While angiography is absolutely essential prior to direct arterial surgery, it does have limitations which must be taken into account. Some of the drawbacks of arteriography are as follows: (1) It is expensive and time consuming. (2) It must be performed with the patient in the hospital. (3) The procedure is uncomfortable and entails some risk. (4) It is frequently difficult to visualize the entire arterial supply to the affected limb. (5) It cannot be performed repeatedly. (6) It does not provide the functional data so essential in determining the extent of the patient's disability.

PHYSIOLOGIC STUDIES

While both clinical evaluation and arteriographic studies provide objective data on the anatomical location of disease, other study techniques are needed to assess the functional effects or pathophysiology of arterial narrowing and obstruction. Atherosclerosis produces changes that disturb the normal pressure-flow relationships, arterial geometry and viscoelastic properties of the wall. Ideally it would be desirable to evaluate these changes at all levels of the circulation, but this is not feasible due to a lack of suitable technology. The traditional approach has depended on measurements of blood pressure, flow and pulse wave recordings. In the future, thorough evaluation of the disease must be made by examining in greater detail the more subtle changes by newly developing techniques.

PRESSURE MEASUREMENTS

Narrowing of the artery lumen will result in an abnormal pressure drop when the reduction in cross-sectional area is sufficient to increase resistance to flow. With narrowing there is a reduction in the pulse pressure distal to the site of involvement.[4, 5] The arterial mean pressure diminishes as well when the artery becomes completely occluded and blood is forced to follow the collateral arteries. The extent to which the mean pressure falls is directly related to the resistance offered by the collateral arteries.

In patients with arterial disease, the traditional methods for measuring arterial pressure (see Fig. 5-5) are not effective, and indirect methods of measurement must be employed.[6, 7, 8] The return of pulsations after deflation of a cuff on the extremity can be registered by several devices such as mercury-filled fine silastic tubes, capacitance pulse pickups or the ultrasonic velocity detector (Fig. 8-2). The determinations should be made by placing a pressure cuff at several levels of the limb (ankle, calf, above knee, upper thigh), with the sensing element over the pedal arteries or about a terminal digit.

The currently available indirect methods measure only the systolic pressure, but this does not appear to be a serious handicap. Since the systolic pressure is the first to decrease with arterial narrowing, it provides a reliable index of the patency of the arterial circulation proximal to the recording site.

Since there is amplification of the pulse pressure as it proceeds distally to the periphery (see Fig. 5-4), the systolic pressure at the ankle should exceed that recorded at the upper arm. If the ankle blood pressure is lower than arm pressure, arterial stenosis or occlusion proximal to the ankle is a certainty (Fig. 8-3). The one situation in which pressure measurements made at rest may not detect disease is

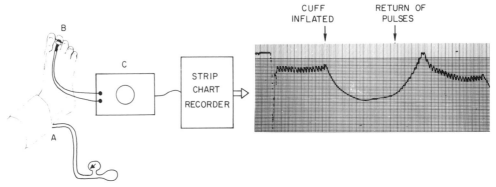

FIGURE 8–2   MEASUREMENT OF SYSTOLIC BLOOD PRESSURE BY A MERCURY-IN-SILASTIC
STRAIN GAUGE

An indirect method of measuring systolic blood pressure using a mercury-in-silastic strain gauge.
A, pneumatic cuff; B, mercury strain gauge; C, impedance matching circuit. With cuff inflation to
above systolic pressure, the digit volume pulses disappear. The point at which pulses reappear with
cuff deflation is recorded as the systolic or opening pressure.

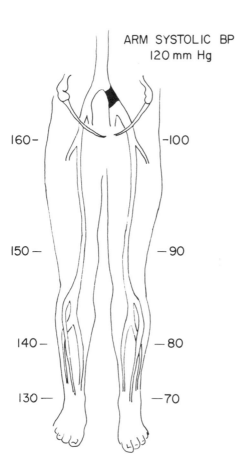

FIGURE 8–3   LOCALIZATION OF ARTERIAL
OCCLUSION BY LIMB BLOOD PRESSURES

The reduced systolic pressures recorded at
all levels of the left limb suggest that the occlusion is located proximal to the inguinal ligament.

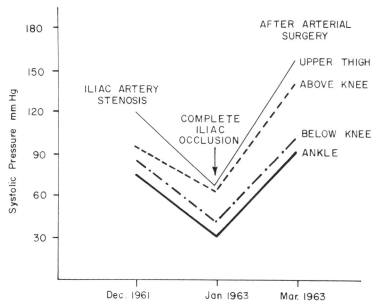

FIGURE 8–4   APPLICATION OF PRESSURE MEASUREMENTS TO FOLLOW DISEASE PROGRESSION

As the stenosis in the iliac artery progressed to a complete occlusion, the systolic blood pressures at all levels decreased. When the occluded segment was opened by direct arterial surgery, the pressures increased to normal levels.

with stenoses that are not sufficient to produce a significant pressure gradient at levels of resting blood flow.

An extremely valuable aspect of the pressure measurements made at the ankle is that it may be used to follow both disease progression and improvement in collateral artery function. With new disease or further narrowing of an existing stenosis, the abnormal pressure gradient will increase and further reduce the systolic pressure distal to the area of involvement (Fig. 8–4).

Measurement of the ankle systolic blood pressure after exercise provides an additional useful test of arterial function. Normally, with moderate exercise, the ankle systolic pressure remains the same or increases. With arterial obstruction proximal to the origin of the sural artery, the ankle blood pressure falls often to unrecord-

able levels, requiring several minutes to return to the pre-exercise level (Fig. 8–5). The basis for the postexercise ankle pressure decrease is not completely understood but the decrease is probably due to several factors: (1) The collateral arteries having an abnormally high resistance cannot provide enough blood flow to prevent ischemia. (2) The ischemia in the exercising muscle results in a marked fall in arterial resistance. (3) The marked fall in arterial resistance in the muscle results in shunting of blood away from the non-muscular components, i.e., the foot, resulting in a marked decrease in skin blood flow.

The major advantage of the resting pressure and postexercise determinations is that the results provide a profile for each patient which may be used for future comparison. The combination of these determinations pro-

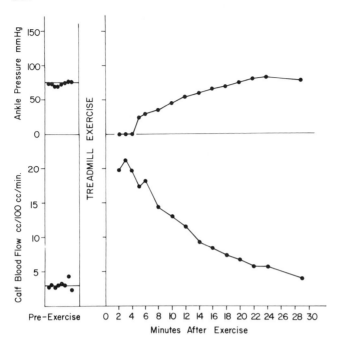

The relationship between the postexercise ankle blood pressure and calf blood flow in a patient with a superficial femoral artery obstruction.

vides the most sensitive methods currently available for objectively following, on a long-term basis, the patient with arterial disease.

FLOW MEASUREMENTS

Plethysmography. The most widely applied method for measuring limb blood flow is venous occlusion plethysmography. The aim of the technique is to briefly arrest venous outflow completely without interfering with arterial inflow. With brief obstruction of venous outflow, the initial rate of volume change is considered to represent the rate of arterial inflow.[9, 10] There are several types of plethysmographs and associated recording equipment available which may be used.[11] These include water-filled and air-filled plethysmographs which directly measure the volume change of the enclosed part. Tiny silastic tubes filled with mercury undergo changes in electrical resistance as they change in

length and may be used to measure the changes in limb girth.[12] Changes in limb circumference are presumed to be linearly related to the volume change. The air- and water-filled instruments are particularly suited for measurements of flow to the foot or hand, which can be completely enclosed in the surrounding jacket.

Indicator-Dilution Methods. The dye-dilution method has been extensively applied in the measurement of cardiac output (see Fig. 3–21). Indicator-dilution techniques have only recently been applied to the measurement of limb blood flow.[13, 14, 15] This method can give accurate results only if complete mixing occurs at some point between the injection and sampling site. Hobbs, *et al.*[15] investigated the method experimentally and concluded that the technique was valid if (1) all the injectate entered the vascular bed being evaluated; (2) the volume of the injectate was sufficiently small so that none was lost in branches proximal to the site of injection; and (3) complete mixing occurred.

While the technique does appear to be valid for estimating total limb blood flow, it does have serious limitations in patient studies. First, it can be applied only to patients with disease distal to the inguinal ligament. Second, the measured flow contribution consists of two components—the normal contribution to the thigh muscles and that which passes through the collateral arteries to supply the limb distal to the site of occlusion. Third, studies can only be made with the patient in the supine position. Fourth, direct needle puncture of both the femoral artery and vein is required, which adds to the potential hazard and limits the number of times the study can be safely repeated.

Isotope Clearance Methods. Kety[16] was the first to propose the measurement of flow by determining the clearance rate of an isotope injected directly into muscle. The validity of this method is based upon three assumptions: (1) The tissue is homogeneous so that no concentration gradients of the isotope exist. (2) The equilibrium between the blood and tissue is immediate. (3) The isotope is removed only by blood flow from the site of injection. Sodium-24 was first used but proved unsatisfactory because of its hydrophilic nature which did not permit ready transfer across the cellular membrane. Lassen[17] investigated Xenon-133, a lipophilic particle, which passed the cellular membrane readily. Its advantages over Sodium-24 can be summarized as follows: (1) The reflux of Xenon-133 back along the needle track is less since it diffuses so quickly. (2) It does not contaminate the needle or skin surface since it diffuses rapidly into the atmosphere. (3) Being a gas and soft gamma emitter, it is easier to handle without contami-

nation of the equipment or laboratory space. (4) The low radiation energy and rapid elimination from the body permits a low radiation dose.

Electromagnetic Flowmeters. Kolin[18] employed the principle of magnetic induction that an electrical current is produced when a conductor moves across the lines of force of a magnetic field (see Fig. 2–20A). Using this principle, blood velocity can be measured using small electromagnetic coils embedded in a plastic head which may be placed about the vessel to be studied.[19, 20] The types of instruments available are classified by the type of current pulse, which are square wave, sine wave or trapezoidal wave.[21]

These flow measuring devices have had their greatest application in animal research for both acute studies on exposed vessels and chronic implantation. At the present time their use in humans is greatly limited because of the necessity for operative exposure of the artery. The electromagnetic flowmeter has been most frequently used in measurements before and after completion of direct arterial surgery.[22, 23]

Ultrasonic Flow Sensors. In recent years flow sensors utilizing ultrasound have been developed, based on two different principles. The transit time flowmeter is based upon the fact that sound waves move faster in the direction of flow than when traveling against the flow stream. Using this principle, it has been observed that blood flow velocity can be registered in terms of the difference in the transit time between two barium titanate crystals mounted across a plastic cylinder enclosing a vessel.[24]

The second and more widely useful type of flow sensor for clinical studies employs the familiar Doppler effect.[25] With this instrument the frequency of the sound beam which is directed into the blood stream is shifted by an amount proportional to flow velocity.

Transcutaneous Applications of Ultrasound. With the exception of plethysmography, the other available methods of measuring flow have the disadvantage that either operative exposure of the artery is required or needles must be inserted into the lumen of the vessel or muscle. With the possible exception of plethysmography and the isotope clearance methods, repeat studies on a routine basis to follow disease progression or the results of therapy are not feasible. The ideal flowmeter would be one that can be used externally at all levels of the limb to measure both instantaneous and mean flow in specific arteries. To do this requires some method of introducing energy into the body which can then be analyzed in terms of the alteration in the energy as it occurs. While it is easy to generate the energy, such as ultrasound, the problems that remain and require a solution are as follows: (1) The vessel's cross-sectional area must be known; (2) the change in cross-sectional area over the pulse cycle should be known and (3) the flow direction and its time-course relationships should be measurable.

The progress that has been made to date can be considered under the following instruments developed: (1) the continuous wave nondirectional ultrasonic velocity detector[25] and (2) the continuous wave directional instrument.[26]

The currently available continuous wave systems employ either a 5 or 10 MHZ signal which is beamed through the skin, subcutaneous tissue and blood vessel. The particles in the moving stream shift the frequency of the transmitted signal by an amount proportional to velocity. A receiving crystal detects the backscattered sound which is mixed with the transmitter frequency to produce a frequency spectrum in the audible range. The output of the instrument may be presented as an audible signal or an analogue output derived by either a spectral density analysis or using a zero-crossing circuit.[27]

Although this simple continuous wave system has proved valuable for clinical studies, it fails to distinguish forward from reverse flow. McLeod[26] developed a phase detector to discriminate between flow going in opposite directions relative to the probe position. It is now possible to record simultaneously either forward or reverse flow on separate recorder channels or to combine the two outputs to give a composite waveform.[28] Simultaneous recording of forward and reverse flow on separate channels has considerable advantages over the differential output since it permits a very accurate estimation of the time-course relationships as they occur in both the arterial and venous systems. (Fig. 8–6).

RESULTS OF FLOW MEASUREMENTS IN ARTERIOSCLEROSIS OBLITERANS

To elicit evidence of restricted blood flow from the abnormality produced by chronic major artery occlusion, it is usually necessary to stress the collateral circulation by either exercise or timed arrest of the arterial inflow. Generally the only useful flow measurements are those made during the postexercise period. Immediately after exercise the limb blood flow normally reaches its peak, with a rapid return to the pre-exercise level. In patients with arteriosclerosis obliterans, even minimal exertion is usually sufficient to bring out blood flow patterns which are easily distinguished

BRACHIAL ARTERY

FIGURE 8–6 BRACHIAL ARTERY
VELOCITY PATTERN

With the continuous wave directional velocity detector, forward and reverse flow may be simultaneously recorded. With occlusion of a side-side radial artery-vein fistula, there is considerable flow reversal in the brachial artery. With release of the fistula compression, mean flow velocity increases considerably with disappearance of flow reversal.

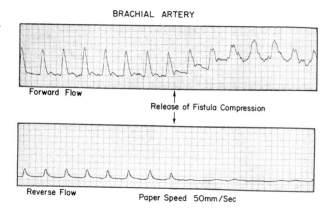

from normal. The type of postexercise flow response that is observed is related to the location and extent of the occlusive disease.[29, 30] With a single segment occlusion proximal to the blood supply to the calf, the initial postexercise blood flow is well above baseline levels but only slowly returns to baseline levels (see Fig. 8–5). With multiple levels of occlusion and limited collateral circulation, the initial postexercise flow may be very low, in some cases below resting levels, increasing very slowly over several minutes to reach a peak level. In these cases the period of postexercise hyperemia may exceed 30 minutes.

When timed arrest of the circulation is used, the level of the peak flows achieved is also useful and indicative of arterial occlusion. Hillestad[31, 32] found that with 5 minutes of occlusion, peak flows of less than 15 ml./min./100 ml. of tissue were indicative of arterial occlusion.

Flow measurements have been made at the time of operation with electromagnetic flowmeters to assess the immediate effectiveness of the result. In most instances the measurements have been made before and after completion of the procedure. A major problem in assessing the flow

changes that occur during operation relates to the conditions under which the measurements are made. Anesthesia in itself tends to produce profound cardiovascular changes which cannot be dismissed lightly.[33] Cardiac output is reduced and peripheral resistance increases, resulting in flows that are undoubtedly well below those measured even in the resting, awake state.[36] While a marked increase in flow after arterial surgery is reassuring, a word of caution is in order. Mannick and Jackson[23] showed that the relative increase in blood flow recorded from femoropopliteal vein grafts was extremely variable and bore little relationship to the postoperative results.

The ultrasonic Doppler velocity detector can be applied to the skin surface to qualitatively examine the flow velocity in those arteries outside the thorax, abdomen and cranial cavity. Since ultrasound at the safe power levels employed cannot penetrate bone or air-containing structures, it has its greatest application to the extremities and neck. Velocity signals can be obtained readily from the level of the subclavian artery to the digital arteries in the arm and the iliac artery to the pedal arteries in the leg.

In order to properly apply the instrument to the clinical evaluation of arteriosclerosis obliterans, certain basic rules should be followed. First, it is important to keep the transducer-artery angle relatively constant. For practical applications, an angle of 45 degrees is relatively easy to maintain. Second, the examiner must be familiar with the normal location of the major vessels. Third, the physician must familiarize himself with the type of velocity signals that are associated with particular pathologic states.

The examination procedure can be varied depending upon the intended application but in general the following sites should be examined: (1) external iliac and common femoral arteries, (2) superficial femoral artery, (3) popliteal artery and (4) posterior tibial-dorsalis pedis arteries at the ankle. Although it is not possible to examine the abdominal aorta or common iliac arteries regularly, it is possible to obtain inferential information about the more proximal arteries from the velocity signals detected at the groin level.

The normal arterial velocity signal consists of two or three components (Fig. 8–7). The first and highest frequency (about 3 to 4 KHZ) coincides with systole. If flow reversal is present, a second sound may be heard occurring in early diastole. The third component when heard occurs later in diastole and is undoubtedly related to a slight amount of forward flow. The second and third sounds are of lower frequency (500 c.p.s. to 1 [KHZ]). If flow reversal is not present, then only two sounds will be heard. The detection of signals of the type just described is sufficient to rule out the presence of arterial occlusion or marked narrowing proximal to the recording site.

In regions of arterial narrowing, the flow velocity is increased and the resulting frequency shift is much greater. The audible signal may reach a frequency of 8 to 10 KHZ, with flow being continuous throughout the pulse cycle (Fig. 8–7).

When the blood flow has traversed a collateral bed, the peak frequencies recorded are often quite low (1 to 2 KHZ), and the second and third sounds are no longer audible (Fig. 8–7). Absence of a signal over a large artery is certain evidence of occlusion.

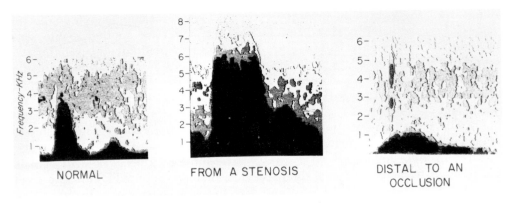

NORMAL   FROM A STENOSIS   DISTAL TO AN OCCLUSION

FIGURE 8–7   SPECTRAL DENSITY ANALYSES

The spectral density analyses indicate the type of signals that may be recorded from normal and diseased peripheral arteries. (See text for detailed explanation.)

The same may not be true over the anterior and posterior tibial arteries at the ankle. At this level, flow velocity may be so low (less than 6 cm./sec.) as to be undetectable with the current instruments. However, if a signal is detected from one pedal artery but not from the other, the vessel is either occluded or congenitally absent.

While the information presented to the examiner is qualitative and does require some experience in interpretation, it can be used to provide the following information: (1) localization of arterial obstruction; (2) determination of patency of the "run-off" vessels so important to the vascular surgeon; (3) assessment of the immediate results of bypass grafts or endarterectomy; (4) evaluation of complaints suggestive of the thoracic outlet syndromes; (5) establishment of the diagnosis of congenital arteriovenous fistulas; (6) indirect measurement of limb blood pressure when return of palpable pulses or Korotkoff sounds cannot be used.

THROMBOPHLEBITIS

Occlusion of venous channels in the arms and legs generally results from inflammation of the vein walls (phlebitis). The cause is not known. The process usually results in thrombosis of the involved vein. The clinical manifestations vary greatly depending upon the location of the involvement, its extent and the associated systemic symptoms and signs. The greatest danger of phlebitis is that it has its highest incidence in the seriously ill, the patient with malignancy and those patients hospitalized and at bed rest for prolonged periods of time. The first warning that a deep vein is occluded may be the appearance of a life-threatening or fatal pulmonary embolus. Early diagnosis is often difficult because of the paucity of physical findings and the lack of readily applicable diagnostic methods. The diagnostic considerations can best be discussed under the headings of acute thrombophlebitis and the postphlebitic syndrome.

ACUTE THROMBOPHLEBITIS

When thrombophlebitis develops, there may be present the usual physical signs that are associated with any inflammatory process. These include local swelling (edema), increased temperature at the site of involvement, tenderness, induration and venous thrombosis. If the process involves the superficial veins, the diagnosis can easily be made by inspection and palpation of the involved segment.[34]

The problem can be much more subtle and difficult to detect if it involves the deep veins of the lower extremity. If the inflammatory process is not sufficient to produce edema or local tenderness, the process usually goes unrecognized. An important point to keep in mind in regard to swelling of the limb is that it is directly related to the site and extent of the thrombosis that occurs. If it is confined to the deep veins below the knee, there is often no edema at all. When the process either propagates or starts in the more proximal deep veins, swelling nearly always occurs. As a general rule, the more proximal the occlusion, the greater the edema. For example, acute thrombosis of the iliofemoral venous segments of the deep system nearly always results in swelling of the entire limb.[34]

PROBLEMS IN CLINICAL EVALUATION

If the acute inflammatory process involving the vein wall is sufficient to produce the characteristic symptoms and signs, the diagnosis is rarely difficult to establish. The one entity which may be difficult to distinguish from phlebitis is bacterial cellulitis. The ultrasonic velocity detector can be helpful in distinguishing cellulitis from nonbacterial phlebitis. This is based upon the observation that thrombosis of the involved vein is an integral part of the phlebitic process. If it can be shown that the deep veins in the area involved with cellulitis are patent, it can be reasonably assumed that the process is not thrombophlebitis.

At this point it is necessary to consider in some detail the use of the velocity detector in the evaluation of venous dynamics. The salient features of the technique are as follows:

(1) Vessels accessible for examination. The major deep veins from the level of the subclavian vein to the wrist and external iliac vein to the ankle can be examined with the velocity detector. The superficial veins can also be examined to determine their patency.

(2) Normal findings. Since the venous dynamics are primarily dependent upon cardiac and respiratory events under resting conditions, it is relatively simple to ascertain the normality of the venous flow dynamics. In the external iliac and femoral veins,

for example, venous flow is phasic with the respiratory cycle. With inspiration, the diaphragm descends and intra-abdominal pressure increases, resulting in either a transitory decrease or cessation of venous flow (Fig 8–8). The opposite occurs with the major deep veins of the upper extremity in that inspiration is normally accompanied by an increase in venous inflow.[21]

(3) Technique of examination. As a rule it is best to begin the examination with the most proximal veins. It is essential to understand their anatomic relationships to the major arteries since the arterial signal may be used as an identifying landmark. Normally, there should be little difficulty in detecting the flow signal from the subclavian-brachial veins and the iliac, femoral and popliteal veins. In cases in which the signal may be inaudible initially, it may be necessary to augment flow velocity by a sudden compression of the limb distal to the site of examination. The augmentation procedure transiently increases the flow velocity, bringing it into an audible range.[33]

In those veins distal to the elbow and below the knee, the venous flow velocity may or may not be detectable at the levels observed under resting

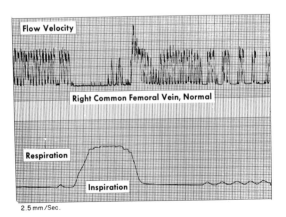

Flow Velocity

Right Common Femoral Vein, Normal

Respiration

Inspiration

2.5 mm/Sec.

FIGURE 8–8 EFFECTS OF RESPIRATION ON FLOW VELOCITY IN FEMORAL VEIN

Respiratory motion was monitored using a strain gauge fixed to the thorax. With inspiration, the intra-abdominal pressure increases as the diaphragm descends. This results in a transient cessation of flow in the femoral vein.

conditions. Thus, if the venous velocity signal from the posterior tibial vein is inaudible, foot compression should be carried out. Failure to elicit a signal with foot compression is certain evidence of occlusion of the vein being studied. Another method of transiently augmenting venous flow to assess patency is to digitally occlude the major vein proximal to the site of examination. With release, the venous flow velocity will transiently increase, permitting detection (Fig. 8–9).

(4) Interpretation of findings. In localizing the site of acute venous obstruction, it is necessary to follow a few simple rules. Absence of a velocity signal from a major deep vein, particularly with augmentation procedures, is certain evidence of occlusion of the vein being studied. When examining veins distal to the site of an acute occlusion, the signal usually loses its

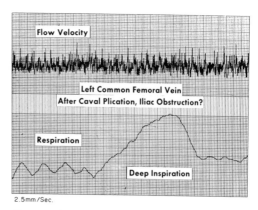

FIGURE 8–10   VELOCITY SIGNAL DISTAL TO OCCLUSION

The flow recorded from a major vein distal to a point of occlusion may be continuous and not be influenced by normal respiration.

normal phasic characteristics and becomes continuous in nature, not influenced by normal respiration (Fig. 8–10).

While venography may provide the same information, there are compelling reasons for not advocating its use particularly with an acute process. First, if cellulitis of a bacterial origin is present, this technique may serve as an avenue for extension of the process. Second, the possible hazards of introducing contrast material into veins already damaged by the inflammatory process should not be underestimated. Third, the test may not be used repetitively to follow the progress of the phlebitic process.

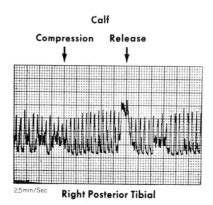

FIGURE 8–9   METHOD FOR TRANSIENT AUGMENTATION OF VENOUS FLOW

The recording illustrated is from the posterior tibial artery and vein at the ankle. Under resting conditions venous flow was not detectable until the medial side of the calf was transiently compressed, impeding venous outflow. With release of the compression, the venous flow transiently increases into the detectable range, thus verifying venous patency at that point.

THE POSTPHLEBITIC SYNDROME

The most serious after-effect of acute deep thrombophlebitis is the chronic venous stasis which follows the thrombosis and destruction of the venous valves. The importance of the valvular mechanism in preventing the long-term complications is clearly evi-

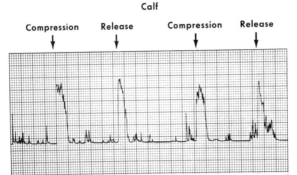

Flow Velocity Through Incompetent Perforating Vein 25 mm/Sec

FIGURE 8–11 BIDIRECTIONAL FLOW WITH INCOMPETENT VENOUS VALVES

When a perforating vein has a competent valvular mechanism, venous flow should occur in one direction only. In the patient illustrated, flow was detectable both during proximal compression and release. This maneuver establishes with certainty both the location and competency of the perforating veins.

dent when their functional integrity is disrupted. In the standing position the pressure in the veins of the foot is on the order of 100 mm. Hg (see Chapter 7). With exercise this pressure rapidly falls to a range of 0 to 5 mm. Hg. The reduced pressure with exercise can be attributed to the competence of the valves which permit unidirectional flow only.

When the valves are incompetent, muscular contraction tends to force blood proximally, distally and through the communicating vessels to the subcutaneous veins. The venous pressure in the foot in this situation does not decrease but actually may increase during the act of walking. The incompetent perforating veins lead to the so-called "high pressure leaks" which result in dilatation and rupture of the smaller superficial veins. These repeated episodes lead to the deposition of hemosiderin pigment within the skin (stasis pigmentation). The skin ultimately becomes thin and prone to ulcerate when subjected to even minor trauma. Once established the so-called stasis ulcers heal very poorly. The predilection for the skin changes along the medial aspect of the lower leg can be attributed to the location of the major perforating veins in this region.

The postphlebitic syndrome is characterized by two major pathological features, deep venous occlusion and valvular incompetence. The examination with the ultrasonic velocity detector looking for areas of occlusion is the same as with acute venous occlusion. A word of caution is in order with reference to the type of signals heard distal to an area of chronic obstruction. Since the occlusion is chronic, the venous dynamics may be normal relative to the respiratory cycle, particularly if the collateral veins are large. The absence of continuous venous flow does not rule out proximal venous occlusion.

In establishing valve incompetence it is necessary to demonstrate a bidirectional flow. This can be done by suddenly manually compressing the limb proximal to the site being examined. Normally there is no velocity signal heard with compression but only upon release. When incompetent valves are present, velocity signals are heard during both limb compression and release (Fig. 8–11).

REFERENCES

1. MITCHELL, J. R. A., and SCHWARTZ, C. J. Arterial Disease. Philadelphia, F. A. Davis Co., 1965.
2. KELLY, W. A., and STRANDNESS, D. E., JR. The subclavian steal syndrome. Pp. 570–

582, in *Collateral Circulation in Clinical Surgery*. D. E. Strandness, Jr., Ed. Philadelphia, W. B. Saunders Co., 1969.

3. CURRY, J. L., and HOWLAND, W. J. *Arteriography: Principles and Techniques*. Philadelphia, W. B. Saunders Co., 1966.

4. KEITZER, W. F., FRY, W. J., KRAFT, R. O., and DeWEESE, M. S. Hemodynamic mechanism for pulse changes seen in occlusive vascular disease. *Surgery*, 57: 163–174, 1965.

5. SCHULTZ, R. D., HOKANSON, D. E., and STRANDNESS, D. E., JR. Pressure-flow relations and stress-strain measurements of normal and diseased aortoiliac segments. *Surg. Gynec. Obstet.*, 124:1267–1276, 1967.

6. CARTER, S. A. Indirect systolic pressures and pulse waves in arterial occlusive disease of the lower extremities. *Circulation*, 37:624–637, 1968.

7. STRANDNESS, D. E., JR., and BELL, J. W. Peripheral vascular disease. Diagnosis and objective evaluation using a mercury strain gauge. *Ann. Surg.*, 161 (Suppl.): 1–35, 1965.

8. WINSOR, T. Influence of arterial disease on the systolic blood pressure gradients of the extremity. *Amer. J. Med. Sci.*, 220:117–126, 1950.

9. LANDOWNE, M., and KATZ, L. N. Critique of plethysmographic method of measuring blood flow in extremities of man. *Amer. Heart J.*, 23:644–675, 1942.

10. WILKINS, R. W., and BRADLEY, S. E. Changes in arterial and venous blood pressure and flow distal to cuff inflated on human arm. *Amer. J. Physiol.*, 147:260–269, 1946.

11. GREENFIELD, A. D. M., WHITNEY, R. J., and MOWBRAY, J. F. Methods for the investigation of peripheral blood flow. *Brit. Med. Bul.*, 19:101–109, 1963.

12. WHITNEY, F. J. The measurement of volume changes in human limbs. *J. Physiol. (London)*, 121:1–27, 1953.

13. AGRIFOGLIO, G., THORBURN, G. D., and EDWARDS, E. A. Measurement of blood flow in human lower extremity by indicator-dilution method. *Surg. Gynec. Obstet.*, 113:641–645, 1961.

14. FOLSE, R. Application of the sudden injection dye dilution principle to the study of the femoral circulation. *Surg. Gynec. Obstet.*, 120:1194–1206, 1965.

15. HOBBS, J. T., AGRIFOGLIO, G., and EDWARDS, E. A. Measurement of femoral artery blood flow using the indicator-dilution method. An evaluation in the dog. *J. Surg. Res.*, 2:386–396, 1962.

16. KETY, S. S. Quantitative measurement of regional circulation by the clearance of radioactive sodium. *Amer. J. Med. Sci.*, 215:352, 1948.

17. LASSEN, N. A. Muscle blood flow in normal man and in patients with intermittent claudication by simultaneous Xe^{133} and Na^{24} clearances. *J. Clin. Invest.*, 43:1805–1812, 1964.

18. KOLIN, A. An alternating field induction flowmeter of high sensitivity. *Rev. Sci. Instrum.*, 16:109, 1945.

19. DENISON, A. B., JR., SPENCER, M. P., and GREEN, H. D. A square wave electromagnetic flowmeter for application to intact blood vessels. *Circ. Red.*, 3:39–46, 1955.

20. RICHARDSON, A. W., DENISON, A. B. JR., and GREEN, H. D. A newly modified electromagnetic blood flowmeter capable of high fidelity flow registration. *Circulation*, 5: 430–436, 1952.

21. YANOF, H. M. *Biomedical Electronics*. Philadelphia, F. A. Davis Co., 1965.

22. GOLDING, A. L., and CANNON, J. A. Application of electromagnetic blood flowmeter during arterial reconstruction. Results in conjunction with papavarine in 47 cases. *Ann. Surg.*, 164:662–675, 1966.

23. MANNICK, J. A., and JACKSON, B. T. Hemodynamics of arterial surgery in atherosclerotic limbs. I. Direct measurement of blood flow before and after vein grafts. *Surgery*, 59:713–720, 1966.

24. FRANKLIN, D. K., BAKER, D. W., ELLIS, R. M., and RUSHMER, R. F. A plused ultrasonic flowmeter, *IRE Trans. Med. Electronics*, ME-6:204–206, 1959.

25. RUSHMER, R. F., BAKER, D. W., and STEGALL, H. F. Transcutaneous Doppler flow detection as a nondestructive technique. *J. Appl. Physiol.*, 21:554–566, 1966.

26. MCLEOD, F. D. JR. A directional Doppler flowmeter. *Proc. 20th Ann. Conf. Engr. in Med. & Biology*, Vol. 9, Nov. 1967, Boston.

27. STRANDNESS, D. E., JR., SCHULTZ, R. D., SUMNER, D. S., and RUSHMER, R. F. Ultrasonic flow detection: A useful technic in the evaluation of peripheral vascular disease. *Amer. J. Surg.*, 113:311–320, 1967.

28. STRANDNESS, D. E., JR., KENNEDY, J. W., JUDGE, T. P., and MCLEOD, F. D., JR. Transcutaneous directional flow detection: A preliminary report. *Amer. Heart J.* (in press).

29. SUMNER, D. S., BAKER, D. W., and STRANDNESS, D. E., JR. The ultrasonic velocity detector in a clinical study of venous disease. *Arch. Surg.*, 97:75–80, 1968.

30. SUMNER, D. S., and STRANDNESS, D. E., JR. The relationship between calf blood flow and ankle blood pressure in patients with intermittent claudication. *Surgery*, 65: 763–771, 1969.

31. HILLESTAD, L. K. The peripheral blood flow in intermittent claudication. V. Plethysmographic studies. The significance of the calf blood flow at rest and in response to timed arrest of the circulation. *Acta Med. Scand.*, 174:23–41, 1963.

32. HILLESTAD, L. K. The peripheral blood flow

in intermittent claudication. VI. Plethysmographic studies. The blood flow response to exercise with arrested and with free circulation. *Acta Med. Scand.*, 174: 671–685, 1963.

33. SHACKMAN, R., GRABER, G. L., and MELROSE, D. G. The hemodynamics of the surgical patient under general anesthesia. *Brit. J. Surg.*, 40:193–201, 1952.

34. HALLER, J. A., JR. *Deep Thrombophlebitis.* Philadelphia, W. B. Saunders Co., 1967.

35. SIGEL, B., POPKY, G. L., WAGNER, D. K., BOLAND, J. P., ESMOND, McD. M., FEIGL, P. A Doppler ultrasound method for diagnosing lower extremity venous disease. *Surg. Gynec. Obstet.*, 127:339–350, 1968.

36. STRANDNESS, D. E., JR., DICKSON, A. H., PARRISH, D., and BELL, J. W. Effects of the depth of anesthesia on peripheral vascular dynamics. *Angiology*, 15:479–484, 1964.

CHAPTER 9

THE CORONARY SYSTEM

By Michel G. Nasser, M.D.

The maximum capacity for sustained physical exertion or work is ultimately limited by the maximum rate of oxygen delivery to the tissues. A major component of this cardiovascular reserve capacity is the ability of the heart to increase its output of useful work in terms of the volume ejected each minute against the pressure in the major arterial trunks. The heart must be supplied with sufficient oxygen and metabolic fuels to replace continuously the energy expended both as useful work and as energy lost because the heart is less than perfectly efficient as a pump. The metabolic mechanisms which supply energy through oxidative and anaerobic processes must be understood to appreciate the significance of insufficient blood flow to contracting myocardium.

If the ventricular myocardium releases more energy than is restored during each cycle, the cardiac output must soon diminish until a balance between energy expenditure and energy restoration is again established. The myocardium exists in an environment of low oxygen tension at all times, judging by the very low oxygen content of blood leaving the heart in the coronary veins. Increased oxygen de-

livery must be attained primarily by increased coronary blood flow since the oxygen extraction is so complete under normal resting conditions.

METABOLISM OF THE NORMAL HEART

The myocardium utilizes energy produced by enzymatic degradation of substrates and trapped in the phosphate bond of ATP. This chemical energy is transformed into mechanical work; also, it supports a variety of anabolic activities such as synthesis of glycogen, lipids, proteins and enzymes. To understand the alterations in metabolism which underlie disease states, it is essential to first appreciate the normal metabolic pathways and the mechanisms influencing transport across cellular membranes.

Under normal conditions cardiac metabolism is entirely oxidative. Carbohydrates, fat, fatty acids and aminoacids are completely metabolized into carbon dioxide and water. Substrates are initially degraded in the cytoplasm of the myocardial cell, leading to small molecules which readily enter the citric acid cycle. Pyruvate is

261

the most common of these key molecules. The chemical reactions leading to its formation differ: anaerobic glycolysis for carbohydrates, hydrolysis for fat, deamination and other chemical transformations for aminoacids. It then enters the citric acid cycle as acetyl CoA and is oxidyzed into carbon dioxide and water. This process is carried out exclusively in the mitochondria and provides the heart with the major part of metabolic energy.

CELLULAR METABOLISM

The breakdown of carbohydrates without the intervention of oxygen is the initiating step in carbohydrate metabolism.[1] Anaerobic glycolysis is not a very effective source of energy: only two molecules of ATP are formed for each molecule of glucose. ATP is formed by direct transfer of a high energy phosphate to ADP through phosphorylations which result in pyruvate, then acetyl CoA. This anaerobic glycolysis assumes extreme importance in coronary insufficiency when the oxidative processes of the citric acid cycle are blocked as a result of inadequate oxygen delivery. At this time the anaerobic breakdown of carbohydrates becomes probably the only source of energy available to the ischemic myocardium. The survival of cardiac muscle deprived of oxygen depends on the stores of carbohydrates in the form of glycogen, on the ability of glucose to cross the cell membrane and on the capacity of the glycolytic enzymes to accelerate anaerobic glycolysis. This phase of carbohydrate metabolism is effectively controlled by phosphofructokinase, an enzyme which is inhibited by ATP and activated by ADP, AMP and inorganic phosphate.[1]

The oxidations which occur within the citric acid cycle are coupled with phosphorylation of ADP to form ATP, hence the term oxidative phosphorylation (Fig. 9–1).[2] Electrons are released by these oxidations and transferred to an electron acceptor by a highly organized system of enzymes and coenzymes, the electron transport system.[3,4] Oxygen is the final electron acceptor with which they combine to form water. Energy is captured by esterification of inorganic phosphate in the high energy bond of ATP. The net energy yield is high since thirty molecules of ATP are produced for one molecule of glucose consumed.

VALIDITY OF BALANCE STUDIES IN THE INTACT HEART

The study of myocardial balance of ions and substrates across the left ventricle requires sampling from the coronary sinus and from an arterial sampling site. The validity of data can be evaluated only by recognizing some inherent limitations. (1) The chemical composition of coronary sinus blood has been commonly used in animal and in man as an index of changes in metabolism of the left ventricle, together with left coronary artery inflow. The validity of such an approach has been demonstrated in the dog, in which the recovery of left coronary arterial inflow in the coronary sinus varies from 80 to 90 per cent.[5] The contamination of coronary sinus content by blood from the right ventricle is only 2 to 3 per cent.[5,6] Corresponding experimental evidence is completely lacking for the human left ventricle. (2) Arteriovenous differences must be interpreted with caution in the presence of a changing arterial level of substrate since a general rule appears to be that myocardial extraction of a substrate is directly related to its arte-

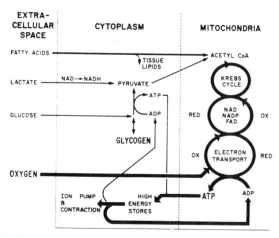

FIGURE 9–1   ENERGY PATHWAYS IN THE WELL-OXYGENATED MYOCARDIUM

When the heart is supplied with adequate amounts of oxygen, the rates of electron transport and oxidative phosphorylation are governed by the supply of ADP. The citric acid cycle utilizes acetyl CoA which is the product of degradation of carbohydrates and lipids. Note that lactate is extracted and converted into pyruvate and that the majority of fatty acids is converted into acetyl CoA. Glycogen is in a relatively steady state, being neither rapidly formed nor utilized. The electron transport system oxidizes reduced flavin and adenine coenzymes formed in citric acid cycle dehydrogenation. The rates of utilization and formation of energy are closely coupled and control the speed of substrate catabolic pathways. (From Scheuer, J.: Myocardial metabolism in cardiac hypoxia. Amer. J. Cardiol., 19:385–392, 1967.)

rial concentration. (3) The traditional method of sampling by syringe may be inadequate when small arteriovenous differences are to be measured, especially so when they are changing rapidly.[7]

METABOLISM OF SUBSTRATES

The heart extracts glucose, lactate, pyruvate and fatty acids and to a lesser extent ketone bodies and aminoacids. Each substrate shares in the total oxygen consumption (see Table 9–1), but its myocardial extraction is a function of its arterial concentration. This essential feature of myocardial extraction of substrates bears two implications: (1) the ability of the heart to gear precisely specific enzymic activities toward the provision of energy from available substrates, and (2) because of this adaptability of the heart to the available substrates, car-

diac function is fulfilled despite wide variations in the nutritional states of the body.

The contribution of glucose to the total oxygen consumption of the heart is about 18 per cent and that of all carbohydrates about 35 per cent (see Table 9–1). Myocardial glucose uptake is limited by its rate of transport across the cell membrane and its rate of utilization by the heart in the glycolytic pathways and in the glycogen synthesis.[8, 9] Both these factors are enhanced by insulin.[10, 11] Under steady state conditions, glucose is not taken up below an arterial level of 60 mgm./100 ml.[12]

The well-oxygenated heart utilizes lactate, extracting about 30 per cent of the quantity in the arterial blood.

The contribution of fatty acids to the economy of the human heart muscle is much higher than that of glucose,

Table 9-1. *RELATIVE CONTRIBUTION OF CARBOHYDRATES AND NONCARBOHYDRATES TO TOTAL MYOCARDIAL OXYGEN USAGE*

CARBO-HYDRATE	PER CENT	NONCARBO-HYDRATE	PER CENT
Glucose	17.90	Fatty acids	67.0
Pyruvate	0.54	Aminoacids	5.6
Lactate	16.46	Ketones	4.3
Total	34.90	Total	76.9

67 per cent of the total oxygen consumption (see Table 9–1) in the postabsorptive state and even more after a high fat intake.[13] In some subjects the fatty acid oxygen extraction ratio is seen to exceed 100 per cent, suggesting storage of fat in the human heart muscle.

The contribution of aminoacids to aerobic metabolism can increase up to 40 per cent of the total cardiac oxygen consumption after an infusion of aminoacids.[13] The increase in their extraction is, however, not directly proportional to their arterial level. This discrepancy may result from incorporation of aminoacids into proteins[14] or conversion into carbohydrates.[15]

THE DIABETIC HEART

The diabetic patient with an otherwise normal coronary circulation has an adequate total myocardial oxygen consumption, but the relative contribution of substrates to total myocardial oxygen usage is disturbed. The most significant defect in diabetics appears to be a depression of carbohydrate utilization by the diabetic myocardium.[16] At equally high arterial glucose concentrations, myocardial usage of this substrate is unexpectedly low in the diabetic as compared to the normal heart.[17] This decrease in the capacity of the myocardium to utilize glucose is probably secondary to lack of insulin. Lactate utilization is also markedly depressed and is not a direct function of arterial lactate concentration as would be the case in normal hearts.[17]

To compensate for this decreased source of energy supply, the heart of the diabetic patient extracts increased amounts of fatty acids from the arterial blood.

METABOLIC CHANGES DURING MYOCARDIAL ISCHEMIA

Extensive experimental data derived from experiments on myocardial ischemia in animals is being confirmed by corresponding measurements on man. When oxygen delivery to the myocardial cell is inadequate, the last electron carrier of the electron transport system is not oxidized (Fig. 9–2). If the state of hypoxia is persistent, reduced enzymes and coenzymes accumulate in the mitochondria, progressively blocking the citric acid cycle and inhibiting ATP formation by oxidative phosphorylation. Disruption of the mitochondria of ventricular muscle in animals and atrial muscle in man is evident after 15 minutes of hypoxia, but restoration of adequate supply of oxygen results in rapid mitochondrial regeneration.[18, 19] The hypoxic heart resorts to anaerobic metabolism when deprived of oxidative phosphorylation, its most powerful source of energy. The rate of glucose uptake is accelerated.[20] Glycogen and ATP are rapidly depleted, and hexosemonophosphate and alpha phosphorylase, the enzyme controlling glycogen utilization, are activated.[21] Energy made available from anaerobic glycolysis is only 6 per cent of that derived from oxidative metabolism.[22] Anaerobic glycolysis is therefore a poor means to compensate for inadequate oxygen supply.[23]

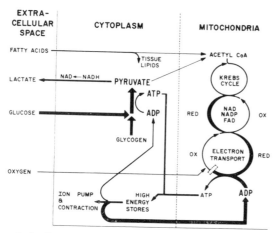

FIGURE 9-2   ENERGY PATHWAYS IN THE HYPOXIC MYOCARDIUM

When oxygen delivery to the myocardial cell cannot meet metabolic demands, there is relative blockage of the electron transport system. Oxidative phosphorylation is inhibited and high energy phosphate stores decline. Reduced substances such as flavin and adenine coenzymes accumulate, and citric acid cycle degradation of acetyl CoA cannot proceed at a normal rate. Under these conditions, the utilization of glucose and glycogen is accelerated and pyruvate accumulates. The mitochondrial and cytoplasmic NAD to NADH ratios decline, and the lactate-pyruvate reaction is reversed. Fatty acids are deposited in tissues as lipids. Increased glycogen breakdown provides an inadequate compensatory mechanism for the formation of ATP. (From Scheuer, J.: Myocardial metabolism in cardiac hypoxia. *Amer. J. Cardiol.*, 19:385–392, 1967.)

Lactate Metabolism During Myocardial Ischemia.   The hypoxic heart's lactic acid production from either glucose or endogenous glycogen is a well-established criterion of myocardial ischemia, and it has been widely recognized in the animal[23, 24] and in man during angina[25] and cardiogenic shock.[26] Reduced lactate extraction has also been reported in man[27] and in the animal[28, 29] as the early disturbance in lactate metabolism during established myocardial ischemia. The significance of this early disturbance in lactate metabolism is more evident when the concentration of lactate in the coronary sinus during myocardial ischemia is viewed in terms of a mixture of contributions from the ischemic portion of myocardium which is producing lactate and from the adequately oxygenated portion of myocardium which is extracting lactate. The net result of this could be a reduction in either lactate extraction or lactate production, depending on the amount of lactate produced (that is, on the area which is ischemic) and that being extracted. In other terms, the ratio of lactate produced to that being metabolized could represent the ratio of ischemic to nonischemic myocardium. When C-14 lactate is injected into a partially ischemic myocardium, it is recovered in the coronary sinus as $C_{14}O_2$[30] simultaneously with lactate production, suggesting that oxidative and anaerobic metabolism occur at the same time in the heart when it is not totally ischemic.

The subendocardium is more vulnerable than the epicardium to ischemia and is probably the first part of the heart to become ischemic during reduction of total coronary flow. A gradient in lactate concentration is present across the ventricular wall during myocardial ischemia as it is much higher in the subendocardial layers than in the outer half.[31]

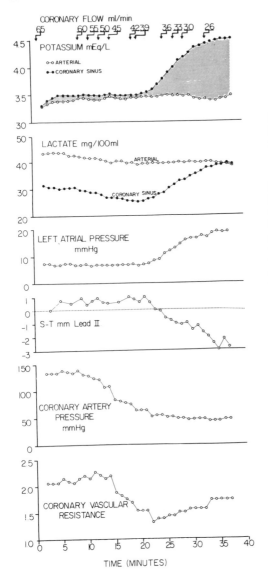

FIGURE 9–3 TIME SEQUENCE OF METABOLIC
EVENTS, CARDIAC AND CORONARY CIRCULA-
TORY DYNAMICS IN EXPERIMENTAL MYOCAR-
DIAL ISCHEMIA

Changes in potassium and lactate metabolism are illustrated during step-wise reduction of coronary flow to the perfused left main
coronary artery. When left atrial pressure rises
from 8 mm. Hg to 20 mm. Hg, there is a progressive rise in coronary sinus lactate which
exceeds arterial lactate during the last two
minutes. There is collateral evidence of myocardial ischemia in that an efflux of potassium
from the heart occurs simultaneously with the
rise in coronary sinus lactate and elevation of
left atrial pressure. S-T segment is depressed at
the same time as coronary sinus lactate rises.
The depression of S-T segment occurs as a "J"
depression first with heart rate relatively constant, 174 ± 0.6 during the control period and
180 ± 0.9 during myocardial ischemia. Coronary arterial pressure and calculated coronary
vascular resistance reach a minimum at the time
metabolic events of ischemia are evident. This
calculated coronary vascular resistance reaches
minimal levels at the onset of ischemia. (From
Case, R. B., Nasser, M. G., and Crampton, R. S.:
Biochemical aspects of early myocardial ischemia. *Amer. J. Cardiol.*, 24:766–775, 1969.

POTASSIUM ION EXCHANGE

The ratio of intracellular to extracellular potassium is generally maintained within narrow limits by an
energy dependent process linked to
ATP.[32, 33] It would appear, therefore,
reasonable that intracellular potassium
is reduced when this energy dependent process is disturbed by hypoxia.

Experimental myocardial ischemia is consistently characterized
by potassium loss from the ischemic
myocardium.[28, 34, 35]

Flow to the cannulated left main
coronary artery of the dog was reduced
in a step-wise fashion until the point
of myocardial ischemia.[28] Using an
automated technique for continuous
sampling,[7] special emphasis was
placed on the time sequence of metabolic and dynamic events (as seen in
Fig. 9–3).[28]

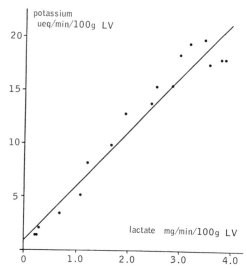

FIGURE 9–4 COMPARISON OF POTASSIUM EFFLUX AND LACTATE PRODUCTION IN EXPERIMENTAL MYOCARDIAL ISCHEMIA

Comparison of potassium loss from the heart and of lactate production shows a linear relationship, suggesting that the amount of potassium loss is directly related to the degree of ischemia.[28] The correlation coefficient of this relationship is 0.96. On a molar basis, approximately one milliequivalent of potassium is lost with each 2 millimoles of lactate produced. (Case, R. B., Nasser, M. G., and Crampton, R. S.: Biochemical aspects of early myocardial ischemia. *Amer. J. Cardiol.*, 24:766–775, 1969.

A significant myocardial potassium loss is evident at the onset of myocardial ischemia as it occurs simultaneously with the onset of reduction in lactate extraction, rise in left atrial pressure and depression of the electrocardiographic S-T segment. Calculated coronary vascular resistance drops progressively during the control period but remains steady as myocardial ischemia is initiated, suggesting that the coronary bed is totally dilated at this time.

Of special interest is a linear relationship between myocardial lactate production and potassium loss (see Fig. 9–4), suggesting that the amount of potassium lost is directly related to

the degree of ischemia.[28] During the postischemic period when coronary flow has been restored, potassium is taken up spontaneously[28] and the rate of uptake at this time is flow dependent until the myocardial potassium has been restored. This particular situation is not encountered during the control period. Indeed, at this time the rate of exchange of potassium ions across the heart is independent of coronary flow as long as the potassium content has not been altered and the oxygen supply is adequate to meet myocardial requirements.

The mechanism for the conservation of intracellular potassium is remarkably resistant to hypoxia. If coronary perfusion is eliminated in a nonbeating dog's heart for a duration up to 45 minutes, restoration of coronary perfusion is followed promptly by pronounced potassium uptake.[36]

METABOLISM OF THE NONBEATING HEART

In open heart surgery, metabolic requirements of the noncontracting heart must be met to assure restoration of normal myocardial function during the recovery period.

ANATOMY OF THE CORONARY ARTERIES

The coronary arteries encircle the heart like a crown ("corona") on the brow of the ventricles. They originate at ostia which are situated 0.7 to 1.0 cm. above the roots of the semilunar cusps so that they are never occluded by the opening of the aortic valve during systole. The main trunks of the right and left coronary arteries pass toward their respective atrioventricular grooves and turn circumferentially about the base of the heart. The coronary trunks are distributed on the epicardial surface, then plunge into the myocardial mass, where they divide sequentially giving rise to a rich network of capillaries.

THE LEFT CORONARY ARTERY

The left coronary artery arises from the left aortic sinus and divides almost immediately into two branches. The anterior descending branch gives off several branches to the anterior septum as it passes along the anterior interventricular groove toward the apex of the heart. The left circumflex branch courses around the base of the left ventricle along the coronary sulcus and terminates in the posterior descending branch. The branches of the left coronary artery supply the entire left ventricle (except for the posterior base of the free ventricular wall), the anterior two thirds of the interventricular septum, the anterior left margin of the free wall of the right ventricle, the apex, the lower half of the interatrial septum and the left atrium.

THE RIGHT CORONARY ARTERY

The right coronary artery originates in the right aortic sinus, reaches the posterior interventricular groove by way of the coronary sulcus at the base of the right ventricle. From the coronary ring, a number of branches descend to supply the ventricular walls. It supplies the anterior and posterior (diaphragmatic) walls of the right ventricle (except for the apex of the right ventricle, which is supplied by the left descending artery), the right atrium and the sinus node, the posterior one third of the interventricular septum, the atrioventricular node, the upper half of the interatrial septum

and the posterior base of the left ventricle.

The right coronary artery presents an advantage over the left in that it is readily accessible on the anterior surface of the heart. This is an advantage to the surgeon who must perform thromboendarterectomy, vein patch grafting or segmental arterial resection.

An accessory coronary ostium exists in 50 per cent of cases, giving rise to the conus artery which supplies the left anterior aspect of the outflow tract of the right ventricle at the level of the pulmonary valve orifice. This artery joins branches from the left coronary artery and forms the arterial circle named after Vieussens, who described it early in the eighteenth century.[37]

The sinus node is supplied by the right atrial artery[38] which arises in most cases from the right coronary artery. Occasionally it is a branch from the left circumflex artery.

The atrioventricular node is supplied by a branch of the same name which takes off from the right coronary artery at the crux.[39, 40] In dogs, the interventricular septum receives a fairly rich vascular supply from septal branches that arise near the origins of the main coronary channels. The conus and septal branches may have great importance in supplying blood flow to vascular beds below obstructions in the main coronary arteries. The profuse networks of coronary vessels supplying the walls of the heart can be most readily appreciated by injecting plastic into the vessels and dissolving away the myocardium (Fig. 9–5).[41, 42] The pattern of distribution is somewhat variable, particularly in the posterior aspect of the ventricular walls and septum. Schlesinger[43] has described three general patterns of coronary distribution: (1) right coronary preponderance, (2) a balanced distribution

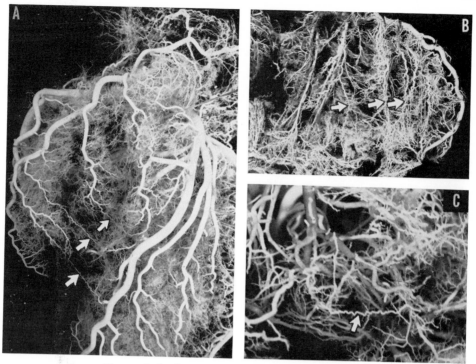

FIGURE 9–5 CORONARY ARTERIES AND COLLATERALS

Casts of the coronary arteries disclose the complex branching and the density of the vascular distribution throughout the walls of the heart. Helical collateral vessels connecting different arterial ramifications are indicated by arrows. These photographs are presented through the courtesy of Dr. Giorgio Baroldi, Instituto di Anatomia Patological, University of Milan, Milan, Italy.

and (3) left coronary preponderance (Fig. 9–6). When the right coronary artery supplies the posterior aspect of the left ventricle, the term of right coronary dominance is applied. Conversely the left coronary supplies some of the contiguous right ventricle in left coronary preponderance.

Data from autopsy and injection studies in human hearts show anatomic predominance of the right over the left coronary artery in a majority of cases (up to 48 per cent) and balanced distribution in 34 per cent.[43, 44] Although it has no functional implication in the normal heart, this anatomic distribution acquires its significance in the outcome of coronary artery disease. For example, sudden occlusion

of a large right coronary artery could be fatal, whereas occlusion of a small right coronary artery which takes no part in the blood supply of the left ventricle would cause no significant myocardial damage. Patients with left coronary preponderance are more apt to succumb to coronary occlusion. The anatomic pattern of right dominance is a pattern of the normal heart and is not a compensatory result of coronary artery disease. Regardless of this anatomic preponderance, the flow to the left coronary artery is always greater than to the right as this was demonstrated in perfusion studies of human hearts postmortem.[44] This preponderance of left coronary artery flow is probably related to the amount

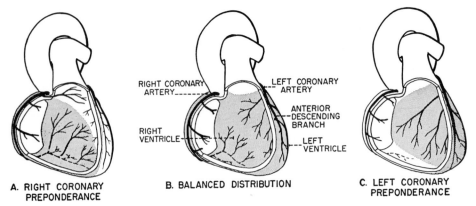

A. RIGHT CORONARY PREPONDERANCE **B. BALANCED DISTRIBUTION** **C. LEFT CORONARY PREPONDERANCE**

FIGURE 9–6 DISTRIBUTION OF THE CORONARY ARTERIES TO THE VENTRICULAR WALLS

A, The posterior portion of the interventricular septum and part of the posterior aspect of the left ventricle were supplied by coronary artery in about 48 per cent of a series of postmortem examinations. This distribution has been classified as right coronary preponderance.

B, Balanced coronary distribution occurred in about 34 per cent of specimens.

C, Left coronary preponderance (left coronary artery supplying some of the contiguous right ventricle and virtually the entire interventricular septum) occurred in 18 per cent. Patients with left coronary preponderance appear to be more susceptible to coronary occlusions with myocardial infarction. (From Schlesinger, M. G.: *Arch. Path.,* 30:403–415, 1940.)

of muscle mass supplied by the left coronary artery.

MYOCARDIAL CAPILLARY CIRCULATION

Branches from the main coronary vessels descend toward the apex, giving off penetrating branches which divide into dense anastomotic capillary networks roughly paralleling the courses of the myocardial bundles. The distribution of scars following occlusion of specific coronary branches suggests that each bundle of myocardial fibers has an individual blood supply although many communicating channels connect these vascular networks. The capillary networks in the ventricular myocardium have been found to contain metarterioles with smooth muscle cells at irregular intervals along their length. True capillaries, consisting of endothelial tubes, arise as branches of the metarterioles. Cuffs of smooth muscle or precapillary sphincters are situated at the origins of

the true capillaries.[45] Thus, the coronary capillary network has an organization comparable to that of corresponding small vessels in other tissues (see Fig. 4–5).

The ratio of capillaries to myocardial fibers in the newborn is approximately 1:4; it approaches 1:1 in the human adult.[46] The distribution of the capillaries is quite uniform in the human left and right ventricles, reaching 4000 per sq. mm. of tissue. The maximum distance necessary for diffusion is calculated to be 8μ. These values appear to be relatively constant throughout life. Interestingly enough, this uniformity of distribution is not shared by all parts of the heart: the interventricular septum has less capillary density than the ventricles. The atrioventricular node has a rather scanty supply of capillaries.[47] As a result of this dispersed capillary network the diffusion distance within the conducting system is much greater than that to the ventricular myocardium, making it more vulnerable to ischemia.

COLLATERAL CIRCULATION

Arterial channels connecting different branches of the same coronary artery (homocoronary anastomoses) or branches of two different coronary arteries (intercoronary anastomoses) have been found in all normal hearts in an extensive study by Baroldi and Scomazzoni.[42] The homocoronary anastomoses were found in large numbers in widely dispersed locations in the ventricular walls, connecting branches smaller than 500 to 1000 μ in diameter. The intercoronary arteries are found in the areas adjacent to two coronary arteries (see Fig. 9–5). Both types are found throughout the full thickness of the ventricular walls except the layers just under the epicardium. In the normal heart, the flow through such collateral channels would be small or unpredictable in amount and have little functional significance since the driving pressure at the two ends of the channels should be almost equal. However, obstruction to one branch or coronary artery would cause a profound reduction in pressure at that end of the channel which would then carry blood from the patent artery into the peripheral distribution of the occluded artery. Thus, the collateral channels have extremely great importance for the survival of individuals with acute coronary occlusion.

THE VENOUS CIRCULATION

Venous drainage is distinctly different in the two ventricles. The right ventricular veins drain into the anterior cardiac veins which empty individually into the right atrium just above the A-V valves;[6] the venous system from the left ventricle is collected into one single channel, the coronary sinus.[48] The implication of this basic difference has prompted the conduct of metabolic studies in the left ventricle in the animal and in man. The deep muscle layers are drained into the right atrial and ventricular cavities by the Thebesian veins.[6] Direct communications between the small vessels of the coronary circulation and the ventricular chambers have received a great deal of attention in the past. Injection studies of the coronary arteries indicated that some small branches from the terminal arteries penetrate directly through the endocardium (arterioluminal vessels), or join larger channels (arteriosinusoidal vessels) which empty into the right or left ventricular chambers. Thebesian veins pass from the venous end of capillaries or from deep coronary veins, to the endocardial surface. The main coronary venous drainage tends to retrace the course of the coronary arteries, passing toward the atrioventricular groove and terminating in the coronary sinus, which empties into the right atrium through its posterior wall.

CORONARY BLOOD FLOW

Flow in any system is based upon the perfusing pressure and resistance to flow. The perfusing pressure in the coronary system is the difference between the left main coronary artery pressure (same as that in the aorta) and right atrial pressure. Resistance to flow varies indirectly with the fourth power of the mean caliber of the peripheral coronary vessels.

MEASUREMENT OF CORONARY FLOW

The ability to measure coronary flow is an essential prerequisite to an evaluation of function of the coronary circulation. Devices for measuring coronary flow have undergone continuous transformations and improvements during the last decades from crude methods, such as collecting flow from the coronary sinus into a graduated glass tube, to more complex but more precise devices applicable to man. Much of our knowledge of the physiology of coronary circulation has been derived from animal experiments using a variety of flowmeters. These methods have been largely covered in a previous chapter.

Most available data on coronary flow in man have been obtained by indirect methods using the Fick principle (see Figs. 2–21, 2–22). If a substance is taken up by an organ, its rate of uptake is proportional to the organ's blood supply and to its arteriovenous difference. Or, in the case of the heart:

Rate of uptake=
   coronary flow × (A-V) difference, or

$$\text{Coronary flow} = \frac{\text{Rate of Uptake}}{\text{(A-V) difference}}$$

A substance suitable for these determinations must diffuse freely in and out of the myocardium and must not alter myocardial performance or coronary vascular resistance. Any substance which meets these requirements evidently can be used in the determination of flow through the myocardium.

The nitrous oxide method introduced by Kety[49] has furnished us with most available data regarding coronary flow in man. A 15 per cent nitrous oxide mixture is breathed by a subject for a period of seven to ten minutes while multiple simultaneous samples for nitrous oxide analysis are collected from the coronary sinus and any arterial sampling site. As the myocardium

takes up this substance, an arteriovenous difference develops. Clearly, the only limitation to the rate of uptake of nitrous oxide is its degree of saturation in the myocardium. When the cardiac muscle becomes fully saturated, coronary arteriovenous difference reaches equilibrium. At this point the coronary venous tension of nitrous oxide is assumed to be identical to the mean tissue tension of nitrous oxide. Mean coronary flow can, therefore, be calculated from the ratio of nitrous oxide tension in the coronary sinus and the area between the arterial and coronary sinus curves (Fig. 9–7). The expression of this ratio is

Mean Coronary Flow per 100 grams left ventricle = Rate of
   Uptake of Nitrous Oxide
   per 100 grams left ventricle

$$\int_0^T \text{(A-V) dt}$$

It is actually equally valid to determine coronary flow from the desaturation curve obtained after cessation of nitrous oxide breathing. Flow changes which occur within the period of determination cannot be detected with this method. Sources of error include the presence of arteriovenous shunts, pericardial effusions and the assumption that coronary sinus flow in man comes entirely from the left ventricle. Compared with direct flow measurements in the dog, the nitrous oxide method shows considerable differences, extremes varying between plus 21 per cent and minus 21 per cent with an average variation of plus 12.4 per cent. For this reason it was regarded as semiquantitative. Perhaps the nitrous oxide method is most reliable when it is used to compare repeated determinations in the same patient. However, because of limitations in a manual sampling technique, its reproducibility may not prove satisfactory.

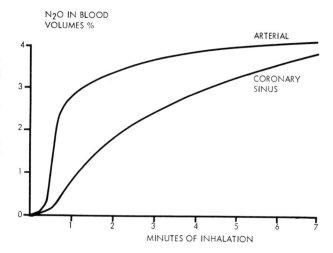

N₂O IN BLOOD VOLUMES %

FIGURE 9–7 DETERMINATION OF CORONARY FLOW IN MAN BY THE NITROUS OXIDE TECHNIQUE

A difference is evident in arterial and coronary sinus nitrous oxide content during inhalation of the gas. This difference serves as a basis for the calculation of coronary flow. (From Case, R. B.: Cardiovascular Disorders. Philadelphia: F. A. Davis & Co., 1968, p. 111.)

MINUTES OF INHALATION

The use of an automated sampling technique[7] will undoubtedly improve the reproducibility of the nitrous oxide method.

As an extension of the Fick principle, several methods employing a variety of indicators (Kr^{85}, Rb^{86}, Rb^{84}, Xe^{133}, NaI^{131}, I^{131}Iodo-antipyrine cold saline) have been developed within the past few years. Some of them have simplified the task of measuring coronary flow, but nearly all require cardiac catherization and measure coronary flow per 100 grams of left ventricle.

Another popular approach depends on the rate of disappearance of a tracer substance; Kr^{85} is injected into the left coronary artery[51] and a scintillation counter detects through the chest wall the rate of disappearance of radioactivity which, in turn, is related to the rate of capillary blood flow. One determination of coronary flow takes two to three minutes. The problem of recirculation of the tracer substance is avoided since Kr^{85} is 95 per cent cleared from the blood during its first passage through the lungs. Compared with direct flowmeter studies in the unanesthetized animal,

the method has proven accurate and reproducible. Its use in conjunction with coronary arteriography provides correlation of flow together with the pathology of vessels. A direct application of this method is the measurement of local coronary flow during surgery by an injection into the myocardium of a solution of Kr^{85} or Xe^{133}.

Using an inert radioactive substance which is not excreted by the lungs, coronary flow was obtained according to the principle of Kety. The substance I^{131}Iodo-antipyrine[52] is infused intravenously and taken up subsequently by the myocardium. Full saturation is reached within two minutes. This method, which requires arterial and coronary sinus sampling, has shown good correlation with the nitrous oxide method. When I^{131}Iodo-antipyrine is used intravenously, precordial monitoring displays a third peak which is thought to be due to coronary flow because it follows the left ventricular peak. The area under the curve is considered to represent coronary flow. However, the presence of radioactivity from noncardiac sites and the fact that noncardiac vessels are included in the area monitored during precordial counting make the validity of this method questionable. Interestingly enough, the third peak which is attributed to coronary flow disappears when the isotope is excluded from the coronary circulation. Data obtained in man with this method do not compare with the nitrous oxide technique.

Another type of coronary flow determination, which does not require cardiac catheterization, uses a peripheral intravenous infusion of Rb[86] and a precordial monitor. Rb[84] is similarly used with coincidence counting.[53] When two monitors are used, the accuracy of recording is increased. However, many assumptions are made and the reliability of this method remains to be demonstrated.

The indicator-dilution principle has found application in the intracoronary injection of cold blood with continuous recording of blood temperature in the coronary sinus. Total coronary flow is obtained and can be determined several times in a minute.

A flowmeter based on the Doppler principle or the alteration in frequency of backscattered sound wave by a moving object has become available recently. Ultrasound reflected from moving particles in the blood (red blood cells) is shifted in frequency by an amount proportional to the velocity of the moving particles (see Fig. 2–20). Most recently a catheter-tip Doppler flowmeter, using a continuous wave meter, has become available for recording phasic arterial flow. Analysis of the frequency spectrum of the reflected signal gives mean flow velocity. It has been recently shown that the backscattered power holds a direct relationship with the number of scatterers (that is, red blood cells). When properly processed, this may yield quantitative indication of volume flow. Catheterization of the coronary artery or coronary sinus may someday provide useful information using this method.

PHYSICAL DETERMINANTS OF CORONARY FLOW

The cyclic pattern of coronary flow is governed by (1) the aortic pressure pulse and (2) the impedance to flow resulting from physical compression of the coronary vessels by myocardial contraction. The instantaneous pattern at any time during systole is determined by the resultant of these two forces. Until recently, coronary flow was believed to cease completely during the early part of systole as a result of extravascular compression. But recent electromagnetic flowmeter studies have indicated that coronary flow in unanesthetized dogs does continue during systole and contributes to about 7 to 45 per cent of total flow (see Fig. 9–8). This wide variation in systolic flow reflects the changes which take place in the vigor of myocardial contraction in the same individual. The perfusing pressure during diastole is most effective in determining coronary flow. At this time coronary vessels released from myocardial compression can open or constrict as needed in order to admit more or less blood flow, depending on the degree of vasoconstriction or dilation at the sites of controlled resistance in the microcirculation. The normal heart does not experience myocardial ischemia during tachycardia even though diastolic time may be significantly shortened.

PHYSIOLOGIC DETERMINANTS OF CORONARY FLOW

The physiologic determinants which drive coronary flow are pre-

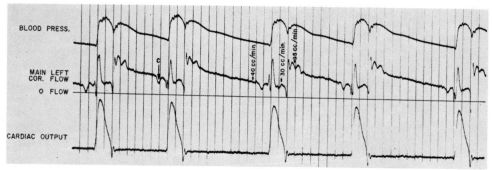

FIGURE 9–8 PHASIC FLOW IN THE MAIN LEFT CORONARY ARTERY

From the Resting Animal: Record showing phasic aortic pressure and phasic flow in the main left coronary artery and ascending aorta obtained by means of a strain gauge and electromagnetic flowmeters. Solid line is true zero. Vertical time lines, 0.1 second. (From Gregg, D. E., Khouri, E. M., and Rayford, C. R.: Systemic and coronary energetics in the resting unanesthetized dog. *Circulat. Res.*, 16:102–113, 1965.)

cisely those which alter myocardial oxygen requirements and consumption. In experimental investigation, coronary flow is shown to increase with greater arterial pressure, heart rate, ventricular wall tension, the maximum rate of pressure generation in the left ventricle, $\left(\dfrac{dp}{dt} \max.\right)$. Similarly it falls when these factors are reduced. This linear relationship can be expressed otherwise as the ratio: $\dfrac{\text{Myocardial Oxygen Supply}}{\text{Myocardial Oxygen Requirements}}$ Measured in the human left ventricle by the nitrous oxide technique[54, 55] coronary flow averages 80 to 100 ml. per 100 grams per minute. But a more pertinent determination would be that of total coronary flow since it can be notably increased in cases of left ventricular hypertrophy while coronary flow per 100 grams of left ventricle remains normal.

REGULATION OF CORONARY FLOW

The primary determinant of coronary flow is believed to be myocardial oxygen tension (pO_2). When more oxygen is consumed than is readily available, myocardial oxygen tension decreases. This is associated with a fall in coronary vascular resistance resulting in prompt increase in coronary flow and restoration of myocardial pO_2 to its previous value. A precise autoregulatory mechanism alters coronary vascular resistance to increase flow by the amount exactly needed, so that coronary sinus pO_2 remains remarkably constant despite wide variations in myocardial oxygen consumption. When coronary perfusion pressure is increased abruptly while myocardial oxygen requirements (see Chapter 4) are maintained constant, flow increases slightly but returns promptly to its control value despite the maintenance of coronary perfusion pressure at the new high level. The reverse happens when coronary perfusion pressure has been lowered. Autoregulation is abolished when coronary perfusion pressure is lowered below 50 mm. Hg or raised above 180 mm. Hg presumably because the coronary tree is maximally dilated or maximally constricted and behaves like a rigid tube. At this time flow bears a linear relationship to pressure. Another way to illustrate

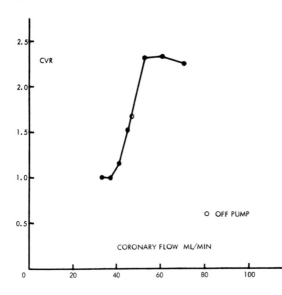

FIGURE 9-9   VASCULAR REACTIVITY IN THE
CORONARY VESSELS

When coronary flow is reduced to the perfused left ventricle with constant oxygen requirements, coronary vascular resistance is seen to fall sharply from its peak values to reach a minimum level representing maximal arteriolar dilatation. The upper plateau of coronary vascular resistance represents maximal arteriolar constriction. Perfusion at normal aortic pressure (open circle) indicates that in normal situations, coronary vascular resistance is maintained midway between maximal constriction and maximal dilatation. The steep slope of the curve at this point demonstrates the sensitivity of response in either direction to an increased or decreased oxygen delivery. (From Case, R. B., and Roven, R. B.: Some considerations of coronary flow. *Prog. Cardiov. Dis.* 6:45–55, 1963.)

vascular reactivity in the coronary circulation is shown in Figure 9–9. When the left main coronary artery is cannulated and perfused from a pump while the heart is working at a constant level of myocardial oxygen consumption, the changes imposed on coronary flow (see Fig. 9–9) induce in the coronary circulation constriction or dilation depending on the direction of change of flow. These changes in coronary vascular resistance are reflected in the recorded coronary perfusion pressure. Such an intervention can be repeated at various levels of myocardial oxygen requirements obtaining a family of curves, each one having a range of coronary vascular resistance, the two extremes being total coronary reserve. Perfusion at aortic pressure (off pump in Fig. 9–9) is near the center of the functional range.

DETERMINANTS OF MYOCARDIAL OXYGEN CONSUMPTION

The ventricular myocardium extracts 75 per cent of the arterial oxygen content. This property of extracting such a high proportion of the arterial oxygen means that a higher coronary flow is the principal means by which this organ can meet an increase in oxygen demand. Myocardial oxygen consumption is directly related to coronary flow, and this relationship is constant in the same individual. Experimental investigation in the animal with controlled aortic pressure, heart rate and cardiac output indicates that myocardial oxygen consumption is not related to the mechanical work of the ventricle but related to the pressure developed by the ventricle and the frequency with which it creates this pressure.[56, 57] The product of the area beneath the ventricular pressure curve and the heart rate, referred to as Tension-Time index, is also linearly related to oxygen consumption. More recently it was found that myocardial oxygen consumption is almost completely determined by the time the ventricular pressure has reached its peak.[58] In other terms, the product of systolic aortic pressure and heart rate could give a reliable indication of myocardial oxygen consumption. When cardiac output is increased by only increasing stroke volume with heart rate being maintained constant, myocardial oxygen consumption is not altered. This experimental situation is, however, rarely encountered clinically since cardiac output is not efficiently increased except through an acceleration in heart rate, so that a rise in cardiac output is usually associated with an increase in myocardial oxygen requirement. But this association must not be viewed as a direct cause and effect relationship. It is tachycardia, which must occur in most cases, which is responsible for the increase in myocardial oxygen consumption.

Myocardial oxygen consumption also is affected by the rate of pressure development in the left ventricle.[59] Drugs which affect left ventricular dp/dt are expected to affect myocardial oxygen requirement beyond that which is expected from pressure and heart rate alone. Another important factor affecting myocardial oxygen requirements is the size of the ventricular chamber, since tension, according to Laplace's law, is directly related to the square of the radius.[60] The actual mass of ventricular muscle bears a direct relationship with coronary flow. During left ventricular hypertrophy and failure, the increase in ventricular size and mass is an important determinant of total myocardial oxygen consumption.

CORONARY FLOW IN THE DISEASED HEART

CORONARY RESERVE

The concept of coronary reserve relates to the maximum ability of the coronary vessels to increase blood flow in response to myocardial oxygen needs (see also Chapter 15). The maximum coronary capacity in the normal individual is a 400 to 500 per cent increase in flow. Coronary reserve represents a truly valid means of assessing the function of the coronary circulation, more so when it is balanced against the efficiency with which the heart utilizes oxygen.

In the chronic hypoxic heart, coronary reserve indicates the extent to which coronary flow is impaired and provides correlation between the clinical course and the functional changes in the coronary circulation.

No methods to determine coronary reserve are currently available. Those using the electrocardiographic changes or the disturbance in lactate metabolism during exercise indicate only the point at which the capacity of coronary circulation is exhausted. Myocardial revascularization procedures and exercise therapy in patients with coronary artery disease will be best assessed if total coronary reserve can be objectively measured.

New techniques to evaluate the function of coronary circulation are obviously needed and will lead to a better and more complete understanding of coronary circulation.

VENTRICULAR HYPERTROPHY

During normal growth and development, the size of the coronary artery grows linearly in relation to the mass of the left ventricle. In all hypertrophied hearts, regardless of the cause of their hypertrophy, this relationship is absent. The cross-sectional area of the coronary artery is smaller than expected when compared to the mass of muscle supplied. Inadequacy of coronary flow has been ascribed to the large diffusion distance of oxygen or to discrepancy between the size of the coronary ostium and the left ventricular mass. There remains a third possibility relating coronary insufficiency to an exhaustion of the ability of the coronary arterioles to dilate (see also Chapter 15).

There is actually little experimental evidence to substantiate the presence of coronary insufficiency in ventricular hypertrophy. Angina does occur in aortic stenosis and insufficiency, but in both conditions perfusion pressure is inadequate. Hypertension is also associated with angina, but the coronary arteries are involved with atheromatous deposits. Right ventricular hypertrophy is rarely associated with angina, a condition in which neither the perfusion pressure nor the coronary vessels are disturbed.

CARDIAC FAILURE

Coronary flow and myocardial oxygen consumption per 100 grams of left ventricle are normal in the patient with cardiac failure.[60, 61, 62] This value indicates the state of adequacy of coronary flow but gives no indication of the degree of ventricular hypertrophy for which total coronary flow must be known. Total oxygen consumption of the failing left ventricle may increase markedly depending on the mass of ventricular muscle and, interestingly, may account completely for the increase in metabolic rate observed in patients with heart failure. In seven patients who died of chronic heart failure, total myocardial oxygen consumption was found to average 42 ml. per minute,[60] a value which represents a 350 per cent increase when compared to the normal of 12 ml. per minute.

The ratio of oxygen consumption per unit of mass to pressure developed is greatly increased in the failing left ventricle. This inefficiency is further enhanced when the heart is acutely stressed as in exercise, hypoxia, post-atropine tachycardia or in disease states such as hyperthyroidism. Cardiac output is slightly increased in response to exercise. In fact, mechanical efficiency can be reduced to the extent that patients with cardiac failure are incapable of the slightest exertion and are literally bedridden.

The normal heart responds to exercise by increasing its output as needed. But beyond this increase in mechanical efficiency of the normal heart during exercise, more significant in so far as true myocardial efficiency is concerned, is the decrease in the ratio of oxygen consumption per unit mass to pressure developed.

The left ventricular end-diastolic pressure is basic in the alteration of myocardial efficiency in response to exercise. In the failing heart, the rise in the left ventricular end-diastolic pressure which occurs during exercise reflects a larger left ventricle which results in a greater tension and a greater oxygen consumption, whereas the normal left ventricle becomes smaller during exercise, thus developing pressure at a lower oxygen consumption per unit mass. Oxygen extraction is normal in patients with heart failure and normal coronary circulation, and it remains constant during exercise.[63] Patients who are in failure and do have impaired coronary circulation increase their myocardial extraction and produce lactate during exercise.

AORTIC VALVE DISEASE

The striking feature in aortic valve disease is the presence of coronary insufficiency without pathological involvement of the coronary artery.

AORTIC STENOSIS

It is well known that angina and sudden death occur in patients with severe aortic stenosis despite normal coronary vessels. In this disorder the left ventricle must rely for its oxygen supply on essentially arteriolar dilatation. Resistance to flow during systole is especially severe because of the high intraventricular pressures which are developed by a left ventricle contracting against a stenotic orifice. A normal heart is at an advantage because a high intraventricular pressure which requires more oxygen consumption is accompanied by a high systolic aortic pressure and similar coronary perfusion pressure. In aortic stenosis, systolic aortic pressure is always lower than systolic intraventricular pressure and the heart is left with arteriolar dilatation as the only means for a larger oxygen supply.

AORTIC INSUFFICIENCY

It is well known that angina occurs in luetic aortic insufficiency with narrowing of the coronary ostia. A large percentage of patients with severe rheumatic aortic insufficiency have classical angina, yet they display normal coronary vessels.[64] An incidence of sudden death was observed in 10 per cent of these patients, suggesting a rather advanced state of coronary insufficiency. A large spectrum of physiologic aberrations ranging from an abnormal increase in myocardial oxygen requirement to a compromised coronary perfusion pressure is present in aortic insufficiency.

The dilated left ventricle which usually accompanies this disorder results in a larger tension and a greater oxygen consumption. The left ventricle must continuously eject a larger stroke volume; this larger stroke volume is useless since part of it is bound to regurgitate into the left ventricular cavity. It is to be pointed out that this rise in stroke volume does not affect in itself myocardial oxygen requirements, but it is the higher systolic pressure which accompanies it which is directly related to myocardial oxygen consumption. In a series of 100 patients suffering from severe aortic insufficiency,[64] systolic aortic pressure averaged 155 mm. Hg. Diastolic pressure is of paramount importance in determining coronary perfusion during diastole. In these patients it was found to average only 37 mm. Hg.[64] This situation in which a high myocardial oxygen requirement and low coronary perfusion pressure occur simultaneously is ideal for the development of angina.

HYPERTENSION

Coronary flow and myocardial oxygen consumption per 100 grams of left ventricle are normal in the hypertensive patient,[61, 65] but total flow and oxygen consumption are increased owing to the intraventricular pressures generated and to ventricular hypertrophy.

MITRAL STENOSIS, RIGHT VENTRICULAR HYPERTROPHY AND PULMONARY STENOSIS

Angina is rare in mitral stenosis, occurring in only 8.5 per cent in a series of 400 patients.[66] Sixty-two per cent of those patients who exhibited classical anginal symptoms were under 37 years of age. The coronary vessels were found normal at autopsy in a number of patients.

In the normal heart, the contraction of the right ventricle does not have the same obstructive effect on right coronary flow as does the left ventricle on left coronary flow. Right coronary flow persists throughout systole in the normal heart, but when the right ventricle is subjected to a chronic pressure load, it hypertrophies and assumes a shape similar to that of the left ventricle. Total oxygen consumption of the right ventricle must then be increased as a result of the high pressure generated. It is a situation somewhat similar to the left ventricle in systemic hypertension insofar as coronary circulation is concerned. The reports on oxygen consumption and coronary flow to the left ventricle in mitral stenosis are contradictory. They have been found to be reduced[67] or normal.[55] In the situation where they were reduced,[67] arterial pressure and heart rate were also reduced but not enough to account for the reduction in oxygen consumption. In those patients cardiac output was lower than normal. The discrepancy between oxygen consumption and that which would be accounted for by arterial pressure and heart rate must be viewed in terms of a reduction of the left ventricular end-diastolic volume resulting in a lower tension and a lower oxygen consumption.

Coronary circulation to the right ventricle is further compromised in the patient with severe pulmonary stenosis because of the low right coronary perfusion pressure during systole in addition to the chronic pressure load imposed on the right ventricle by a stenosed pulmonary valve orifice.

HYPERTHYROIDISM

Hyperthyroidism is usually associated with manifestations of increased metabolic rate such as tachycardia, increased output and increased pulse pressure. Myocardial oxygen consumption was increased by 33 per cent and 37 per cent in various reports.[68, 69]

Heart rate was increased by 30 per cent and systolic arterial pressure by 7 per cent. This increase in coronary flow evidently is the result of the hemodynamic changes accompanying hyperthyroidism. The nonfailing hyperthyroid heart appears to behave like the heart in acute stress as in exercise.

CORONARY ARTERY DISEASE

The principal cause of restricted coronary flow results directly or indirectly from atherosclerosis. Although its cause has not yet been determined, atherosclerosis is no longer considered a degenerative process to be expected with advancing age. It is now regarded as a metabolic disturbance of lipid metabolism, for which specific therapy may be ultimately developed. This change in attitude is a most important development for future progress.

THE NATURE OF CORONARY ATHEROMATA

Atherosclerosis occurs with greatest frequency in the aorta and in the cerebral and coronary arteries. In Figure 9–10, the pathogenesis of atherosclerotic lesions in the coronary arteries is illustrated schematically in accordance with the sequence of events described by Moon and Rinehart.[70] In early lesions the intima is diffusely thickened by accumulated mucoid ground substance and a proliferation of subendothelial fibroblasts. The internal elastic membrane is fragmented by focal areas of degeneration. Accumulation of lipids is not always demonstrable in early lesions, and its localization—in the intima, in the media or in both—is somewhat unpredictable.

When coronary atherosclerosis is well developed, the intima is thickened by fibrous proliferation, the advancing borders of the plaques being composed of loosely arranged fibroblasts and mucoid ground substance

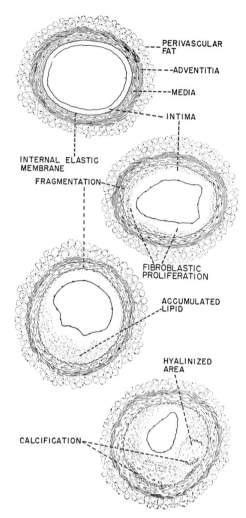

FIGURE 9-10 PATHOGENESIS OF CORONARY
ATHEROSCLEROSIS

In the normal coronary artery, the intima is uniformly thin and composed of collagenous connective tissue. The early stages of coronary atherosclerosis are characterized by fragmentation of the internal elastic membrane and thickening of the intima due to fibroblastic proliferation associated with accumulation of mucopolysaccharide. In the early phases of the process, accumulation of lipid may or may not be demonstrable. As the intima becomes thickened, lipids (e.g., cholesterol) tend to accumulate at the junction of the intima with the media. Finally, areas of the atherosclerotic plaque degenerate and become hyalinized. Calcium is deposited predominantly at the edges of hyaline areas and at the junction of intima and media. The lumen of the vessel is greatly restricted, and may even become completely occluded, by progressive expansion of the atheroma.

(mucopolysaccharide) resembling the early lesions. Lipid accumulates as fine and coarse droplets, principally at the base or center of the plaque and least along the endothelial border. The intimal plaques often encroach upon the media.

Advanced stages of atherosclerosis are characterized by hyaline degeneration at the base or center of the plaques where the concentration of lipid is greatest. Calcification usually begins at the junction of the intima and media, or in the hyalinized areas. The elastic tissue suffers extreme degeneration and fragmentation. Infiltration of the adventitia with lymphocytes is frequently observed. The histologic appearance of atherosclerotic lesions is illustrated by the photomicrographs in Figure 9-11.

INCIDENCE OF CORONARY ATHEROSCLEROSIS

The initial stages of coronary atherosclerosis are observed in nearly all adults. If rigid criteria are used, only very young children are completely free of any stigmata. The incidence and severity of atherosclerotic lesions in the coronary arteries increases with age. White, Edwards and Dry[71] tabulated the degree of coronary atherosclerosis observed during 100 consecutive autopsies on men whose ages were distributed through the six decades between 30 and 89 years. Some results of this study are summarized in Figure 9-12. The average severity of the lesions increased very rapidly from age 30 through 49 years. The lesions in the right main coronary artery and in the two main branches of the left coronary artery (anterior descending and circumflex) were comparable. On the average, the plaques were less extensive in the smaller branches of the

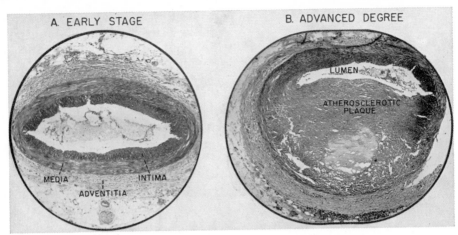

FIGURE 9–11   HISTOLOGY OF CORONARY ATHEROSCLEROSIS

Two photomicrographs of a main coronary artery (on the right) and a small branch of the same vessel (on the left) illustrate the histologic appearance of early and advanced coronary atherosclerosis.

A, The intima is irregularly thickened to a very slight degree. Slight fragmentation of the internal elastic media is present but not effectively reproduced in this photomicrograph. In other respects the vessel is normal.

B, The lumen of this large coronary artery is greatly reduced by a large atherosclerotic plaque. Fusiform vacuoles in the intima remain where lipids were dissolved away. The intima is grossly thickened by processes illustrated in Figure 9–10. A hyalinized area appears in the basilar portion of the plaque. Lymphocytes have infiltrated a region around the periphery of the adventitia at the bottom of the photomicrograph.

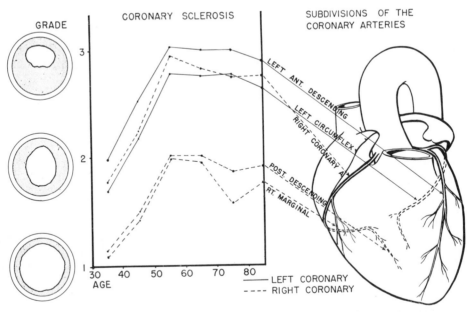

FIGURE 9–12   DEVELOPMENT AND DISTRIBUTION OF CORONARY ATHEROSCLEROSIS

The most severe atherosclerotic lesions in each subdivision of the coronary arteries were determined in 100 consecutive postmortem examinations on men in each decade from 30 through 89 years. The average grade of the most severe lesion was plotted for each decade of life in each segment of the arterial tree. Similar degrees of atherosclerotic changes were noted in the right main coronary artery and in the anterior descending and circumflex branches of the left coronary artery. Smaller branches of the right coronary artery had less severe lesions. (After White, Edwards and Dry.[71])

right coronary artery (posterior descending and right marginal). This study indicates that the severity of atherosclerotic lesions tends to remain fairly constant after the fifth decade. About 70 per cent of the men who had passed their fifth decade had sclerosis of grade 3 or more somewhere in the distribution of the coronary arterial system.

FUNCTIONAL EFFECTS OF CORONARY OBSTRUCTION

Expanding atheromatous plaques seriously restrict the lumen of the coronary arteries (Figs. 9-10 and 9-11). The diminished lumen increases the resistance to the flow of blood past the site of atherosclerotic lesions. Thus, the pressure drop along the vessel is greater than normal and the perfusion pressure in the distal branches is diminished. Since the pressure gradient is very shallow in large arteries, their lumens can be considerably diminished without a significant reduction in the pressure head beyond the obstruction. In small arteries, the same reduction in the lumen produces a much greater pressure drop. Coronary atherosclerosis is usually not an isolated lesion but a number of lesions scattered throughout the coronary arterial tree. Some of the arterial pressure head is lost as the blood passes each obstruction. Vadodilatation of the small coronary vessels helps compensate for increased resistance upstream. However, the compensatory dilatation of the coronary bed is limited, so that encroachment on the lumen of an artery beyond some critical degree will produce progressive diminution in blood flow.

Atherosclerosis develops gradually and may completely occlude a large branch of a coronary artery without causing destruction of the myocardium because collateral channels from adjacent branches expand and carry additional blood to maintain the viability and function of the affected area. Widespread coronary atherosclerosis is occasionally observed in postmortem examination of patients who had no previous disability attributable to insufficient blood flow to the heart. Experimental coronary occlusion has clearly indicated the importance of the rate at which obstruction develops.

Experimental Coronary Obstruction. The functional effects of acute coronary occlusion have been investigated in unanesthetized dogs fully recovered from implantation of recording devices of the sort described in Chapter 3. Little effect was noted following acute occlusion of one major coronary artery (i.e., anterior descending or circumflex) by means of an externally activated snare. By ligating the anterior descending branch at the time of surgery and occluding the circumflex artery one or two weeks later, profound effects in left ventricular function developed within 20 beats.[72] By injecting Isuprel before and after the experimental coronary occlusion, it was possible to demonstrate that the ventricular response to this stress was both smaller and shorter than during the control period. This suggests that the coronary reserve had been significantly depleted.

The changes produced by coronary occlusion were characterized by tachycardia, more gradual outflow acceleration to a lower peak, slightly reduced ventricular systolic pressure with more gradual upslope and downslope and increased ventricular filling pressure (Fig. 9-13).

From such observations stemmed the concept that the ventricles act like impulse generators, imparting energy very rapidly to the flowing blood more like a mallet striking a piston than like

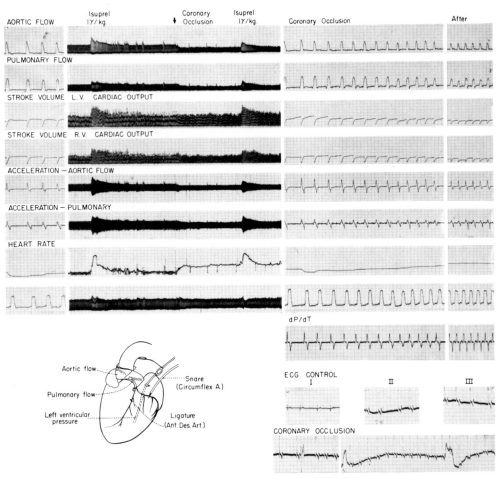

FIGURE 9-13   ACUTE OCCLUSION OF THE CIRCUMFLEX CORONARY ARTERY

Acute occlusion of the circumflex coronary artery (anterior descending artery previously ligated) produced prompt reduction in pulmonary artery and aortic flow velocity and acceleration of flow. The center panel shows the right and left ventricular outputs, obtained by integrating aortic and pulmonary flow over 2.5-second intervals. Reduced stroke volume was offset by sustained tachycardia, maintaining cardiac output. Changes in left ventricular ejection patterns are illustrated by records on the right (paper speed 25 mm./sec.). (From Rushmer, R. *et al. Amer. Heart J.* 66:530, 1963.)

a hand squeezing an orange. The initial acceleration of blood out of the ventricle during each contraction appeared to be the most sensitive and significant feature of the ventricular function when depressed by coronary occlusion and by other experimental procedures known to reduce the dynamic performance of the heart.[73]

If a major branch of the coronary arteries in a dog is gradually occluded over a period of weeks or months, neither histologic evidence of myocardial damage nor reduced ventricular performance may be demonstrable.[74] Progressive occlusion of two main coronary branches may also be well tolerated. Dogs which survived this procedure ran at 3 m.p.h. on a grade of 25 degrees for 30 minutes without difficulty. One animal survived successive ligation of all three major branches of the coronary arteries. The septal and conus arteries must have been the principal remaining source of blood to the ventricles. A similar degree of coronary obstruction has been seen in man.[75] In about half of human hearts, an artery arises from a separate ostium near the right coronary artery to supply the pulmonary conus.[75] This artery may provide substantial collateral flow when the other vessels are more seriously afflicted with atherosclerosis.

Even moderate degrees of atherosclerosis presumably limit the cardiac reserve. Since coronary venous blood contains very little oxygen, a reduction in the arteriovenous oxygen difference would do little to remedy the deficiency (see Chapter 15). Complete occlusion of one or more major branches of the coronary arteries must diminish the total coronary reserve even though collateral channels dilate to serve myocardium deprived of its blood supply. Since atherosclerotic plaques are usually not restricted to one or two coronary branches (Fig. 9–12), collateral channels generally connect vascular networks with varying degrees of sclerosis.[76] In view of the fact that atheromata usually appear in several coronary trunks, the degree of coronary sclerosis which can develop without seriously limiting the exercise tolerance is almost unbelievable.[75, 76] The disparity between the extensive pathologic involvement of the coronary arteries and the limited degree of functional disability is difficult to explain. However, such discrepancies between organic disease of the heart and its powers of compensation are not only commonplace, but a constant source of difficulty in predicting the course of cardiovascular disease.

ANGINA PECTORIS

The most common symptom of impaired coronary flow is precordial pain. Patients with coronary atherosclerosis may develop a syndrome consisting of a fairly specific, constricting type of pain, which seems to originate behind the sternum and frequently radiates over the left precordium and along the inner surface of the left arm. The term "angina pectoris" is applied to this particular type of pain. It characteristically occurs in paroxysms of relatively brief duration, brought on most commonly by exertion or any other activity which increases the cardiac output. Walking rapidly uphill against a cold wind is perhaps the most frequently cited set of circumstances precipitating an attack. The discomfort is often accompanied by a sensation of impending doom, causing the patient to stop in his tracks until the pain recedes.

ETIOLOGY OF ANGINA PECTORIS

Myocardial ischemia is the logical precipitating cause of angina pectoris. Anginal pain is usually compared to the pain produced by exercising the muscles of the forearm when their blood supply is cut off by an inflated cuff. Acid metabolites tend to accumulate in contracting muscles receiving too little oxygen, and these substances may stimulate pain endings directly or through changes in pH.

Inadequate blood flow through the coronary arteries is the principal underlying feature of the disease and may result from (a) increased resistance to coronary flow, (b) reduced perfusion pressure, (c) increased oxygen requirements of the myocardium or (d) a combination of these factors. Increased resistance to coronary blood flow stems from coronary atherosclerosis, coronary spasm or both. Coronary spasm is generally assigned an important role in angina pectoris because of its brief duration, and because of the facts that strong emotions may precipitate an attack, the pain disappears with rest, and clinical signs may be absent between attacks. The relief of pain after administration of nitroglycerin also indicates that coronary spasm existed during the attack.

In general, angina pectoris can be produced by any set of conditions which simultaneously impose a load on the heart and impede coronary blood flow. However, the picture is not as clear as this statement implies. Many patients have severe angina, apparently without sufficient changes in coronary vessels, and others have no angina even after attacks of acute coronary occlusion. Furthermore, not all patients have the typical retrosternal pain with radiation to the left arm. The pain may be referred to different regions over the precordium or back and to more distant sites. These deviations from the typical response must be related to the perception and radiation of pain from the heart.

CHARACTERISTICS OF VISCERAL PAIN FROM THE HEART

The pain of angina pectoris is described variously as a constriction, a burning sensation, a fullness or tightness in the chest, a choking sensation or an uncomfortable aching discomfort. Most commonly, the pain seems to be centered just behind the mid-portion of the sternum, radiating predominantly to the left precordium but occasionally extending to the epigastrium, the root of the neck, the jaw, the shoulder, the back and down the arms

(usually the left). In contrast with somatic sensations of touch or pain evoked from the skin, visceral sensation is characteristically poorly localized. Somatic pain in many regions of the body is recognized as coming from a very discrete area; this can be easily demonstrated by pricking the finger or tongue with a pin. Conversely, pain produced by a needle thrust through the skin into skeletal muscles or into a blood vessel may produce a diffuse, deep, aching sensation which involves a large area, even an entire arm or leg. Inaccurate localization and diffuse distribution of pain from viscera are the basis for the radiation of pain in angina pectoris.

Radiation of anginal pain may raise problems in the differential diagnosis of coronary atherosclerosis and diseases in other viscera such as the gallbladder. In patients with cholecystitis or peptic ulcer, angina may be ameliorated by eliminating the source of irritation in the gallbladder or the stomach, but it rarely disappears. Since most attacks of angina pectoris are transient, differentiation between this condition and chronic cholecystitis or peptic ulcer should not be difficult. It is important to keep in mind the fact that pain in these distant regions may be associated with disease of the coronary arteries.

Even relatively slight intensities of visceral pain are peculiarly distressing and intolerable. Not only is the pain subjectively disagreeable, but stimulation of visceral afferents is prone to elicit powerful autonomic reflex activity often resulting in profuse sweating, epigastric uneasiness, bradycardia, hypotension and syncope.

A diagnosis of angina pectoris is not complete until the other sources of precordial pain are excluded and the etiology of myocardial ischemia has been determined as accurately as possible. Bean[77] listed more than one hundred different conditions which had been improperly diagnosed as angina pectoris or coronary occlusion. If the angina results from coronary atherosclerosis, acute massive myocardial infarction with sudden death could conceivably occur at any time.

MYOCARDIAL INFARCTION

ACUTE CORONARY OCCLUSION

Coronary arteries are most frequently occluded abruptly by thrombi formed in the lumen of the vessel. Roughening of the endothelial surface over atheromatous plaques and encroachment on the arterial lumen produce eddy currents beyond the obstruction and contribute to thrombus formation. Fragments of atheromatous plaques may break off and lodge at some point farther on. Inflammatory process in the arterial wall theoretically might play a role in some cases. In recent years formation of hematomas within atheromatous plaques has received considerable attention. Sudden expansion of the hematoma may occlude the arterial lumen without rupture of the intimal lining. Differentiating between such a condition and a mural thrombus at postmortem examination is difficult, but the evidence for intramural hemorrhage is becoming more convincing. Embolic obstruction of coronary arteries has been reported but is a rare phenomenon.

DIAGNOSIS OF MYOCARDIAL INFARCTION

Any particular patient with acute myocardial infarction may present either no definitive symptoms or, more frequently, a combination of a great many complaints. The incidence of various symptoms in a group of cases studied by Bean[78] is indicated in Table 9–2. These signs and symptoms can be arranged in a functional grouping which provides a rational approach to responses of different patients (Table 9–3).

Pain with Myocardial Infarction. The origin of pain in myocardial infarction is presumably the same as that in angina pectoris. Pain from infarction is usually more severe and persists for longer periods of time, being unre-

Table 9–2.   INCIDENCE OF SIGNS AND SYMPTOMS OF MYOCARDIAL INFARCTION*

	FIRST ATTACK PER CENT	SECOND ATTACK PER CENT
1. Dyspnea	95	96
2. Enlarged heart	83	85
3. Weak heart sounds	85	82
4. Rales	83	82
5. Cyanosis	77	86
6. Cough	70	84
7. Pallor	69	79
8. Pain	75	66
9. Orthopnea	68	63
10. Sweating	60	60
11. Vomiting	59	59
12. Ankle edema	55	54
13. "Shock"	57	45
14. Restlessness	44	49
15. Tachycardia (rate over 100)	42	39
16. Systolic murmur	38	71
17. Cheyne-Stokes respiration	24	42
18. Ascites	26	33
19. Cloudy sensorium	26	23
20. Enlarged liver	18	27
21. Gallop rhythm	12	4
22. Prodromal phenomena	21	15
23. Bradycardia (rate below 80)	16	20
24. Angor animi	12	11
25. Pericardial friction rub	15	14
26. Pulsus alternans	9	8
27. Precordial hyperesthesia	8	10

*From Bean, W. B.: Infarction of the heart. II. Symptomatology of acute attack. *Ann. Intern. Med.*, 11:2086–2108, 1938.

Table 9–3. *FUNCTIONAL GROUP-
ING OF SIGNS AND SYMPTOMS OF
MYOCARDIAL INFARCTION*

I. Pain
II. Autonomic Effects
   A. Pallor   E. Syncope
   B. Sweating   F. Tachycardia
   C. Vomiting   G. Shock
   D. Bradycardia H. Disturbed Sensorium
III. Diminished Myocardial Contractility
   A. Congestive Heart Failure
     1. Left ventricular 2. Right ventricular
       failure   failure
      a. Dyspnea   a. Peripheral
                   congestion
      b. Orthopnea b. Enlarged liver
      c. Cough   c. Edema
                   d. Cyanosis
   B. Cardiac Signs
     1. Weak heart tones 6. Paradoxical
     2. Gallop rhythm   pulsation
     3. Systolic murmur 7. Pericardial
     4. Pulsus alternans   friction rub
     5. Ventricular   8. ECG alterations
       enlargement

In some patients, acute myocardial infarction may not be accompanied by any pain, but there is disagreement on how often this occurs. Bean[78] reported 28 per cent of attacks without pain while Kennedy[79] found only 4 per cent. In reviewing the literature, Pollard and Harvill[80] found the reported incidence of painless myocardial infarction to vary from 61 per cent to 4 per cent. The actual incidence probably lies somewhere between these figures, but no value can be stated with confidence. When myocardial infarction occurs without pain, some combination of the other possible symptoms and signs can generally be discovered (Table 9–3). These "substitution symptoms" are particularly important in the absence of the typical precordial pain.

lieved by cessation of physical exertion. Indeed, many attacks occur when the patient is at rest or even asleep. A wide variety of descriptive words is used by different patients to indicate the type of pain they experienced (Table 9–4). In general, these terms are the same as those used to describe anginal pain, to which about half of the patients have been subject prior to their first attack of acute myocardial infarction.

Table 9–4. *TYPES OF PAIN IN
MYOCARDIAL INFARCTION**

	PER CENT
Crushing pressure	44
Squeezing, constricting, vise-like	29
Choking, smothering, suffocating	18
Sharp, stabbing, knife-like	11
Sore, aching, dull	11
"Excruciating"	7
Burning	5

*From Bean, W. B.: Infarction of the heart. II. Symptomatology of acute attack. *Ann. Intern. Med.*, 11:2086–2108, 1938.

SUMMARY

Myocardial ischemia occurs whenever the coronary blood flow is insufficient in relation to the oxygen requirements of the myocardium. Many types of cardiac disease simultaneously increase the requirements for myocardial energy release and interfere with delivery of oxygen to the myocardium. For this reason, myocardial ischemia can be an important limitation on the cardiac reserve in virtually all types of heart disease.

Direct interference with the coronary blood flow most commonly results from coronary atherosclerosis, which develops to a significant degree in more than 70 per cent of men over 50 years of age. Moderate coronary sclerosis can be compensated for by peripheral vasodilation in the terminal coronary arterial tree and by expansion of collateral vessels. Progressively increasing coronary obstruction usually affects several branches of the coronary tree, and the coronary flow reserve is depleted. Characteristic pain in the precordium (angina pectoris), often radiating to other regions, occurs during exertion in some patients with coronary atherosclerosis and disappears quite promptly with rest. Spasm of the coronary vessels is probably important in the production of this type of precordial pain.

Gradual occlusion of coronary vessels provides time for collateral circulation to develop, and destruction of myocardial tissue is thereby avoided. However, a sudden occlusion of a coronary artery produces both dysfunction and death of myocardium deprived of its blood supply. A surprisingly large proportion of hearts showing infarction at postmortem examination have no obvious signs of recent coronary occlusion. The principal signs and symptoms of myocardial infarction can be considered in terms of (*a*) intense radiating precordial pain, (*b*) severe autonomic responses, (*c*) heart failure from diminished ventricular contractility, (*d*) changes in heart sounds and blood pressure, (*e*) roentgenographic findings and (*f*) electrocardiographic signs. Although interpretation of the electrocardiographic signs of myocardial infarction is somewhat empirical, serial records coupled with careful clinical studies usually indicate the diagnosis. Since the electrocardiographic changes are rather nonspecific, a number of other conditions can produce similar patterns (e.g., ventricular strain patterns). For this reason, the diagnosis must depend upon sound judgment applied to the total clinical picture.

REFERENCES

1. Ui, M. A role of phosphofructokinase in pH dependent regulation of glycolysis. *Biochim. Biophys. Acta*, 124:310–322, 1966.
2. Ziegler, D. M., Green, D. E., and Doeg, K. A. Studies on the electron transfer system. XXV. The isolation and properties of a lipoflavoprotein with diaphorase activity from beef heart mitochrondria. *J. Biol. Chem.*, 234:1916–1921, 1959.
3. DeBernard, B. Studies on the terminal electron transport system. V. Extraction of a soluble DPNH cytochrome C reductase from the electron transport particle. *Biochim. Biophys. Acta*, 23:510–515, 1957.
4. Hatefi, Y., Lester, R. L., Crane, F. L., and Widmer, C. Studies on the electron transport system. XVI. Enzymic oxido-reduction reactions of coenzyme Q. *Biochim. Biophys. Acta*, 31:490–501, 1959.
5. Rayford, C. R., Khouri, E. M., Lewis, F. B., and Gregg, D. E. Evaluation of use of left coronary artery inflow and oxygen content of coronary sinus blood as a measure of left ventricular metabolism. *J. Appl. Physiol.*, 14:817–822, 1959.
6. Gregg, D. E. The coronary circulation in health and disease. Philadelphia, Lea & Febiger, 1950.
7. Nasser, M. G., Wachter, M., and Case, R. B. A continuous automated sampling technique. *J. Appl. Physiol.*, 26:501–503, 1969.
8. Morgan, H. E., Randle, P. J., and Regen, D. M. Regulation of glucose uptake by muscle. 3. The effects of insulin, anoxia, salicylate and 2:4-dinitrophenol on membrane transport and intracellular phosphorylation of glucose in the isolated rat heart. *Biochem. J.*, 73:573–579, 1959.
9. Morgan, H. E., Henderson, M. J., Regen, D. M., and Park, C. R. Regulation of glucose uptake in muscle. 1. The effects of insulin and anoxia on glucose transport and phosphorylation in the isolated, perfused heart of normal rats. *J. Biol. Chem.*, 236:253–261, 1961.
10. Stadie, W. C. Current concepts of the action of insulin. *Physiol. Rev.*, 34:52–100, 1954.
11. Feller, D. D., Chaikoff, I. L., Strisower, E. H., and Searle, G. L. Glucose utilization in the diabetic dog, studied with C-14 glucose. *J. Biol. Chem.*, 188:865–880, 1951.
12. Bing, R. J., Siegel, A., Vitale, A., Balboni, F., Sparks, E., Taeschler, M., Klapper, M., and Edwards, S. Metabolic studies on the human heart in vivo. 1. Studies on carbohydrate metabolism of the human heart. *Amer. J. Med.*, 15:284–296, 1953.
13. Bing, R. J., Siegel, A., Ungar, I., and Gilbert, M. Metabolism of the human heart. II. Studies on fat, ketone and amino acid metabolism. *Amer. J. Med.*, 16:504–515, 1954.
14. Schoenheimer, R. The dynamic state of body constituents. Cambridge, Mass., Harvard University Press, 1942.

15. BALLARD, F. B., DANFORTH, W. H., NAE-
GLE, S., and BING, R. J. Myocardial metabolism of fatty acids. *J. Clin. Invest.*, 39:
717–725, 1960.

16. UNGAR, I., GILBERT, M., SIEGEL, A., BLAIN,
J. M., and BING, R. J. Studies on myocardial metabolism. IV. Myocardial metabolism in diabetes. *Amer. J. Med.*, 18:385–
396, 1955.

17. BING, R. J., SIEGEL, A., VITALE, A., BAL-
BONI, F., SPARKS, E., TAESCHLER, M.,
KLAPPER, M., and EDWARDS, S. Metabolic studies on the human heart in vivo.
I. Studies on carbohydrate metabolism of
the human heart. *Amer. J. Med.*, 15:284–
296, 1953.

18. BURDETTE, W. J., and ASHFORD, T. P. Structural changes in the human myocardium
following hypoxia. *J. Thorac. Cardiov.
Surg.*, 50:210–216, 1965.

19. COPELAND, J., KOSEK, J. C., and HURLEY,
E. J. Early functional and ultrastructural
recovery of canine cadaver hearts. *Circulation*, 37, Suppl. II:188–200, 1968.

20. BRACHFELD, N., and SCHEUER, J. Metabolism of glucose by the ischemic dog heart.
Amer. J. Physiol., 212:603–606, 1967.

21. DANFORTH, W. H., NAEGLE, S., and BING,
R. J. Effect of ischemia and reoxygenation
on glycolytic reactions and adenosine triphosphate in heart muscle. *Circulat. Res.*,
8:965–971, 1960.

22. GREEN, D. E., and GOLDBERGER, R. F. Pathways of metabolism in heart muscle.
Amer. J. Med., 30:666–678, 1961.

23. SHEA, T. M., WATSON, R. M., PROTROWSKI,
S. F., DERMKSIAN, G., and CASE R. B.
Anaerobic myocardial metabolism. *Amer.
J. Physiol.*, 203:463–469, 1962.

24. HUCKABEE, W. E. Relationship of pyruvate
and lactate during anaerobic metabolism.
V. Coronary adequacy. *Amer. J. Physiol.*,
200:1169–1176, 1961.

25. PARKER, J. O., CHIONG, M. A., WEST, R. O.,
and CASE, R. B. Sequential alterations in
myocardial lactate metabolism, S-T segments, and left ventricular function during
angina induced by atrial pacing. *Circulation*, 40:113–131, 1969.

26. MUELLER, H., GREGORY, J., AYRES, S.,
GIANNELLI, S., CONKLIN, E., and GRACE,
W. Myocardial metabolic adaptations to
coronary (CS) and noncoronary (NCS)
cardiogenic shock. *Circulation*, 38, Suppl.
VI:143, 1968.

27. COHEN, L. S., ELLIOTT, W. C., KLEIN, M.
D., and GORLIN, R. Coronary heart disease: clinical, cinearteriographic and
metabolic correlations. *Amer. J. Cardiol.*,
17:153–168, 1966.

28. CASE, R. B., NASSER, M. G., and CRAMPTON,
R. S. Biochemical aspects of early myocardial ischemia. *Amer. J. Cardiol.*,
24:766–775, 1969.

29. NASSER, M. G., and CASE, R. B. Early

30. GRIGGS, D. M., JR., NAGANO, S., LIPANA,
J. G., and NOVACK, P. Myocardial lactate
oxidation *in situ* and the effect thereon of
reduced coronary flow. *Amer. J. Physiol.*,
211:335–340, 1966.

31. LEUNISSEN, R. L. A., PIATNEK-LEUNISSEN,
D. A., NAKAMURA, Y., GRIGGS, D. M., JR.
Regional metabolism of the heart during
reduced coronary flow. *Circulation*, 34,
Suppl III:155–156, 1966.

32. GARRAHAN, P. J., and GLYNN, I. M. Uncoup-
ling the sodium pump. *Nature*, 207:1098–
1099, 1965.

33. WOODBURY, J. W. P. 237 in: *Handbook of
Physiology, Section II: Circulation, Vol. 1.*
Baltimore: Williams and Wilkins, 1962.

34. GERLINGS, E. D., MILLER, D. T., and GIL-
MORE, J. P. Oxygen availability: A deter-
minant of myocardial potassium balance.
Amer. J. Physiol., 216:559–562, 1969.

35. CASE, R. B., ROSELLE, H. A., and CRAMP-
TON, R. S. Relation of S-T depression to
metabolic and hemodynamic events.
Cardiologia, 48:32–41, 1966.

36. NASSER, M. G., McCORD, C. W., CATER, P.,
HUTCHINSON, J., and CASE, R. B. Myocardial metabolic studies in the revived
canine cadaver heart. *Circulation*, 38,
Suppl. VI:147, 1968.

37. VIEUSSENS, R. Nouvelles découvertes sur le
coeur. Paris, 1706.

38. JAMES, T. N., and BURCH, G. E. The atrial
coronary arteries in man. *Circulation*, 17:
90–94, 1958.

39. JAMES, T. N., and BURCH, G. E. Blood supply of the human interventricular septum.
Circulation, 17:391–396, 1958.

40. JAMES, T. N. The arteries of the free ventricular walls in man. *Anat. Rec.*, 136:371–
384, 1960.

41. WAGNER, A., and POINDEXTER, C. A. Demonstration of the coronary arteries with
nylon. *Amer. Heart J.*, 37:258–266, 1949.

42. BAROLDI, G., and SCOMAZZONI, G. Coronary circulation in the normal and pathologic heart. Office of the Surgeon General, Dept. of the Army, Washington, D.C.,
1967.

43. SCHLESINGER, M. J. Relation of anatomic
pattern of pathologic conditions of the
coronary arteries. *Arch. Path.*, 30:403–
415, 1940.

44. VASKO, J. S., GUTELIUS, J., and SABISTON,
D. C. A study of predominance of human
coronary arteries determined by arteriographic and perfusion technics. *Amer. J.
Cardiol.*, 8:379–384, 1961.

45. PROVENZA, D. V., and SCHLERLIS, S. Demonstration of muscle sphincters as a capillary component in the human heart. *Circulation*, 20:35–41, 1959.

46. ALTMAN, P. L. P. 37 in: *Handbook of Circulation.* Nat. Acad. Sci.–Natl. Research

Council, Philadelphia, W. B. Saunders, 1959.

47. GALLO, O. A study in the topographical and quantitative relations between capillaries and fibers of the conduction system of the heart and on their functional significance. *Cardiologia*, 29:241–253, 1956.

48. TRUEX, R. C., and ANGULO, A. W. Comparative study of the arterial and venous systems of the ventricular myocardium with special reference to the coronary sinus. *Anat. Rec.*, 113:467–484, 1952.

49. KETY, S. S. Measurements of local blood flow by exchange of inert diffusible substance. *Meth. Med. Res.*, 8:228–236, 1960.

50. GREGG, D. E., LONGINO, F. H., GREEN, P. A., and CZERWONKA, L. J. A comparison of coronary flow determined by the nitrous oxide method and by a direct method using the rotameter. *Circulation*, 3:89–94, 1951.

51. HERD, J. A., HOLLENBERG, M., THORBURN, G. D., KOPALD, H. H., and BARGER, A. C. Myocardial blood flow determined with Krypton[85] in unanesthetized dogs. *Amer. J. Physiol.*, 203:122–124, 1962.

52. KRASNOW, N., LEVINE, H. J., WAGMAN, R. J., and GORLIN, R. Coronary blood flow measured by I[131]Iodo-antipyrine. *Circulat. Res.*, 12:58–62, 1963.

53. COHEN, A., ZALESKI, E. J., BALEIRON, H., STOCK, T. B., CHIBA, C., and BING, R. J. Measurement of coronary blood flow using Rubidium[84] and the coincidence counting method. *Amer. J. Cardiol.*, 19:556–562, 1967.

54. BING, R. J., HAMMOND, M. M., HANDELSMAN, J. C., POWERS, S. R., SPENCER, F. C., ECKENHOFF, J. E., GOODALE, W. T., HAFKENSCHIEL, J. H., and KETY, S. S. The measurement of coronary blood flow, oxygen consumption and efficiency of the left ventricle in man. *Amer. Heart J.*, 38:1–24, 1949.

55. FRANK, M. J., LEVINSON, G. E., and HELLEMS, H. L. Left ventricular oxygen consumption blood flow and performance in mitral stenosis. *Circulation*, 31:824–833, 1965.

56. SARNOFF, S. J., BRAUNWALD, E., WELCH, G. H., JR., CASE, R. B., STAINSBY, W. N., and MACRUZ, R. Hemodynamic determinants of oxygen consumption of the heart with special reference to the tension-time index. *Amer. J. Physiol.*, 192:148–156, 1958.

57. KATZ, L. N. The performance of the heart. *Circulation*, 21:483–498, 1960.

58. MONROE, R. G. Myocardial oxygen consumption during ventricular contraction and relaxation. *Circulat. Res.*, 14:294–300, 1964.

59. SONNENBLICK, E. H., ROSS, J., JR., COVELL, J. W., KAISER, G., and BRAUNWALD, E. Velocity of contraction: major determinant of myocardial oxygen consumption. *J. Clin. Invest.*, 44:1099, 1965.

60. LEVINE, H. J., and WAGMAN, R. J. Energetics of the human heart. *Amer. J. Cardiol.*, 9:372–383, 1962.

61. LOMBARDO, T. A., ROSE, L., TAESCHLER, M., TULUY, S., and BING, R. J. The effect of exercise on coronary blood flow, myocardial oxygen consumption and cardiac efficiency in man. *Circulation*, 7:71–78, 1953.

62. LINZBACH, A. J. Heart failure from the point of view of quantitative anatomy. *Amer. J. Cardiol.*, 5:370–382, 1960.

63. MESSER, J. V., WAGMAN, R. J., LEVINE, H. J., NEILL, W. A., KRASNOW, N., and GORLIN, R. Patterns of human myocardial oxygen extraction during rest and exercise. *J. Clin. Invest.*, 41:725–742, 1962.

64. SEGAL, J., HARVEY, W. P., and HUFNAGEL, C. A clinical study of one hundred cases of severe aortic insufficiency. *Amer. J. Med.*, 21:200–210, 1956.

65. ROWE, G. G., CASTILLO, C. A., MAXWELL, G. M., and CRUMPTON, C. W. A hemodynamic study of hypertension including observations on coronary blood flow. *Ann. Intern. Med.*, 54:405–412, 1961.

66. STUCKEY, D. Cardiac pain in association with mitral stenosis and congenital heart disease. *Brit. Heart J.*, 17:397–407, 1955.

67. ROWE, G. G., MAXWELL, G. M., CASTILLO, C. A., HUSTON, J. H., and CRUMPTON, C. W. Hemodynamics of mitral stenosis with special reference to coronary blood flow and myocardial oxygen consumption. *Circulation*, 22:559–562, 1960.

68. LEIGHT, L., DEFAZIO, V., TALMERS, F. N., REGAN, T. J., and HELLEMS, H. K. Coronary blood flow, myocardial oxygen consumption, myocardial metabolism in normal and hyperthyroid human subjects. *Circulation*, 14:90–99, 1956.

69. ROWE, G. G., HUSTON, J. H., WEINSTEIN, A. B., TUCHMAN, H., BROWN, J. F., and CRUMPTON, C. W. The hemodynamics of thyrotoxicosis in man with special reference to coronary blood flow and myocardial oxygen metabolism. *J. Clin. Invest.*, 35:272, 1956.

70. MOON, H. D., and RINEHARD, J. F. Histogenesis of coronary arteriosclerosis. *Circulation*, 6:481–488, 1952.

71. WHITE, N. K., EDWARDS, J. E., and DRY, T. J. The relationship of the degree of coronary atherosclerosis with age, in men. *Circulation*, 1:645–654, 1950.

72. RUSHMER, R. F., WATSON, N., HARDING, D., and BAKER, D. Effects of acute coronary occlusion on performance of right and left ventricles of intact unanesthetized dogs. *Amer. Heart J.*, 66:522–531, 1963.

73. RUSHMER, R. F. Initial ventricular impulse; a potential key to cardiac evaluation. *Circulation*, 29:268–283, 1964.

74. BURCHELL, H. G. Adjustments in the coronary circulation after experimental coronary occlusion. Pp. 139–144 in *Blood, Heart and Circulation*. Publication No. 13, F. R. Moulton, Ed. Washington, D.C., American Association for the Advancement of Science, 1940.

75. ZOLL, P. M. Normal and pathological anatomy of the coronaries. *Trans. Amer. Col. Cardiol.*, 1:29–43, 1951.

76. BLUMGART, H. S., SCHLESINGER, M. J., and DAVIS, D. Studies on the relation of the clinical manifestations of angina pectoris, coronary thrombosis, and myocardial infarction to the pathologic findings. With particular reference to the significance of the collateral circulation. *Amer. Heart J.*, 19:1–91, 1940.

77. BEAN, W. B. Coronary artery disease. Some aspects of the natural history of ischemic heart disease. Chap. 30 in *Diseases of the Chest, Including the Heart*, J. A. Myers, Ed. Springfield, Ill., Charles C Thomas, 1960.

78. BEAN, W. B. Infarction of the heart. II. Symptomatology of acute attack. *Ann. Intern. Med.*, 11:2086–2108, 1938.

79. KENNEDY, J. A. The incidence of myocardial infarction without pain in 200 autopsy cases. *Amer. Heart J.*, 14:703–709, 1937.

80. POLLARD, H. M., and HARVILL, T. H. Painless myocardial infarction. *Amer. J. Med. Sci.*, 199:628–635, 1940.

CHAPTER 10

CARDIOVASCULAR SOUNDS

I. HEART VALVES AND HEART SOUNDS

The contracting ventricles supply the energy for a unidirectional flow of blood around the circulatory system. Efficient pumping action of the ventricles depends upon the effectiveness of heart valves in preventing retrograde flow. To serve this function adequately, the cardiac valves must conform to a number of stringent requirements. The valves must open easily and widely to offer minimal impedance to blood flowing at a high velocity. Otherwise, excessive pressure energy will be dissipated and wasted in propelling blood through restricted orifices. The valves must close completely with minimal leak and minimal displacement because any blood passing in the retrograde direction must be pumped forward again. Thus, the valves must close abruptly and seal promptly. Since the closed valves represent a diaphragm between regions of very high and very low pressure, the valve structure must be able to withstand large stresses. The valve cusps shut and are subjected to stress by these pressures roughly 48,000 times a day for as long as 100 years without interruption for repairs or replacement. Thus, the cardiac valves must be extremely flexible, very strong and highly durable to function during the lifetime of an individual. These requirements are so difficult to meet that no reasonable substitute for natural valves has been devised in spite of our tremendous technological advances of the last half century.

FUNCTION OF ATRIOVENTRICULAR VALVES

The tricuspid and the mitral valves are interposed between the ventricles and atria on the right and left sides of the heart, respectively. Their structural characteristics were summarized in a preceding chapter (see Figs. 2-7 and 2-10). The valve cusps are firmly attached around the circumference of the fibrous valve rings and form an uninterrupted diaphragm which is shaped like a shallow funnel. According to Brock,[1] the area of the orifice at the small end of the mitral "funnel" is not significantly greater than the aortic orifice. The main valve cusps extend quite deeply into the ventricular cavity, and their combined area is about twice the area of the orifice they must occlude.

In spite of their large area, the

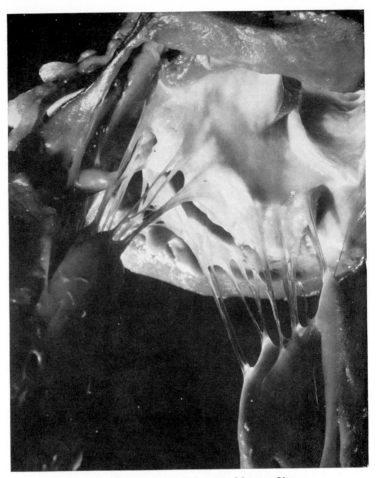

FIGURE 10-1   ANATOMY OF THE MITRAL VALVE

These normal human mitral valves are presented in a postulated position of rest with slight tension being exerted by the chordae tendineae. From this position, slight separation of the valves could admit a rapid flow from the atria or slight movement toward apposition would produce rapid closure with little or no regurgitation.

atrioventricular valves do not function effectively if the chordae tendineae are ruptured or sectioned. The chordae tendineae extend from the papillary muscles to the edge of the valve cusps and continue into the substance of the valve (Fig. 10-1). These tough strands of collagenous fibers contribute much to the strength of the valve cusps. The chordae tendineae appear to function like sheets and clew lines fastened to the edges of square sails. They act to prevent flapping and ever-

sion of the valve cusps that would render the valves incompetent or unable to seal the atrioventricular orifice. Some of the chordae (first order) insert on the edges of the valve cusps; others (second order) insert just beyond the free edge of the cusp; and a few (third order) originate directly from the ventricular wall near the valve ring and insert on the ventricular surface of the valves. The chordae are of unequal length but are so arranged that tension is exerted on all strands when the valve is closed. The valve substance between the insertions of the first-order chordae is very thin and flexible and thus produces a completely watertight seal as soon as the valve edges come into apposition.

CONCEPTS OF VALVE CLOSURE

In 1912, Henderson and Johnson[2] reported a series of most ingenious demonstrations of two different mechanisms for closure of heart valves. The first mechanism is a retrograde flow of blood toward the atria as the ventricles

begin to contract, catching the valves like a pair of sails and flinging them into apposition (Fig. 10–2A). Imagine a door being slammed by a gust of wind. Clearly, this mechanism inevitably involves a large leak before the orifice is closed. The occurrence of such regurgitation is widely acknowledged when the atrioventricular valves are closed by ventricular systole which is not preceded by an atrial contraction, i.e., premature ventricular contraction. The mitral valve normally closes without regurgitation. The forward flow of blood through the mitral orifice during atrial systole must

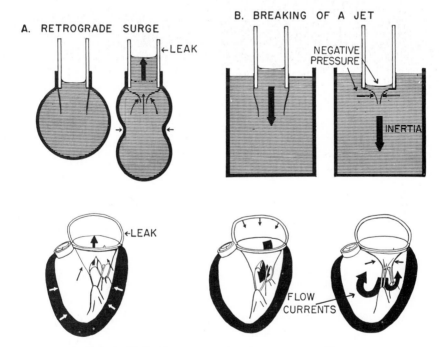

FIGURE 10–2   CLOSURE OF ATRIOVENTRICULAR VALVES

   Two mechanisms for closure of A-V valves are indicated by simple models and by schematic drawings.
   A, A valve, consisting of a section of thin-walled rubber tubing mounted within a rubber bulb, could be closed by a surge of fluid only after considerable leakage past the closing valve. Similarly, if the mitral valves gape wide at the beginning of ventricular contraction, considerable blood would regurgitate into the left atrium during closure of these valves.
   B, If the flow of fluid through a model valve ceases rather abruptly, the inertia of the moving fluid carries it onward, leaving a wake of negative pressure which could close the valve with no regurgitation whatever. Cessation of flow into the ventricle after atrial systole may produce partial closure of the A-V valves by this mechanism, facilitated by currents of flow upward and behind the closing valve cusps (after Henderson and Johnson[2]).

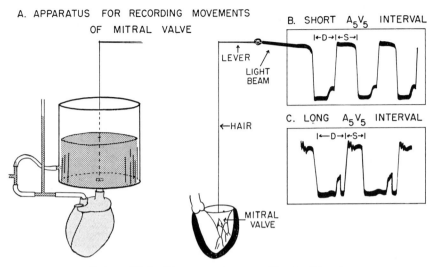

FIGURE 10–3   MOVEMENTS OF THE MITRAL VALVE

Dean's records indicated that during the later part of diastole (*D*) the valve cusps moved toward a position of closure after atrial systole and before ventricular systole (*S*). If the interval between atrial systole and ventricular systole was short, valve closure was initiated before ventricular systole and was completed by the rising ventricular pressure. If this interval was sufficiently long, the valves closed partially and then gaped wide before ventricular contraction ensued (lower record).

bring the valves into partial or complete apposition. Henderson and Johnson[2] also demonstrated that when flow of fluid through an orifice is suddenly arrested, the inertia of the moving blood produces in its wake a negative pressure which closes either simulated or real heart valves (Fig. 10–2*B*). The portion of the valves nearest their base is the first to move inward, and the edges of the flaps are the last to make contact. In this way, the valves close without the slightest regurgitation. Such inrolling during valve closure "invariably occurred under conditions simulating the movements of blood in the normal heart."

Dean[3] connected the edge of a mitral valve cusp to a delicate lever by means of a human hair and recorded the valve movements in isolated, perfused hearts (Fig. 10–3). When the interval between atrial and ventricular

systole was less than 0.147 second, the valve cusps opened wider at a time when blood was flowing through the orifice and, near the end of atrial contraction, moved quickly and markedly toward the atrium but did not close completely. The onset of ventricular contraction at this moment completed closure of the valves as a single movement. A longer interval between atrial and ventricular systole (greater than 0.272 sec.) allowed the valves to move toward apposition and then separate again before ventricular contraction ensued. These observations are clearly consistent with the concepts of Henderson and Johnson.[2]

The concepts proposed by Henderson and Johnson and by Dean promptly achieved wide acceptance and have served as the basis for most interpretations of both valve function and heart sounds.

FAULTY A-V VALVE FUNCTION IN EXPOSED OR ISOLATED HEARTS

Direct observation and motion picture recording of the action of atrioventricular valves[4, 5] in isolated hearts have revealed that during systole the valve cusps tend to bulge upward toward the atrium. Displacement of the valves toward the atrium is basically equivalent to a retrograde leak through the valves so far as the ventricular myocardium is concerned. When it was learned that the exposed or excised heart tends to shrink and function at abnormally small dimensions (see Fig. 3–9), it seemed probable that valve mechanics are distorted under these experimental conditions. The ventricular myocardium shortens as the cardiac chambers shrink, but the fibrous valve rings, valve cusps and chordae tendineae retain their same dimensions. Under these conditions, the valves and their attachments might have a great deal more slack than normal and thus could execute wider excursions. For this reason, the motion of the mitral valves in the intact dog was studied by means of motion pictures of the images produced by x-rays on fluorescent screens (cinefluorography).

CINEFLUOROGRAPHIC STUDIES OF MITRAL VALVE FUNCTION IN INTACT DOGS

To study the displacement of the valves in intact dogs, a probe applicator was devised which could be inserted through the left atrial wall and into the left ventricular cavity. When a plunger was activated, tiny silver clips were crimped to the edge of the valve cusps or to the chordae tendineae near the valve attachments. The location of the mitral valve ring was marked by suturing a delicate silver chain to the atrioventricular groove. The animals recovered from this operation promptly and lived indefinitely. Motion pictures of the movements of the metal markers were obtained days or weeks after the operation.[6]

In such experiments, the excursion of the valves was surprisingly small. Certainly, the valve cusps did not gape wide at any phase of the cardiac cycle. At no time did the valve edges ascend to the plane of the mitral valve ring. In other words, the valve edges were apparently held well down within the ventricular cavity during all phases of the cardiac cycle. To be sure that large valve excursions were not occurring in some other plane, stereoscopic cinefluorographic equipment was developed to study valve motion in three dimensions.[7] These studies merely confirmed that the valve edges moved very small distances apart when open or toward the A-V ring when closed. Both the restricted lateral movement during diastole and the limited motion toward the atrium during systole point to more or less continuous restraint by the chordae tendineae.

The valve action was also studied when the heart was functioning at abnormally small dimensions (either immediately after the operation or after induction of pneumothorax). Under these conditions, the excursion of the valve edges was consistently much wider than that observed when the heart had regained its normal large dimensions in the intact chest.

MECHANISMS OF MITRAL VALVE CLOSURE

The factors responsible for the closure of the atrioventricular valves remain controversial after centuries of study by many different investigators.

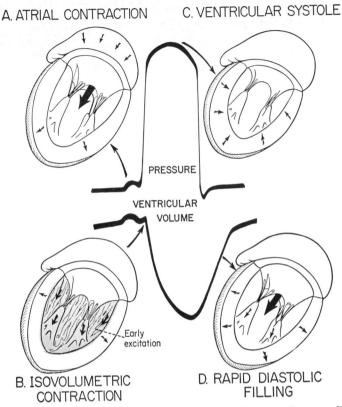

A. ATRIAL CONTRACTION   C. VENTRICULAR SYSTOLE

PRESSURE

VENTRICULAR
VOLUME

Early
excitation

B. ISOVOLUMETRIC   D. RAPID DIASTOLIC
CONTRACTION   FILLING

FIGURE 10–4   ATRIOVENTRICULAR VALVE ACTION DURING CARDIAC CYCLE

At the end of diastole, the distended ventricle applies traction through the chordae tendineae to the valve cusps, drawing them toward apposition. At the end of atrial systole, the jet of flow through the valves is arrested and the valve cusps close, aided by the swirling currents. Ventricular systole seals the valves together by the high internal pressure. The valves gape open promptly as the ventricular myocardium relaxes at the end of systole.

This is due primarily to reliance on pressure measurements for criteria of valve opening and closing. For example, the reversal of pressure gradient between atria and ventricles is not an absolute sign of closure of the valve cusps.[8, 9] The aortic pressure drops slightly below ventricular pressure as outflow slows down during the latter part of systole (see Fig. 2–18). This clearly cannot be interpreted as closure of the aortic valve since outflow from the ventricle continues. Pressure differences are not reliable indicators of the direction of blood flow or of valve closure in the presence of rapidly

changing or fluctuating flow velocities. A description of the sequence of mitral valve closure has been synthesized from the functional anatomy of ventricular contraction. This or any other hypothesis must ultimately be tested by direct measurements of displacements, accelerations and vibrations of blood and heart walls to supplement observations on pressures and pressure gradients.

During the final stages of ventricular filling, the ventricular cavity is well distended with blood. The roots of the papillary muscles are correspondingly displaced toward the apex and away from the atrioventricular valve ring (Fig. 10-4). The chordae tendineae and valve cusps are probably under some tension, drawing the valve edges toward apposition. This is the period of slow filling or diastasis, when little or no blood is flowing through the valve. At the onset of atrial contraction, blood is propelled through the cleft formed by the valve cusps. The valve cusps are then approximated by the negative pressure following the interrupted stream of blood, supplemented by eddy currents flowing back behind the valves (see Fig. 10-2B). The wave of excitation, rapidly propagated by Purkinje fibers, first enters the ventricular myocardium at the roots of the papillary muscle and over the endocardial surface. Ultrasonic displacement sensors indicated that the maximal rate of valve closure ranges between 20 and 40 cm./sec.[10] The early contraction of papillary muscles and trabeculae carneae simultaneously draws the valve edges and valve rings toward the apex and produces a lateral displacement of ventricular walls (see Fig. 2-17). The valves are tightly sealed by the rising ventricular pressure. As ventricular ejection proceeds, the shortening of the ventricular myocardium is accompanied by shortening of the papillary muscles, taking up any slack in the valves that might otherwise develop (Fig. 10-4). At the end of systole the relaxation of the ventricular myocardium (and papillary muscles) releases the tension on the valves, and they can gape open freely as blood pours rapidly from the atrium into the ventricle. At the end of the rapid-filling interval, the ventricle is well distended and the valve cusps are again drawn toward apposition by the traction exerted by the stretched papillary muscles, and the cycle repeats (Fig. 10-4). Although corresponding studies have not been conducted on the tri-

cuspid valves, the similarity in structure and function of the two atrioventricular valves (Fig. 2-10) suggests that they both utilize the same basic mechanisms.

FUNCTION OF SEMILUNAR VALVES

The pulmonary and aortic valves are each composed of three cusps of equal size which resemble flexible cups attached symmetrically around the circumference of the valve orifice (Fig. 10-5). Two valve cusps of equal size would be equally effective in completely closing and sealing off the opening in the valve ring. However, such a bicuspid valve would not open widely and would necessarily obstruct the flow of blood. Occasionally a bicuspid valve develops as a congenital deformity, characteristically producing functional changes corresponding to stenosis of the valve. The normal aortic and pulmonary valves close completely and when open have a triangular orifice which is considerably smaller than the cross-sectional area of the artery (Fig. 10-5). This opening is sufficiently large that the pressure gradient required to force blood through it is negligible even at the highest velocities attained during ejection.

Behind the aortic valve cusps are three outpouchings, the sinuses of Valsalva, which help prevent obstruction of the coronary ostia. If a valve leaflet came in contact with the coronary orifice, shutting off the blood flow from the aorta, the pressure in the coronary artery would fall rapidly as blood passed out of the coronary capillaries. The coronary arterial pressure would approach coronary venous pressure during each diastolic interval while the aortic pressure was continu-

A. BICUSPID VALVE   B. SEMILUNAR VALVES

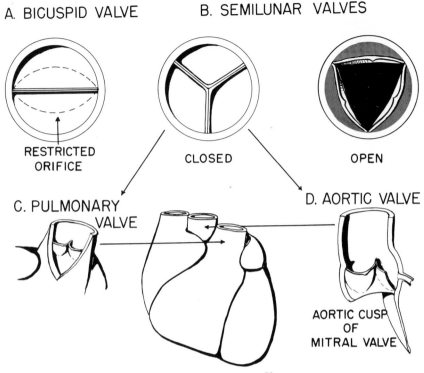

RESTRICTED   CLOSED   OPEN
ORIFICE

C. PULMONARY   D. AORTIC VALVE
        VALVE

                                                          AORTIC CUSP
                                                              OF
                                                         MITRAL VALVE

FIGURE 10–5   SEMILUNAR VALVES

A, Bicuspid valves can close completely but they will not open fully.

B, A valve with three symmetrical cusps can close completely and theoretically could open to the full dimensions of the artery. However, motion pictures of aortic valve action have demonstrated that even normal valve cusps are only partly displaced during systolic ejection, opening a triangular orifice very much smaller in area than the cross section of the artery. (From McMillan, I. K. R., and Daley, R.: The action of human mitral and aortic valves studied postmortem by cinematography, presented at the Second World Congress of Cardiology, Washington, D. C., September 16, 1954.)

C, The pulmonary valve is situated at the junction of the conus region and the pulmonary artery.

D, The aortic valve cusps are in close relation to the orifices of the coronary arteries. The sinuses of Valsalva behind the valve cusps, coupled with the incomplete opening of the cusps, prevent obstruction of the coronary orifices during ventricular systole.

ously maintained at high pressure. Under these conditions, a valve cusp sealing a coronary orifice even momentarily would remain sealed because there appears to be no mechanism which could release it. The sinuses of Valsalva provide a space behind the valve cusps and apparently prevent this unfortunate accident. Flow through hydraulic models suggests that turbulent eddies circle back behind the valve cusps during systolic ejection, holding the valve edges out away from the walls of the sinuses of Valsalva (Fig. 10–6). At the end of ventricular systole, ejection ceases for a brief interval before ventricular relaxation becomes manifest. At that moment, a slight retrograde surge of blood toward the ventricle is abruptly arrested as the valve cusps snap shut. The closure of both atrioventricular and semilunar valves is associated with the development of vibrations or heart

A. SYSTOLE   B. DIASTOLE

FIGURE 10-6 EDDY CURRENTS BEHIND VALVE
                CUSPS

Hydraulic models, simulating the aortic
valve, demonstrate eddy currents that swirl
behind the flexible cusps during rapid flow
through the valve orifice. These currents tend to
prevent the cusps from sealing off the coronary
orifices and stagnation of blood behind the
valves. (Derived from studies by Dr. K. A.
Merendino, Department of Surgery, and Mr.
Wayne Quinton, Medical Instrument Shop,
University of Washington.)

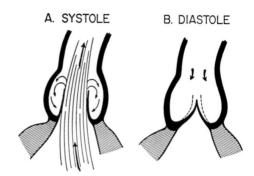

sounds which are easily heard by
listening over the surface of the chest.

HEART SOUNDS

Auscultation is the most sensitive
test of the functional integrity of the
heart. Frequently, murmurs or alterations in the heart sounds are the only
definite signs of organic heart disease,
appearing long before the stress on
the cardiovascular system is sufficient
to produce other signs and symptoms.
As in any sensitive test of physiologic
function, the distinction between
normality and abnormality is difficult
in many borderline cases. Nevertheless, characteristic murmurs and
changes in heart sounds may direct
attention toward the heart as the site of
disease processes. In a few conditions,
a distinctive murmur provides a definite diagnosis of an anatomic lesion at
an early stage in its development.
Clinicians learn to recognize well-
developed, characteristic murmurs by
training and experience. However,
the significance of murmurs and the
subtle changes in heart sounds can be
more fully appreciated with a fairly
clear understanding of the nature of
the sounds, the mechanics of sound
transmission and the characteristics of
auditory perception.

THE NATURE OF SOUNDS

Production of Sounds. Sounds
are subjective interpretations of the
sensations produced by the vibrations
reaching the auditory apparatus. Sound
waves are produced and transmitted
by the vibratory motion of particles
or bodies which are repetitively displaced from their position of equilibrium and then restored by a force of
restitution toward their position of
rest (Fig. 10-7A).

Characteristics of Sounds. Consider a tuning fork with its prongs
vibrating simultaneously (Fig. 10-7B).
During the time that the right prong
moves toward the tube, the air molecules are compressed at the orifice. A
wave of compression moves through
the tube with the velocity of sound in
air (1100 ft. per second). When the
prong moves back, the air molecules
rush back to fill the void and a wave of
rarefaction follows the compression
at the same velocity down the tube.

FREQUENCY. The frequency at
which a system vibrates depends
upon the mass in motion in relation
to the restoring force (elasticity). A
small mass fastened to a stiff spring
vibrates rapidly (Fig. 10-8A). In general, the mass of body tissues is large
in relation to their elasticity, so they
tend to vibrate at low frequencies.

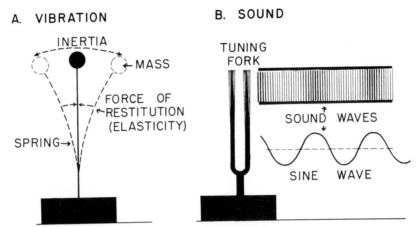

FIGURE 10-7   THE NATURE OF VIBRATIONS

A, Vibration occurs when a mass, held in position by elastic support, is displaced from its position of rest. The spring tension acts to return the mass toward the equilibrium position, but momentum carries it beyond the position of rest. An oscillatory motion of the mass back and forth past the position of rest persists until the energy instilled in the system is dissipated by friction.

B, Sound waves produced by a tuning fork are waves of alternating compression (increased pressure) and expansion (reduced pressure) of the air. The fluctuating pressures from a vibrating tuning fork are recorded from a microphone as a sine wave, indicating that the sound is a pure tone.

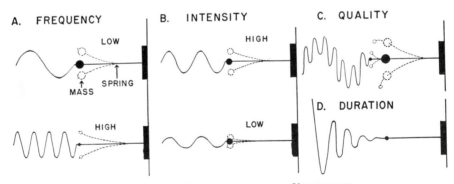

FIGURE 10-8   CHARACTERISTICS OF VIBRATIONS

A, The frequency of vibration (cycles per second) is determined by the relation between the mass and the elasticity of its support; a large mass on a weak spring produces a slow vibration; a small mass on a stiff spring vibrates rapidly.

B, The amplitude of vibrations depends on the amount of displacement from the position of rest (the energy imparted to the system).

C, The quality of vibrations refers to the number of overtones or harmonics, which are schematically represented by two vibrating systems connected in series. When responding to complex sounds, a single structure (e.g., the cone of a loudspeaker) may be simultaneously vibrating at more than one frequency.

D, The duration of a vibration after the source of energy is cut off depends upon the rate at which the energy is dissipated. The greater the frictional resistance to motion, the faster the energy is used up, and the greater the "damping."

Exceptions to this rule are bones and connective tissue structures under high tension (e.g., arterial walls).

INTENSITY. The intensity of the sound depends upon the amplitude of the vibrations, which is determined by how far the vibrating body is displaced. In other words, the intensity of the sound depends upon the amount of energy imparted to the vibrating body as it is displaced from its position of rest (Fig. 10–8B).

QUALITY. A tuning fork is an instrument that produces a pure tone, a sound with but one frequency which is recorded as a sine wave (Fig. 10–7B). Most natural sounds are composed of various frequencies or overtones which combine to determine the quality of the sound (Fig. 10–8C). Distinctive combinations of tones and harmonics allow recognition of different musical instruments, of familiar voices and characteristic heart sounds. The vibrations emitted by the heart should be classed as noises since they are composed of unrelated frequencies with very brief durations.

DURATION. Vibrations tend to die out as the energy originally imparted to the system is dissipated in the form of heat from friction. If the frictional resistance is increased, the vibratory motion persists for a shorter period of time because it is "damped" (Fig. 10–8D). The soft tissues of the body very effectively damp the vibrations of internal structures. For example, heart sounds consist of relatively few vibrations, but sounds of longer duration may persist as long as energy is supplied to the vibrating system (murmurs).

ORIGIN OF HEART SOUNDS

As many as 40 different theories have been proposed to explain the first heart sound.[5] A monograph by McKu-sick[11] contains an excellent historical review of the causes of heart sounds and murmurs. Wide divergence of opinion also characterizes the theories regarding the origin of other sounds and murmurs. This chaotic condition appears to stem from the type of investigation which has been applied to the problem. Virtually every possible mechanical event occurring during the cardiac cycle has, at one time or another, been ascribed a role in the production of heart sounds. For example, different components of the first sound are attributed variously to vibrations of numerous structures including valves, muscular walls and arteries. Since the chambers of the heart are filled with blood, none of these structures can vibrate independently without producing movements of the blood. Similarly, vibrations in the blood must be transmitted to the surrounding structures. If the sounds can be picked up from the external surface of the body, all structures between the heart and the thoracic wall must be vibrating. It is futile to consider vibrations of the heart walls, valves, arterial walls and blood individually when in fact they constitute an interdependent system and all vibrate at the same time. A more realistic approach to the problem results from considering those conditions which lead to vibrations of cardiohemic systems composed of the blood, heart walls and valves.

Vibrations in Fluid-Filled Elastic Systems. Much of the controversy regarding heart sounds and murmurs can be resolved by considering the vibrations in the cardiovascular system as caused by two general mechanisms: (*a*) acceleration or deceleration of blood and (*b*) turbulence developing during rapid blood flow. In the subsequent discussion, vibrations or sounds due to acceleration or deceleration of blood will be classified as heart sounds. Vibrations or sounds due to turbulence in flowing blood will be considered as murmurs.

The characteristics of vibrations are described in terms of a mass supported by a spring (Fig. 10–7). In an elastic chamber completely filled with fluid, the elasticity of the walls is analogous to the spring, and the fluid plus the supporting walls are analogous to the vibrating mass. Imagine a fluid-filled balloon in which any sudden movement (acceleration or deceleration) throws the entire system into vibration (Fig. 10–9). Clearly, no portion of the balloon could vibrate independently, without affecting all other portions of the system. A sharp tap in a very small area produces vibrations affecting all parts of the fluid and the walls. The vibrations result from the momentum of the fluid producing an overstretch of the elastic wall, which recoils and displaces the fluid in the opposite direction. This

sequence is repeated until the residual energy in the system is dissipated. The intensity of the vibrations is determined largely by the rate of change of velocity (the amount of acceleration or deceleration). Their frequency depends upon the relation between the vibrating mass and the elasticity of the walls. In the heart, the combined mass of the blood and the walls of the chambers is very large in relation to the elasticity of the walls, so the vibrations usually have a low frequency. When the ventricles are contracting, the elasticity of the walls should be greater and the vibration frequency increased. Vibrations due to acceleration and deceleration of blood tend to consist of only a few cycles, indicating that they are promptly damped.

Cardiohemic Systems in Heart Sound Production. From a knowledge of the mechanical events of the cardiac cycle, the regions where acceleration or deceleration of blood is

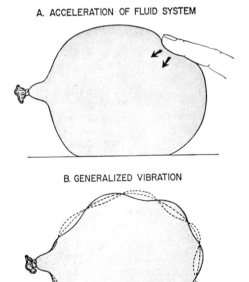

A. ACCELERATION OF FLUID SYSTEM

B. GENERALIZED VIBRATION

FIGURE 10–9   VIBRATIONS IN A FLUID-FILLED BALLOON

Tapping a balloon filled with water throws the entire system into vibrations. Although the deformation was applied at a single point, the vibrations involve all parts of the fluid and walls.

occurring at any particular phase should be readily identifiable. The character of the vibrations is influenced by the nature of the specific *cardiohemic system* which is vibrating. The term *cardiohemic system* has been coined to cover any combination of blood and heart walls which is the site of vibrations produced by changes in velocity of the blood. The vibrations induced within any cardiohemic system may be transmitted in all directions and may be audible if they are transmitted to the thoracic walls with sufficient intensity and at a high enough frequency. From the concept of cardiohemic systems, the etiology of heart sounds can be described logically.

ATRIAL SOUNDS. In the latter part of the diastole, the ventricles are well filled with blood and in direct communication with the atria through the partially open atrioventricular valves. When atrial contraction displaces blood through these valves, the ventricular walls become more distended and stretched, as indicated by the slight increase in the intraventricular pressure. The recoil of the distended ventricles sets the stage for vibrations back and forth between the atria and ventricles. This recoil may also contribute to transient valve closure. Since this cardiohemic system consists of the thin-walled right and left atria and relaxed ventricular walls, it is not surprising that these vibrations consist of a few low-frequency oscillations. They have such low frequency and low intensity that they are inaudible in normal adults.

FIRST HEART SOUND. At the onset of ventricular contraction, blood is accelerated in the ventricle, surging toward the atrioventricular valves. This acceleration of blood, occurring before the valves are sealed and taut, is responsible for the introductory

vibrations of the first heart sound (first component) which precede elevation of the intraventricular pressure. Their frequency is very low and their intensity is slight, presumably because the ventricles remain largely relaxed and the acceleration of blood is not rapid. However, this movement of blood must be sufficient to close, seal and apply tension to the atrioventricular valves before ventricular pressure rises. When this movement of the blood is suddenly arrested, the valves become tense. The second component of the first sound begins as the momentum of the moving blood produces sufficient valvular overstretching to cause a recoil back toward the ventricles (Fig. 10–10A). In this case, the cardiohemic vibrating systems consist primarily of the two ventricular cavities, completely enclosed by valves and contracting myocardium. Thus, the vibrations generated at the onset of ventricular systole have a higher frequency and a greater amplitude than those produced by atrial contraction.

The intensity of the vibrations depends upon the velocity attained by the blood and the abruptness with which it is decelerated. Thus, the sound would be greater if the valves gaped wide at the onset of the ventricular contraction than if they were approximated at this moment, because the blood would attain a higher velocity before complete closure occurred. This concept appears consistent with the observations of Henderson,[2] Dean,[3] Shearn et al.[12] and others.[13-15] Even more reassuring is confirmation of the relationship of heart sounds to acceleration of blood flow.[16]

The third component of the first heart sound begins as ventricular contraction elevates the intraventricular pressure above that in the corresponding artery and blood begins

A. COMPONENTS OF FIRST HEART SOUND

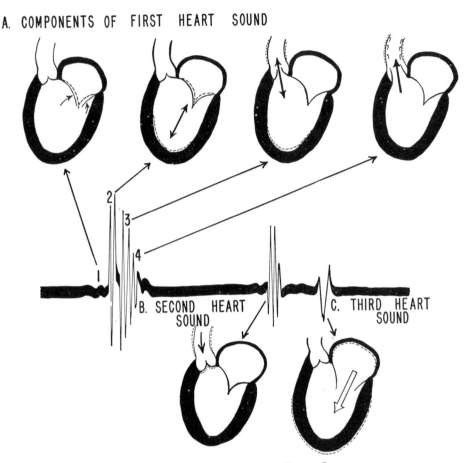

FIGURE 10–10   THE ETIOLOGY OF HEART SOUNDS

Schematic drawings of the causes of various components of the heart sounds based on the concept that the vibrations are induced by acceleration or deceleration of the blood within elastic chambers.

A, The first sound can be divided into four components. The initial vibrations occur when the first myocardial contractions in the ventricle shift blood toward the atrium to approximate and seal the atrioventricular valves. The second component begins with abrupt tension of closed atrioventricular valves decelerating the moving blood. It may represent oscillation of blood initiated by overdistention of the atrioventricular valves, countered by recoil of the contracting ventricular myocardium. The reaction would be similar to tapping a balloon filled with water. The third component may involve oscillations of blood between the distending root of the aorta and the ventricular walls. The fourth component probably represents vibrations due to turbulence in blood flowing rapidly through the ascending aorta and pulmonary artery.

B, The second heart sound is introduced by a few low-frequency vibrations which may accompany the deceleration and reversal of flow through the aorta and pulmonary artery prior to the closure of the semilunar valves. The audible portion of the second sound begins with closure and tensing of the semilunar valves. Although the primary vibrations occur in the arteries, they are also transmitted to the ventricles and atria by movements of the blood, valves and valve rings.

D, The third heart sound occurs at the end of the rapid filling phase. Sudden termination of the rapid-filling phase may throw the entire atrioventricular system into vibrations which have very low frequency because the walls are relaxed.

to move toward the semilunar valves. The inertia of the long columns of blood in the arterial trunks opposes acceleration just as though there were an obstruction a short distance beyond the semilunar valves. Therefore, the first portion of the blood moving out of the ventricles distends the proximal portions of these arteries. Sudden distention of the proximal arterial segments may induce a rebound of blood toward the ventricles. Oscillation of the blood back and forth between the arterial roots and the ventricular chambers would result from a mechanism similar to that associated with closure of the atrioventricular valves (Fig. 10-10A). Since the cardiohemic systems producing the second and third components of the first sound are very similar, their frequencies, intensities and qualities are also similar. Indeed, these two components are usually merged into a single set of vibrations which cannot be differentiated. Splitting or reduplication of the first sound is usually ascribed to asynchronous closure of the tricuspid and then the mitral valves in rapid succession[17]

The fourth component of the first heart sound is probably the result of turbulence in the blood flowing rapidly through the arterial trunks and for this reason will be considered under *Murmurs*.

SECOND HEART SOUND. Near the end of systole, the rate of ejection slows as the ventricular and arterial pressures begin to diminish. Ventricular pressure drops precipitously at the onset of ventricular relaxation. Blood in the roots of the aorta and in the pulmonary artery rushes back toward the ventricular chambers, but this movement is abruptly arrested by closure of the semilunar valves. The momentum of the moving blood overstretches the valve cusps, and the recoil initiates oscillations in both the arterial and the ventricular cavities (Fig. 10-10B). The pitch of the second sound seems higher than that of the first sound. The intensity of the sound, again, depends upon the velocity attained by the blood gushing back toward the ventricle and the abruptness with which the motion is arrested. In systemic or pulmonary hypertension, the velocity should be great and the sounds intensified. In the presence of semilunar valvular stenosis, on the contrary, the amplitude of the second sound should be reduced if the valves are largely approximated before the retrograde flow is well established. Observations reported by Piemme *et al.*[16] suggested the need to postulate a somewhat different cause of the second sound. Their records indicated that the second sound began just before the flow reversal occurred, at the point in time of most abrupt deceleration of forward flow. The second sound ended with the nadir of the flow reversal, apparently having been developed before closure. Studies of various hemodynamic variables by Kusukawa *et al.*[18] revealed that the amplitude of the second heart sound was not directly related to the aortic pressures, pressure differences between aorta and left ventricle or rate of change of these pressures at the time of the dicrotic notch. A high correlation (0.98) was found only with the rate of change in pressure gradient which is theoretically related to "mass acceleration functions" in the aorta. Using a special electrical-contact device,[19] the precise moment of valve closure was found to occur at least 5 to 13 msec. before the notch on the aortic pressure record. Resolution of these differences must await studies which directly measure the exact time of apposition of the semilunar valve cusps.

THIRD HEART SOUND. When intraventricular pressure drops below atrial pressure, the atrioventricular valves swing open before a mass movement of blood into the relaxed ventricular chambers. Inflow is arrested rather suddenly, as is manifest in the rapid transition from the rapid-filling phase to the plateau which indicates slow filling or diastasis.[20] The momentum of the moving mass of blood produces low-frequency vibrations because the chamber walls are all relaxed. Such vibrations would be more likely to occur when the rapid-filling phase terminates abruptly. Because of their low frequency, the vibrations must have considerable amplitude to reach the auditory threshold, particularly if the loss of energy during transmission is great. Third heart sounds are consistently audible in children or in adults during auscultation in sound damped rooms with very low ambient noise levels.

GALLOP RHYTHMS. When three audible heart sounds occur in rapid succession, followed by a pause, the subjective impression is similar to the sounds produced by a galloping horse. Several combinations of heart sounds can produce this impression. The most common form of gallop occurs when the third heart sound is clearly audible. In such instances the three heart sounds occur in sequence and are followed by a relatively silent interval during the remainder of diastole. This type is frequently called the "protodiastolic" gallop, which is a misnomer because the third sound follows the protodiastolic interval. For no very good reason, third heart sounds, commonly heard in normal children, are usually not included among gallop rhythms. A gallop rhythm which develops in the course of heart disease (e.g., myocarditis, congestive failure) signifies alterations in the myocardium. The third heart sound is so

rarely audible in aged individuals without obvious heart disease that the protodiastolic gallop often indicates a serious prognosis. The nature of the myocardial change which accentuates the third heart sound is not clear, but presumably the rapid-filling phase is terminated more abruptly.

If the sounds accompanying atrial systole are intensified and precede the first sound by a sufficient interval to be distinguished, a gallop rhythm is produced which consists of the fourth, first and second heart sounds in succession. Since the abnormal sound occurs in late diastole, this rhythm is called a "presystolic" gallop.

If the heart rate is rapid, the diastolic interval becomes shorter and the third and fourth heart sounds may occur almost simultaneously. The combined intensity of the two sets of vibrations may become audible, and the resulting rhythm is called a *summation* or mid-diastolic gallop.

Transmission of Sounds. The factors that influence the transmission of vibrations are the same as those involved in their production (see Fig. 10–8). The elasticity or restoring force of the transmitting media is very important. Since the mass of vibrating material (the heart, blood and tissues) is great in relation to tissue elasticity, low frequency sounds predominate in both production and transmission. This is most unfortunate because the human auditory mechanism is particularly insensitive to low-pitched sounds (see *Auditory Perception of Heart Sounds*).

The maximum transmission distance from the heart to the surface of the chest is undoubtedly less than a foot, and the cycle length of the vibrations is greater than this distance. For this reason, all the structures involved in the transmission of these vibrations to the surface tend to oscillate together.

Under these conditions, sound waves are not reflected. The most important loss of heart sound energy occurs in compressible tissues (e.g., lung) interposed between the heart and chest wall. Vibrations of the heart wall may be so well damped while passing through a thick cushion of aerated lung tissue that they are poorly transmitted to the chest wall (e.g., in emphysema). Thus, the heart sounds have maximum intensity in those surface areas to which the vibrations are transmitted directly through solid tissues or through a minimal thickness of inflated lung. Layers of fat also attenuate heart sounds because of damping.

To study transmission characteristics of the thorax, Faber and Burton[21] recorded the arrival time of heart sounds at many different points over the precordium and computed the transmission velocity at about 15 meters per second, assuming that the sounds originated from a site within the heart and traveled to the mitral area and then spread over the surface of the chest. The conclusions may be questioned on the basis of evidence by Zalter et al.[22] that the amplitude of the first sound was very uniform when recorded over various areas of the cardiac surface, indicating that the sound source is not well localized but is well distributed throughout the cardiac chambers as would be expected in a cardiohemic system (see Fig. 10-9).

SURFACE LOCALIZATION OF HEART SOUNDS. Sounds emitted from the vicinities of the four valves have maximal intensities at four different surface areas. For example, murmurs from the region of the pulmonary valve are most intense in the *pulmonary area*, centered at the third left intercostal space at the left parasternal line (Fig. 10-11). The *aortic area* lies to the right of the sternum in

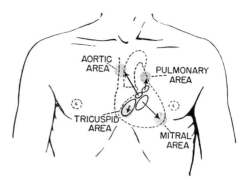

FIGURE 10-11   TRANSMISSION OF SOUNDS AND MURMURS

Although heart sounds are widely transmitted over the precordium, vibrations from the four valves tend to be of maximal intensity at the areas on the precordium indicated by the arrows above. The mitral area on the precordium is near the apex of the heart, the tricuspid area is in the fourth intercostal space on either side of the sternum. The pulmonary area is in either the second or the third intercostal space at the left parasternal line, and the aortic area is in the second right intercostal space but often extends obliquely across the precordium toward the apex (see Fig. 10-17).

the second right intercostal space. The *tricuspid area* is near the right sternal border in the fourth intercostal space, and the *mitral area* is near the apex of the heart. This particular localization of sounds on the surface probably represents the most effective transmission pathways from the original sites of vibration to the surface of the chest. The pulmonary and tricuspid valves are near the precordium, and the corresponding auscultatory areas are close by. The aortic and mitral valves are situated farther from the precordium, and their auscultatory areas do not overlie the valve rings (Fig. 10-11). In the region of the apex, the heart sounds are usually loud because the heart is in direct contact with the anterior wall of the thorax. Vibrations of the ventricular chamber, associated with mitral valvular disease, are frequently localized over the apex. The ascending aorta curves forward and most closely approaches the anterior chest wall near the aortic area. Sounds emitted from the region of the aortic valve may also traverse the right ventricular chamber to appear in the third or fourth intercostal space to the left of the sternum, or follow the left ventricular chamber to a point near the apex.

The fact that both the first and second heart sounds are generally audible at all four areas indicates that their production is not limited to vibrations in the regions of the valves. The wide distribution is consistent with oscillation of cardiohemic systems produced by mass movements of blood.

It is inaccurate to consider the second sound in the pulmonary area to be composed primarily or exclusively of vibrations from the pulmonary valve. In records taken from directly over the A-V valve rings on the surface of the heart, the contribution of one valve cannot be dissociated from that of another. The reason for this becomes apparent when it is recognized that the atria, ventricles, arterial trunks and valves are all firmly fastened to the fibrous skeleton of the heart (Fig. 2–7) and must all be affected by vibrations at any point. Nevertheless, a loud second sound in the pulmonary area on the precordium is frequently a reliable indication of pulmonary hypertension, and its localization permits its differentiation from a loud aortic second sound, which may occur with systemic hypertension.

Auditory Perception of Heart Sounds. Under optimal conditions the ear can detect vibrations with an amplitude less than the diameter of a hydrogen molecule. The energy of barely perceptible sound waves is so slight that it would have to be continued without loss or interruption for more than two million years to elevate

the temperature of 1 gm. of water 1° C.[23] The ear is more sensitive than the finest microphone, so sensitive at 1000 c.p.s. that it is only about 12 decibels above the thermal agitation of molecules.[24]

Although the maximal range of audible frequencies normally lies between 20 and 16,000 c.p.s., the maximal sensitivity of human audition lies within the speech range, about 1000 to 2000 c.p.s.[25] To be perceived, sound with a frequency of 30 c.p.s. must attain energy levels thousands of times those needed by vibrations at 1000 c.p.s. (Fig. 10–12). Heart sounds extend above and below the threshold of hearing, so some are inaudible while others considerably exceed threshold levels. The frequencies of the audible vibrations of the heart probably range from below 20 c.p.s. to above 200 c.p.s. (The frequencies of murmurs may be

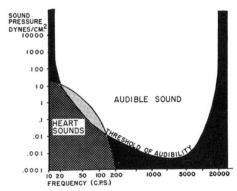

FIGURE   10–12 AUDIBILITY   OF   VARIOUS
                    FREQUENCIES

The threshold of audibility varies for different sound frequencies. The auditory mechanism is far more sensitive to frequencies in the speech range (1000 to 2000 c.p.s.) than to sounds of either higher or lower pitch. The heart sounds are primarily low-frequency vibrations. Only a portion of the vibrations have sufficient intensity to reach the auditory threshold, the remainder being completely inaudible. Certain high-pitched murmurs reach frequencies of 1000 c.p.s. and can be perceived even when the sound energy is relatively slight.

as high as 600 to 1000 c.p.s.) Owing to extreme lack of sensitivity to low-frequency vibrations, the auditory mechanism may perceive relatively weak overtones of heart sounds more clearly than the more intense low-frequency fundamental vibrations. Thus, the low-frequency vibrations, which are most easily recorded electronically, may constitute only a portion of the heart sounds which are heard during auscultation.

When listening to sounds of a particular frequency, the human hearing apparatus responds to sounds of very low and very high energy. At certain frequencies the energy level of the threshold for pain is more than three million times that for the threshold of audibility. This tremendous range of perceptible intensity is possible because the perceived "loudness" is proportional to the logarithm of the stimulus strength. In other words, if the sound intensity is doubled successively, the "loudness" of the sensation increases in equal steps. Thus, the auditory mechanism can respond to a tremendous range of sound energies while retaining sensitivity to sounds of very low intensity.

In complex sounds, the low-pitched tones often seem more prominent because the higher pitched tones become masked. This phenomenon is more marked when the intensity of the low tones is increased. Thus, the quality of sounds may be affected by any factor which alters the intensity.

The human ear can select desired signals from many other frequency patterns, as in detecting the sound of an oboe in a symphony orchestra. The brain can store sound patterns for future recognition so that we can improve our performance on repeated trials.

The remarkable properties of the hearing mechanism are readily demon-strated by merely closing one's eyes and listening to sounds coming from the environment. When one recognizes sounds such as a familiar voice, the click of a door latch, the rustle of paper or the scuff of a shoe on a carpet, one is effortlessly accomplishing functions beyond the most complex computer available.

The higher frequencies found in diastolic murmurs can often be brought out by judicious use of the stethoscope, selectively attenuating the low frequencies.

STETHOSCOPES. Heart sounds can be readily heard by placing the ear directly on the chest of the patient. Stethoscopes are employed for the sake of convenience and propriety rather than to amplify the sound. A critical evaluation[26] disclosed that the Laennec stethoscope (a straight rigid tube) is just as good as modern stethoscopes and may be somewhat better, except for convenience and utilization of both ears.

Sounds are both damped and distorted by stethoscopes. Various types of stethoscopes exhibit marked differences in their efficiency at transmission of cardiovascular sounds,[28] as determined by length of transmission pathway, diameter and stiffness of tubing and especially the seal at the chest wall and in the ear. When an open bell is applied to the chest, the skin forms a diaphragm while the underlying tissues act as a damping medium.[27] If the bell is held firmly against the skin, the low frequencies are attenuated more than the higher frequencies, which seem louder even though their actual sound energy is diminished. A similar effect can be produced by using a Bowles type stethoscope with a plastic diaphragm covering the air chamber. In any case, the presence of a taut diaphragm produces attenuation of the low frequencies which is useful in

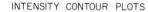

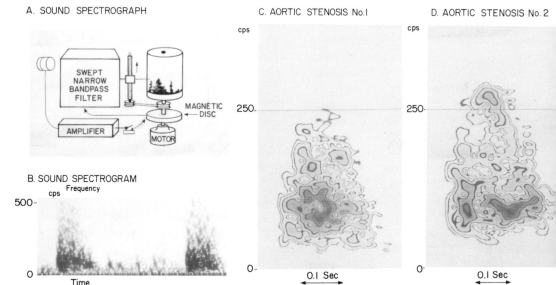

FIGURE 10-13   EXTRACTING INFORMATION FROM SOUNDS

A, To produce a sound spectrogram, a short sample of the sounds are recorded on a magnetic disc and repeatedly rerecorded through a series of filters to produce a record of the sound intensity at different frequencies.

B, The time sequence is on the horizontal axis, the frequency scale is on the vertical axis and the intensity of sound at any time is displayed as gradations of darkness on the record.

Sound intensity contour plots (*C* and *D*) indicate the variations in intensity on a record resembling a contour map to illustrate the differences between murmurs from two different patients with aortic stenosis.

detecting the high-pitched diastolic murmurs but undesirable in eliciting faint, low-pitched murmurs. It is not generally recognized that properly fitting ear pieces on stethoscopes are extremely important since a leak with a diameter approximately five times that of a human hair may markedly reduce perception of heart sounds and murmurs.[29]

Lepeschkin[30] devised a most ingenious quantitative stethoscope with an adjustable orifice in the chest piece so that sound intensity may be graded far more accurately than by purely subjective impression.

Phonocardiography. Verbal descriptions of sounds (e.g., harsh, coarse, ringing) are notoriously inadequate. For this reason, phonocardiography affords a common meeting ground for

the discussion of heart sounds. The temporal relations between the heart sounds and the mechanical events of the cardiac cycle are of paramount importance in the interpretation of the significance of sounds and murmurs. In this sphere, phonocardiography makes its greatest contribution.

The heart sounds are so attenuated and modified by transmission through various media and by the vagaries of auditory perception that it is manifestly impossible to produce heart sound records which match the sounds heard during auscultation.

Typical phonocardiograms are oscillograph recordings (see Fig. 10–10) which are very useful in assessing the time relations of sounds and murmurs. They fail to give any impression of actual sound frequencies or qualities.

More comprehensive sound pattern displays can now be accomplished by sound spectograms which indicate the time-varying fluctuations in both intensity and frequency. The underlying principle of the sound spectrogram is illustrated schematically in Figure 10–13A. The intensity of the various frequencies at any moment in time is indicated by the density of the record. (Fig. 10–13B) More quantitative indication of the intensity is displayed by contour plots which show increasing intensity as contours at 3 or 6 decibel steps (Fig. 10–13C, D). The advantages have been described by Winer et al.[31]

II. MURMURS

Heart sounds which are normal attributes of cardiac function are distinctively different from murmurs with reference to both origin and functional significance. Some murmurs are audible in normal individuals while others are indicators of structural abnormalities in the heart.

In the preceding discussion, the origination of heart sounds has been ascribed to vibrations induced by sudden displacement of blood (acceleration) or by abrupt cessation of flow (deceleration). In contrast, heart murmurs are defined here as the result of turbulence developing in rapidly flowing blood. These definitions provide clear, functional and physical distinctions between the heart sounds and murmurs. Since the causes of turbulence are well known, the source of most murmurs should be explicable simply and logically. The pathologic conditions which predispose toward such turbulence are well established for most types of murmurs. Certain murmurs have no satisfactory explanation at present, simply because we lack essential information concerning conditions in the heart producing these vibrations.

CAUSES OF TURBULENCE IN FLOWING BLOOD

The flow of blood through virtually all vascular channels of the body produces no audible sound unless a constriction of partial occlusion produces disturbances of flow or turbulence. The conditions producing turbulence in fluid flowing through tubes of constant caliber are expressed in the formula RVD/v = critical constant for turbulence (Reynolds' number), where a fluid of viscosity v and density D flows with a mean velocity V through a tube of radius R. This formula indicates that turbulence occurs when fluids of low viscosity flow at high velocity through tubes of large diameter (Fig. 10–14). Since the blood viscosity and the vascular diameter are relatively constant, the major variable is the velocity of blood flow. The critical level of Reynolds' number for turbulence in blood is reported as 970 ± 80. Blood flows rapidly through the largest arterial channels and at the highest velocity in the roots of the aorta and the pulmonary artery. The critical level for turbulence is normally exceeded at these sites during the rapid ejection phase of ventricular systole. On this basis, the vibrations usually classified as the fourth component of the first heart sound are probably caused by turbulence and are actually an early systolic murmur according to the definitions being used here. Thus, virtually all persons have an early systolic murmur, even though its duration and intensity are insufficient for its detection (see *Functional Murmurs*).

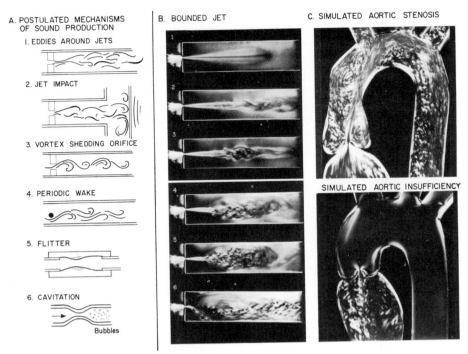

FIGURE 10-14   CAUSE OF MURMURS

A, The mechanisms of sound production most commonly postulated include vibrations from eddies produced by jets, the impact of jets on vascular walls, vortex shedding and periodic wakes. Occurrences of flitter and cavitation have been postulated but are not readily confirmed *in vivo*.

B, The unstable flow and eddy currents produced by jets are displayed by means of a birefringent suspension.

C, The turbulent patterns that might occur with aortic stenosis or insufficiency are indicated by flow models.

Experience has shown that murmurs are most commonly produced just downstream from some sort of obstruction in large vascular channels. However, many different mechanisms have been postulated as sources of murmurs produced within the heart or in major arteries near the heart, based on models or by analogy with various sound sources such as musical instruments, turbulent jets or fluid dynamic phenomena. Some of the most familiar hypotheses are present schematically in Figure 10-14A.

1. By far the most common concept is the sound produced in the vicinity of a rapidly flowing jet of blood emerging from a restricted orifice. Sounds produced by jets tend to be noises composed of random mixtures of frequencies rather than pure tones.

2. A jet impacting a wall or partition can theoretically produce vibrations as might occur on the arterial wall opposite a patent ductus arteriosus or where a regurgitant jet from a faulty mitral valve might strike the atrial wall. Endothelial thickening and patches of atherosclerosis are prone to develop at such sites of impact (Fig. 10-14A2).

3. When liquids flow at relatively slow rates through an orifice, oscillations may develop which produce sounds with a distinct tonal quality. These are ascribed to fluctuations of a jet accompanying shedding vortices.

As trains of vortices are shed, relatively intense tones with fundamental frequencies and harmonics may be produced. They may excite resonance in surrounding structures. When the flow velocity is increased, the tones are replaced by the random frequency noises characterized by high speed jets illustrated in Figure 10–14A1.

4. Liquids flowing around an obstruction in a channel may produce a periodic wake (Fig. 10–14A4) as they alternately flow on either side of such an obstruction. The mechanism is responsible for the Aeolian tones produced in ancient times by the movement of air around cylinders mounted on hilltops. The resulting sounds in air approach pure tones, but corresponding phenomena in the cardiovascular system have not been unequivocally demonstrated. This mechanism could play a role in the production of "musical murmurs," but the suggestion by Bruns[34] that they constitute a general theory of murmur production fails to account for the common types of "noisy" murmurs.

5. The Bernoulli effect on fluids flowing through collapsible tubes may produce a fluttering motion of the walls, called flitter. Such phenomena have been produced in models but corresponding observations have not been made in blood vascular channels.

6. Cavitation can be produced by high speed jets in models. This is a well-known mechanism for producing noise but seems intuitively improbable under conditions found in the cardiovascular system.

To select the most likely causes of murmurs from these diverse postulates requires an appreciation of the characteristics of sounds emitted as murmurs. The most common types of murmurs are highly nonspecific, consisting of noises or random frequencies without obvious fundamental or harmonic frequencies. A most convincing demonstration of this fact can be achieved by the simulation of murmurs by a wide variety of sound sources. For example, a group of freshman medical students were presented with tape recordings of typical heart murmurs from patients with known cardiac lesions. The students were challenged to duplicate these murmurs by any technique of sound production they could conjure up. They found a very large number of procedures that produced tape-recorded sounds that could be distinguished from murmurs with the greatest of difficulty.

Three of the most successful procedures for simulating specific murmurs are illustrated in Figure 10–15. The murmur of ventricular septal defect was quite accurately simulated by holding a contact microphone against the palm and stroking a hand brush across the skin nearby. The "heart" sound was simulated by a light tap of the brush. The closest simulation was attained by artificially interposing the sounds produced by a random noise generator between normal heart sounds by means of special gating techniques. The simulated murmur illustrated in Figure 10–15D was essentially impossible to distinguish by ear from the murmur of aortic stenosis in Figure 10–15C. A "blowing" type murmur was easily simulated by a stream of air blown onto a microphone. This nonspecific character of heart murmurs is the basis for the recent development of heart sound simulators.

Based on such observations, the most likely theory is that heart murmurs develop in the vicinity of turbulent jets produced by liquid flowing at high velocity through narrow orifices. Experiments conducted in this laboratory by Meisner and Rushmer[35, 36] and by Yellin[37] have thrown some light on

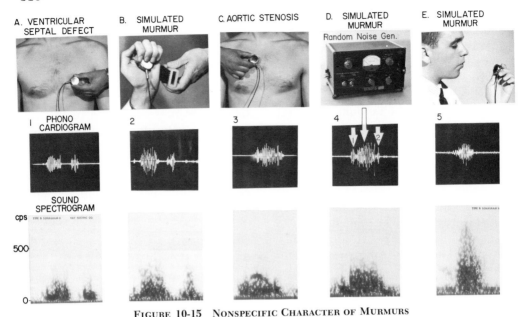

A. VENTRICULAR SEPTAL DEFECT   B. SIMULATED MURMUR   C. AORTIC STENOSIS   D. SIMULATED MURMUR Random Noise Gen.   E. SIMULATED MURMUR

1 PHONO CARDIOGRAM   2   3   4   5

SOUND SPECTROGRAM

cps

500

0

FIGURE 10-15   NONSPECIFIC CHARACTER OF MURMURS

Heart murmurs can be simulated by a variety of techniques, including rubbing a brush on a palm, holding a microphone (B) or by interposing random noise between normal heart sounds (D) or even by blowing on a microphone (E). (See text.)

sound production in liquids. Aqueous suspensions of white Hector bentonite flowing through channels illuminated by polarized light display differences in light intensity in regions of disturbed flow and eddy currents. Fluid flowing through narrow orifices in flat models form an expanding jet. The changes in the shape of the expanding jet and the distribution of the eddies with increasing flow velocity in the channel are shown in Figure 10-14B. As flow velocities increase, the jet expands and attaches to the wall at considerable distances downstream from the orifice.

Yellin[37] used a phonocatheter to record the pressure fluctuations in and around jets of the type visualized in Figure 10-14. The phonocatheter picked up loud signals within and at the boundaries of liquid jets. The signals picked up by the phonocatheter diminished rapidly as it was moved away from the jet. Upstream from the orifice, no signals were detectable. These observations indicate that the possibility that the jet is producing compression waves conducted through the fluid and the vascular walls must be discounted. Compression waves are transmitted over much greater distances through liquids. Instead, the possibility must be considered that vascular noise results from the impact of eddies on the walls downstream from an orifice (Fig. 10-14B4). These fluctuations in local pressure appear to strike the walls in random sequence (like rain on the roof) to produce wall vibrations without dominant frequencies. The local vibrations of vascular walls might then be transmitted through the surrounding tissues to the surface of the body.

In contrast, the rare musical murmurs are probably due to mechanisms like vortex shedding or periodic wake fluctuations which produce tones under special combinations of geometry and flow rates. This would account for their low incidence and distinctive characteristics.

CONSISTENCY IN DETECTION OF MURMURS BY AUSCULTATION

The consistency of the most elemental auscultatory findings reported under controlled conditions by experienced physicians has proved to be unexpectedly poor. For example, Dobrow et al.[39] presented tape-recorded heart sounds from 100 selected patients to five well qualified physicians. The physicians were asked three questions: (1) is a murmur present? (2) is a systolic murmur present? (3) is a diastolic murmur present? The responses, summarized in part in Table 10-1, indicate a surprisingly high proportion of disagreement with a standard. Butterworth and Reppert[40] reported that 523 physicians at an A.M.A. convention correctly identified only about half of 15 of the "simplest examples we could find in our library of heart sounds."

Table 10-1. **PHYSICIAN VARIATION IN HEART SOUND INTERPRETATION** (*After Dobrow* et al.[39])

QUESTION	AGREE-MENT WITH STAND-ARD	FALSE POSI-TIVES	FALSE NEGA-TIVES
Is a murmur present?	74%	21%	44%
Is a systolic murmur present?	71%	22%	44%
Is a diastolic murmur present?	79%	55%	7%

FUNCTIONAL MURMURS

Vibrations during the early ejection phase of ventricular systole occur in virtually all individuals, even though murmurs cannot always be heard (Fig. 10-16A). Early systolic murmurs can be heard in a large proportion of children, particularly those with thin chest walls. In these individuals, all the heart sounds are loud because so little energy is lost in transmission to the surface. The "normal systolic murmur" can be recorded in practically all normal adults at rest if suitable equipment is used in a sound-damped room. Such murmurs are classified as functional and are most commonly heard at the pulmonary area on the precordium. Although the velocity of flow through both the pulmonary artery and the aorta is sufficient to produce turbulence in early systole, certain additional factors present in the outflow tract of the right ventricle are generally overlooked (Fig. 10-16B).

Audible, early systolic murmurs are usually produced by the increased velocity of flow in almost all normal persons following vigorous exercise, particularly if the subject leans forward and holds his breath after a forced exhalation. In patients with anemia, "hemic" murmurs develop because the viscosity of the blood is diminished while the flow velocity is accelerated owing to an increase in cardiac output.

SYSTOLIC MURMURS DUE TO VALVULAR ABNORMALITY

Detection and recognition of heart murmurs is a valuable source of information concerning the function of heart valves. Although the mechanisms producing these sounds are very similar, certain types of valvular dis-

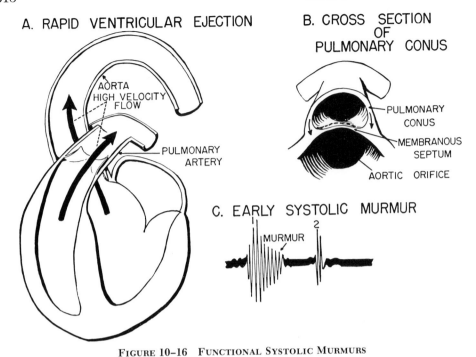

A. RAPID VENTRICULAR EJECTION

B. CROSS SECTION
OF
PULMONARY CONUS

C. EARLY SYSTOLIC MURMUR

FIGURE 10–16 FUNCTIONAL SYSTOLIC MURMURS

A, Under normal conditions, blood flows through the aorta and pulmonary arteries at sufficient velocity to produce turbulence during the rapid ejection phase of ventricular systole. Early systolic murmurs can be heard in many normal children at rest and in nearly any normal subject after exercise.

B, The right ventricular outflow tract has a roughly crescentic cross-sectional area, partly because the membranous portion of the interventricular septum bulges into the lumen. Bundles of myocardial fibers, encircling the conus region, tend to further diminish the cross-sectional area of this channel during systole. For these reasons, turbulence is more likely to develop in the pulmonary artery than in the aorta. Systolic murmurs in normal subjects usually have maximal intensity in the pulmonary area on the precordium.

C, An early systolic "functional" murmur may be regarded as an intensified fourth component of the first heart sound.

ease produce typical sound patterns which can be distinguished on the basis of frequency, transmission and timing.

Aortic Stenosis. The aortic valve lies at a considerable distance from the precordium. Vibrations from this source reach the precordium after transmission directly from the ascending aorta (aortic area), through the pulmonary artery and conus (third left intercostal space) or through the ventricles toward the apex of the heart. Systolic murmurs of aortic origin have been clearly demonstrated in the broad area indicated in Figure 10–17C.

Thus, aortic murmurs may be localized at various points on the precordium along a line paralleling the outflow tract of the left ventricle. Systolic murmurs of early aortic stenosis may be evidenced only in the pulmonary area and may be difficult to differentiate from functional murmurs. Levine[41] emphasized the fact that these murmurs tend to have maximum intensity in the mid-systolic period and used this criterion to differentiate such murmurs from functional, pulmonary or mitral systolic murmurs.

Pulmonary Stenosis. Uncomplicated pulmonary stenosis, either con-

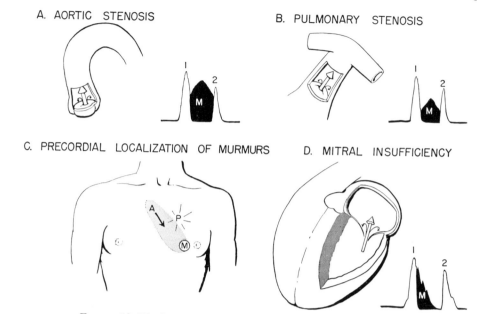

FIGURE 10-17   SYSTOLIC MURMURS FROM VASCULAR DEFORMITY

A, Aortic stenosis produces a membranous obstruction with a small orifice through which blood is ejected at high velocity during systole. The resulting systolic murmur tends to reach maximum intensity in mid-systole and is usually transmitted primarily to the aortic area. In different patients, the region of maximal intensity may occur anywhere in an area extending from the second left intercostal space toward the apex of the heart.

B, Pulmonary stenosis produces a loud systolic murmur extending through the systolic interval, although the intensity is often greatest immediately after the first sound and diminishes progressively. The murmur is transmitted widely over the entire precordium.

C, The surface localization of systolic murmurs originating from various valves is indicated schematically (see also Fig. 10-11).

D, Mitral insufficiency produces systolic murmurs with maximum intensity near the apex of the heart.

genital or acquired, is relatively rare. Fusion of the pulmonary leaflets produces a local constriction beyond which turbulence occurs during systolic ejection from the right ventricle (Fig. 10-17*B*). The resultant loud, harsh, systolic murmur usually resembles the murmur of aortic stenosis. Such murmurs are heard most loudly in the pulmonary area and are widely transmitted over the precordium. Pulmonary stenosis is usually due to a congenital malformation.

Mitral Insufficiency. If for any reason the mitral valve cusps fail to occlude the mitral orifice completely, blood rushes through the defect during ventricular systole, propelled by the large pressure difference between the left ventricle and left atrium. The gap between the valve cusps acts as a local constriction through which the blood squirts at high velocity into the capacious atrial chamber (Fig. 10-17*D*). The resulting turbulence produces an apical systolic murmur which is ordinarily widely transmitted, particularly toward the left axillary region.

DIASTOLIC MURMURS DUE TO VALVULAR ABNORMALITY

Mitral Stenosis. The blood flows rapidly from the atria into the ventricles during the early filling period and during atrial systole. The fact that the diastolic period is normally quiet indicates that the velocity of flow is insufficient to induce significant turbulence and that the mitral and tricuspid orifices do not constitute a local constriction. Thus, diastolic murmurs are rarely encountered unless there is some form of organic disease.

Rheumatic valvulitis may convert the efficient, flexible mitral valves into a rigid funnel with a narrow elliptical orifice. This local constriction between large chambers satisfies all the requirements for the production of turbulence if blood flow attains sufficient velocity (Fig. 10–18A). The sequence of events leading to advanced stenosis will be discussed in Chapter 14. A low frequency murmur which immediately precedes the first sound is the classic finding in mitral stenosis. In the early stages, this presystolic murmur can be easily missed since it is often localized to a very small area at or near the apical region on the precordium. The murmur may be audible only when the patient reclines in the left lateral position or after exertion. The low-pitched "rumble" seems to gather intensity and terminate in an accentuated first sound. Since this murmur frequently disappears in patients who develop atrial fibrillation, its presence has been attributed to rapid flow through the stenosed valve during atrial contraction.

In many cases of mitral stenosis, an early diastolic murmur predominates. This murmur occurs during the phase of rapid filling and attains maximum intensity shortly after the second sound. Thereafter, the murmur usually diminishes in intensity, frequently disappearing during the mid-diastolic period (see Chapter 14).

In many patients, the murmur appears to develop maximum intensity in mid-diastole. This is probably due to two factors: (a) A very slight interval between the second sound and the initial vibrations of the murmur gives a mistaken impression that the peak intensity occurs later than is revealed on heart sound records. (b) In some patients the rapid filling period may be prolonged because resistance is offered by the restricted orifice. The vibrations have such low frequency that they frequently escape detection by auscultation even when the recorded deflections appear large on phonocardiograms.

Pulmonary Insufficiency. Dilation of the pulmonary artery due to sustained pulmonary hypertension may render the pulmonary valves incompetent. When the pulmonary valves fail to approximate, a diastolic murmur becomes audible in the pulmonary area.

Pulmonary valvular insufficiency permits the regurgitation of blood during the diastolic interval, which accounts for the diastolic murmur. The regurgitant stream flows rapidly through slits between the valve cusps and enters a large ventricular chamber (see Fig. 10–18B).

Aortic Insufficiency. Aortic insufficiency without stenosis generally results from cardiovascular syphilis (Fig. 10–18C). Systolic murmurs generally accompany the diastolic murmur because the regurgitation increases the rate and volume of ventricular ejection. Combined systolic and diastolic murmurs resemble the sounds produced by sawing wood with a hand saw, the systolic murmur representing the cutting stroke and the higher pitched diastolic murmur corresponding to the back stroke.

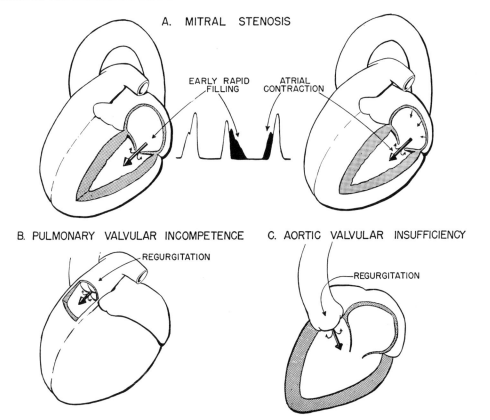

FIGURE 10–18   DIASTOLIC MURMURS FROM VALVULAR DEFORMITY

A, Mitral stenosis produces murmurs occurring primarily during rapid flow through the mitral valve: during rapid ventricular filling in early diastole and during atrial systole. The murmur has a very low frequency and may be difficult to hear even though the sound intensity is great. The early diastolic murmurs tend to be localized fairly discretely at the apex of the heart.

B, Pulmonary insufficiency permits regurgitation of blood into the right ventricle during diastole. The resulting murmur tends to have maximum intensity in the pulmonary area but is often transmitted over a wide area on the precordium.

C, Aortic insufficiency tends to produce high-pitched diastolic murmurs usually heard best in the aortic area but occasionally most intense in the pulmonary area or even near the apex of the heart.

THE SIGNIFICANCE OF PALPABLE THRILLS

Vibrations produced by murmurs occasionally have such great intensity that they may be palpated on the surface of the chest. In comparison to auditory perception, the tactile vibratory sense is extremely insensitive. The palpation of a thrill indicates the great intensity of the vibrations but provides no information of diagnostic significance that is not gained by auscultation.[42]

VARIABILITY IN DETECTION OF HEART MURMURS

Whenever a group of physicians gather beside a patient with cardiac disease, differences of opinion concerning the auscultatory findings almost invariably arise. Such controversies result from differences in auditory acuity, training and the technique of listening, complicated by the extreme difficulty of describing auditory sensations. When examiners are confronted with patients with advanced heart disease, the differences of opinion are lessened but are by no means eliminated. Recognition of the limitations of auscultation is the first step toward its maximal effective use as a diagnostic tool. The most common deficiency is the inability to perceive certain low-frequency sounds. For example, many examiners consistently miss third heart sounds or low-frequency diastolic murmurs. Timing of murmurs by auscultation also presents problems to some clinicians. Although some of the difficulties may result from depressed auditory acuity, an improper approach to auscultation is frequently the source of the trouble.

A SYSTEMATIC APPROACH TO AUSCULTATION

The body is continuously bombarded by sensory stimuli of all kinds, but their entry into consciousness must be restricted to one at a time to make any order out of chaos. It is impossible to listen attentively and still be acutely aware of visual images, odors, proprioceptive stimuli or pain. If an attempt is made to concentrate on two things simultaneously, attention rapidly shifts from one to the other with little detailed information being gained from either source. Thus, the ability to concentrate on a single source of stimuli is an essential characteristic of human perception. Similarly, innumerable complex sound waves impinge continuously upon the ear, but most of these sounds fail to reach consciousness. While you read

these words you are probably ignoring the sounds in your immediate environment.

However, undivided attention is insufficient for accurate auscultation. If an examiner listens to all the noises emitted by the heart, his attention is usually directed toward the most intense sounds, which may not be the most meaningful. It is necessary to utilize a high degree of "selective" attention to gain the maximum information from auscultation. Consider how many common sounds can be identified as coming from a specific source such as a nearby radio, a familiar voice, the sound of a car, the creak of a chair or foot steps. Some of these vibrations are sustained, others are intermittent and still others may occur singly, but if they are familiar, their source can be immediately recognized. The ability to synthesize combinations of complex sound waves and overtones into patterns which can be identified represents an important attribute of audition. As an example, a symphony orchestra emits sound waves having a wide range of frequencies of almost inconceivable complexity. One can listen to the music as a harmonic entity made up of sounds from all the instruments. On the other hand, the sounds produced by a single instrument may be extracted from this mass of complex sound waves by merely directing attention toward them. The conductor is constantly alert to tones which are off beat or out of tune. He can instantly fix the offender with a malevolent glance. By a similar process, heart sounds and murmurs can be analyzed individually and assigned their proper temporal relationship within the cardiac cycle. The following routine has proved valuable in this regard.

SELECTIVE ATTENTION
DURING AUSCULTATION

The most convenient initial step is positive identification of the first heart sound. If the stethoscope is placed near the apex, the timing of the first sound can be correlated with the precordial thrust. When the identity of the first sound is definitely established, attention should be confined to this sound alone during several successive cycles. If the listener voluntarily blanks out all other sounds in the cycle, the first sound can be subjectively isolated. Several characteristics of the first sound should be noted individually and in sequence, including intensity, duration, relative frequency or pitch, splitting and so forth. The loudness of the sound must be interpreted in light of judgment concerning the transmission characteristics and hemodynamic situation of the individual subject. For example, a loud first sound in an obese subject has far greater significance than one of a similar intensity in an asthenic adult or a thin-chested youth. The intensity of the vibrations is also affected by the vigor of the ventricular contraction, the heart rate, the cardiac output, the P-R interval and similar factors. The relative intensity of the first and second sounds provides an additional clue concerning these factors.

The next step is to direct attention solely to the second sound for a period sufficient to establish its characteristics. The loudness of the first sound and second sound can then be compared, but a final decision concerning this observation should be deferred until other areas of the precordium have been examined. At this stage, the first and second sounds at the apex should be so familiar that they can be recognized without reference to the apex beat.

A systematic search for murmurs is initiated by directing attention solely to the interval which follows each first sound. Little experience is required to focus on this interval without actually hearing the first sound. Listening first for low-pitched sounds and then for high-pitched sounds is a good policy because attention is so discrete that involuntary anticipation of low-frequency vibrations may cause one to overlook a high-pitched murmur. Having ascertained that the early systolic interval is either quiet or occupied by a murmur, attention is next directed toward the later portions of systole. If a murmur is present during either of these portions of systole, the attention can then be spread to include the whole of the systolic interval to determine the time at which the murmur reaches maximum intensity. This technique is the best way to differentiate early systolic murmurs from mid-systolic and late systolic murmurs.

The diastolic interval is scanned in the same way. Attention is directed first to the interval immediately following the second sound. Focusing the attention on the early diastolic interval during a succession of beats is extremely important because it provides the only hope of detecting third heart sounds or early diastolic gallop, the "opening snap" of mitral stenosis and certain early diastolic murmurs. It is even more important to listen for both low-pitched and high-pitched sounds during this interval.

The period just preceding the first sound is then selectively analyzed. For many individuals this is the most difficult step of all because there is no specific stimulus for "turning on" the attention during each cycle. If

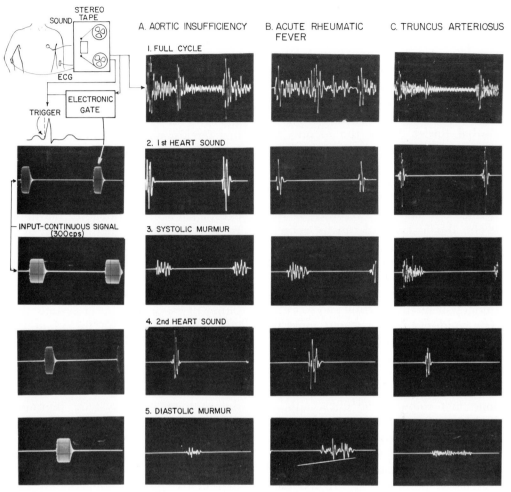

FIGURE 10–19   TIME SAMPLING BY ELECTRONIC GATING

Selective auscultation can be simulated by an electronic gate triggered by the electrocardiogram and set to open at a particular time in each cardiac cycle allowing the observer to hear in turn the heart sounds and murmurs in systole and diastole as illustrated in cases of (A) aortic insufficiency, (B) acute rheumatic fever and (C) truncus arteriosus.

the heart is beating regularly, this difficulty can be easily overcome because the rhythm is established. With practice, the presystolic interval can be scanned even in the presence of arrhythmia. Similarly, the process of directing selective attention to a particular interval while voluntarily blanking out all others is more difficult during tachycardia. This technique is not only applicable but absolutely essential when the heart is beating rapidly or irregularly.

When a detailed analysis of the heart sounds and murmurs at the apex has been completed, the same process is repeated in the pulmonary, the aortic and the tricuspid areas. If a murmur is recognized in any of the intervals, the region of maximum intensity and the extent of transmission should be established. By limiting attention only to the murmur in question, these characteristics can be determined very quickly by systematically listening over a sequence of points around the primary areas. It is frequently desirable to establish the relative intensities of the heart sounds and murmurs by going back over each area in quick succession, evaluating each sound in turn. This is accomplished rapidly if the sounds have become familiar during the more careful analysis in each area.

The process of selective auscultation can be simulated by an adjustable electronic gate which can be triggered by the electrocardiogram and opened at any desired time in each successive cardiac cycle.[43] By adjusting the opening time of this "gate" the observer can hear in sequence the first heart sound, the second heart sound, early or late systole and early or late diastole as illustrated in Figure 10–19.

When this technique is recommended to medical students, they commonly express concern regarding their ability to accomplish this task. In most cases, these doubts can be alleviated by suggesting that they produce schematic drawings of what they hear. It is very helpful to compare such drawings with phonocardiograms at first. Even experienced examiners agree that the process of schematically drawing subjective impressions of sounds and murmurs can be a valuable experience.

A second objection to systematic auscultation of the type described is the increased expenditure of time. There is no doubt that this technique is more time-consuming, particularly at first. However, routine use of the method rapidly improves proficiency. After a few weeks of concentrated effort, analysis of heart sounds and murmurs can become complete and accurate with little wasted time. With experience it is possible to scan each phase of the cardiac cycle in turn by listening to only a few cycles during each step. The time and effort spent are amply rewarded by striking improvement in accuracy of auscultatory diagnosis. After many years of unsystematic auscultation, many examiners begin to recognize certain types of murmurs for the first time by taking advantage of dormant ability to focus attention on specific intervals of time.

SUMMARY

Heart sounds and murmurs are audible vibrations emitted from the heart and great vessels. Since the walls of the heart cannot vibrate without setting the blood into vibration, and vice versa, the origin of heart sounds was described in terms of oscillations induced by abrupt changes in velocity of the blood (due to closure of valves and so forth). Heart murmurs occur in rapidly flowing blood and can be attributed to turbulence. Turbulence occurs in fluids of low viscosity flowing rapidly through tubes of large caliber. The velocity required to induce turbulence is greatly diminished by local obstructions in a tube, causing fluid to flow through a small orifice into a large channel or chamber. Most heart murmurs can be readily explained on the basis of high velocity flow or abrupt changes in caliber of the vascular channels. These mechanisms obviously apply to systolic and diastolic murmurs, produced by valvular deformities.

REFERENCES

1. BROCK, R. C. The surgical and pathological anatomy of the mitral valve. *Brit. Heart J.*, 14:489–513, 1952.
2. HENDERSON, Y., and JOHNSON, F. E. Two

modes of closure of the heart valves. *Heart*, 4:69–82, 1912.

3. DEAN, A. L., JR. The movements of the mitral cusps in relation to the cardiac cycle. *Amer. J. Physiol.*, 40:206–217, 1916.

4. ESSEX, H. E., SMITH, H. L., and BALDES, E. J. Origin of the heart sounds (motion picture with sound recording). *Fed. Proc.*, 12:40, 1953.

5. SMITH, H. L., ESSEX, H. E., and BALDES, E. J. A study of the movements of heart valves and of heart sounds. *Ann. Intern. Med.*, 33:1357–1359, 1950.

6. RUSHMER, R. F., FINLAYSON, B. L., and NASH, A. A. Movements of the mitral valve. *Circulat. Res.*, 4:337–342, 1956.

7. RUSHMER, R. F., ELLIS, R. M., and NASH, A. A. Stereo-cinefluorography. Motion roentgenography in three dimensions. *Radiology*, 64:191–196, 1955.

8. DI BARTOLO, G., NUNEZ-DEY, E., MUISAN, G., MACCANON, D. M., and LUISADA, A. A. Hemodynamic correlates of the first heart sound. *Amer. J. Physiol.*, 201:888–892, 1961.

9. BROCKMAN, S. K. Mechanism of movements of atrioventricular valves. *Amer. J. Cardiol.*, 17:682–690, 1966.

10. YOSHITOSHI, Y., SEKIGUCHI, H., MACHII, K., MISHINA, Y., and OHTA, S. Measurement of the maximal velocity of mitral-valve closure and of the anterior ventricular wall movement by ultrasonic Doppler's method. *Digest of 6th Internatl. Conf. Med. Electronics and Biol. Eng.*, 35–36, 1965.

11. MCKUSICK, V. A. *Cardiovascular Sounds in Health and Disease.* Baltimore, The Williams and Wilkins Co., 1958, vii, 570 pp.

12. SHEARN, M. A., TARR, E., and RYTAND, D. A. The significance of changes in amplitude of the first heart sound in children with A-V block. *Circulation*, 7:839–846, 1953.

13. WOLFERTH, C. C., and MARGOLIES, A. The influence of auricular contraction on the first heart sound and the radial pulse. *Arch. Intern. Med.*, 46:1048–1071, 1930.

14. RYTAND, D. A. The variable loudness of the first heart sound in auricular fibrillation. *Amer. Heart J.*, 37:187–204, 1949.

15. LITTLE, R. C., and HILTON, J. G. Effect of ectopic ventricular contractions on the first heart sound. *Fed. Proc.*, 12:89, 1953.

16. PIEMME, T. E., BARNETT, G. O., and DEXTER, L. Relationship of heart sounds to acceleration of blood flow. *Circulat. Res.*, 18:303–315, 1966.

17. LEATHAM, A. Splitting of the first and second heart sounds. *Lancet*, 2:607–614, 1954.

18. KUSUKAWA, R., BRUCE, E. W., SAKAMOTO, T., MACCANON, E. M., and LUISADA, A. A. Hemodynamic determinants of the amplitude of second sound. *J. Appl. Physiol.*, 21:938–946, 1966.

19. MACCANON, E. M., AREVALO, F., and MEYER, E. C. Direct detection and timing of aortic valve closure. *Circulat. Res.*, 14:387–391, 1964.

20. DUNN, F. L., and DICKERSON, W. J. Third heart sound: possible role of pericardium in its production. *Circulat. Res.*, 3:51–55, 1955.

21. FABER, J. J., and BURTON, A. C. Spread of heart sounds over the chest wall. *Circulat. Res.*, 11:96–107, 1962.

22. ZALTER, R., HARDY, H. C., and LUISADA, A. A. Acoustic transmission characteristics of the thorax. *J. Appl. Physiol.*, 18:428–436, 1963.

23. FOLEY, A. D. *College Physics*, 3rd ed. Philadelphia, The Blakiston Co., 1941.

24. WIRT, L. S. The perfect instrument. *Instrument Control Syst.*, 38:136–139, 1965.

25. STEVENS, S. S., and DAVIS, H. *Hearing, Its Psychology and Physiology.* New York, John Wiley & Sons, Inc., 1938, 489 pp.

26. ERTEL, P. Y., LAWRENCE, M., BROWN, R. K., and STERN, A. M. Stethoscope acoustics I. The doctor and his stethoscope. *Circulation*, 34:889–908, 1966.

27. RAPPAPORT, M. B., and SPRAGUE, H. B. Physiologic and physical laws that govern ausculation, and their clinical application. The acoustic stethoscope and electrical amplifying stethoscope and stethograph. *Amer. Heart J.*, 21:257–318, 1941.

28. GROOM, E. Comparative efficiency of stethoscopes. *Amer. Heart J.*, 68:220–226, 1964.

29. RAPPAPORT, M. B., and SPRAGUE, H. B. The effects of improper fitting of stethoscope to ears on ausculatory efficiency. *Amer. Heart J.*, 43:713–715, 1952.

30. LEPESCHKIN, E. A quantitative stethoscope and its clinical applications. *Amer. Heart J.*, 43:881–888, 1952.

31. WINER, D. E., PERRY, L. W., and CACERES, C. A. Heart sound analysis: a three dimensional approach. *Amer. J. Cardiol.*, 16:547–551, 1965.

32. COULTER, N. A., JR., and PAPPENHEIMER, J. R. Development of turbulence in flowing blood. *Amer. J. Physiol.*, 159:483–491, 1949.

33. WISKIND, H. K., and TALBOT, S. A. Physical basis of cardiovascular sound; an analytical survey. U.S. Air Force Off. Sci. Res. Tech. Rep. No. TR. 58–160, 1958.

34. BRUNS, D. L. A general theory of the causes of murmurs in the cardiovascular system. *Amer. J. Med.*, 27:360–374, 1959.

35. RUSHMER, R. F., and MORGAN, C. L. Meaning of murmurs. *Amer. J. Cardiol.*, 21:722–730, 1968.

36. MEISNER, J. E., and RUSHMER, R. F. Eddy formation and turbulence in flowing liquid. *Circulat. Res.*, 12:455–463, 1963.

37. MEISNER, J. E., and RUSHMER, R. F. Production of sounds in distensible tubes. *Circulat. Res.*, 12:651–658, 1963.

38. YELLIN, E. L. Sound production in bounded jets. *Biomedical-Fluid Mechanics Symposium.* New York, The American Society of Mechanical Engineers, 1966.

39. DOBROW, R. J., CALATAYUD, J. B., ABRAHAM, S., and CACERES, C. A. A study of physician variation in heart-sound interpretation. *M. Ann. District of Columbia,* 33:305, 1964.

40. BUTTERWORTH, J. S., and REPPERT, E. H. Auscultatory acumen in the general medical population. *J.A.M.A.*, 174:32, 1960.

41. LEVINE, S. A., and HARVEY, W. P. *Clinical Auscultation of the Heart.* Philadelphia, W. B. Saunders Co., 1949, 327 pp.

42. COUNIHAN, T. B., RAPPAPORT, M. B., and SPRAGUE, H. B. Physiologic and physical factors that govern the clinical appreciation of cardiac thrills. *Circulation,* 4:716–728, 1951.

CHAPTER 11

THE SIZE AND CONFIGURATION OF THE HEART

By J. R. Blackmon

ESTIMATION OF HEART SIZE

All significant cardiac lesions eventually place the heart under stress which causes hypertrophy or dilatation of the cardiac chambers. The major purpose of this chapter is to review the methods for determining heart size since cardiomegaly is a frequent and important sign of heart disease. The recognition of cardiomegaly is, therefore, of critical importance in the detection of cardiac disease. A characteristic pattern of enlargement often suggests the diagnosis of a specific lesion.

In this chapter the great vessels will be included in consideration of the configuration of the heart since many diagnostic clues are provided by the aorta, pulmonary artery and vena cavae.

As is so common in discussions of methodology, each method has its criteria for normality and abnormality and none of the methods is entirely accurate because of wide variations in the normal. Therefore, a definitive diagnosis of heart disease should not

328

be based on a single method of examination. Even after all methods of examination have been made, a few individuals may be considered borderline normal or abnormal. In this situation the physician must await the appearance of critical signs before making a definitive diagnosis of normal or abnormal. Annual follow-up of these individuals over a period of several years will usually provide the necessary information to distinguish abnormality.

ORIENTATION OF THE HEART WITHIN THE THORAX

A major source of variation in apparent heart size is the fact that the heart occupies an asymmetrical position within the thorax. The septa which divide the atria and ventricles are oriented between the sagittal and frontal planes of the thorax. A frontal view of the heart (Fig. 11-1A) discloses the right atrium, right ventricle, pulmonary artery and aortic arch with a small portion of the left ventricle appearing on the left border. On the

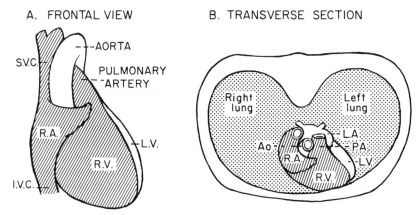

A. FRONTAL VIEW   B. TRANSVERSE SECTION

FIGURE 11–1   THE ORIENTATION OF THE HEART WITHIN THE THORAX

A, In the frontal view, the right atrium forms the usually convex right side of the cardiac silhouette. The right ventricle is anterior. A small portion of the left ventricle appears as the left border. The superior vena cava, aorta and pulmonary artery are grouped above the heart in the superior mediastinum.

B, Viewed from above, the heart occupies an oblique position within the thorax with the right ventricle making contact with the anterior thoracic wall to the left of the midline. The left atrium forms the posterior wall of the heart.

posterior aspect of the heart lie the remainder of the left ventricle, the left atrium and a portion of the right atrium. A transverse section through the thorax (Fig. 11–1B) indicates the relation of the heart and the thoracic walls. The cardiac chambers are separated from the anterior and lateral thoracic walls by varying amounts of lung tissue except near the apex of the heart. Here the right ventricle near the interventricular groove makes contact with the thoracic wall.

PHYSICAL EXAMINATION OF THE HEART

The eye, the hand and the ear are essential tools in determining size and configuration of the heart by experienced clinicians and may provide more information about heart size and function than any single tool or method.

Inspection. Inspection of the precordium includes observation from the suprasternal notch down to the epigastrium and from right to left anterior axillary lines. The point of maximal impulse (PMI) may be a visible or palpable local displacement and in normal persons lies within the mid-clavicular line in the fifth intercostal space and occupies an area no larger than a quarter (Fig. 11–2A). This impulse in the normal is due to the impact of the right ventricle against the chest wall during systolic contraction and displacement (Fig. 11–1B). This represents an important clue to the location of the left border of the heart and should be noted in every examination.

When right ventricular hypertrophy occurs, the anteriorly-oriented right ventricle contacts the chest wall just to the left of the sternum. A diffuse impulse may be seen along the left sternal border and even in the epigastrium (Fig. 11–2B). In children with congenital heart disease or in adults with chronic heart disease, the precordium in this area may be protuberant since right ventricular enlargement has been present from birth. The precordial aspects of the superior media-

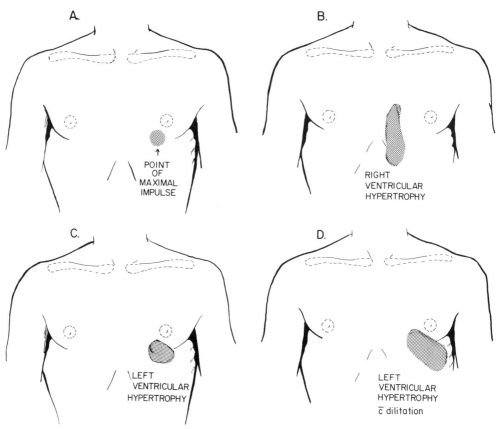

FIGURE 11–2   DISPLACEMENT OF THE CARDIAC IMPULSE BY VENTRICULAR OR GREAT VESSEL
ENLARGEMENT

A, During each cardiac contraction, a thrust can be observed and palpated in a small area on the precordium, located in the fifth intercostal space at or medial to the mid-clavicular line.

B, The right ventricle enlarges anteriorly and produces a diffuse impulse along the left sternal border and into the epigastrium.

C, Left ventricular hypertrophy causes the point of maximal impulse to enlarge and be displaced slightly to the left and downward.

D, Left ventricular hypertrophy with dilatation causes a more diffuse impulse which is markedly displaced to the left and downward.

stinum are observed for pulsations which arise from the aorta, pulmonary artery and left atrial appendage. The use of a "goose-necked" adjustable light which is positioned to reflect shadows is of considerable help in discerning these subtle pulsations on the chest wall. This is particularly true in examining normal subjects. In making the examination, it is important to assess thoracic wall thickness since the thinner the chest wall the

more pulsations will be seen. Conversely, emphysematous lungs and adiposity diminish apparent pulsations.

When the left ventricle enlarges, the point of maximal impulse changes in location and size. In pure left ventricular hypertrophy, the observed impulse is more obvious and may extend beyond the mid-clavicular line (Fig. 11–2C). When left ventricular enlargement is due to both hypertrophy and dilatation, the point of maximal impulse occupies a larger area and is always to the left of the mid-clavicular line (Fig. 11–2D). This indicates that left ventricular enlargement is indeed present.

Palpation. Palpation of the precordium is used to confirm inspection in most cases but adds an additional dimension to the examination since the force of pulsations is more easily perceived by tactile than visual sensation. In palpating the precordium, the hand should be placed on the chest wall and the fingers should be aligned in the intercostal spaces for greater tactile perception of impulses. In the normal person, palpation discloses the point of maximal impulse at or within the mid-clavicular line and is usually perceived as a gentle systolic tap.

In pure left ventricular hypertrophy, the point of maximal impulse may be slightly larger and displaced to the left but is now a forceful thrust. Hypertrophy without dilatation is usually associated with high ventricular systolic pressures (pressure overload), such as hypertension or outflow tract obstruction from a variety of causes.

In left ventricular enlargement with both hypertrophy and dilatation a diffuse heaving displacement of the left precordium is perceived, commonly observed in patients with lesions causing sustained increase in stroke volume (volume overload) of the left ventricle such as aortic or mitral regurgitation or arteriovenous fistulas of the systemic circulation.

Right ventricular enlargement is also caused by pressure or volume overload but cannot be as well differentiated by inspection and palpation as can left ventricular enlargement. Electrocardiographic and radiographic signs help make this distinction.

In addition to palpating precordial impulses arising from the heart, it is important to palpate over the area of the great vessels, i.e., pulmonary artery and aorta. In normal hearts, pulmonic valve closure may be felt during expiration.

In abnormal hearts, the exploring fingers or palm may sense vibrations of the chest wall called systolic or diastolic thrills. Vibrations due to valve closure may be felt over the pulmonary artery and suggest that the pulmonary artery is enlarged in patients with pulmonary hypertension. Contraction of the left atrial appendage may be felt when the left atrium is enlarged and contracting synchronously.

Percussion. Percussion brings in another human sensor, the ear, in combination with tactile sensation. Percussion is most useful in outlining on the chest wall the location and configuration of the borders of the heart and great vessels. The technique of percussion was originated by Leopold Auenbrugger (1761) as a result of the observation that the quantity of wine in a barrel can be estimated by tapping the end and noting the resonance.[3] When a sharp tap is delivered to the thoracic wall, the underlying tissues are suddenly displaced. Due to their elasticity, they rebound and oscillate while the imparted energy is dissipated. The ensuing vibrations have four characteristics important in percussion: (1) frequency, (2) quality, (3) duration and (4) intensity. The frequency of vibration depends upon the elasticity of the structures in relation to the mass of tissue in vibration, which in this case includes tissues of varying density and elasticity (e.g., muscle, fat, bone, lung).

The vibrations produced by percussion over a well-inflated lung appear to have relatively high intensity (loudness), low frequency (pitch) and

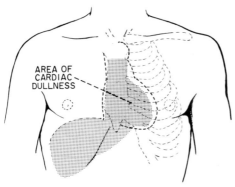

AREA OF
CARDIAC
DULLNESS

FIGURE 11-3   PERCUSSION OF THE HEART
BORDERS

The size of the heart can be approximated by skilled percussion over the precordium. The region of dullness to percussion is always smaller than the actual size of the heart because of its rounded contour (see Fig. 11-1B). Severe cardiac enlargement consistently produces expansion of the area of dullness, but minor degrees of enlargement cannot be reliably detected.

long duration (resonance). A region of "absolute dullness" may be outlined over the precordium (Fig. 11-3). The percussion note over this area has relatively low intensity, high pitch and short duration (reduced resonance). Extending beyond the region of absolute dullness is an area of relative dullness which approximately delineates the heart borders (Fig. 11-3). The area of relative dullness is not sharply defined. The rounded surfaces of the heart do not conform to the anterior thoracic wall (see Fig. 11-1B) and the heart borders outlined by percussion tend to be smaller than the silhouette observed on roentgenograms by 1.0 to 1.5 cm. or more. Percussion is best accomplished by placing the left hand parallel with the ribs, with the middle finger in an intercostal space, and sharply tapping the middle finger of the left hand with the tip of the middle finger of the right hand. One should avoid percussing too heavily since this causes a loss of discrimination by causing too many vibrations which

tend to diminish accuracy in determining initial heart borders represented by dotted lines in Figure 11-3. Actually, the vibrations perceived by the finger are as important as the sound picked up by the ear. With experience, percussion can be successfully accomplished in a noisy room.

It is apparent that the eye, the hand and the ear can provide considerable information regarding the size and shape of the heart. Certainly one can always tell when the heart is grossly enlarged and deformed. One can usually tell when the heart is normal if the body is not deformed. In the borderline cases or when there is marked deformity of the chest or spine, other techniques of estimating the size of the heart and great vessels are necessary.

The bare essentials in a complete examination of the heart include the physical examination, radiography and electrocardiography.

ROENTGENOGRAPHIC EXAMINATION OF THE HEART

When x-rays penetrate the chest, absorption of the radiation depends upon the radiodensity of the tissues lying in the path of each ray. Bone has the greatest radiodensity in the chest, thus the spine and ribs are most apparent, then the heart, blood vessels and finally lung tissue. Medical science adopted this radiographic principle very early in its inception and has made frequent modifications of the technique to enhance its applicability and safety both to the patient and physician.

Methods of Roentgenography. Four methods of roentgenography are depicted in Figure 11-4. Each has a specific function. However, all serve to show the size and configuration of the heart and great vessels in a single plane.

A. TELEROENTGENOGRAPHY

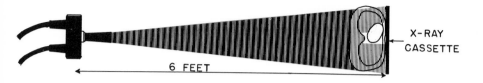

X-RAY CASSETTE

6 FEET

B. FLUOROSCOPY

C. CINEFLUOROGRAPHY

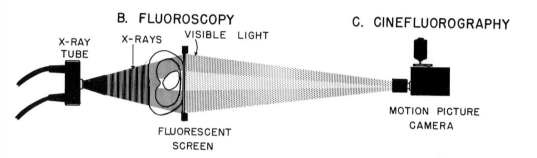

X-RAY TUBE   X-RAYS   VISIBLE LIGHT

MOTION PICTURE CAMERA

FLUORESCENT SCREEN

D. IMAGE INTENSIFIER

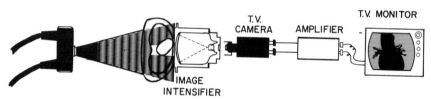

T.V. CAMERA   AMPLIFIER   T.V. MONITOR

IMAGE INTENSIFIER

FIGURE 11–4 METHODS OF ROENTGENOGRAPHY

As x-rays penetrate the body, the tissues absorb the rays in relation to their radiodensity. The rays which penetrate the body delineate the border of internal organs on either x-ray film or the surface of a fluorescent screen.

A, Teleroentgenograms are x-ray plates exposed with the tube six feet from the x-ray film. At this distance the distortion of the heart size by the diverging rays is minimized.

B, Fluoroscopy is accomplished by observing directly the visible light emitted by fluorescent screens exposed to x-rays. The tube is close to the screen, and the image of the heart is enlarged by the diverging rays.

C, Cinefluorography, commonly termed cineradiography, involves motion picture photography of images on fluorescent screens.

D, The image intensifier utilizes low energy radiation converting it to light then to an electron density pattern which is accelerated and refocused producing an image several thousand times brighter than the conventional fluorescent screen. By means of an optical lens system, the image can be viewed directly or picked up by a television camera, and displayed on a television monitor. The image can be captured by motion picture film or videotape.

Teleroentgenography produces static films of the silhouette of the heart and great vessels with excellent resolution, little distortion and minimal x-ray exposure. The films can be studied in detail and repeatedly in this,

the most common radiologic examination of the heart.

Fluoroscopy and cinefluorography are included primarily for historical interest only. The disadvantages of straight fluoroscopy include poor resolution and greater x-ray exposure to patient and physician. It requires a darkened room and dark adaptation by the viewer which is time consuming and inconvenient.

Image intensification alleviates the disadvantages of fluoroscopy and has become standard in radiologic examination for observing dynamic features of the beating heart. The resolution is improved, there is minimal x-ray exposure and a dark room or dark adaptation is not required. The tube to screen distance is small, producing an apparent increase in heart size by about 25 per cent. This image can be viewed directly or on a television monitor and can be recorded on tape or photographic film.

Standard Positions for Cardiac Roentgenography. Radiographic signs of abnormality are based on changes in the size and configuration of the silhouette of the heart and great vessels. It is obvious from our previous discussion of the orientation of the heart within the thorax, Fig. 11–1A, that all chambers and great vessels cannot be seen in any one view. For this reason, four standard projections have been used in an attempt to better delineate each specific chamber. In addition, a suspension of barium can be swallowed to outline the course of the esophagus and delineate more readily the posterior wall of the heart (Fig. 11–5).

The Posteroanterior Position (Fig. 11–6A). The superior vena cava forms the right border of the cardiac silhouette in the superior part of the chest, but in the normal individual only the spine is usually seen. The right atrium is on the right border in the lower portion of the cardiac silhouette. The inferior vena cava is not usually seen in the normal heart. The right ventricle does not appear on the cardiac silhouette in this view. The

ascending aorta is well within the heart shadow and is not seen on the right border in the normal. The aortic knob appears as a rounded bulge high on the left border of the cardiac silhouette. Below the aortic knob the pulmonary artery protrudes slightly. The lower half of the left cardiac border is the left ventricular wall which slopes toward the diaphragm. A small triangular shadow of lesser density often appears at the junction of the left ventricle and diaphragm and represents the epicardial fat pad.

Thus, the posteroanterior view in the normal shows right atrium, aortic knob, pulmonary artery, left ventricle and the epicardial fat pad. This view is particularly useful for observing signs of right atrial enlargement, left ventricular enlargement, pulmonary artery enlargement and dilatation of the aortic arch and descending thoracic aorta. In addition, both superior vena cava and inferior vena cava may extend beyond the normal borders of the silhouette when they become enlarged. Left atrial enlargement is also evident in this view as a double density in cardiac silhouette and by elevating the left main stem bronchus which is visible in this view. The posteroanterior view is by far the most useful single view of the heart and great vessels.

Lateral Position (Figs. 11–6B and 11–7B). The straight lateral position shows the right ventricle and left atrium to advantage since the right ventricle forms the anterior border and the left atrium forms the posterior border of the heart. The barium filled esophagus lies against the posterior wall of the heart. The pulmonary artery can be seen on end and the ascending aorta in silhouette. When either the right ventricle or left atrium is enlarged, it is more easily recognized than the normal chamber.

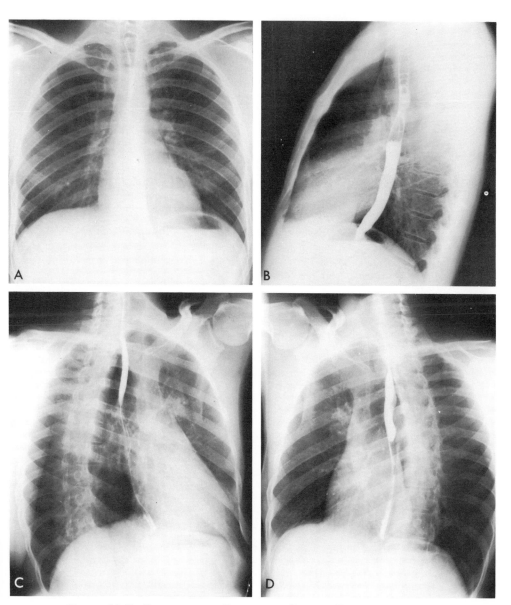

FIGURE 11–5   CONVENTIONAL FILMS FROM CARDIAC ROENTGENOGRAPHY

The four conventional films from cardiac roentgenography are (A) the posteroanterior view, (B) the left lateral view, (C) the right anterior oblique view and (D) the left anterior oblique view. All with barium filled esophagus.

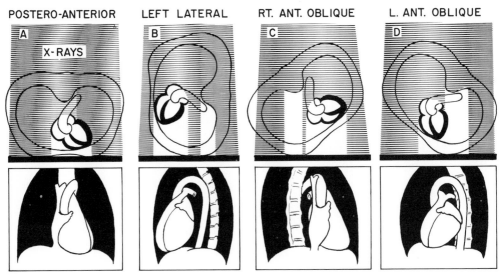

FIGURE 11-6   **FOUR STANDARD POSITIONS FOR CARDIAC ROENTGENOGRAPHY**

The conventional roentgenographic examination of the heart records the cardiac silhouette in four positions. The orientation of the heart in each position is indicated schematically in a transverse section and on a teleroentgenogram. For labels, see Figure 11-7.

A, In the posteroanterior position the sagittal plane of the body is parallel with the cassette.

B, In the left lateral position the sagittal plane of the body makes a 90-degree angle with the cassette.

C, In the right anterior oblique position the right shoulder is rotated toward the cassette until the sagittal plane of the body makes an angle of 45 degrees.

D, In the left anterior oblique position the left shoulder is rotated toward the cassette until the sagittal plane of the body makes an angle of 45 degrees.

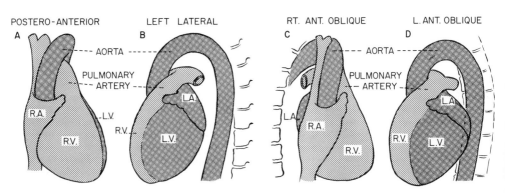

FIGURE 11-7   **THE ORIENTATION OF THE HEART IN FOUR STANDARD POSITIONS**

A, In the posteroanterior position the borders of the right atrium and left ventricle are displayed. The right ventricle and the left atrium are not visible on the borders of the silhouette.

B, In the lateral position, the silhouette of the right ventricle is seen anteriorly and the left atrium posteriorly.

C, In the right anterior oblique position the right ventricle and left atrium are again seen in silhouette.

D, In the left anterior oblique the right and left ventricle are seen in silhouette. The left atrium can be discerned in this projection.

The two oblique positions (Figs. 11-6C, D and 11-7C, D), while in common usage, do not provide a great deal of information regarding the heart size not contained in the posteroanterior and lateral views.

Quantitative appraisal of chamber size is difficult because the precise angle of observation is never known to the observer; overlying structures obscure heart borders; and the separation of the chambers by the septae cannot be distinguished. Oblique views are sometimes helpful in delineating expanding great vessels.

SOURCES OF VARIATION IN THE CARDIAC SILHOUETTE

Roentgenographic interpretation is complicated by a number of factors which are not necessarily related to cardiac size or function. Certain of these conditions cause the normal heart to appear large. Others tend to cause an enlarged heart to appear normal in size. For this reason it is convenient to speak of the "apparent" size when considering the sources of variation in the cardiac silhouette. The sources of variation in the cardiac silhouette can be divided into two main categories: (a) individual variation and (b) technical variation. By careful standardization of the roentgenographic technique, technical variation can be partially eliminated. Individual variation must be recognized by the physician and evaluated in each case.

Individual Variation. The most important initial step in the roentgenographic examination of a patient is to visualize the "normal" range of cardiac size and configuration for a person with his particular habitus and extracardiac conditions. Proficiency in this essential feature of the examination is gained only through experience. Sound judgment can be developed simply by taking advantage of every opportunity to correlate the roentgenographic appearance of the heart with the habitus and cardiac condition of patients.

HABITUS. In asthenic individuals, the thoracic cavity is long and narrow so that the long axis of the ventricles approaches a vertical orientation (Fig. 11-8). The cardiac silhouette is narrow, and the left border may lie several centimeters inside the midclavicular line. Enlargement of the heart tends to restore the apparent cardiac size toward the normal configuration. In patients of this sort, a considerable degree of left ventricular enlargement is required to bring the left border of the heart to the midclavicular line, which is within the "normal" range for the average individual. For this reason, early ventricular enlargement is frequently overlooked in patients in whom the resting position of the diaphragm is lower than average.

In contrast, a patient with a stocky build characteristically has an elevated diaphragm (Fig. 11-8). When the longitudinal axis of the heart approaches a horizontal position, even a heart of normal size may appear enlarged. In such a patient the pulmonary markings are accentuated, the cardiovascular angle is more acute and the apex of the heart is displaced toward the left. In short, such a normal individual could easily be mistaken for a patient with left ventricular enlargement. Thus, an important step in roentgenographic interpretation is determining the habitus of the patient and the relative height of the diaphragm. For this purpose, it is convenient to establish the level of the dome of the diaphragm in relation to the costovertebral junctions (Fig. 11-8).

VARIATION IN PATIENTS WITH THE SAME HABITUS. Individual vari-

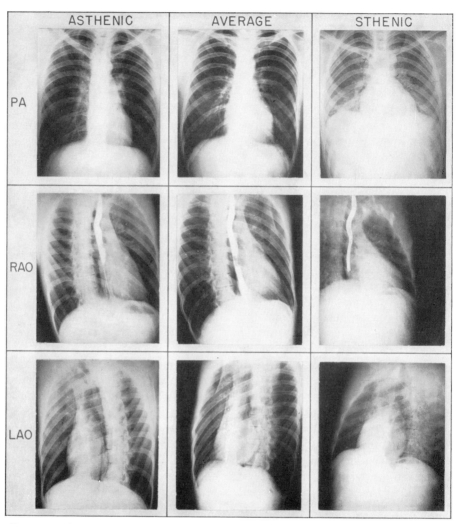

FIGURE 11-8   THE EFFECTS OF HABITUS AND POSITION ON THE CARDIAC SILHOUETTE

Roentgenograms obtained on three normal individuals of different habitus indicate the variation in the shape and apparent size of the normal cardiac silhouette.

In asthenic individuals the thorax is long and narrow so the heart assumes a vertical position. The cardiac silhouette is so narrow that severe enlargement of the heart may be overlooked in such patients.

If all patients had average habitus, criteria for enlargement of the individual chambers could be easily established and slight changes could be consistently detected.

In sthenic individuals, the high diaphragm supports the heart in a horizontal position. The wide cardiac silhouette gives the impression of left ventricular enlargement, and accentuation of the pulmonary vascular markings suggests pulmonary congestion. These factors must be constantly evaluated in analyzing roentgenographic images.

Note that the right dome of the diaphragm in the three individuals is at the level of the eleventh, tenth and eighth costovertebral junctions, respectively.

ation is a constant problem in anatomy, physiology and clinical medicine. The cardiac silhouettes of different patients of similar age, sex, habitus and physical condition may vary rather strikingly. These changes may be explained in terms of the orientation of the heart within the thorax or of developmental variations of the heart, lungs or thoracic cage. Obviously, individuals in different age groups with the same type of habitus may have significantly different cardiac silhouettes. Again, wide experience is the most important factor in this type of evaluation.

THE PHASE OF THE CARDIAC CYCLE. Teleroentgenograms are generally exposed during a very brief period of time (e.g., one fifth to one sixtieth of a second). Since the diastolic interval is somewhat longer than the duration of systole, more than half of a series of teleroentgenograms will be exposed during diastole. However, more than one third of the teleroentgenograms are exposed during some phase of systole. Fortunately, the change in the size and shape of the cardiac silhouette during the cardiac cycle is rarely sufficient to produce any serious error from this source.

THE PERICARDIAL FAT PAD. In many normal individuals, a triangular shadow appears at the apex of the heart which is due to the accumulation of fat in this region. Elongation of the left ventricular outflow tract and displacement of the apex downward and to the left might be erroneously suspected unless the region is carefully scrutinized. It is generally possible to detect the apical border passing through the shadow of the pericardial fat pad.

DISPLACEMENT OF THE HEART. The heart does not always occupy its normal position within the thorax. For example, the heart may be displaced toward the left either by atelectasis in the left lung or pressure pneumothorax in the right pleural cavity. In either case, the left border of the heart moves toward the left and the right border may overlie the spine. If the pulmonary condition is unrecognized, cardiac enlargement may be incorrectly suspected.

DEFORMITIES OF THE THORAX. If the lower end of the sternum is depressed (funnel chest), the distance between the sternum and the vertebral spine is reduced. The heart may be compressed in its posteroanterior dimension and displaced toward the left. The left border of the heart may become rounded, giving the impression of ventricular enlargement.

In kyphoscoliosis, the abnormal curvature of the vertebral spine may produce cardiac displacement as well as a change in the "apparent" cardiac configuration. The border of the curved vertebral spine may be confused with the cardiac silhouette, giving an impression of cardiac enlargement.

INACCURATE POSITIONING OF THE PATIENTS. If the patient is correctly placed in the posteroanterior position, the manubrium of the sternum should be centered over the vertebral bodies. If the patient is rotated even slightly from this position, the apparent configuration of the heart may be significantly altered. Similarly, the configuration of the heart and its position in relation to the thoracic spine are seriously distorted by either inadequate or excessive rotation of the patient to obtain oblique views of the heart. Standardization of patient positioning is essential for accurate evaluation of teleroentgenograms. This problem need not arise during fluoroscopy because the examiner can view the heart from all angles and control the positioning during visualization.

RESPIRATORY ACTIVITY. The

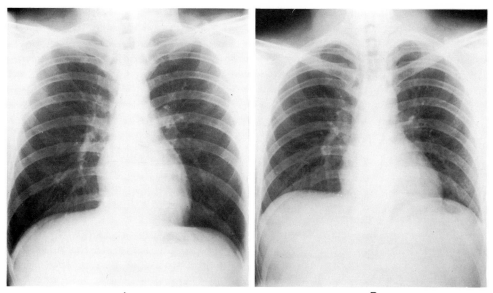

A   B

FIGURE 11–9   INSPIRATORY AND EXPIRATORY FILMS

Inspiratory and expiratory films illustrating difference in size and shape of the heart. In the in-spiratory film the diaphragm is at the level of the tenth rib and in the expiratory film the ninth rib.

level of the diaphragm is influenced by the phase of respiration in which the teleroentgenogram is exposed. If the x-ray technician instructs the patient to take a deep breath prior to exposing the x-ray plate, the level of the diaphragm is depressed and the longitudinal axis of the heart assumes a more nearly vertical position (Fig. 11–9A). On the other hand, the patient may be instructed to press against the x-ray cassette, in which case he may forcibly exhale, elevating the level of the diaphragm. Changes in the level of the diaphragm due to respiratory activity may seriously distort the apparent cardiac size (Fig. 11–9B).

THE VALSALVA MANEUVER. A patient instructed to hold his breath may inadvertently or unconsciously raise the pressure within the thorax—the Valsalva maneuver. The increased intrathoracic pressure impedes the blood flow into the thorax and causes a progressive reduction in the size of the heart. Under these conditions, the actual size of the cardiac silhouette may be significantly reduced.[7] The sources of variation due to respiratory activity and the Valsalva maneuver can be largely eliminated by well trained technicians (Fig. 11–10).

MEASUREMENTS OF THE CARDIAC SILHOUETTE

Detection of cardiac enlargement is generally a more or less subjective judgment in view of the numerous causes of variation described previously. A more scientific approach to roentgenographic interpretation has been attempted by measuring various dimensions of the cardiac silhouette. Information concerning the length or width of the individual ventricular chambers would be most helpful. However, the position occupied by the atrioventricular valve rings cannot be accurately identified, with the result that most of the measurements include

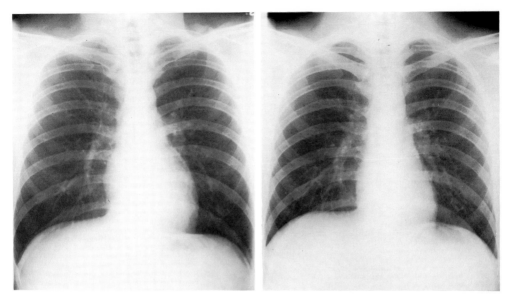

FIGURE 11–10   VALSALVA MANEUVER

This pair of films illustrates the reduction in the heart size due to the Valsalva maneuver.

both atrial and ventricular dimensions. Further, the dense shadows cast by abdominal organs largely obscure the inferior margin of the cardiac silhouette. The transverse diameter is the most common measurement in current use. To determine this dimension, a vertical line is inscribed over the vertebral spine on a teleroentgenogram exposed in the posteroanterior position. The point on the right border of the heart which is farthest from the midline is selected by inspection (in the midportion of the right atrial border). From this point a line is drawn perpendicular to the vertical reference line. In the same way a perpendicular is erected from the point on the left border of the heart which is most distant from the midline. The sum of the two horizontal segments is called the transverse diameter (Fig. 11–11).

In view of the extreme variation in different individuals, this measurement has no significance without reference to the habitus of the individual.

A fairly common practice is to divide the transverse diameter of the heart by the width of the thorax (the cardiothoracic ratio). It is frequently stated that a cardiothoracic ratio of more than 0.5 indicates cardiac enlargement. This assumption may have some validity among individuals of average body build. However, a vertically placed heart may be considerably enlarged before reaching a cardiothoracic ratio of 0.5. If the long axis of the heart approaches the horizontal, the cardiothoracic ratio may exceed 0.5 without any cardiac enlargement. The cardiothoracic ratio has little value and may be seriously misleading.

To overcome this deficiency, Ungerleider et al.[2, 3] measured the transverse diameter of a large group of "normal" individuals and devised tables by which it is possible to predict the transverse diameter of an individual according to his weight, height, age and sex. If the measured transverse diameter of a patient exceeds the pre-

A. TRANSVERSE DIAMETER

B. CARDIOTHORACIC RATIO

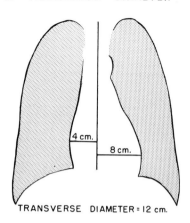

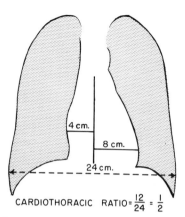

FIGURE 11–11 CARDIAC MEASUREMENTS

A, The transverse diameter of the cardiac silhouette is measured from a vertical line along the vertebral spine. The maximum distances from this line to the right and left borders of the heart shadow are added to measure this dimension. Although neither of these points of measurement is particularly appropriate for detecting chamber enlargement, no other dimension has proved more revealing.

B, The quotient obtained when the transverse diameter is divided by the width of the thoracic cage at its widest point is termed the cardiothoracic ratio. This device is intended to correct for differences in habitus among patients. If the ratio exceeds 0.5, cardiac enlargement is said to be present. The extent to which this measurement can be misleading is indicated by a glance at Figures 11–8 and 11–9.

dicted dimension by more than 10 per cent, he "probably" has an enlarged heart.

Before using the transverse diameter as a criterion of cardiac enlargement, one must recognize the following limitations: (a) the measurement includes both the right atrium and the left ventricle; (b) the ventricular chambers do not enlarge primarily along a horizontal axis; (c) elongation of the outflow tract of the left ventricle would be detected but there is no representation by the right ventricle in this measurement; and (d) the application of the measurement presupposes that the sources of variation other than habitus, age and sex have been eliminated or controlled. If these restrictions are recognized, the tables of Ungerleider and Clark may serve a useful purpose.

NORMAL HEART CHAMBERS

By this time, it should be obvious that the evaluation of cardiac size by use of teleroentgenography is largely a subjective, intuitive appraisal without real quantitative measurements. In experienced hands, however, the teleroentgenogram is extremely helpful in estimating overall heart size and specific chamber enlargement.

The normal right atrium forms the right border of the heart silhouetted against the radiolucent lung in posteroanterior projection, usually projecting slightly to the right of the vertebral column.

The normal right ventricle is not seen in the posteroanterior projection but forms the anterior border of the heart in lateral projection.

The normal left atrium forms the

POSTEROANTERIOR

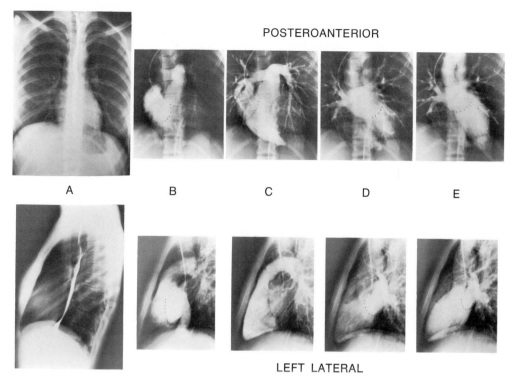

A   B   C   D   E

LEFT LATERAL

FIGURE 11–12   ROENTGENOGRAPHY AND ANGIOCARDIOGRAPHY OF NORMAL HEART

A, Shows the posteroanterior and left lateral chest films on the left with frames from biplane angiocardiograms illustrating the intracardiac chambers on the right.

The dotted lines approximate the location of the A-V valves.

B, The right atrium is filled with contrast material.

C, The right ventricle is seen in the posteroanterior view filled with contrast material and seen to advantage in the lateral projection.

D, The contrast-filled left atrium is best seen in the lateral view. Note the reduction in size due to atrial contraction in E.

E, The contrast-filled left ventricle can be seen in both the posteroanterior and lateral projections.

posterior border of the heart but does not cause posterior displacement of the barium filled esophagus.

In the normal, the left ventricle is responsible for the left border of the cardiac silhouette and has a rather straight slope from the area of the pulmonary artery to the maximum curve of the left cardiac silhouette.

Figure 11–12 shows contrast material sequentially filling the four cardiac chambers in both the anteroposterior and lateral views in a normal heart.

SPECIFIC CHAMBER ENLARGEMENT

Enlargement of the right atrium is most commonly due to right ventricular failure or tricuspid valvular disease. When the right atrium enlarges, its border is displaced to the right and can fill a large portion of the right chest as viewed in posteroanterior projection (Fig. 11–13A). Superior vena caval enlargement always accompanies gross enlargement of the right atrium.

Right ventricular enlargement usu-

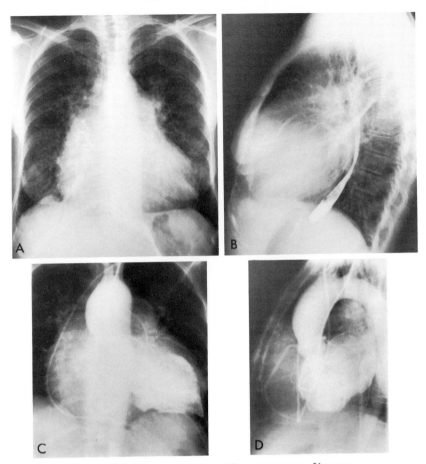

FIGURE 11–13 RIGHT HEART ENLARGEMENT – VOLUME

A, Posteroanterior film shows a large right atrium protruding into the right chest and prominent pulmonary artery.

B, Lateral projection shows the right ventricle impinging on the sternum and filling the superior retrosternal space.

C, D, A set of biplane angiocardiograms illustrates the left ventricle and left atrium filled with radiopaque dye for comparison with the large right heart which contains no contrast media. In the lateral projection the left ventricle is displaced posteriorly by the large right ventricle. The right coronary artery can be well seen sweeping around the right ventricle. In the frontal angiocardiogram the large pulmonary artery appears to the right of the dye filled aorta.

ally does not change the size and shape of the cardiac silhouette in the posteroanterior view. The right ventricle is located on the diaphragmatic and anterior surfaces of the heart. Early or mild enlargement is easily missed which reinforces the idea that roentgenograms should be supplemented by a physical examination and electrocardiograms.

The right ventricle enlarges in response to either pressure and volume overloads. With a chronic pressure overload, the right ventricle elongates and rotates the long axis of the heart toward the left. The left ventricle is displaced posteriorly, and the left border of the cardiac silhouette can be formed by the right ventricle. The pulmonary artery may or may not be en-

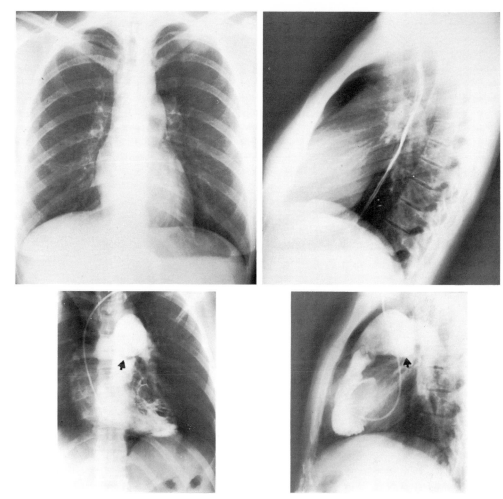

FIGURE 11–14   RIGHT VENTRICULAR ENLARGEMENT – PRESSURE

Posteroanterior and lateral chest films (above) and the anteroposterior and lateral biplane angio-cardiograms (below) in a patient with valvular pulmonic stenosis. In the posteroanterior chest film only the pulmonary artery is prominent. However, in the lateral film the right ventricle can be seen to impinge on the sternum. In the anteroposterior angiocardiogram a large pulmonary artery is noted and the arrow points to the stenotic valve. Poststenotic dilatation of the pulmonary artery is well seen in the lateral angiocardiogram.

larged depending on the lesion (Fig. 11–14).

In the presence of volume overload, the right ventricular chamber elongates longitudinally, rotates to the left and enlarges transversely giving a "mitral configuration" in the postero-anterior view (Fig. 11–13A, B) with left ventricle located posteriorly (Fig. 11–13C, D). The pulmonary artery is always enlarged and most readily observed in the frontal views (Fig. 11–13A–C). Pressure and volume overload patterns can also be confirmed by electrocardiography.

Left atrial enlargement is usually due to mitral valvular disease or left ventricular failure. Enlargement occurs in three directions: posteriorly, causing indentation in the barium

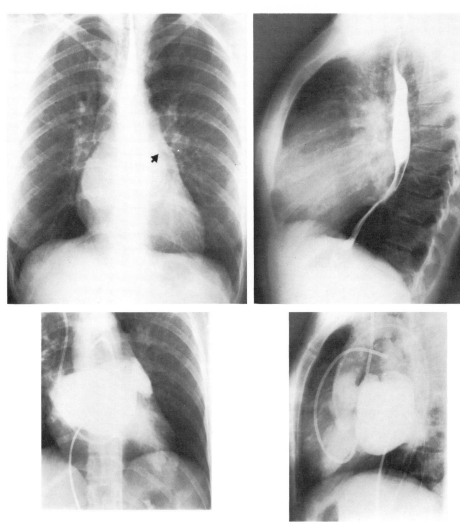

FIGURE 11–15   LEFT ATRIAL ENLARGEMENT

The posteroanterior and lateral chest films (above) and anteroposterior and lateral biplane angio-cardiography (below) in a patient with mitral stenosis. In the posteroanterior view the arrow points to the elevated left main stem bronchus and a double border is seen over the right atrium showing that the left atrium is enlarging superiorly and to the right. In the lateral view the barium filled esophagus is pushed posteriorly by the large left atrium. The angiocardiogram below shows the left atrium filled with contrast material. In the frontal angiocardiogram the left atrial appendage is seen to participate in the straightening of the left heart border.

filled esophagus; superiorly, elevating the left main stem bronchus; and to the right, causing a double shadow over the right atrial border. The left atrial appendage appears below the pulmonary artery straightening the superior portion of the left cardiac border. The

left atrium enlarges in response to both pressure and volume overload, but there is no specific pattern. In general, long standing volume overload produces a massive enlargement, resulting in the "giant" left atrium. The right border of the heart or total cardiac silhouette may represent the extent of the left atrium. Enlargement of the left atrium is best seen in the posteroanterior and lateral projections (Fig. 11–15).

LEFT VENTRICLE

The left ventricle also responds in different ways to pressure and volume stresses. The uncomplicated pattern of each will be described, but in actual practice most lesions are mixed or have a component of myocardial failure complicating the picture.

Systolic Overload. Hypertension or obstructed left ventricular outflow are major causes of systolic (pressure) overload of the left ventricle. The left ventricle shows some elongation which is usually not appreciated because of its extension below the diaphragm in the posteroanterior view. With considerable experience, one may discern a more rounded appearance to the left ventricular silhouette apparent as a "shouldering" or bulbous contour as concentric hypertrophy develops. This is best seen in the posteroanterior view (Fig. 11–16).

Diastolic Overload. The left ventricle elongates markedly and enlarges to the left in the posteroanterior view with dilation of the chamber. The cardiothoracic ratio becomes abnormal (Fig. 11–17) in patients with aortic regurgitation, mitral regurgitation, left-to-right shunt (at the ventricular or systemic arterial level) or myocardial failure. With marked left ventricular enlargement, the right border may be involved in the transverse widening of the cardiac silhouette by being crowded to the right without involving right atrial enlargement.

Configuration of the Aorta and Pulmonary Artery. Both the aorta (Fig. 11–16) and pulmonary artery (Fig. 11–14) enlarge in response to jet lesions, pressure and volume stresses, inherent disease of the vessel walls or trauma. The pulmonary artery may be enlarged without apparent cause (idiopathic dilatation). These expansions of the great arteries are usually seen in the posteroanterior view. However, the oblique views are sometimes helpful in delineating expanding vessels.

ELECTROCARDIOGRAPHY

In judging heart size, the electrocardiogram is an integral part of the examination of each patient. The electrocardiogram frequently reveals specific chamber enlargement that may not be clearly picked up by physical examination or chest x-rays. The electrocardiographic criteria for both atrial and ventricular enlargement are given in detail in Chapter 12.

ANGIOCARDIOGRAPHY

Angiocardiography is a technique whereby the radiodensity of the blood stream is greatly enhanced by injection of iodinated contrast materials. Rapid filming of the great vessels and cardiac chambers by several techniques gives a graphic record of the internal architecture and anatomy of the heart and great vessels.

In the past few years, great strides have been made in perfecting the technique of angiocardiography. Better contrast materials, catheters, injectors, filming equipment and well-trained physicians have reduced the hazards and made this procedure acceptable for routine diagnostic work in both children and adults.[4]

QUALITATIVE ANGIOCARDIOGRAPHY

Angiocardiography is the *sine qua non* of diagnosis in the infant or child

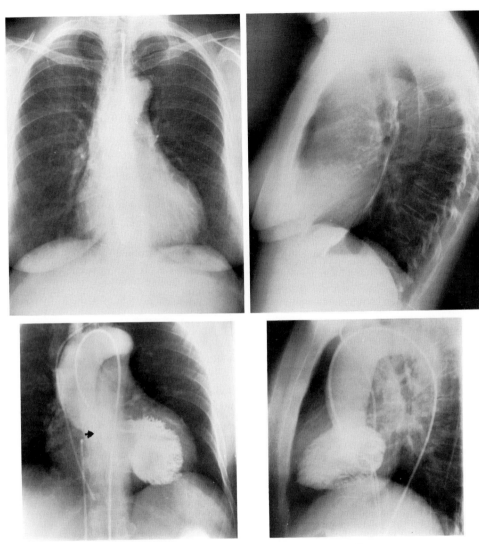

FIGURE 11–16   LEFT VENTRICULAR ENLARGEMENT – PRESSURE

The posteroanterior and lateral chest films (above) and anteroposterior and lateral biplane angio-cardiograms (below) in patient with aortic stenosis. The left ventricle shows a bulbous contour in the posteroanterior chest film. In the frontal angiocardiogram, the chamber volume is normal but the wall is thick. The arrow points to the thickened stenotic valve. Poststenotic dilatation is present on the angiogram but not appreciated on the plain chest films.

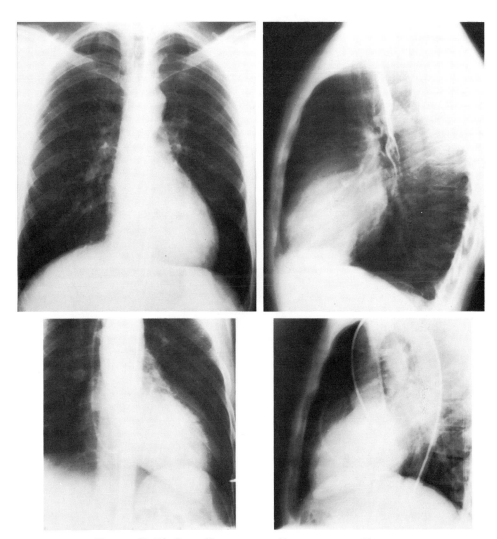

FIGURE 11-17   LEFT VENTRICULAR ENLARGEMENT — VOLUME

Posteroanterior and lateral chest films (above) and the anteroposterior and lateral biplane angiocardiograms (below) in a patient with aortic regurgitation. The left ventricle is elongated in both the
chest film and angiocardiogram in the frontal projection. The volume of the left ventricle is large in
contrast to that in aortic stenosis (Fig. 11–16).

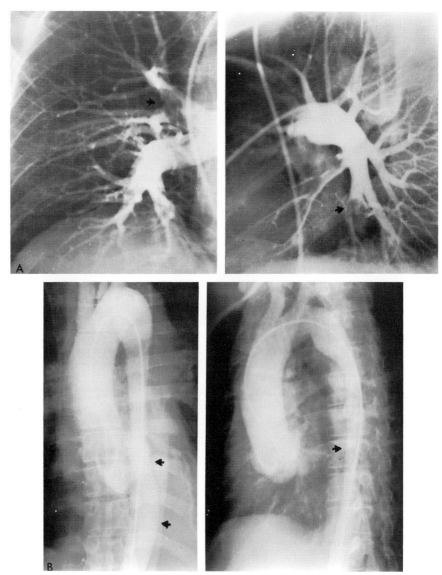

FIGURE 11–18   PULMONARY EMBOLI AND DISSECTING ANEURYSM

A, Selective pulmonary arteriograms in a patient with pulmonary emboli. The arrows point to obvious intravascular filling defects.

B, The anteroposterior and oblique aortogram in a patient with a dissecting aneurysm of the aorta. The arrows point to the dissection plane between the true and false channels.

with cyanotic congenital heart disease. It enables the physician to follow the circulation of the blood showing the abnormal relationships between cardiac chambers and the great vessels (see Chapter 13).

In less complex lesions, angiocardiography provides anatomic confirmation of physiologic data obtained during cardiac catheterization (i.e., with simple congenital heart lesions such as atrial septal defects, including A-V communis defects, ventricular septal defects, patent ductus arteriosus and pulmonic stenosis). It is equally true in acquired forms of heart disease such as valvular stenosis of regurgitation, diseases of the coronary arteries and differential diagnosis or outflow tract obstruction.

At the present time, pulmonary angiography is probably the most sensitive way of detecting pulmonary emboli and their resolution (Fig. 11–18A). Angiography also identifies aneurysmal dilatation of the great vessels. Frequently a dissection plane in the aorta can be seen which is helpful to the surgeon (Fig. 11–18B).

QUANTITATIVE ANGIOCARDIOGRAPHY

Early studies by Rushmer,[5] Arvidson[6] and Dodge[7] utilized angiocardiographic methods to determine left ventricular configuration and volumes.

The method we shall briefly describe is the length-area method of Dodge et al.[7] utilizing biplane filming. This method makes the assumption that the left ventricular chamber is best represented by an ellipse of rotation and that the volume can be calculated by the formula for the volume of an ellipsoid.

$$\text{Volume} = \frac{4\pi}{3} \times \frac{L_i}{2} \times \frac{L_{ii}}{2} \times \frac{L_{iii}}{2}$$

L_i, L_{ii}, L_{iii} are the major axes of the ellipsoid. The longest length is obtained from the films directly, and the two minor axes are derived from the planimetered area of the chamber in both the anteroposterior and lateral views. Two correction factors are used, one for x-ray distortion and the other from a regression formula for predicted and actual volumes. Figure 11–19 shows a set of angiocardiograms on which major axes and wall dimensions have been outlined and volumes and mass calculated. Normal values in adults for end-diastolic volume (EDV), end-systolic volume (ESV), stroke volume (SV) and systolic action fraction (SV/EDV) have been reported by Kennedy and colleagues[8] and Sanmarco and Bartle.[9]

Rapid filming techniques enable construction of left ventricular volume curves over several cardiac cycles (Fig. 11–20). This technique, when used in patients without shunts or regurgitation gives results comparable to Fick or dye dilution stroke volumes.[10] The two major disadvantages to this method are (1) it is a somewhat laborious technique and (2) repeated angiographic injections cannot reliably produce the initial results because of the changes in myocardial function following injection of contrast materials.[11]

In addition to determining left ventricular volumes, left ventricular mass can be calculated by the method of Rackley et al.[12] If the volume of the chamber is subtracted from the volume of the chamber plus the wall thickness, the difference between the two volumes multiplied by the specific gravity of cardiac muscle (1.050) gives left ventricular mass in grams. This method assumes that the ventricular septum is part of the left ventricle and the ventricular wall is of the same dimension throughout. Comparison of

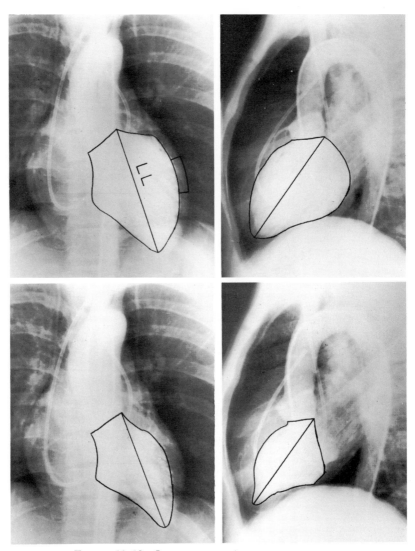

FIGURE 11–19   QUANTITATIVE ANGIOCARDIOGRAPHY

This set of anteroposterior and lateral biplane angiocardiograms at end-diastole and end-systole represent the basic material necessary to calculate left ventricular volumes and mass. The area of the chambers are outlined and the longest lengths drawn. In the upper left a 2 cm. length of left ventricular myocardium is outlined for wall thickness.

End-diastolic volume = 156 ml
End-systolic volume = 56 ml

Stroke volume   = 100 ml
Heart rate   = 59 beats/min
Angiocardiographic
    cardiac output   =   5.9 L/min
Left ventricular mass = 80 grams/M²

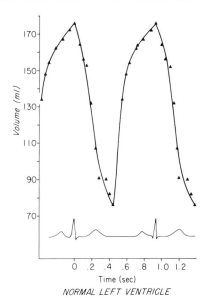

NORMAL LEFT VENTRICLE

FIGURE 11–20 NORMAL LEFT VENTRICULAR VOLUME CURVE

Normal left ventricular volume curve obtained from biplane angiocardiograms during successive cardiac cycles. Maximum volume is at the peak of the QRS with minimum volume after the T-wave. (Courtesy of M. M. Figley, M.D.)

angiocardiographic and postmortem left ventricular weights showed an excellent correlation (r = 0.97).[13]

The use of volume and mass measurements are extremely helpful in determining the presence of cardiomegaly and in quantitating the degree of abnormality (see also Chapter 15).

INDICATOR-DILUTION TECHNIQUES

Indicator-dilution techniques commonly include dye dilution and thermodilution although isotopes have also been used as indicators in determining ventricular end-diastolic volume. These techniques require recording of distortion-free washout curves from the ventricle. The method assumes rapid injection, complete mixing in the ventricular chamber, stable sampling site and rapid sampling. It is well known that complete mixing does not occur in the ventricular chamber.[14, 15] The results vary if the sampling catheter changes position, and it is necessary to use another method to determine stroke volume.

Comparative studies show poor agreement between angiocardiographic volumes and volumes obtained from indicator dilution techniques.[9] Recent reviews by Carleton et al.[16] and Rolett and colleagues[17] detail the problems with this technique.

REFERENCES

1. VIAMONTE, M. JR., and PARKS, R. E. *Progress in Angiography.* Chapter 2, Springfield, Ill., Charles C Thomas, 1964.
2. UNGERLEIDER, H. E., and CLARK, C. P. A study of the transverse diameter of the heart silhouette with prediction table based on the teleroentgenogram. *Amer. Heart J.*, 17:92–102, 1932.
3. UNGERLEIDER, H. E., and GRUBNER, R. Evaluation of heart size measurements. *Amer. Heart J.*, 24:494–510, 1942.
4. BRAUNWALD, E. and SWAN, H. J. C., Eds. Cooperative study on cardiac catheterization. *Circulation*, 37 (Suppl. 3), May, 1968.
5. RUSHMER, R. F., and CRYSTAL, D. K. Changes in configuration of the ventricular chambers during the cardiac cycle. *Circulation*, 4:211–218, 1951.
6. ARVIDSON, H. Angiocardiographic determination of left ventricular volume. *Acta Radiol.*, 56:321–339, 1961.
7. DODGE, H. T., SANDLER, H., BALLEW, D. W., and LORD, J. D., JR. The use of biplane angiocardiography for the measurement of left ventricular volume in man. *Amer. Heart J.*, 60:762–776, 1960.
8. KENNEDY, J. W., BAXLEY, W. A., FIGLEY, M. M., DODGE, H. T., and BLACKMON, J. R. Quantitative angiography I. The normal left ventricle in man. *Circulation*, 34: 272–278, 1966.
9. BARTLE, S. H., and SANMARCO, M. E. Comparison of angiocardiographic and thermal washout technics for left ventricular volume measurement. *Amer. Jour. Cardiol.*, 18:235–252, 1966.
10. DODGE, H. T., HAY, R. E., and SANDLER, H. Angiocardiographic method for directly

determining left ventricular stroke volume in man. *Circulat. Res.*, 11:739–745, 1962.

11. FRIESINGER, G. C., SCHAFFER, J., CRILEY, J. M., GAERTNER, R. A., and ROSS, R. S. Hemodynamic consequences of the injection of radiopaque material. *Circulation*, 31:730–740, 1965.

12. RACKLEY, C. E., DODGE, H. T., COBLE, Y. D., JR., and HAY, R. E. A method for determining left ventricular mass in man. *Circulation*, 29:666–671, 1964.

13. KENNEDY, J. W., REICHENBACK, D. D., BAXLEY, W. A., and DODGE, H. T. Left ventricular mass. A comparison of angiocardiographic measurements with autopsy weight. *Amer. J. Cardiol.*, 19:221–223, 1967.

14. IRISAWA, H., WILSON, M. F., and RUSHMER, R. F. Left ventricle as a mixing chamber. *Circulat. Res.*, 8:183–187, 1960.

15. SWAN, H. J. C., and BECK, W. Ventricular nonmixing as a source of error in the estimation of ventricular volumes by the indicator dilution technique. *Circulat. Res.*, 8:989–998, 1960.

16. CARLETON, R. A., BOWYER, A. F., and GRAETTINGER, J. S. Overestimation of left ventricular volume by the indicator dilution technique. *Circulat. Res.*, 18:248–256, 1966.

17. ROLETT, E. L., SHERMAN, H., and GORLIN, R. Measurement of left ventricular volume by thermodilution: an appraisal of technical errors. *J. Appl. Physiol.*, 19:1164–1174, 1965.

CHAPTER 12

ELECTRICAL ACTIVITY OF THE HEART

By Warren G. Guntheroth

I. BIOPHYSICAL BACKGROUND

Electrical potentials associated with waves of excitation which spread through the heart can be recorded from electrodes applied to the surface of the body. Some form of galvanometer is essential to demonstrate the variation in potential between two electrodes. The record of cardiac potentials, varying with time, is called an electrocardiogram (ECG).

Although complete electrocardiographic diagnosis may require considerable experience, much useful information can be obtained from the electrocardiogram with little training or experience. In particular, the diagnosis of certain arrhythmias at the bedside may be lifesaving and cannot be postponed for an electrocardiographer's interpretation. Also, the attending physician has the benefit of clinical information about the patient, without which a clinical diagnosis of heart disease cannot be made, regardless of the electrocardiographic findings. The ECG does not permit a unique diagnosis since the potentials on the body surface could be produced by an infinite variety of internal electrical sources (superposition principle).

Fortunately, there is a normal sequence of excitation and a fixed conduction system in the heart, and this knowledge, taken with data on the normal range of voltage and the anatomic distribution of the voltages, provides a great deal of information about the disorders of rhythm, disturbances of conduction and sequence of excitation and ventricular hypertrophy.

The sources of the cardiac potentials, the sequence of excitation and the method and theory of recording are important background for electrocardiographic diagnosis.

THE SOURCE OF CARDIAC POTENTIALS

The variations of potentials at the body surface recorded as the electro-

355

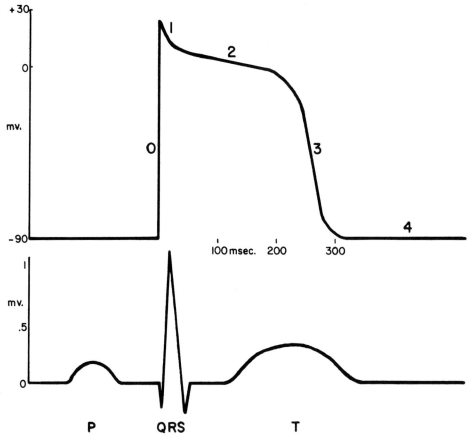

FIGURE 12-1   INTRACELLULAR AND CONVENTIONAL ELECTROCARDIOGRAM

The upper record represents the ventricular, intracellular potential during a complete cardiac cycle, and the lower record represents a standard electrocardiographic lead. The numbers on the upper trace are used to designate phases in the cycle: the upstroke, the brief spike, the plateau, the rapid recovery and electrical diastole, respectively. (From Guntheroth, *Pediatric Electrocardiography*, W. B. Saunders Co., 1965.)

cardiogram originate in a great number of individual cardiac cells. The electrical phenomena in cardiac cells resemble the phenomena in other excitable tissues such as skeletal muscle, smooth muscle and nerves. The time course of an intracellular recording made by direct puncture of a cardiac cell with a high impedance, ultramicroscopic electrode, and its relation to the body surface electrocardiogram is shown in Figure 12–1. At

rest, there is a difference in potential between the inside and outside of the myocardial fiber of approximately 75 to 90 millivolts, depending upon the cell type and species.[2] The potential exists because the cell wall is a semipermeable membrane with a marked difference in concentration of sodium and potassium ions inside and outside the cell. The diffusion potential is related not only to the difference in concentration of the ions but also to the permeability of the cell membrane to the specific ion and to the variation of permeability and concentration gradient of the ions with excitation and recovery.[3] The concentration of potassium inside the cell is much greater than outside, and the concentration of sodium inside the cell is much less than outside. At rest, the cell membrane is relatively permeable to potassium and inpermeable to sodium; consequently, the electromotive force of the resting cell is generated by the potassium diffusion potential. With excitation of the cardiac cell, there is a sudden marked increase in permeability of the membrane to sodium, greatly exceeding the permeability of potassium. Thus, depolarization is dominated by the diffusion potential of sodium and the intracellular potential becomes positive with respect to the outside of the cell (Phase 1). Whereas depolarization utilizes the potential energy of concentration gradients, repolarization restores these gradients in an uphill fashion, requiring energy expenditure by an "ion pump."[4] The energy source ultimately is oxidative metabolism in the cell, and consequently the repolarization process, reflected in T-wave changes in the surface electrocardiogram, is quite sensitive to hypoxia.

The surface electrocardiogram differs from the monophasic action potential of the individual cardiac cell because the former records only the *moving* boundaries of depolarization (P wave for the atria, QRS for the ventricles) and repolarization (T-wave). The conventional ECG lead does not record the resting cellular potential (Phase 4) or the cellular potential between activation and recovery (early Phase 2). Although the resting cell is polarized such that there are positive charges externally and negative charges internally, the exploring electrode sees[*] both near and far walls of the cell. The outer surface of the near wall is positively charged, but this effect is cancelled by the negative charge of the inner surface of the far wall (Fig. 12–2). Similarly, a completely depolarized cell would have a negative external charge on the wall facing the electrode and positive internal charge on the remote wall. A net positive charge is seen only when a depolarization wave is advancing toward the electrode, or a repolarization wave is receding from the electrode.

SEQUENCE OF EXCITATION

The heart beat normally is initiated by specialized pacemaker cells of relatively high rhythmicity in the sinus node. Intracellular recordings from pacemaker cells are distinguished by a prepotential, a gradually increasing potential in Phase 4 (Fig. 12–3). When the potential in Phase 4 reaches a threshold, there is spontaneous depolarization of the pacemaker cells.[5] Cells of the A-V node also demonstrate spontaneous depolarization during Phase 4, but the slope is lower, insuring a firing sequence lower than that of the sinus node, avoiding interference with the atrial beats.

Normally, the sinoatrial activation wave is propagated from its origin to the atrioventricular node by contiguous spread. The S-A node is at the junction of the superior vena cava and the right atrium, and the A-V node is near the tricuspid valve ring, above the ventricular septum; consequently, the vector orientation for atrial excitation

---

[*]Correctly, the potential at the electrode is proportional to the solid angle formed by joining the electrode to the boundary of the active membrane. The solid angle equals area/radius^2.

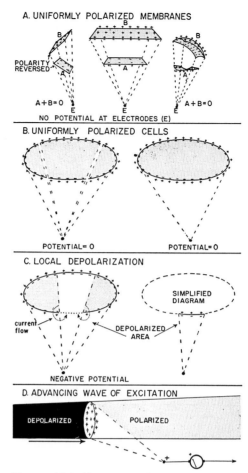

FIGURE 12-2   POLARIZED CELL MEMBRANES

A, The potentials from pairs of uniformly polarized membranes will cancel if they present the same solid angles and the orientation of the charges is reversed. In each of the three examples, the potential at the electrode is zero because the negative charges of one membrane are precisely balanced by the positive charges of its mate.

B, If a uniformly polarized cell is considered in three segments, the principle illustrated in part *A* applies. In each of the three solid angles, the proximal portion of the membrane has positive charges and the more distant portion has negative charges facing the electrode. Since the near and distant portions of the membrane subtend the same solid angle and the charges are oriented in opposite directions, their effects cancel and the potential at the electrode is zero. Thus, a uniformly polarized (or uniformly depolarized) cell produces no potential which can be recorded by an external electrode. In other words, if the membrane is uniformly polarized, there is no potential difference and no flow of electrical current, and no potential can be recorded.

C, When a region of a polarized cell becomes partially or completely depolarized, electrical currents flow from the polarized regions into the depolarized zone. A potential can then be recorded by a distant electrode; the magnitude of the potential is determined by the solid angle subtended by the depolarized area. On the far side of the cell, negative charges are not balanced by opposite charges in the depolarized region, so the electrode records a negative potential. On the right, a suitably charged membrane conforming to the depolarized area is comparable to the more complicated picture on the left, since the solid angle is the same.

D, The advancing wave of excitation can be visualized as though a suitably charged membrane were placed at the junction between polarized and depolarized regions (as in *C,* above). Since the outside of the polarized area is positive in relation to the inside, an electrode records a positive potential when a wave of excitation advances toward it and a negative potential when a wave of excitation is moving away.

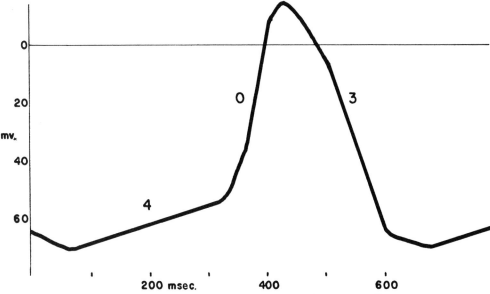

FIGURE 12-3   INTRACELLULAR RECORDING FROM SINOATRIAL PACEMAKER

Intracellular recording from sinoatrial pacemaker tissue. Note the gradually increasing potential in phase 4 as compared to the lack of any activity in this phase in Figure 12-1. (From Guntheroth, *Pediatric Electrocardiography*, W. B. Saunders Co., 1965.)

(p-wave) is to the left and inferior. The repolarization wave of the atrium is not ordinarily seen because of its negligible amplitude.

After the wave of atrial excitation, there is a delay of 60 msec. or greater before ventricular activation is recorded by the ECG. This interval, the P-R interval, is not without electrical activity, but the current produced by cells of the A-V node is too small to be recorded except by special techniques.[6,7] Most of the interval is consumed by transmission through the junctional cells between the atrial cells and the upper A-V node. These cells have numerous small filaments which are presumed to reduce the action potential as well as the velocity of conduction, and for these reasons, A-V conduction is vulnerable to partial or even complete failure.

Transmission is very rapid, once the electrical impulse enters the main body of the A-V node and the bundle of His. The bundle divides near the upper ventricular septum into right and left branches. The right bundle continues with little arborization toward the apex, where it crosses the right ventricular cavity in the moderator band, a recognizable structure. The left bundle branch divides almost immediately into two major divisions: one anterior and superior, and the second posterior and inferior. In both ventricles, the Purkinje fibers continue as a subendocardial network, penetrating a relatively short distance into the myocardium, and excitation proceeds thereafter through myocardial cells, from endocardium to epicardium.

The sequence of activation of the ventricles was worked out by Scher and Young,[8] with miniature multipolar electrodes distributed along a central shaft, inserted through the walls of the right and left ventricles and the sep-

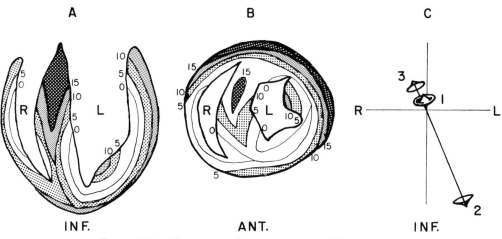

FIGURE 12-4   EXCITATION SEQUENCE OF THE MYOCARDIUM

A and B, Cross-sectional views of the canine heart, coronal and horizontal projections, indicating the sequence of excitation of the myocardium as determined by miniature electrodes. The numbers indicate the intervals in milliseconds after the earliest excitation. The shading increases in darkness with increasing length of intervals. The segments of myocardium excited last are the posterior free walls of the two ventricles and the uppermost part of the ventricular septum.

C, The general sequence of excitation has been averaged as a (1) initial, (2) major and (3) terminal vector. (From data in Scher and Young, 1956.) (From Guntheroth, *Pediatric Electrocardiography*, W. B. Saunders Co., 1965.)

tum. Figure 12–4 is drawn from their data in the dog, although the general sequence in man is similar.[9] From this figure, it is apparent that there are islands of simultaneous activity and the ECG is the resultant, at any instant, of the electrical forces produced by these areas of activity. Figure 12–4C is a vectorial presentation of the sequence of activation for the (1) initial, (2) major and (3) terminal portions of the QRS. The average forces of ventricular activation begin in an anterior direction, and slightly to the right and superior. The major forces are directed, in the adult heart, to the left, posterior and inferior, which reflects the relative thickness of the two ventricles. The velocity of excitation is the same for the myocardium of both ventricles, and the thinner right ventricle is completely activated at a time of continued spread of the activation front in the left ventricle. The last

segments of the myocardium to be activated are the upper septum and the high, posterior wall of the right and left ventricles, resulting in a terminal vector directed posteriorly, and slightly to the right and superior.

Although ventricular depolarization produces a characteristic QRS complex in an individual because of an anatomically defined conduction system, repolarization is not a propagated wave following a fixed pathway. Consequently, the orientation of the T wave is the most variable of electrocardiographic parameters and has the least specific significance. Although repolarization is inherently opposite to depolarization in polarity, the T wave is not, as expected, opposite the QRS complex in direction. On the contrary, the T wave is normally similar to the QRS in direction, suggesting that the sequence of repolarization is opposite to that of depolarization. Pressure and temperature gradients between the endocardium and epicardium have been proposed as explanations of the apparent sequence of repolarization from the epicardium to the endocardium.

THE CARDIAC GENERATOR AS AN EQUIVALENT DIPOLE

It may be difficult to understand how such a large, complex generator of electromotive force could be simplified to a single, instantaneous vector. The simplification is valid to the extent that the source approximates a dipole, a fixed, single point current source. Over 85 per cent of cardiac potentials measured at the body surface in a normal subject can be attributed to a simple dipole.[10, 11] A dipole is a single pair of positive and negative poles, infinitely close together, whose orientation in space may be described in terms of its projection onto three orthogonal axes, X, Y and Z. The reduction of the relatively large, complex electrical generator described in the previous section, into an equivalent dipole source, rests in part on cancellation of opposing electromotive forces. At least 90 per cent of all the potential generated by ventricular fibers is cancelled because of excitation waves moving in opposite directions.[12] In addition, blood within the heart has a conductivity ten times greater than that of the lungs, favoring internal short circuiting and reducing the apparent size of the generator. Although nondipolar information is available in the ECG, particularly from the precordium,[13] its detection requires extremely precise recording techniques and computer analysis.[13, 14] Interpretation of the ECG by vector analysis was introduced by Einthoven[15] in 1913 and popularized by Robert Grant.[16] In this method, the components of the ECG are summarized as a vector or force with magnitude and orientation in space. This approach seems preferable to pattern recognition which requires the student to memorize numerous disease patterns in 12 or more electrocardiographic leads.

TRANSMISSION CHARACTERISTICS

Clinical electrocardiography is based on variations in electrical potential at the body surface, which are determined not only by the electrical signal generated by the heart, but by the conducting properties of the tissues between the heart and the body surface. Fortunately, the body behaves as a simple resistive medium,[17] for the frequencies involved in the electrocardiogram,[18] and no significant distortions of wave forms are introduced in transmission to the body surface.

LEAD SYSTEMS

An electrocardiographic lead is a specific array of electrodes connected to the two inputs of a galvonometer. A lead may consist of an electrode on the left arm versus an electrode on the right arm (standard limb lead 1), and is then called a bipolar lead because both electrodes experience significant variations in potential with the heart beat, and the recorded potential is the instantaneous difference between the two electrodes. A unipolar lead combines an exploring electrode, which experiences considerable potential variation with an indifferent electrode which experiences relatively little change. Usually, the latter is achieved by a sufficient remoteness from the

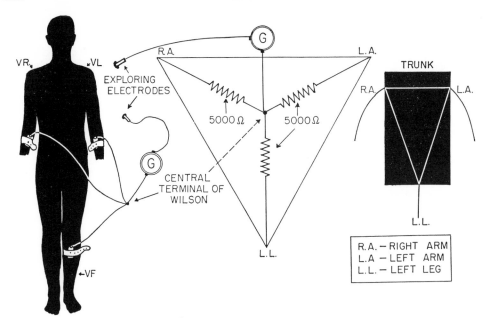

FIGURE 12-5   CENTRAL TERMINAL OF WILSON

Accurate unipolar recording of cardiac potentials requires an indifferent electrode which is un-affected by potentials developed by the heart. If electrodes on all three extremity leads are connected through 5000 ohm resistors to a single terminal (the central terminal of Wilson) the potentials at the extremities almost completely cancel out to provide a fairly reliable indifferent electrode. The heart is not exactly equidistant from each electrode, since it is situated toward one end of a roughly rectangular volume conductor, but the resulting errors have not proved too serious for practical purposes.

generator, but in clinical use, the indifferent electrode is apt to be formed in a manner introduced by Wilson for his central terminal[19] (Fig. 12–5).

The first lead system, three bipolar limb leads, remains the bedrock of present clinical electrocardiography. This system is diagrammed in Figure 12–6A as Einthoven's "equilateral triangle." Actually, the limb leads would not record equal voltages if a standard signal from the heart were transmitted with equal intensity, parallel to each of the three leads. Berger's triangle (Fig. 12–6B) illustrates the distortion introduced by several physical factors, particularly the eccentric location of the heart in the chest, and the nature and extent of the conductor interposed between the heart and the surface electrodes. These transmission characteristics may be determined experimentally and are summarized as the transfer impedance; they are incorporated in the lead field concept of McPhee and Johnston.[20]

The conventional precordial leads, introduced by Wilson,[19] have the exploring electrode placed in specific anatomic locations and use the central terminal of Wilson as the indifferent electrode (Fig. 12–7). Although the unipolar limb leads and precordial leads are quite useful in vector analysis of the electrocardiogram, these leads were popularized under a mistaken applicaion of theory and experimental evidence. It was assumed that these leads recorded predominantly,

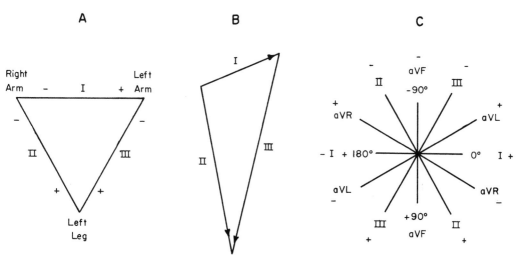

FIGURE 12-6 LIMB LEAD SYSTEMS

A, Einthoven's equilateral triangle.

B, Burger's triangle, summarizing the effects of transfer impedance on the limb leads of Einthoven.

C, Hexaxial reference system, placing all 6 limb leads concentrically through the electric center of the heart, the "equivalent dipole" location. (From Guntheroth, *Pediatric Electrocardiography*, W. B. Saunders Co., 1965.)

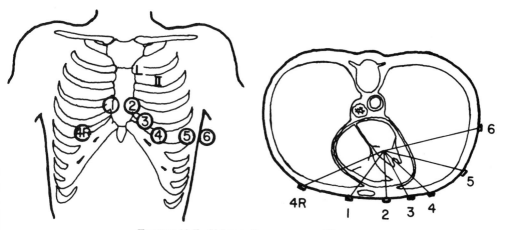

FIGURE 12-7 V-LEAD POSITIONS OF WILSON

Frontal and horizontal cross-sectional views of the thorax in relation to the precordial V-lead positions of Wilson. In the former, "L" indicates the angle of Louis, immediately below which is the second intercostal space, "II." V_1 and V_2 are in the fourth I.S., V_4 is in the fifth I.S. at the midclavicular line, and V_3 is half way between V_2 and V_4. V_5 and V_6 are on the same level as V_4; V_5 is at the anterior axillary line and V_6 is at the midaxillary line. V_{4R} is comparable to V_4, but over the right hemithorax. (From Guntheroth, *Pediatric Electrocardiography*, W. B. Saunders Co., 1965.)

if not exclusively, the subjacent myocardium, and therefore were able to detect local changes, such as myocardial infarcts. Although local information is, in fact, contained in these unipolar leads, it is a small percentage of the total potential recorded at that site, in relation to the large potential variations introduced by imprecise positioning of the electrodes in clinical practice.

Unipolar limb leads are composed of an exploring electrode on one limb versus the central terminal of Wilson, usually modified by deleting from the central terminal the input from the limb which is recorded. This combination is referred to as an augmented unipolar limb lead,[21] and designated as aVR, aVL or aVF, for the right arm, left arm and foot, respectively.

The unipolar leads, as well as the precordial leads, may be used for vector analysis in a manner identical with the bipolar leads. For convenience of analysis, a triaxial or hexaxial system is commonly used (Fig. 12–6C). The transformation of the triangular system to the triaxial system is justifiable by vector analysis of the electrical forces. A vector is unchanged by any maneuver as long as its direction and magnitude are unchanged. Therefore, a vector with a force of 2 mV directed horizontally to the left is the same, whether it is visualized at the level of the shoulders (standard limb lead 1) or at the heart level (triaxial system). Although the unipolar limb leads are redundant in terms of informational content, nevertheless, they are useful clinically in breaking down the frontal plane into 30-degree sectors for rapid analysis.

Although Einthoven used graphic vectorial analysis for the ECG by plotting the magnitude and direction of ten instantaneous vectors for a complete QRS cycle, vectorcardiography was held back until the development of the cathode ray tube, or oscilloscope. The first popular system was Wilson's equilateral tetrahedron, which added an anterior-posterior lead for the Z-axis to Einthoven's triangle supplying the inputs for the X and Y axes.[22] The newer lead systems are designed to minimize distortions produced by varying body build and variations in the position of the equivalent dipole[23, 24, 25] and are referred to as corrected lead systems. The cost and availability of equipment for vectorcardiograms has limited their application in clinical medicine, but vectorcardiography has had a major impact on the approach to the conventional 12 lead electrocardiogram.

RECORDING EQUIPMENT

The modern electrocardiographic recorder is usually a compact, transistorized amplifier with a heated stylus, writing on heat sensitive paper. Unfortunately, many of the recorders in use today are inadequate in their frequency response.[26] Both an underdamped and overdamped galvanometer can produce serious distortions in a record (Fig. 12–8). In most clinical situations, overdamping is a more common problem. The instruments should have a frequency response of 50 cycles per second or greater.[27] Gross distortions can be determined by inspection of the recording produced by the built-in calibration apparatus. For more precise analysis of the frequency response, the rise time for the calibration square wave should be less than .01 second. (The rise time is the time required for the deflection of the stylus to travel between the tenth and ninetieth percentage points of the ascent.[28]) The frequency response is roughly .40 divided by the rise time.

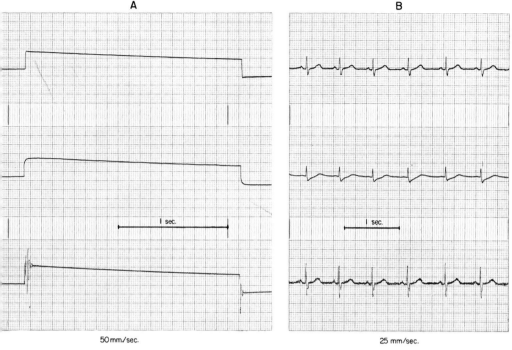

FIGURE 12-8   GALVANOMETER DISTORTIONS

A, From above downward, square waves produced by the calibration voltage of 1 mv. applied to properly damped, overdamped, and underdamped recorders. In the properly damped record there is a minimal overshoot; the slow descent of the plateau is due to the time constant of the machine.

B, Lead II was fed simultaneously to the three recorders demonstrated in A. Note particularly the apparent S-T segment depression in the overdamped (middle) record, and the factitious increase in amplitude of the S wave in the underdamped record. (From Guntheroth, *Pediatric Electrocardiography*, W. B. Saunders Co., 1965.)

Needless to say, a faster paper speed than the conventional paper speed of 25 mm. per second is helpful in analyzing the frequency response of the recorder. Many of the modern recorders have both 25 and 50 mm. per second paper speeds, and the higher paper speed facilitates precise reading of the duration of various complexes, particularly in the presence of tachycardia.

The method of coupling the leads from the patient to the recorder affects the slower components of the electrocardiogram, the P and T waves and the S-T segment. Frequently, there are relatively large potential differences between various electrodes in the ECG leads which would have to be balanced by an elaborate adjustment for each patient if the leads were directly coupled, and the balancing would have to be repeated many times during the routine recording in order to keep the stylus on the paper. These difficulties are overcome in the modern instrument by accepting the input from the patient through a resistor-condensor coupling, which tends to restore the stylus to the center of the paper in a relatively short time. The values of the condensor and resistor are selected to achieve a time constant of 3 seconds; i.e., when a one mV square wave is added to the input by the calibration device, the deflection will decay toward the baseline, so that in 3 seconds, the galvonometer deflection will be only one third of the original calibration deflection. This type of decay is seen in Figure 12–8. Other time constants are used in other recorders and those with a very short time constant may introduce serious artifacts by eliminating the slower components. For example, fetal electrocardiograms are sometimes recorded with an electroencephalographic recorder which employs a very short time constant, effectively eliminating both maternal and fetal P and T waves.[29]

Proper grounding of the recorder is essential not only for records free of noise but also for safety, particularly in situations involving the use of pacemaker units, where remarkably small stray currents can induce ventricular fibrillation.[30]

II. ROUTINE INTERPRETATION

Considerable training and experience may be necessary to fully appreciate all of the information contained in the electrocardiogram. However, every physician should be familiar with the technique to the point of recognizing disorders of rate and rhythm. This requires some familiarity with the conventions of electrocardiographic recording.

The calibration device on most recorders introduces a one mV signal which, with normal amplification, produces a deflection of 1 cm. of paper, or 10 small squares (Fig. 12–8). At the ordinary paper speed of 25 mm. per second (Fig. 12–8B), each millimeter of paper, or one square, represents .04 seconds. There is a heavier line every fifth square at .20 second, consequently, one second is equivalent to 25 small squares, or five of the large squares. The heart rate may be determined by dividing an average cycle length in seconds (the R-R interval) into 60, or by counting the number of cardiac cycles in three seconds (15 large squares) and multiplying by 20. Many physicians use special rulers designed to read off the rate at an interval of three heart beats.

DISORDERS OF RATE AND RHYTHM

Ordinarily, the heart rate is between 60 and 100 beats per minute for the adult, and each beat begins in the sinus node and produces a normally oriented P-wave which is followed after a normal interval by the QRS and the T-wave. If these criteria are met, the subject has a normal sinus rhythm (Table 12–1). A subject in whom the heart rate is over 100 but otherwise meets these criteria, is defined as having sinus tachycardia, and if the rate is under 60, sinus bradycardia.

RAPID RATE, REGULAR RHYTHM

The range of sinus tachycardia is great, particularly for infants in whom rates of as much as 210 are found with stressful situations. At these rates, there is frequently some superimposition of the P-waves on the T-waves, and it may be difficult at times to be certain that the origin of the P-wave is in the sinus node, a fact suggested by an upright P-wave in all three of the standard limb leads. Extremely rapid

Table 12–1.   *DISORDERS OF RATE,*
MECHANISM, AND RHYTHM

NORMAL RATE, MECHANISM, AND RHYTHM
  Regular sinus rhythm

RAPID RATE, REGULAR RHYTHM
  Sinus tachycardia
  Ectopic tachycardias (atrial, A-V nodal, and
    ventricular)
  Atrial flutter

SLOW RATE, REGULAR RHYTHM
  Sinus bradycardia
  A-V nodal rhythm with S-A block or com-
    plete A-V block
  Idioventricular rhythm with S-A block or
    complete A-V block
  2:1 A-V block

NORMAL RATE, REGULAR RHYTHM, ABNORMAL
MECHANISM
  Wandering pacemaker
  Ectopic atrial pacemaker
  First degree A-V block
  Moderate nodal tachycardia
  Atrial tachycardia with 2:1 A-V block

ARRHYTHMIAS, SINGLE OR INFREQUENT BEATS
  Extrasystole (atrial, A-V nodal, and ven-
    tricular)
  A-V dissociation with interference
  Second degree A-V block (occasional
    dropped beats)

REGULAR ARRHYTHMIAS
  Sinus arrhythmia
  Wenckebach phenomenon
  Bigeminy (atrial, A-V nodal, and ventricular)
  Trigeminy
  Reciprocal rhythm
  Parasystole

IRREGULAR ARRHYTHMIAS
  Atrial flutter with variable A-V block
  Atrial fibrillation
  Ventricular fibrillation

ASYSTOLE
  Sinoatrial arrest
  Complete A-V block with no escape

rates suggest atrial tachycardia or atrial flutter.[31] By definition, atrial tachycardia does not originate in the sinus node and therefore represents an abnormal mechanism as well as an abnormal rate. (The term mechanism is used in electrocardiographic texts to designate the anatomic origin of an electrocardiographic deflection. It also is used to designate disorders of conduction between the atria and ventricles.) The rhythm is characteristically unvarying with atrial tachycardia, and it is difficult to be certain of the origin or presence of the P-waves. In the latter instance, the arrhythmia may be labeled as a supraventricular tachycardia since A-V nodal tachycardia may occur with unusually high rates. The clinical characteristics are helpful in making a diagnosis of paroxysmal atrial tachycardia (PAT), a disorder with abrupt onset and termination. A record of such an abrupt conversion to sinus rhythm is seen in Figure 12–9. If supraventricular tachycardia is associated with abnormal ventricular conduction, it is very difficult, if not impossible, to differentiate with ordinary electrocardiographic means, ventricular tachycardia from the more benign supraventricular tachycardias. One condition which is prone to develop repeated episodes of PAT is the Wolff-Parkinson-White syndrome, or pre-excitation syndrome. This syndrome shows marked ventricular conduction disturbances of a special type and is illustrated in Figure 12–10. An example of a true ventricular tachycardia is seen in Figure 12–11. The diagnosis rests upon the independence of the ventricles from the atria, in addition to the wide, slurred QRS complexes with secondary T-wave changes.

SLOW RATE, REGULAR RHYTHM

Sinus bradycardia may be sufficiently slow to permit the A-V node to escape from the control of the sinus node (Fig. 12–12C). In this subject there was only a slight variation in the R-R interval and no apparent arrhy-

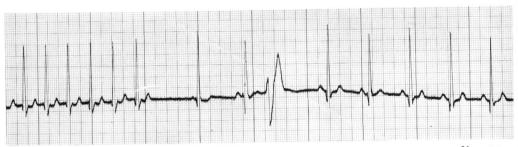

**FIGURE 12-9   SPONTANEOUS CONVERSION FROM PAROXYSMAL ATRIAL TACHYCARDIA TO NORMAL
SINUS RHYTHM**

ECG recorded during spontaneous conversion from paroxysmal atrial tachycardia to normal sinus
rhythm. The last ectopic atrial beat is not conducted. The next beat is an aberrantly conducted beat
originating in the atrium, and the third beat after conversion appears to be a ventricular extrasystole,
although it may represent an aberrantly conducted atrial beat. (From Guntheroth, *Pediatric Electrocardiography*, W. B. Saunders Co., 1965.)

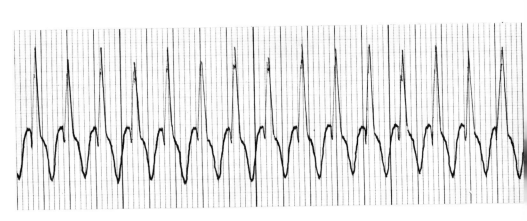

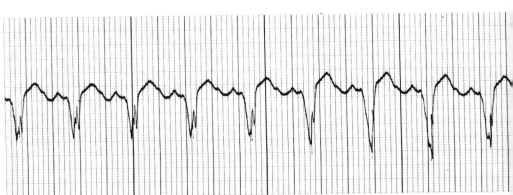

FIGURE 12-10   WOLFF-PARKINSON-WHITE SYNDROME WITH P.A.T.

Above, Paroxysmal atrial tachycardia in a patient with pre-excitation syndrome (Wolff-Parkinson-
White syndrome), more evident in the lower record. The upper record is practically indistinguishable
from ventricular tachycardia. (From Guntheroth, *Pediatric Electrocardiography*, W. B. Saunders
Co., 1965.)

I

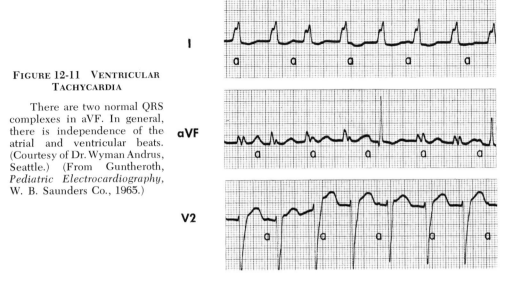

aVF

V2

FIGURE 12-11 VENTRICULAR TACHYCARDIA

There are two normal QRS complexes in aVF. In general, there is independence of the atrial and ventricular beats. (Courtesy of Dr. Wyman Andrus, Seattle.) (From Guntheroth, *Pediatric Electrocardiography*, W. B. Saunders Co., 1965.)

A

B

C

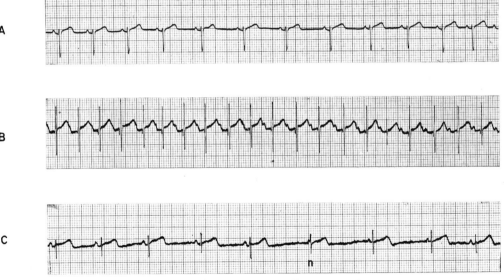

FIGURE 12-12 ECG's FROM NORMAL PREMATURE INFANTS

A, Sinus arrhythmia.
B, Sinus tachycardia.
C, Sinus bradycardia with nodal escape (n) for one beat. The complex with the escape is a fusion beat, since atrial excitation had begun just prior to the independent firing of the A-V node. (From Guntheroth, *Pediatric Electrocardiography*, W. B. Saunders Co., 1965.)

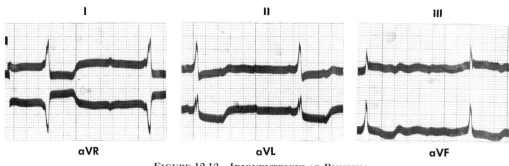

FIGURE 12-13   IDIOVENTRICULAR RHYTHM

Idioventricular rhythm in a patient with diphtheritic myocarditis. Note the independence of the atria and ventricles, and the wide, slurred QRS complexes suggestive of left bundle branch block. (From Guntheroth, *Pediatric Electrocardiography,* W. B. Saunders Co., 1965.)

thmia because there were no dropped beats.[32] The beat following the nodal escape originated from the sinus node, which depolarized early enough to recapture the A-V node. This is a form of A-V dissociation. To avoid ambiguity, this term should be reserved for dissociation of the atrial and ventricular beats due to the rate of the A-V node exceeding that of the sinus node and should not be used in those situations involving failure of A-V conduction (A-V block). It follows that A-V dissociation will rarely be associated with slow rates or regular rhythm. If there is intact A-V conduction and an active, if slower, sinus node, it is a mathematical certainty that the sinus node will occasionally capture and produce a mild irregularity of the rhythm. True A-V block, in contrast, is characterized by a remarkably constant rate, since there is no interference from the sinus pacemaker.

An even slower rate is present in the very uncommon idioventricular rhythm seen in Figure 12–13, from a patient with diphtheritic myocarditis.[33] The rate is very slow, the QRS complexes are broad and bizarre in configuration, with no regular association with P-waves, and there are marked T-wave changes.

These several levels of automaticity in the heart comprise a safety feature. In the event of sinus arrest or a complete A-V block there are two lower levels of possible pacemaker activity, the A-V node and the ventricles. Normally, competition between the centers is avoided by the higher rate of automaticity of the sinus node and the lack of protection for the lower centers from waves transmitted from the sinus node. In other words, the lower centers are depolarized by the propagated wave from the sinus node before the lower centers spontaneously depolarize. In addition, there is a decreasing influence of the effects of vagal stimulation in the lower centers (A-V node and ventricle), enhancing the possibility of escape by these centers from excessive vagal inhibition.

Another example of relatively slow rate and regular rhythm is seen in Figure 12–14, with a ventricular rate of 75 and an atrial rate of 150. Only every other sinus beat is conducted, resulting from a 2:1 A-V block, one type of a larger class of second degree A-V block. (First degree block is defined as slowed A-V conduction but with all sinus beats conducted to the ventricles. In second degree block, some, but not

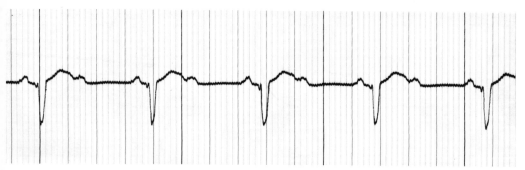

FIGURE 12-14   SECOND DEGREE A-V BLOCK

A particular type of second degree A-V block, 2:1 block. (From Guntheroth, *Pediatric Electrocardiography*, W. B. Saunders Co., 1965.)

all, atrial beats are dropped, and in third degree block there is no A-V conduction whatsoever.)

NORMAL RATE, REGULAR RHYTHM, BUT ABNORMAL MECHANISM

These are subtle disorders, diagnosed almost exclusively by the ECG.

A P-R interval prolonged beyond normal limits for age and rate (Table 12–2) is defined as first degree A-V block. The great majority of children with this electrocardiographic finding have no heart disease, although it occasionally serves as a subtle indication of myocardial disorders. There is nothing specific about P-R prolongation in relation to rheumatic fever, however; similar findings occur with a variety of infectious diseases.[37] In fact, the P-R interval is second in lability only to the T-wave. P-R prolongation, however, is a very useful early sign of digitalis intoxication in children, and for this reason, a control ECG is mandatory before digitalization.[38]

Nodal tachycardia of modest degree may produce a normal heart rate, even though the rate would represent a tachycardia relative to the usual automaticity of the A-V node. Similarly, atrial tachycardia with a 2:1 A-V block may produce a ventricular rate within the limits of normal.

ARRHYTHMIAS: SINGLE OR INFREQUENT BEATS

Extrasystoles are very common and are probably a universal experience at one time or another. If the premature contraction begins with a P-wave, it is probably an atrial extrasystole (Fig. 12–15). Usually, the P-wave will be different from the normal sinus node beat, and the P-R interval will vary, depending upon the refractory state of the A-V node. With the atrial extrasystole, all of the atrium, including the sinus node, is depolarized, and the normal pacemaker cells are reset so that the next beat occurs at the normal P-P interval. Consequently, there is no compensatory pause after the extrasystole. Occasionally, these atrial premature beats will be associated with abnormal ventricular conduction, such as that produced in the first atrial extrasystole in Figure 12–15, resulting in a complex which is difficult to distinguish from a ventricular extrasystole. Similarly,

Table 12–2.   *CYCLE LENGTH, HEART RATE, AND Q-T INTERVAL AVERAGE (AND UPPER LIMITS)*[36]

CYCLE LENGTH (SEC.)	HEART RATE PER MIN.	AVERAGE Q-T (SEC.)	CYCLE LENGTH (SEC.)	HEART RATE PER MIN.	AVERAGE Q-T (SEC.)
1.50	40	0.45(0.49)	0.85	70	0.36(0.38)
1.40	43	0.44(0.48)	0.80	75	0.35(0.38)
1.30	46	0.43(0.47)	0.75	80	0.34(0.37)
1.25	48	0.42(0.46)	0.70	86	0.33(0.36)
1.20	50	0.41(0.45)	0.65	92	0.32(0.35)
1.15	52	0.41(0.45)	0.60	100	0.31(0.34)
1.10	55	0.40(0.44)	0.55	109	0.30(0.33)
1.05	57	0.39(0.43)	0.50	120	0.28(0.31)
1.00	60	0.39(0.42)	0.45	133	0.27(0.29)
0.95	63	0.38(0.41)	0.40	150	0.25(0.28)
0.90	67	0.37(0.40)	0.35	172	0.23(0.26)

P-Q (P-R) INTERVAL, WITH RATE AND AGE: AVERAGE (AND UPPER LIMITS OF NORMAL)[34-36]

RATE	0-1/12 YEAR	1/12-6/12 YEAR	6/12-1 YEAR	1-3 YEARS	3-8 YEARS	8-12 YEARS	12-16 YEARS	ADULT
<60						0.16 (0.18)	0.16(0.19)	0.17(0.21)
60- 80					0.15 (0.17)	0.15 (0.17)	0.15(0.18)	0.16(0.21)
80-100	0.10(0.12)				0.14 (0.16)	0.145(0.16)	0.15(0.17)	0.15(0.20)
100-120	0.10(0.115)			(0.15)	0.13 (0.155)	0.145(0.15)	0.15(0.16)	0.15(0.19)
120-140	0.10(0.11)	0.105(0.14)	0.11 (0.14)	0.12(0.14)	0.125(0.15)	0.14 (0.15)		0.15(0.18)
140-160	0.09(0.11)	0.10 (0.13)	0.105(0.13)	0.11(0.14)	0.12 (0.14)			(0.17)
160-180	0.10(0.11)	0.10 (0.12)	0.10 (0.12)	0.10(0.12)				
>180	0.09	0.09 (0.11)	0.10 (0.11)					

QRS DURATION: AVERAGE (AND UPPER LIMITS) FOR AGE[34]

Years:	0-1/12	1/12-6/12	6/12-1	1-3	3-8	8-12	12-16	ADULT
Seconds:	0.05(0.065)	0.05(0.07)	0.05(0.06)	0.06(0.07)	0.07(0.08)	0.07(0.09)	0.07(0.10)	0.08(0.10)

A-V nodal extrasystoles may be associated with abnormal conduction and will be even more difficult to distinguish from ventricular extrasystoles, since they are not preceded by atrial waves.

Ventricular extrasystoles frequently are not conducted in a retrograde fashion into the atria, and consequently the next normal sino-atrial impulse finds the ventricles refractory, and this beat is dropped. There is no further activity until the next sinus beat which occurs at the normal P-P interval and is followed by a normal QRS complex, but the R-R interval is unusually long, called a compensatory pause (Figs. 12–9 and 12–15). Figure 12–15 also demonstrates a nodal premature beat which failed to excite the atria and was associated with a compensatory pause. It is possible for either nodal or ventricular extrasystoles to be conducted retrogradely into the atria and reset the sinus node and thereby eliminate the compensatory pause. Therefore, the absence of a compensatory pause is

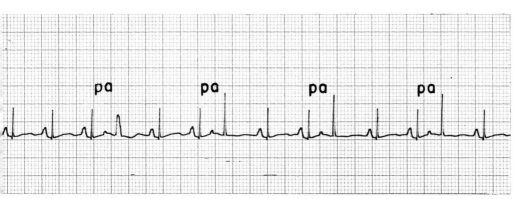

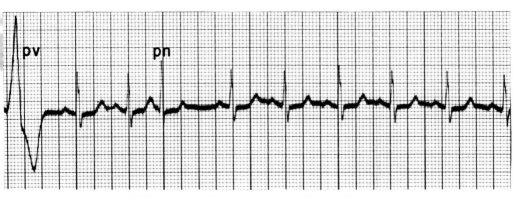

FIGURE 12-15   ATRIAL, VENTRICULAR AND NODAL EXTRASYSTOLES

Above, Frequent atrial extrasystoles or premature atrial contractions (pa). The succeeding sinoatrial beat is only slightly delayed, and there is no compensatory pause. In the first atrial extrasystolic beat, the QRS is somewhat broadened, indicating aberrant ventricular conduction. In the lower record, ventricular extrasystole or premature ventricular beat (pv) is the first complex, followed by a compensatory pause prior to the next, normal sinoatrial beat. The beat labeled "pn" is a premature nodal beat or nodal extrasystole, with no retrograde conduction to the atria, suggested by the compensatory pause. (From Guntheroth, *Pediatric Electrocardiography*, W. B. Saunders Co., 1965.)

more common with atrial extrasystoles but does not rule out a nodal or ventricular source.

Interference dissociation may produce arrhythmias with only infrequent irregularity in a basically regular rhythm. Figure 12–16*B* illustrates an ECG with a regular R-R interval of .53 seconds and a single premature beat with an R-R interval of .42 second. This premature beat is preceded by a P-R interval of .21 second, and it may be seen that most of the other beats have a random relationship between the P and QRS waves. The basic mechanism is an A-V nodal tachycardia, producing the dissociation by virtue of its higher rate, 113, compared to the sinus node rate of 107. The single premature beat here is an instance in which the sinoatrial impulse arrived at a time when the A-V node was receptive, and there was capture by the sinoatrial mechanism for one beat. This is referred to as interference dissociation. This is not a benign disorder, as contrasted to the simpler type of A-V dissociation seen with in-

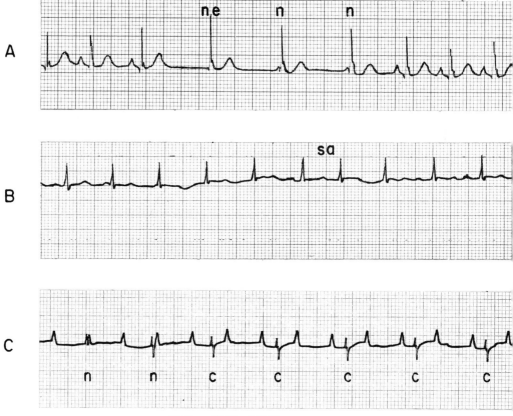

FIGURE 12-16   A-V DISSOCIATION

A, Sinus arrhythmia with nodal escape (ne).

B, Nodal tachycardia producing A-V dissociation with interference by sinoatrial capture for one beat (sa).

C, 2:1 A-V block with nodal tachycardia is the basic rhythm; most atrial beats are conducted (c), but occasionally the A-V nodal pacemaker is sufficiently rapid to take over (n). (From Guntheroth, *Pediatric Electrocardiography*, W. B. Saunders Co., 1965.)

creased vagal tone and slow rate, illustrated in Figure 12–16A. The type of A-V dissociation illustrated in Figure 12–16B, associated with A-V nodal tachycardia, is frequently a sign of more severe disturbance; in this case the patient had active rheumatic fever with carditis. Figure 12–16C represents another form of A-V dissociation, producing a fairly regular R-R interval. The fundamental rhythm is a 2:1 A-V block, but occasionally the A-V node ("n") escapes and becomes the pacemaker. The first of these two beats is a fusion beat resulting from superimposition of the P and QRS complexes, indicating the dissociation of the two complexes.

Some forms of second degree block will produce a mild arrhythmia by dropping an occasional ventricular response due to failure of some sinoatrial beats to be conducted.

REGULAR ARRHYTHMIAS

The most common of all arrhythmias is illustrated in Figure 12–12A, sinus arrhythmia. Although the varia-

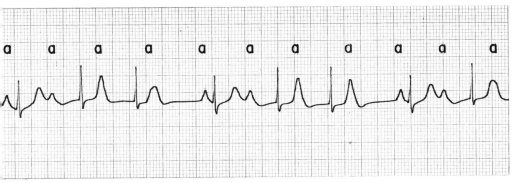

FIGURE 12-17   WENCKEBACH PHENOMENON

Wenckebach phenomenon, a special form of second degree A-V block. Every fourth or fifth atrial beat is not conducted. (From Guntheroth, *Pediatric Electrocardiography*, W. B. Saunders Co., 1965.)

tion between beats can be very marked, there is a regular acceleration of rate with inspiration and a slowing with expiration, and all QRS complexes are preceded by P waves with a normal P-R interval.

Figure 12–17 is another cyclical arrhythmia but with definite pathologic significance. There is a dropped beat every fourth or fifth beat. The first beat after the dropped beat has a normal P-R interval, but the P-R interval increases progressively with each beat thereafter until a QRS is dropped and the cycle begins again. Another characteristic of this disorder known as Wenckebach phenomenon is the progressive shortening of the R-R interval with each beat after the dropped beat. This specific form of second degree A-V block represents an A-V conduction disorder which is rate-related. In a healthy heart, a sufficiently rapid atrial stimulus can produce A-V block.[39] In an A-V node which is disturbed by rheumatic carditis, hypoxia or other disorders, the rate at which the A-V node fatigues will be lower. In the Wenckebach phenomenon, the dropped beat allows an interval sufficient for recovery of the A-V node and the following P-R in-

terval is normal. However, the next sinus beat occurs before complete recovery and again results in a delay in A-V conduction. This delay is further increased in the following beats until the sinoatrial wave encounters the A-V node during its refractory period and no ventricular response is seen, and the cycle begins again.

An easily recognizable regular arrhythmia is ventricular bigeminy or coupling (Fig. 12–18). In this disorder, there is a regular alternation between normal sinus beats and ventricular extrasystoles. Coupling can also occur from either atrial or nodal foci.

Another form of regular coupling is seen in Figure 12–19. Every third beat is a ventricular extrasystole. Although many texts describe this as ventricular trigeminy, this term probably should be reserved for the situation when two extrasystoles follow a single normal beat.[40] (At any rate, "three twins" is a questionable compound.) The clinical distinction of the two states is of some importance, since two consecutive extrasystoles represents an ominous condition, frequently progressing to ventricular tachycardia, whereas the disorder

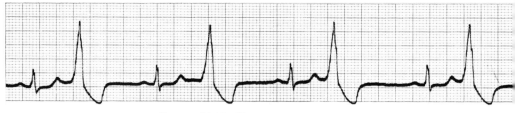

FIGURE 12-18   VENTRICULAR BIGEMINY

Ventricular bigeminy or coupling. (From Guntheroth, *Pediatric Electrocardiography*, W. B. Saunders Co., 1965.)

illustrated in Figure 12–19 is less worrisome than bigeminy.

Another arrhythmia which closely resembles bigeminy is illustrated in Figure 12–20. This rhythm represents sinoatrial block with an A-V nodal pacemaker, followed in most instances by a coupled atrial beat. This type of rhythm is frequently called echo or reciprocal rhythm, or return extrasystole.[41] The return extrasystole is thought to originate through retrograde conduction from the A-V nodal beat into the atrium, although in the usual instance, this produces a P-wave which is different in polarity from that which would be expected. An alternate possibility is simple mechanical stimulation of the atria by the initial A-V nodal contraction.

An uncommon arrhythmia is parasystole. This arrhythmia appears to be merely an occasional ventricular extrasystole, but on close inspection with the aid of a pair of calipers and a long ECG strip, it is apparent that there is a systematic occurrence of the extrasystoles at regular intervals, with no fixed relationship to the normally conducted beats.[40] This is in contrast to the usual form of ventricular extrasystoles which have a relatively fixed coupling with the normal beats. Because of its characteristic independence of the influence of the normal sinus beats, an entrance block is inferred. The entrance block is thought to result from ischemic tissue with a slowed recovery, which fails to be depolarized by the normally conducted beat. The parasystolic focus then fires and finds the tissue on its periphery recovered sufficiently to conduct the extrasystole back to the normal tissue.

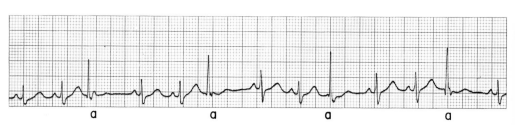

FIGURE 12-19   REGULAR EXTRASYSTOLES

Ventricular extrasystoles occurring every third beat. (From Guntheroth, *Pediatric Electrocardiography*, W. B. Saunders Co., 1965.)

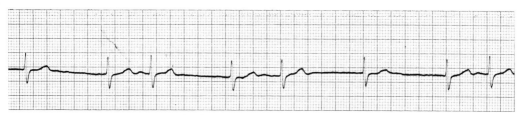

FIGURE 12-20   SINOATRIAL BLOCK WITH ECHO RHYTHM

Sinoatrial block with reciprocal rhythm or return extrasystoles. This form of coupling occurs here after the second, third and fifth A-V nodal beats. (Courtesy of Dr. Philip G. Deane, Mercer Island, Washington.) (From Guntheroth, *Pediatric Electrocardiography*, W. B. Saunders Co., 1965.)

IRREGULAR ARRHYTHMIAS

Completely irregular arrhythmias involve either chaotic electrical activity (fibrillation) or very rapid pacemaker activity, with varying ventricular response. The former type is illustrated in Figure 12–21 from a patient with atrial fibrillation. Figure 12–22 represents atrial flutter with variable ventricular response. More often, flutter is associated with a fixed 2:1, 3:1 or 4:1 ventricular response, but in this patient the varying A-V block is comparable to the Wenckebach phenomenon. The abnormal atrial focus in this patient was capable of slowing down to normal rates with sleep at which time his A-V conduction improved, to the point of a 1:1 response with a normal P-R interval. The transition in this patient between the widely varying atrial rates, from 70 up to 250, adds clinical grounds to the experimental evidence presented by Scherf,[42]

that atrial flutter is not due to circus movement but to rapid firing of a single ectopic pacemaker. The alternate theories of atrial flutter are diagramed in Figure 12–23. A similar dispute exists as to the mechanism involved in atrial fibrillation: circus waves, or multiple ectopic pacemakers. There is evidence that both mechanisms may operate, depending on the given patient. Figure 12–24 demonstrates the ultimate in electrocardiographic chaos, ventricular fibrillation. The fatal consequence of this arrhythmia lies in the resultant failure of cardiac output and therefore of coronary arterial perfusion. Recovery is impossible without prompt resuscitative measures such as electrical countershock, or cardiac massage.[43] The patient presented in this illustration was successfully resuscitated without countershock, but with cardiac massage.

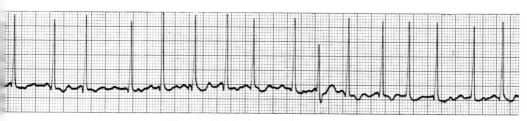

FIGURE 12-21   ATRIAL FIBRILLATION

Atrial fibrillation in a 15-year-old girl with advanced rheumatic mitral stenosis. (Courtesy of Dr. Beverly C. Morgan, Seattle, Washington.) (From Guntheroth, *Pediatric Electrocardiography*, W. B. Saunders Co., 1965.)

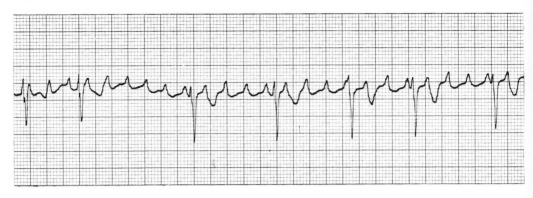

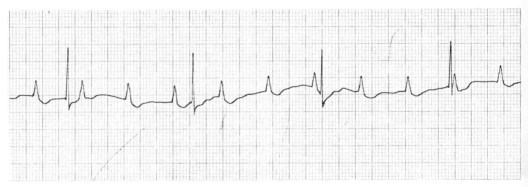

FIGURE 12-22   ATRIAL FLUTTER

Above. Atrial flutter with variable ventricular response.
Below, Same patient as above, but with much slower atrial rate and with a slow, regular ventricular rate indicating complete A-V block. (From Guntheroth, *Pediatric Electrocardiography,* W. B. Saunders Co., 1965.)

ASYSTOLE

The other highly lethal form of arrhythmia is ventricular asystole. This can result from either a sinoatrial arrest or complete A-V block with no nodal or ventricular escape. Spontaneous recovery is possible if the lower centers escape, but if persistent ventricular asystole occurs, cardiac massage is essential. Figure 12–25 illustrates atrial tachycardia with complete A-V block, resulting in ventricular standstill. The two complexes at the end of the tracing represent initial resuscitative efforts with closed chest massage, which were successful in reviving the patient.

INTERVAL MEASUREMENTS

Although the most urgent and widespread requirement of ECG interpretation involves the arrhythmias, there is a great deal of additional information contained in the electrocardiogram and vectorcardiogram. In a systematic fashion, measurements are made and recorded of the heart rate, the P-R interval, QRS duration and the Q-T interval (Fig. 12–26). The initial deflection of the QRS complex in any scalar lead is either a Q or an R wave. If the initial deflection is negative (below the isoelectric or baseline) it is a Q wave, and if it is positive, an R

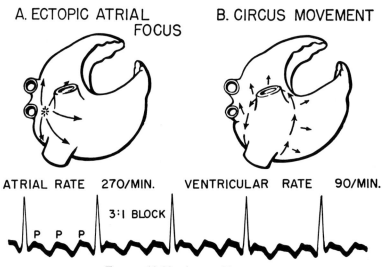

A. ECTOPIC ATRIAL FOCUS   B. CIRCUS MOVEMENT

ATRIAL RATE 270/MIN.   VENTRICULAR RATE 90/MIN.

3:1 BLOCK

P P P

FIGURE 12-23   ATRIAL FLUTTER

Atrial flutter is characterized by repetitive atrial excitation occurring at such a rapid rate that all waves of excitation are not transmitted through the A-V node into the ventricles. Thus, there may be two P waves for each QRS complex (2:1 block), three P waves to one QRS (3:1 block) or even 4:1 block.

A, According to one theory, the rapid atrial rate results from the rapid firing of an ectopic focus in the atrial musculature, similar to atrial paroxysmal tachycardia except for the failure of the A-V node to transmit all the impulses.

B, According to another theory, atrial flutter occurs when a wave of excitation encircles the roots of the superior and inferior vena cava at a rate determined by the conduction velocity of the myocardium. Waves of excitation spread from the circular pathway to the remainder of the atrial musculature. Circus movements of this type can be produced experimentally.

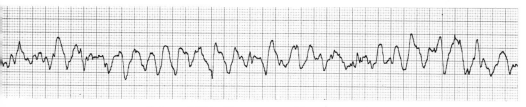

FIGURE 12-24   VENTRICULAR FIBRILLATION

(From Guntheroth, *Pediatric Electrocardiography*, W. B. Saunders Co., 1965.)

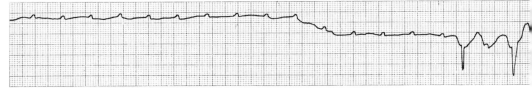

FIGURE 12-25   VENTRICULAR ASYSTOLE

Complete A-V block with atrial tachycardia, and no nodal or ventricular escape. Ventricular asystole is interrupted by external cardiac massage producing the two QRS complexes at the end of the strip. (From Guntheroth, *Pediatric Electrocardiography*, W. B. Saunders Co., 1965.)

wave. A negative deflection after the R wave is an S wave. An entire ventricular complex which has no discernible R wave is referred to as a QS complex. A secondary positive deflection after the S wave is labeled R′, and a secondary negative wave after the R′ is S′. By convention, capital letters are used when the component is the major deflection, or is at least one-half the amplitude of the major deflection. Minor components with less than one-half the amplitude of the major deflection are written in lower case letters. For example, the complex in Figure 12–26 is written qRs.

The P-R interval is measured between the start of the P wave to the beginning of the QRS complex. Although this interval might logically be called the PQ interval, by convention, it is referred to as the P-R interval.

The duration of the QRS, like other components of the electrocardiogram, is distributed in a more or less normal fashion and increases somewhat with age (Table 12–2).

The Q-T interval is measured from the onset of the Q to the end of the T wave. When measuring the Q-T interval, or the P-R or QRS duration, lead II is ordinarily utilized because there is frequently a recognizable Q wave in lead II, permitting reasonable certainty that all of the QRS complex can be identified. If a lead were selected in which the initial part of the QRS complex was isoelectric, a systematic error would be introduced. The Q-T interval represents the re-

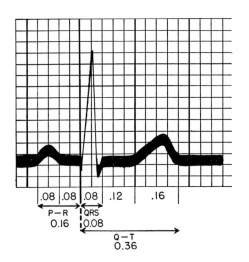

FIGURE   12-26   DURATION OF WAVES AND INTERVALS

The P-R interval, QRS interval and Q-T interval are among the most common values measured during routine electrocardiographic interpretation. Arrows indicate the basis for determining their respective duration.

polarization time and may be the only indication of a metabolic disturbance of the myocardium. There is a normal Q-T interval for any heart rate, which may be obtained from tables such as the one in Table 12–2, or a correction may be made for rate by dividing the measured Q-T interval by the square root of the cycle length. The corrected QT or QTc should not exceed .425 second.[44] When measuring the Q-T interval, some care must be taken to separate the terminal portions of the T wave from the U wave, a positive wave immediately following the T wave. The U wave has no consistent clinical significance, with the exception of hypokalemia.[45]

DIRECTION AND MAGNITUDE OF ELECTRICAL FORCES

Additional interpretation of the electrocardiogram rests upon analysis of the magnitude and spatial orientation of the electrical forces and the sequence of these forces during a cardiac cycle. Although it is unwise to make literal anatomic inferences from electrical phenomena, it is essential to keep in mind the cardiac anatomy, in addition to the normal sequence of activation, and the orientation of the commonly used ECG leads. A particular anatomic relationship of paramount importance is that the right ventricle is anterior and to the right, and the left ventricle is posterior and to the left. If the right ventricle is hypertrophied, the total muscle mass is increased, and the total electrical forces generated by this muscle mass will cause a deviation in the average electrical force toward the right and anterior. The left ventricle is the dominant ventricle in the normal adult, performing more than five times as much work as the right ventricle. Conse-

quently, the great majority of electromotive force generated by the adult heart is produced by the left ventricle, and left ventricular hypertrophy will not necessarily alter the orientation of the normal mean vector, which is directed to the left and posterior. The only criteria available for hypertrophy in this instance are voltage criteria. Increased voltage in left ventricular hypertrophy is found in leads which are more or less parallel to the average vector, namely the R waves in leads I, aVL, V_5 and V_6, and the S wave in V_1 and V_2. Tables of normal values should be consulted for the upper limits of normal for the various leads (Table 12–3).

Orientation of the electrical forces in the frontal plane is determined from the limb leads. Figure 12–27 and 12–28 represent a normal electrocardiogram and the derived mean electrical axis from this recording. This presentation is essentially the same as that introduced by Einthoven with the substitution of a triaxial reference system for the triangular coordinates originally used. As in Einthoven's original method, leads I and III are utilized. The net amplitude of lead I is the amplitude of the positive deflections minus the amplitude of the negative deflections. For lead I the Q wave is .5 mm. and the R wave is 7, with a net deflection of +6.5 mm. Lead III has an equal R and S, with a net deflection of zero. If perpendiculars are dropped from leads I and III at +6.5 and 0 units respectively, the intersection will define the direction of the mean electrical axis (MEA), +30 degrees, and the magnitude of the vector will be 7.5 units, or in this case, 7.5 mm. It is permissible to use any two limb leads in calculating the mean electrical axis, and leads I and aVF are somewhat more convenient since they are perpendicular to each other. When the

Table 12–3.   R VOLTAGES ACCORDING TO LEAD AND AGE: MEAN (AND UPPER LIMITS)[34] (MEASURED IN MILLIMETERS, WHEN 1 mv = 10 mm. PAPER)

LEAD	0-1/12 YEAR	1/12-6/12 YEAR	6/12-1 YEAR	1-3 YEARS	3-8 YEARS	8-12 YEARS	12-16 YEARS	YOUNG ADULTS
I	4 (8)	7 (13)	8 (16)	8 (16)	7 (15)	7 (15)	6 (13)	5.5(13)
II	6 (14)	13 (24)	13 (27)	12.5(23)	12.5(22)	13.5(24)	13.5(24)	9 (25)
III	8 (16)	9 (20)	9 (20)	9 (20)	9 (20)	9 (24)	9 (24)	5.5(22)
aVR	3 (7)	3 (6)	2.5(6)	2 (6)	1.5(5)	1.5(4)	1.5(4)	1 (4)
aVL	2 (7)	4 (8)	4.5(10)	4.5(10)	3 (10)	2.5(10)	2.5(12)	2.5(9)
aVF	6.5(14)	9.5(20)	9.5(16)	8 (20)	10 (19)	10 (20)	11 (21)	5 (23)
V_1	15 (25)	11 (20)	10 (20)	9 (18)	7 (18)	6 (16)	5 (16)	3 (14)
V_2	21 (30)	21 (30)	19 (28)	16 (25)	13 (28)	10 (22)	9 (19)	6 (21)
V_5	12 (30)	17 (30)	18 (30)	19 (36)	21 (36)	22 (36)	18 (33)	12 (33)
V_6	6 (21)	9.5(20)	13 (20)	12 (24)	13.5(24)	14 (24)	13.5(22)	10 (21)

S VOLTAGES ACCORDING TO LEAD AND AGE: MEAN (AND UPPER LIMITS)

LEAD	0-1/12 YEAR	1/12-6/12 YEAR	6/12-1 YEAR	1-3 YEARS	3-8 YEARS	8-12 YEARS	12-16 YEARS	ADULT
I	4.5(10)	3.5(9)	3.5(9)	3 (8)	2 (8)	1.5(8)	1.5(8)	1 (6)
V_1	10 (20)	7 (18)	8 (16)	13 (27)	13.5(30)	16 (26)	15 (24)	9.5(23)
V_2	20 (35)	16 (30)	17 (30)	21 (34)	23 (38)	23 (38)	23 (48)	14 (36)
V_6	3.5(12)	2 (6)	2 (4)	1.5(4)	1 (4)	1 (4)	1 (5)	1 (13)

R/S RATIO ACCORDING TO AGE: MEAN, LOWER AND UPPER LIMITS OF NORMAL[34]

LEAD	0-1/12 YEAR	1/12-6/12 YEAR	6/12-1 YEAR	1-3 YEARS	3-8 YEARS	8-12 YEARS	12-16 YEARS	ADULT
LLN*	0.5	0.3	0.3	0.5	0.1	0.15	0.1	0.0
V_1 Mean	1.5	1.5	1.2	0.8	0.65	0.5	0.3	0.3
ULN†	19	S=0	6	2	2	1	1	1
LLN	0.3	0.3	0.3	0.3	0.05	0.1	0.1	0.1
V_2 Mean	1	1.2	1	0.8	0.5	0.5	0.5	0.2
ULN	3	4	4	1.5	1.5	1.2	1.2	2.5
LLN	0.1	1.5	2	3	2.5	4	2.5	2.5
V_6 Mean	2	4	6	20	20	20	10	9
ULN	S=0	S=0	S=0	S=0	S=0	S=0	S=0	S=0

*Lower limits of normal.
†Upper limits of normal.

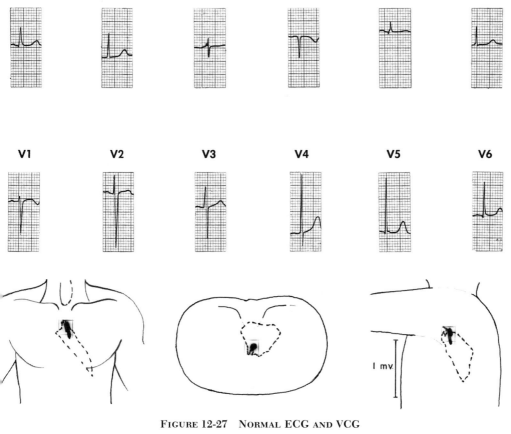

| I | II | III | aVR | aVL | aVF |

| V1 | V2 | V3 | V4 | V5 | V6 |

I mV.

FIGURE 12-27 NORMAL ECG AND VCG

ECG and VCG from a normal 9-year-old girl. (From Guntheroth, *Pediatric Electrocardiography*, W. B. Saunders Co., 1965.)

mean electrical axis is directed toward the patient's left and superiorly, the angle is designated in negative numbers from 0 to −90 degrees, with 0 degrees as the horizontal and −90 degrees as the vertical. If the MEA is directed inferiorly to either right or left, the axis is given in positive degrees. By convention, the normal electrical axis is from 0 to +90 degrees; from 0 to −90 degrees is designated as left axis deviation, and from +90 to +180 degrees is right axis deviation. If the average forces are directed to the patient's right and in a superior direction, the axis is designated as indeterminate. Actually, the normal electrical axis varies more than 90 degrees, even in the adult (Figure 12–29).

A quick and reasonably accurate method of determining the axis in the frontal plane is to inspect the limb leads for that lead which has the greatest amplitude, either positive or negative. The mean electrical axis will be parallel to that lead, and the direction will depend upon whether the deflection is positive or negative. Another method is to find a lead which has an equal R and S wave; the mean electrical axis will be perpendicular to that lead (e.g., lead III in Fig. 12–27).

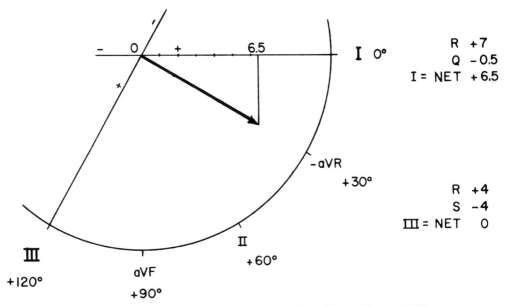

FIGURE 12-28   DERIVED MEAN ELECTRICAL AXIS FROM NORMAL ECG

Derivation of mean QRS vector from leads I and III of Figure 12-27. See text for discussion. (From Guntheroth, *Pediatric Electrocardiography*, W. B. Saunders Co., 1965.)

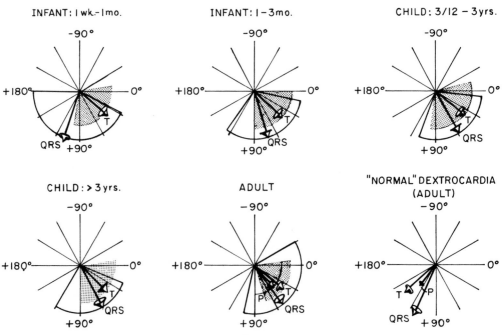

FIGURE 12-29   NORMAL RANGES FOR QRS AND T VECTORS ACCORDING TO AGE

(From Guntheroth, *Pediatric Electrocardiography*, W. B. Saunders Co., 1965.)

FIGURE 12-30 SPATIAL ORIENTATION OF THE
MEAN QRS VECTOR

Drawing of a model for determining and displaying the spatial orientation of the mean QRS vector. The shaft of the arrow is aligned according to the frontal plane axis relative to the triaxial lead system. The disk which is perpendicular to the shaft is then adjusted to project onto the precordial V-leads which show equal R and S complexes (the transition zone). The model here is adjusted for a mean electric axis of +30 degrees and a transition zone close to V_3, reflecting a slightly posterior orientation. (From Guntheroth, *Pediatric Electrocardiography*, W. B. Saunders Co., 1965.)

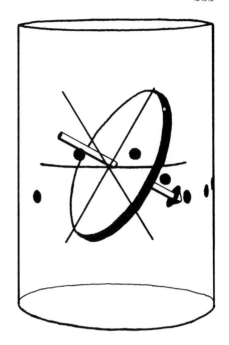

Further refinements are possible by comparing complexes of adjacent leads, and extrapolating between them. Since the limb leads are separated by 30 degrees, an accuracy of at least ±15 degrees is possible.

Determination of the anterior-posterior relationship of the mean cardiac vector is subject to more inaccuracies than the determination of the mean electrical axis in the frontal plane. The precordial leads of Wilson are not spaced at regular intervals, and none of these leads present pure anterior-posterior projections of the cardiac vector, although V_2 is the closest single lead (see Fig. 12–7). If the R wave is greater than the S in V_2, the mean vector is generally anterior. If the S is dominant, the mean vector is posterior, and if the R and S waves are equal, the mean vector is approximately perpendicular to V_2. The only situation in which major errors are introduced by this method is in marked right axis deviation, when a deep S is sometimes found in V_2 in the absence of posterior forces (determined by a vectorcardiogram with a corrected lead system).

Another method of determining the orientation of the mean vector in space is the null contour method popularized by Grant.[46] An equivalent dipole would produce an electrical field on the body surface which could be divided into two large areas of positivity and negativity, separated by a more or less narrow band of equiphasic QRS potentials (equal R and S complexes). This line of equiphasic potentials, the null contour, represents the intersection with the torso of a simple plane perpendicular to the long axis of the QRS vector (Fig. 12–30). This plane usually intersects the anterior chest wall somewhere between the conventional precordial electrode positions. (This intersection was referred to as the transition zone in unipolar theory, because it was thought to represent a transition between "right" and "left ventricular" potentials.) Devices such as that illustrated in Figure 12–30 are useful for the null contour method. Viewing the cylinder from the front, the shaft of the arrow is aligned with the mean electrical axis of the frontal plane. Then, maintaining this relationship, the disc perpendicular to the shaft is adjusted so that it projects onto the precordial lead positions to satisfy the null contour suggested by the precordial leads. In Figure 12–30, the plane of the disc intersects the precordium at the V_3 position, the site of the average transition zone.

A combination of these two methods is quite satisfactory. Lead V_2 is used as the initial indication of anterior or posterior orientation, but the null contour method is used to check its validity. If, for example, S is dominant in V_2, but V_3 shows an equiphasic QRS complex, it is clear that the mean vector is only slightly posterior, and is almost perpendicular to V_2. It is thus possible to refine the location of the mean vector in the anterior-posterior relationship.

A method of approaching the precordial leads which has empiric usefulness, is the R/S progression. Scanning the relationship of the R to the S wave of each of the precordial leads as it progresses from the right precordium toward the left, there should ordinarily be a smooth progression in the adult from an rS pattern in V_1 through an equiphasic R and S in V_2 and V_3 and a qRs in V_4 through V_6. In newborn infants this R/S progression is reversed so that there is a dominant R in the right precordial leads and a dominant S in V_5 and V_6. Between the ages of one month and two years of age, a partial reversal of the adult R/S progression is normally present, with a dominant R in V_1 as well as in V_6. In the adult, failure of a smooth progres-

sion from the right to the left suggests the possibility of an abnormality of the sequence of activation, which may be produced by an anterior myocardial infarction.

In a few electrocardiograms, particularly those involving serious disturbances in ventricular conduction, there may be two major vectors, frequently in almost opposite directions. It is obvious that averaging two divergent vectors will not only result in the loss of valuable information, but may actually produce a meaningless value. In these instances, Grant suggested that the two vectors be graphically represented separately and, specifically, he suggested the use of an initial .04 second vector and a terminal vector. In many instances, it is simpler and more logical to use merely the first half and second half of the total QRS duration.

The T wave can also be analyzed in terms of its average orientation in space. In general, the QRS and the T vector are relatively close to each other, which can be seen in the similarity in ranges of the normal in Figure 12–29. The QRS-T angle, formed by the angle between the two vectors, is normally less than 60 degrees and an angle greater than 90 degrees almost always indicates a pathological state. Also, the T vector tends to remain in the normal sector (0 to +90 degrees), or at least between the QRS vector and the normal sector. In other words, in the presence of left axis deviation of the QRS complex, the T axis will usually be closer to 0 degrees than will the QRS axis, and in right axis deviation, the T axis should be closer to +90 degrees than the QRS axis. Figure 12–31 represents a graphical presentation of the characteristic disorders of QRS and T vectors.

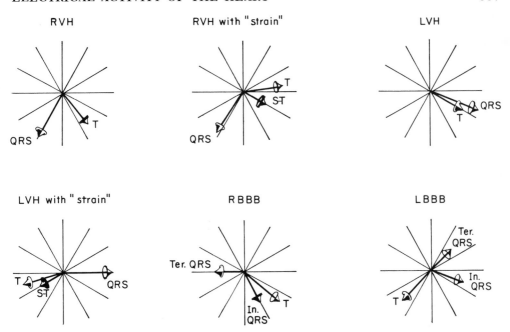

FIGURE 12-31   CHARACTERISTIC DISORDERS OF QRS AND T VECTORS

Characteristic disorders of QRS and T vectors associated with major categories of hypertrophy and conduction disturbances. Magnitudes of the vectors are not proportional. (From Guntheroth, *Pediatric Electrocardiography*, W. B. Saunders Co., 1965.)

VECTORCARDIOGRAPHY TERMINOLOGY AND CRITERIA

True vectorcardiograms, photographs of an oscilloscope trace, are being used increasingly in larger medical centers, and they will be discussed here briefly because it assists in understanding what is recorded in the ordinary ECG. Figure 12–32 relates scalar electrocardiographic leads with the vector presentation and also demonstrates the terminology commonly used to describe the vectorcardiogram. The corrected, orthogonal leads of the Frank system are represented by X, Y and Z in Figure 12–32A, and on the left side of each of these torso figures, there is the comparable lead from the conventional ECG. Although the voltage is different, the relative proportions of the QRS cycle are in agreement.

When the X and Y leads of Frank are combined, the frontal vector loop is inscribed. The horizontal plane is produced by combining the X and Z leads, and the saggital is composed of Y and Z leads. Although the third plane is redundant, it is frequently useful because superimposition of some of the parts of the loop may obscure details in one of the planes. The comet-shaped dots occur at 2 millisecond intervals (.002 second). The loop is inscribed in the direction in which the comets are heading; for example, in the frontal plane the loop is inscribed in a clockwise fashion.

The E point is the vectorcardiographic equivalent of the baseline or isoelectric line of the conventional ECG. There is no precise separation of initial forces from major forces, but the distinction is drawn from a sub-

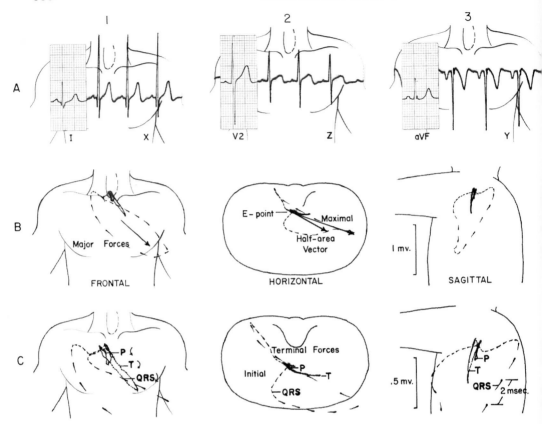

FIGURE 12-32   SCALAR AND VECTOR COMPONENTS

A, Comparison of scalar ECG leads I, V₂ and aVF with the corresponding orthogonal inputs X, Z and Y of the Frank corrected lead system. Except for differences in amplification and polarity, the complexes of the two systems are remarkably similar.

B, Three planes of the VCG at an average amplification (calibration is indicated in B-3). The frontal plane is inscribed in a clockwise direction, and the horizontal and sagittal planes are counterclockwise.

C, The three planes at double the normal amplification, permitting recognition of the P and T loops. Note the normal slowing of the initial and terminal portions of the loops, indicated by the closeness of the comet-shaped dots which are at 2 millisecond intervals. (From Guntheroth, *Pediatric Electrocardiography*, W. B. Saunders Co., 1965.)

stantial change in the direction of the loop. Usually the initial and terminal portions of the loops are inscribed relatively slowly, and the dots will be closely spaced, whereas the major forces are inscribed at a time when the instantaneous vector is moving rapidly and the dots are widely spaced.

A range of amplifications is commonly used in recording the vector loops, and the actual magnitude of

deflection must be judged against a calibrated signal, usually a 1 millivolt signal. Routine measurements which are commonly used are the greatest loop diameter in any plane expressed in millivolts. When the total development of the loop to the right of the E-point is greater than 1 millivolt, right ventricular hypertrophy is usually diagnosed, and when the sum of the loop's extensions to the left and poste-

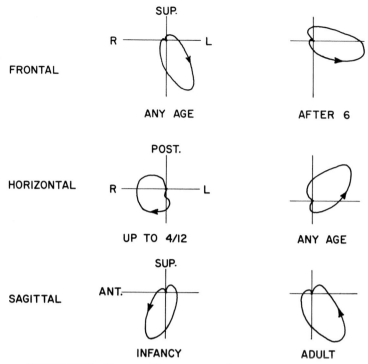

FIGURE 12-33   NORMAL DIRECTION OF INSCRIPTION OF LOOPS

Pairs of loops for the frontal, horizontal and sagittal planes indicating the normal direction of inscription of loops at different ages. In the frontal plane, a clockwise loop is found normally up to age 6 years; 30 per cent of adults show a counterclockwise loop. The sagittal loop is normally CCW at all ages. (From Guntheroth, *Pediatric Electrocardiography*, W. B. Saunders Co., 1965.)

rior exceeds 3.5 millivolts, left ventricular hypertrophy is probable.[47] As in the interpretation of the scalar ECG, hypertrophy is generally diagnosed on the basis of orientation of the forces and the potentials exceeding the limits of normal. Additional useful information is found in the direction of inscription of the loops, clockwise or counterclockwise, related to the age of the patient. Figure 12–33 indicates the normal direction of inscription of the loops in the three planes. For example, a clockwise loop in the frontal plane is normal at any age, but a counterclockwise loop prior to the age of 5 to 6 years is usually associated with a tendency toward left axis deviation and probable left ventricular hypertrophy.

On the other hand, a clockwise loop in the horizontal plane suggests right ventricular dominance which is normal only in early infancy. The sagittal loop is almost always counterclockwise. Conduction disturbances in the vectorcardiogram are more or less specific and will be discussed under that heading.

NORMAL TRENDS WITH AGE

At birth, the right ventricle is only slightly greater than the left in mass. This reflects the increased pressure work which the right ventricle performs in fetal life. With the first breath, after birth, there is a profound fall in the pulmonary vascular resistance and an increase in the systemic vascular resistance resulting in an increased workload for the left ventricle and a diminished workload for the right. By one month of age, the ratio of muscle mass of the two ventricles has reversed and the adult ratio of left/right ventricular mass is achieved. The electrical evidence of right ventricular domi-nance persists for the first month, and up until one to two years of age there is normally more evidence of right ventricular potentials than are present in the older child or the adult.

The QRS mean vector progresses from the right and anterior direction of the first neonatal month to the adult orientation to the left and posterior. The T vector moves more anteriorly with age.

III. ABNORMAL ELECTROCARDIOGRAPHIC CRITERIA

HYPERTROPHY

Hypertrophy requires a decision that the ECG is abnormal because of the orientation of the mean vector or voltages which exceed the limits of normal, or both. Inherent in the choice of criteria are the problems of sensitivity versus specificity. A criterion for hypertrophy that is sensitive enough to predict *all* instances of hypertrophy will catch too many normal subjects in the same net. Conversely, a criterion which will yield no false positives will probably miss many pathological states. Clinical judgment is essential in deciding which kind of error can best be tolerated in a given situation. For a robust, asymptomatic child with no cardiac enlargement and no murmur, the diagnosis of ventricular hypertrophy is unjustified on the basis of voltages which are slightly beyond two standard deviations of normal. On the other hand, an infant in congestive failure with a large heart almost certainly has ventricular hypertrophy, and the desired clinical information is merely which ventricle is involved, and a sensitive criterion would be appropriate.

ATRIAL HYPERTROPHY

The characteristic changes of atrial hypertrophy involve changes in the morphology and the voltage of the P wave. Right atrial hypertrophy produces a tall, peaked P wave known as p-pulmonale (Fig. 12–34A). In adults, a P wave greater than 2.5 mm. is usually abnormal, but in infants, a 3 mm. deflection is the upper limit of normal. When present, this pattern is usually seen in leads II, V_1 and V_2. A broad notched P wave, greater than .10 second in duration, is characteristic of p-mitrale, or left atrial hypertrophy (Fig. 12–34B). This is most often seen in leads I and V_5 and V_6. Combined atrial hypertrophy (Fig. 12–34C) involves combinations of the two previously listed abnormalities of the P waves, an increase in amplitude and an increase in duration.[48] It should be admitted that these patterns, particularly p-pulmonale, can appear and disappear very rapidly, suggesting that the pattern is not literally diagnostic of hypertrophy of the atrial muscle, although in general the patterns are associated with either overload or hypertrophy.

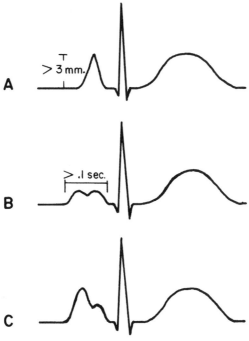

FIGURE 12-34   ATRIAL HYPERTROPHY

A, P-pulmonale or right atrial hypertrophy.
B, P-mitrale or left atrial hypertrophy.
C, Combined atrial hypertrophy. (From Guntheroth, *Pediatric Electrocardiography*, W. B. Saunders Co., 1965.)

RIGHT VENTRICULAR HYPERTROPHY

The mean QRS vector in right ventricular hypertrophy (RVH) falls to the right of and anterior to the normal orientation for age and exceeds the normal limits for potentials in leads reflecting this orientation. There are myriad additional criteria for RVH, some of which are selected and presented in Table 12-4. In right ventricular hypertrophy, the QRS vector may deviate to the right greater than normal as judged by the mean electrical axis, or anteriorly in excess of normal as judged by the R/S ratio in V_2 (Table 12-3). When the abnormal deviation is both anterior and rightward, the diagnosis is more secure. If, in addition, there is an S-T segment and T vector shift (Fig. 12-31), the specificity of the diagnosis of RVH is enhanced. This combination of RVH with S-T and T wave changes is frequently referred to as RVH with "strain pattern." Although some authorities have belittled the use of "strain" because it is a term from mechanical physics applied to an electrical phenomenon, it is no more illogical than the inference of hypertrophy from the same electrical phenomenon.

Both rightward and anterior orientation of the QRS vector are reflected in V_1 and an R/S ratio greater than normal in this lead is an important criterion of RVH, particularly if the R wave is greater than 5 mm. in amplitude.[49] The S in V_6 also reflects forces directed to the right and anterior, and an R/S ratio less than 1 after the first

Table 12–4.   *SELECTED CRITERIA FOR DIAGNOSIS OF VENTRICULAR HYPERTROPHY*

A. RIGHT VENTRICULAR HYPERTROPHY
    1. Orientation Criteria
        a. Right QRS deviation, greater than normal for age (mean electric axis)
        b. Anterior QRS deviation, greater than normal for age (R/S ratio in V_2)
        c. Wide QRS-T angle with S-T and T vector posterior and leftward ("strain")
        d. R/S ratio in V_1 or V_2 greater than normal for age
        e. R/S ratio in V_6 less than 1 after 1 month
        f. Clockwise loop in horizontal plane after 6 months
        g. Vector loop anterior/posterior ratio greater than 1.5 after 1 year
    2. Voltage Criteria
        a. R in V_1, V_2, or aVR greater than normal for age
        b. S in I or V_6 greater than normal for age
        c. Vector loop greater than 1 mv. to right of E-point
    3. Interval Criterion
        VAT in V_1 greater than normal with normal QRS duration
B. LEFT VENTRICULAR HYPERTROPHY
    1. Orientation Criterion
        a. Left QRS deviation, greater than normal for age (mean electric axis)
        b. Posterior QRS deviation, greater than normal for age (R/S ratio in V_2)
        c. Wide QRS-T angle with S-T and T vector rightward and anterior ("strain")
        d. R/S ratio in V_1 or V_2 less than normal for age
        e. Counterclockwise loop in the frontal plane before the age of 6 years
    2. Voltage Criteria
        a. R in I, II, aVL, aVF, V_5, or V_6 greater than normal for age
        b. S in V_1 or V_2 greater than normal for age
        c. Vector loop potential greater than 2 mv. overall
        d. Leftward + posterior potential greater than 3.5 mv.
    3. Interval Criterion
        VAT in V_6 greater than normal with normal QRS duration
C. COMBINED VENTRICULAR HYPERTROPHY
    1. Orientation Criteria
        a. Equiphasic QRS complexes in over half of limb leads
        b. Equiphasic QRS complexes in V_2
        c. "Fat" vector loops in two or more planes
        d. Two major vectors in frontal or horizontal planes
    2. Voltage Criteria
        a. Positive voltage criteria for right and left VH
        b. Positive voltage criteria for right or left VH and relatively large voltages for the other ventricle

---

month of life is another useful criterion of RVH.

The vector orientation in right ventricular hypertrophy accounts for certain characteristics of the VCG loops. If the mean vector is sufficiently anterior, the loop in the horizontal plane will be inscribed in a clockwise fashion, diagnostic of right ventricular hypertrophy after the age of six months. In extreme anterior deviation, a clockwise loop may occur even in the saggital plane.

Voltage criteria of RVH of partic-ular merit are those relating to leads aVR, V_1 and V_2 in terms of R waves, and leads I and V_6 in terms of abnormally deep S waves for age. For vector loops, deviation of the loops more than 1 mV to the right is diagnostic of right ventricular hypertrophy, and an anterior/posterior ratio greater than 1.5 after the age of one year.

All the above criteria and those listed in Table 12–4 may occur as isolated findings in normal infants and children. The occurrence of all of them in one individual would make the

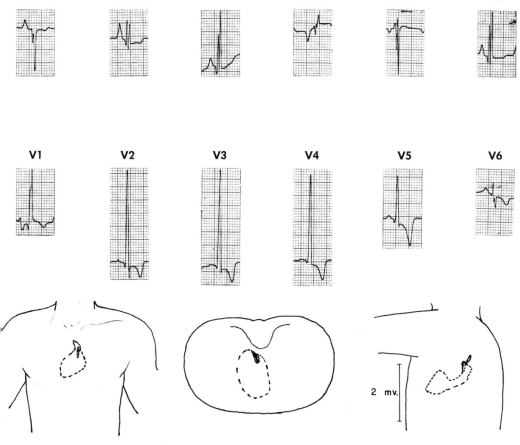

FIGURE 12-35   SEVERE RIGHT VENTRICULAR HYPERTROPHY

RVH with "strain" and p-pulmonale in a 3-year-old with severe, isolated pulmonic stenosis. VCG amplification is one-half average. (From Guntheroth, *Pediatric Electrocardiography*, W. B. Saunders Co., 1965.)

probability of RVH almost a certainty. Figure 12–35 is an example of severe right ventricular hypertrophy which satisfies most of these criteria.

LEFT VENTRICULAR HYPERTROPHY (LVH)

After the first few months of life, there is normally left ventricular dominance, and the spatial orientation of the QRS vector is to the left and posterior. Consequently, in left ventricular

hypertrophy, voltage criteria may be the only basis for diagnosis. In fact, Grant[16] pointed out that marked left axis deviation in the frontal plane is usually associated with conduction disturbances and not due to hypertrophy per se. Moderate left axis deviation, however, is a valid clue to left ventricular hypertrophy, particularly the type involving some degree of enlargement of the left ventricle. Quantification of the posterior deviation of the QRS vector is of little value due to the enormous spread of the normal values. The average vector direction for an adult in the horizontal plane is 37 degrees posterior, or counterclockwise, to the X axis, but two standard deviations exceed 160 degrees.[50] Satisfactory data are available on the R/S ratio in V_2, which is related to the degree of posterior direction of the QRS vector. If the R/S ratio in V_2 is less than the lower limits of normal, statistically abnormal posterior deviation is present, and left ventricular hypertrophy is probable. The major reservation for this criterion is the presence of marked right axis deviation which will sometimes be projected as a deep S in V_2, not associated with a true posterior orientation of the QRS vector as demonstrated by corrected lead vectorcardiography. The presence of abnormal T vectors, wide QRS-T angles and S-T segment shifts increases the specificity of the diagnosis of LVH and usually indicates a more severe degree of the disorder. This "strain pattern" in LVH characteristically results in a T vector directed to the right and anteriorly, and an S-T segment shift in the same direction (Fig. 12–31).

The voltage criteria for LVH (Table 12–4) are for leads which, because of their ability to reflect leftward and posterior forces, will exhibit abnormally tall R waves (leads I, AVL, V_5 and V_6), or abnormally deep S waves (V_1 and V_2). In addition, AVF and lead II may be useful to detect left ventricular hypertrophy, particularly in patients with moderate degrees of abnormal pressure overload, such as aortic stenosis. For vector loops, an overall loop magnitude in excess of 2 mV, most of which is directed posteriorly and leftward, suggests LVH. Another vector criterion of LVH is the sum of leftward and posterior potentials greater than 3.5 mV.[47]

Figure 12–36 is an example of se-

vere LVH with "strain" from an 18-month-old child with severe aortic stenosis.

COMBINED VENTRICULAR HYPERTROPHY (CVH)

Although many cardiac disorders involve an increased load for both ventricles, particularly in congenital heart disease, the electrocardiographic diagnosis of combined ventricular hypertrophy may be difficult, due in part to cancellation of opposing forces. Fortunately, most clinical conditions which produce anatomic CVH may be easily recognized as significant heart disease, and in such instances, a normal ECG would suggest CVH. If, in the presence of clear-cut LVH by customary criteria, there are additional substantial forces to the right and anterior, it may be argued that cancellation of some of the right ventricular electromotive force by the oppositely directed left ventricular forces has prevented the full expression of RVH. In such a situation, a diagnosis of CVH with left ventricular dominance may be made. For relative certainty of the diagnosis of CVH, however, several criteria for the diagnosis of both right and left ventricular hypertrophy should be present.

One criterion for CVH is the Katz-Wachtel phenomenon, equiphasic QRS complexes in at least two of the three limb leads.[51] This phenomenon subsequently has been extended to the precordial leads (V_2-V_4) as an additional diagnostic criterion for CVH, but this is a weaker one, because of the common occurrence of this pattern in the normal.[52] However, the manifestation of large forces, both anteriorly and posteriorly, as well as rightward and leftward, is logically suggestive of CVH. In vectorcardiograms, this is demonstrated by either "fat" loops

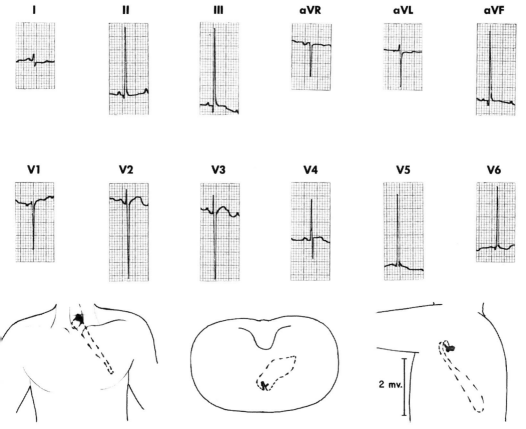

FIGURE 12-36 SEVERE LEFT VENTRICULAR HYPERTROPHY

Severe LVH with "strain" in a 18-month-old with severe aortic stenosis. VCG amplification is one-half average. (From Guntheroth, *Pediatric Electrocardiography*, W. B. Saunders Co., 1965.)

(Fig. 12–37) or loops with two major components (Fig. 12–38). In either instance, it should be apparent that a single, mean vector is not an adequate representation of the ECG. Empirically, deep Q waves in V_5 and V_6 are frequently associated with CVH, as seen in Figure 12–37.

"OVERLOAD" PATTERNS

In an attempt to predict abnormal hemodynamics from electrocardiographic changes, Cabrera and Monroy[53] developed criteria for systolic and diastolic overload. Their criteria for right ventricular overload patterns are reasonably valid, but the criteria for the left ventricle are frequently misleading. Most electrocardiographers continue to use the older terminology of hypertrophy rather than overload, but we will briefly summarize the overload patterns.

Systolic overload of the right ventricle (RVSO) is produced by abnormal pressure work for the right ventricle, such as pulmonic stenosis. This will produce an increase in amplitude of the R wave in V_1. Right ventricular diastolic overload (RVDO) is due to abnormal volume work for the right

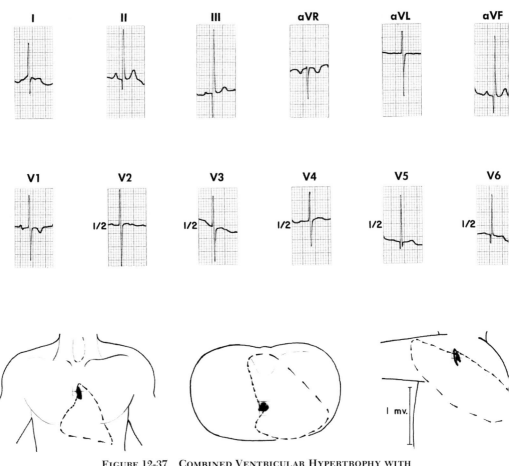

FIGURE 12-37   COMBINED VENTRICULAR HYPERTROPHY WITH
LEFT VENTRICULAR DOMINANCE

CVH and left ventricular dominance in a 1-year-old with a ventricular septal defect. (From
Guntheroth, *Pediatric Electrocardiography*, W. B. Saunders Co., 1965.)

ventricle, which distends the heart in diastole, as in atrial septal defect, "causing" right bundle branch block (see under *Disorders of the Sequence of Excitation*). The electrocardiogram shows broadening of the QRS complex, in relation to the normal duration of the QRS (Table 12–2) and some slowing and slurring of the terminal portions of the QRS complex, seen as slurred S waves in leads I and V_6, and slurred or notched R waves in leads III and V_1.

Left ventricular systolic overload (LVSO) was originally described as altered patterns in the repolarization process with prolongation of the Q-T interval and changes in the S-T segment and T wave in V_5 and V_6. This category would correspond to the earlier ECG term of left ventricular "strain" and severe aortic stenosis is an example. Left ventricular diastolic overload (LVDO) would be produced by aortic regurgitation, for example, and was thought to be characterized by a deep S wave in V_2 and a tall R wave in V_5 and V_6, with a relatively

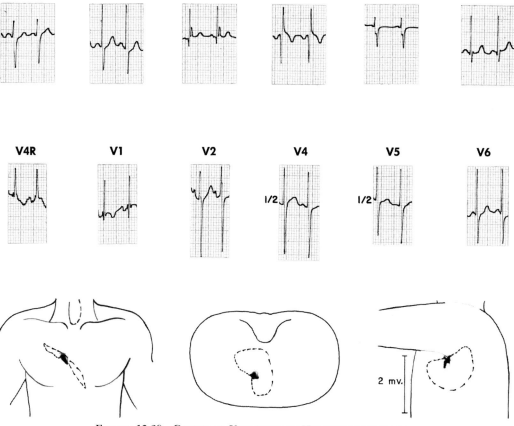

FIGURE 12-38   COMBINED VENTRICULAR HYPERTROPHY WITH RIGHT VENTRICULAR DOMINANCE

CVH and right ventricular dominance in a 17-month-old with a ventricular septal defect with moderate pulmonary hypertension. VCG amplification is one-half average. (From Guntheroth, *Pediatric Electrocardiography*, W. B. Saunders Co., 1965.)

normal QRS-T angle. Other authors subsequently have added to this group of criteria a deep Q wave over the left precordium as evidence of LVDO.

In general, the overload patterns have not proved sufficiently specific to recommend them as replacement for the older terminology.

DISORDERS OF THE SEQUENCE OF EXCITATION

This group of disorders includes diverse anatomic and functional en-

tities such as bundle branch block, pre-excitation and myocardial infarction.

DEXTROCARDIA AND VENTRICULAR INVERSION

Dextrocardia produces a sequence of excitation which is the mirror image of the normal sequence. Only the right-left relationships are reversed, and the anterior-posterior relationships are unaltered (Fig. 12–29). The most common "cause" of dextrocardia in the frontal plane is the misapplication of

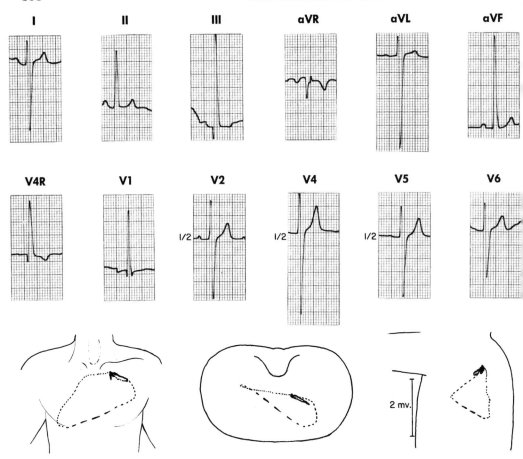

FIGURE 12-39   VENTRICULAR INVERSION

Congenitally corrected transposition of the great vessels in a 17-year-old boy, an example of ventricular inversion in a "pink tetralogy." The records show RVH and RBBB. The VCG amplification is one-half average. Note the characteristic qR in V_4R and absent q in V_6. (From Guntheroth, *Pediatric Electrocardiography*, W. B. Saunders Co., 1965.)

the right arm lead to the left arm and vice-versa. This error can be detected by inspection of the precordial leads. In the presence of true dextrocardia, "RVH" or hypertrophy of the pulmonic ventricle will produce deviation of the QRS vector toward the left and anterior, whereas dominance or hypertrophy of the systemic ventricle would produce a vector oriented to the right and posterior.

Inversion of the ventricles may occur with a relatively normal heart position, creating an entity of congenitally corrected transposition of the great vessels, and in a few patients with transposition of the great vessels. Thus, the posterior ventricle will have the characteristic anatomic and electrical features of the normal right ventricle, and the anterior ventricle will have features of the normal left or systemic ventricle. In this condition, overall septal activation proceeds from right to left (Fig. 12–39). The anterior-posterior sequence of septal activation is not reversed, as might be expected, and the initial vector is directed simply to the left. The orientation of these initial forces produces a characteristic Q wave over the right precordium and an absence of a Q wave in V_5 and V_6. The major forces in corrected transposition are not appreciably affected by the ventricular inversion, and will reflect ventricular hypertrophy as accurately as in the normally oriented heart. Not all patients with this pattern have corrected transposition, however. Occasionally, a normal individual will have an unusual degree of leftwardness of the initial forces, which will produce an ECG pattern indistinguishable from those with inversion of the ventricles.

RIGHT BUNDLE BRANCH BLOCK (RBBB)

The original criteria for right bundle branch block were a QRS exceeding 0.10 second and a wide, slurred S in lead I and R in lead III. With introduction of the precordial leads the definition was extended to include the pattern of RSR' in V_1. The duration criteria have frequently been neglected in the pediatric age group, but it seems reasonable to require that the QRS duration be at least the upper limits of normal for age before this diagnosis is made. Earlier, a QRS complex with a duration greater than .12 second was called complete right bundle branch block, and those with duration of .10 to .12 were described as incomplete. Grant[16] objected to the distinction between these two and recommended using the term right bundle branch block without qualification.

The orientation of forces is normal for the initial portions of the QRS complex in RBBB (Fig. 12–31). In addition, the orientation of the major forces is altered relatively little by

RBBB in a subject with an otherwise normal heart. However, asynchronous excitation of the two ventricles lessens the normal cancellation of the divergent electromotive forces of the two ventricles and allows a greater manifest potential for both ventricles. The effect of asynchronous excitation is more obvious in patients who have right ventricular hypertrophy. The terminal forces are characteristically changed in RBBB, almost invariably rightward and usually anterior. In addition, there is a slowness of movement of the instantaneous vector in the terminal portion of the QRS, manifested by slurring of the QRS in the ECG, in contrast to the normally sharp, narrowed deflections, and by abnormally close spacing of the dots on the VCG. There is always some closeness of the dots in the VCG in the initial and terminal parts of the loop, but this is normally quite limited. There are no exact criteria for normal limits of slurring of the complexes or slowing of the VCG loops, and the decision is usually based on a "gestalt" impression. From the orientation of the terminal forces, it may be seen that the scalar ECG will show a wide QRS complex, with a slurred S in leads I and V_6 and a slurred R' in leads III, aVR and V_1 (Fig. 12–40). The VCG may show a two-vector pattern, particularly in the horizontal plane with the loop crossing through or anterior to the E-point and ending in a slow terminal loop to the right and anterior. Usually, the T vector is not altered.

A particularly marked form of RBBB is found in Ebstein's anomaly, commonly associated with a p-pulmonale pattern. It is not uncommon in this condition to have voltage in the P waves exceed that of the QRS complex in some leads.

Inherent in the statement about

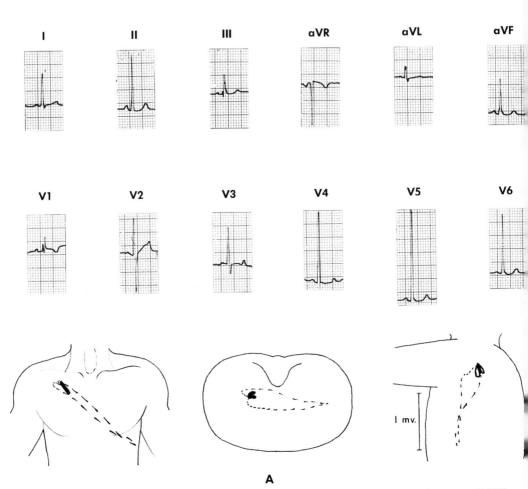

A

FIGURE 12-40   ECG AND VCG BEFORE AND AFTER RIGHT VENTRICULOTOMY: ACQUIRED RBBB

A, Preoperative ECG and VCG in a 5-year-old with a moderate sized ventricular septal defect; the diagnosis is CVH.

B, Post-right ventriculotomy; the diagnosis is now RBBB. (From Guntheroth, *Pediatric Electrocardiography*, W. B. Saunders Co., 1965.)

Figure continues on opposite page.

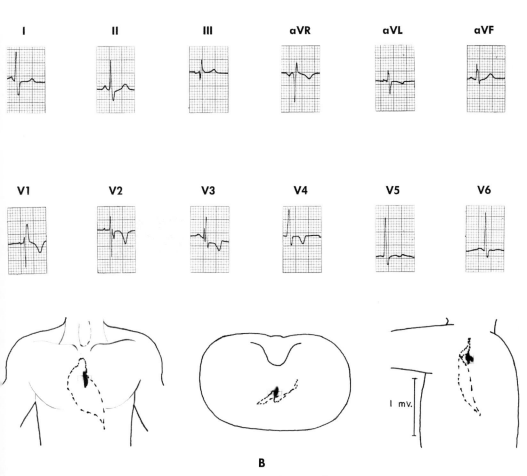

B

FIGURE 12-40   *Continued*

cancellation is the warning that ventricular hypertrophy should be diagnosed with caution in the presence of marked conduction disturbances.

LEFT BUNDLE BRANCH BLOCK (LBBB)

Left bundle branch block is more rare than right bundle branch block, and has a more serious implication, particularly in younger subjects. It is extraordinarily rare in the pediatric age group. Part of the explanation for its rarity may be found in the anatomy of the left main bundle which divides shortly after its origin into two major divisions, an anterior-superior division and a posterior-inferior division. If only one of these divisions is blocked, the total QRS duration will not necessarily be prolonged, although the orientation of the major forces will change. This is the case in left ventricular parietal block, which is thought to be the cause of most instances of left axis deviation in adults.[54] However, if a lesion involves the left main bundle before its bifurcation, the QRS complex will be prolonged and the initial forces due to septal activation will necessarily be altered (Fig. 12–31). The initial forces in LBBB are directed more markedly to the left, and somewhat posteriorly, and the terminal half of the QRS is directed superiorly, leftward and posteriorly. There is usually a wide separation of the QRS and T vectors, with the T vector characteristically directed anteriorly and to the right (Fig. 12–41). The characteristic changes in the initial vector of LBBB produce a loss of Q waves in leads I, V_5 and V_6. As contrasted to RBBB, in which there is a wide separation of the initial and terminal halves of the vectors, there is a relatively narrow angle between the two halves of the QRS vectors in LBBB.

INTRAVENTRICULAR BLOCK

In diffuse myocardial disease and in some metabolic disorders, gross prolongation of the QRS duration may occur without the characteristic changes of either right or left bundle branch block. In this situation, intraventricular block may be diagnosed, assuming that each beat originates from the sinus node, and the P-R interval is relatively normal.

PARTIAL BUNDLE BRANCH BLOCK

The intermittent appearance of a conduction disturbance, which when present satisfies the duration and orientation criteria of bundle branch block, is called partial bundle branch block, right or left, depending upon the terminal forces. This is most often seen in association with arrhythmias involving atrial premature beats.

PRE-EXCITATION SYNDROME (WOLFF-PARKINSON-WHITE)

This is a diagnosis based entirely on the electrocardiogram, although its presence may be suggested by the frequent occurrence of paroxysmal atrial tachycardia. The pre-excitation syndrome consists of a short P-R interval and a long QRS duration, both of which are due to partial "short-circuiting" of the normal delay in A-V conduction. The initial part of the QRS complex is slurred and is called the delta wave. Ordinarily, the duration of the rest of the QRS complex is not necessarily involved, permitting a relatively normal P-J interval, i.e., the interval between the onset of the P and the end of the QRS complex. However, most instances of pre-excitation syndrome demonstrate considerable

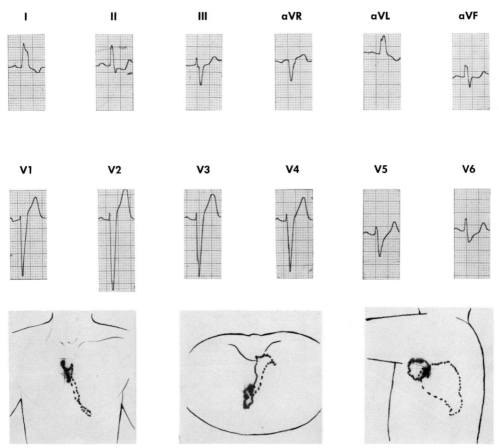

FIGURE 12-41   LEFT BUNDLE BRANCH BLOCK

Left bundle branch block in a 58-year-old male. The QRS duration is 0.12 seconds. The initial vector is leftward, causing a loss of the normal Q in leads I and V_6. The terminal vector is of relatively small amplitude and is directed to the left and superiorly. There are marked secondary changes in the S-T segment and T waves.

alteration in the direction and amplitude of the QRS vector, apart from the delta wave. Consequently, it is not possible to diagnose ventricular hypertrophy with any certainty in the presence of pre-excitation. Figure 12–42 is an example of a patient with pre-excitation syndrome. There are subgroups of patients with pre-excitation syndrome, based on the spatial orientation of the delta wave, but these subdivisions are of largely academic interest.

ENDOCARDIAL CUSHION DEFECTS

Endocardial cushion defects (synonymous with persistent A-V canal) produce a characteristic, abnormal sequence of activation. Whereas ventricular hypertrophy alone rarely causes a superior deviation, the mean QRS vector in cushion defects is oriented superiorly, initially to the left and terminally to the right. The leftward and superior orientation of the mean QRS vector will produce left

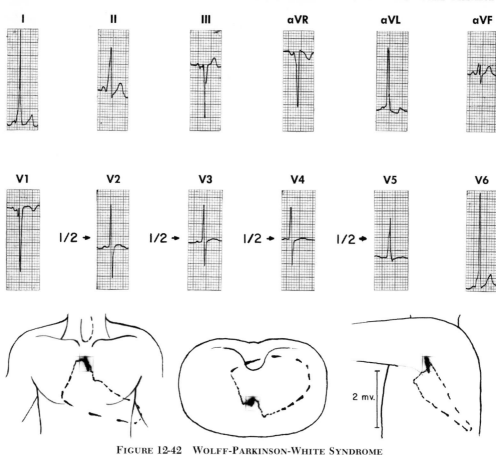

FIGURE 12-42   WOLFF-PARKINSON-WHITE SYNDROME

Pre-excitation syndrome, Grant's second type, or Rosenbaum's Type B. VCG amplification is one-half average. (From Guntheroth, *Pediatric Electrocardiography*, W. B. Saunders Co., 1965.)

axis deviation, and a counterclockwise loop in the frontal plane (Fig. 12–43). Curiously, the precordial leads are very little affected by this disorder of excitation, and ventricular hypertrophy criteria based on the precordial leads or the anterior/posterior relationship of the VCG are reasonably accurate.

MYOCARDIAL INFARCTION AND FIBROSIS

Myocardial infarction, by definition, produces an area of dead myocardium, which cannot be excited by the normally propagated wave of excitation. The endocardium is normally excited from the Purkinje system and the depolarization spreads from the endocardium toward the epicardium. When infarction occurs, there is interference with the normal sequence of excitation resulting in a deflection of the initial vector away from the area of infarction. The clinically apparent infarction almost always occurs in the left ventricle or septum, and the initial vector will tend to point away from some aspect of the left ventricle. This accounts for the preoccupation of "pattern" electrocardiographers with Q waves in leads II, III and aVF. In particular, the duration of Q waves usually exceeds .04 second. If the infarction occurs near either of the subdivisions of the left bundle branch, a delay of excitation of the noninfarcted myocardium peripheral to the infarction may produce a late vector directed toward the infarction. The initial .04 second vector will be away from the infarction, and the terminal half will be toward the infarction. This type of infarction will produce a widely sepa-

rated initial and terminal vector, over 100 degrees, and the delay is called peri-infarction block.[16] Peri-infarction block occurs in almost one half of myocardial infarctions (Fig. 12–44).

In addition to the QRS changes, there are characteristic changes in the ST and T waves, and there is a characteristic sequence of events involving these components of the ECG (Fig. 12–45). Ischemic but functional myocardium will produce changes in the T vector, and the T vector will generally be directed away from the area of ischemia. Tissue which is more seri-

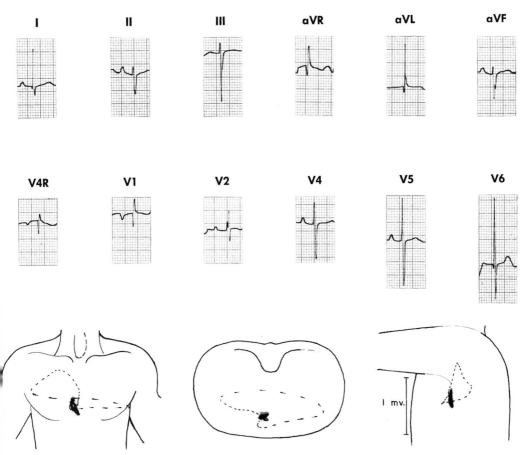

FIGURE 12-43 EXCITATION SEQUENCE OF THE ENDOCARDIAL CUSHION TYPE

Excitation sequence of the endocardial cushion type, with LVH in a 4-year-old boy. (From Guntheroth, *Pediatric Electrocardiography*, W. B. Saunders Co., 1965.)

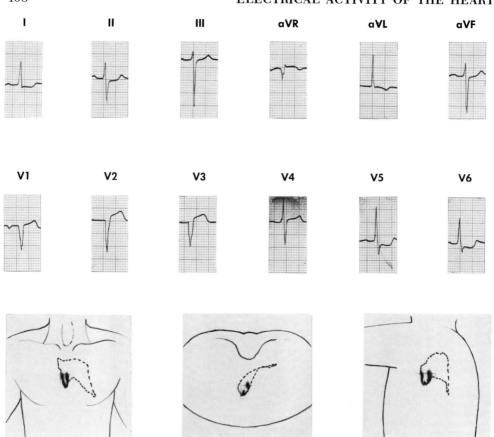

FIGURE 12-44   ANTEROLATERAL INFARCTION WITH PERI-INFARCTION BLOCK

Anterolateral infarction with peri-infarction block in a 54-year-old man. The QRS duration is not prolonged (QRS duration of 0.10 second). There are two widely divergent vectors in the frontal plane: the first half is to the left and inferior, the terminal half is superior and leftward. The anterior forces have not developed, producing an absent R-wave in the first three V-leads, and the concave loop seen in the horizontal vector loop (middle panel). The patient was also on digitalis.

ously injured, but not infarcted, will produce a "current of injury" which will change the S-T segment, and when represented by a vector, the S-T vector is shifted toward the injured myocardium. After recovery from the infarction, the only permanent change in the electrocardiogram may be in the QRS complex, which reflects the altered sequence of excitation due to the dead myocardium.

Localization of infarction has been of interest to electrocardiographers for many years, although the clinical significance and the accuracy of localization are not particularly strong. Two categories have existed for many years, the so-called anterior myocardial infarction and the posterior myocardial infarction. To understand the terminology, it should be known that, for the adult, the anterior part of the left ventricle is the interventricular septum, and an anterior infarction involves the septum, rather than the right ventricle. Grant suggested the use of five areas of the left ventricle for localization of infarction.[16] An infarction of the

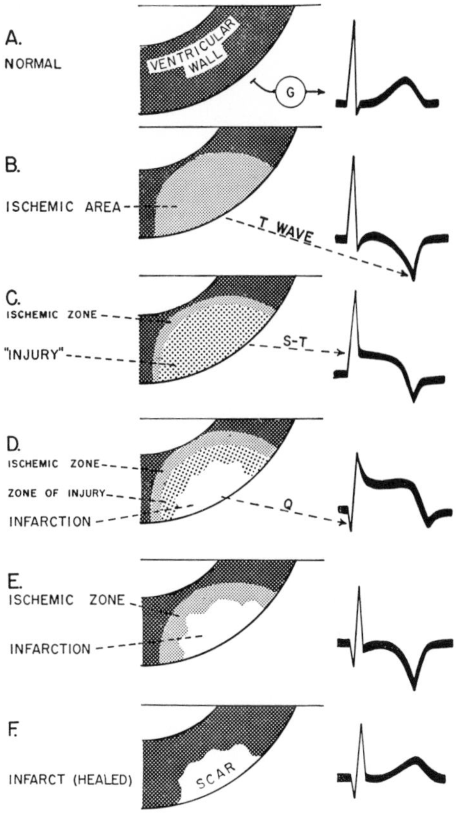

FIGURE 12-45 ELECTROCARDIOGRAPHIC SE-
QUENCE OF MYOCARDIAL INFARCTION

The sequence of electrocardiographic patterns recorded from unipolar electrodes over the site of a developing infarct is presented as reconstructed by Bayley.[55]

A, A normal electrocardiographic pattern recorded from a precordial electrode is illustrated for comparison.

B, Immediately after occlusion of a coronary artery, the myocardium served by the vessel becomes ischemic. A change in the rate of repolarization in the area produces a sharply inverted T wave.

C, Within a short time myocardial hypoxia interferes with the repolarization process to the point that the affected myocardium fails to polarize to the normal extent. Incomplete repolarization produces an "injury" current. The S-T segment assumes a different level than the T-Q segment; this is generally described as a displacement of the S-T segment.

D, Within the center of the ischemic region, some of the myocardium dies and fails to contribute to the potentials during either systole or diastole. Under these conditions, a Q wave appears because the proximal tissue fails to balance the potentials in more distant regions where the wave of excitation is moving away from the electrode.

E, The myocardium in the zone of injury either dies or is incorporated in the ischemic zone, so the "injury" current disappears and the S-T segment returns to the baseline. The ischemic zone persists, as indicated by the sharply inverted T wave.

F, In a healed infarct, the ischemic zone is supplied by collateral vessels and returns to normal. The only residual sign is the Q wave, which is attributed to the presence of electrically inactive scar tissue.

inferior aspect of the left ventricle is called a diaphragmatic infarct and produces an initial .04 second vector which is directed superiorly and leftward (Fig. 12–46); frequently there is peri-infarction block, with a terminal vector directed inferiorly and rightward. An infarction of the superior aspect of the left ventricle is called anterolateral and produces an initial .04 second vector directed rightward and inferiorly, and a terminal vector in the opposite direction due to peri-infarction block. A strictly anterior infarction usually alters only the initial .04 second vector, allowing it to shift posteriorly and slightly leftward (Fig. 12–47). A strictly posterior infarction is associated with an initial .04 second vector that is anterior and leftward. This direction is not abnormal except for the duration of this initial vector. Normally, the vector remains anterior for only about .01 to .02 second, and the average of the initial .04 second vector is normally somewhat posterior and leftward. Finally, an apical infarction would produce an initial .04 second vector directed rightward and superiorly. This would produce the "classic" infarction pattern of a broad Q in leads I, II and III.

It must be emphasized that disorders that produce fibrosis from

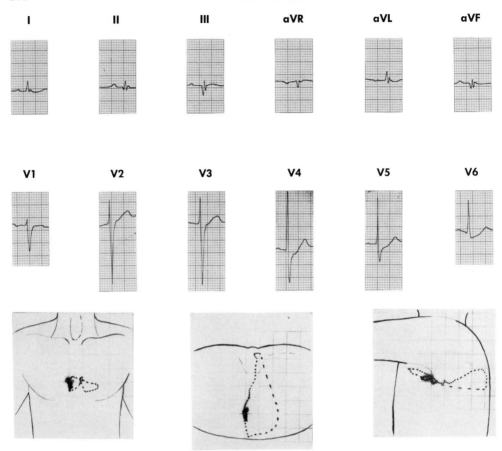

FIGURE 12-46 INFERIOR MYOCARDIAL INFARCTION

A diaphragmatic, or inferior myocardial infarction, in a 58-year-old male on digitalis. There is a deep and wide Q in III and to a lesser degree in aVF. The precordial R/S progression is relatively normal. Although peri-infarction block is common with diaphragmatic infarction, it is absent here.

causes other than infarction will produce changes in the QRS orientation which may be indistinguishable from the patterns observed in infarction.[56]

DISORDERS OF REPOLARIZATION

The diagnosis of disorders of repolarization rests upon the Q-T interval and the direction and voltage of the T vector. The methods of assessment have been discussed earlier and will be reviewed here in relation to specific disorders. However, specific disorders do not produce specific changes in repolarization, and intelligent interpretation of these changes requires explicit knowledge of the patient's age, clinical diagnosis and drug treatment. The repolarization process is undoubtedly the most labile part of the cardiac cycle, manifesting the earliest changes of metabolic and myocardial disorders. Similarly, rather dramatic changes may occur in the S-T segment and T vector in benign conditions. In addition, the T vector may undergo marked changes secondary to QRS changes produced by conduction disturbances which must be distinguished from primary repolarization disorders on the basis of the relationship of the T vector to the QRS vector.

PHYSIOLOGICAL FACTORS

Exercise changes the repolarization process in both normal and abnormal hearts, but the differences between the two groups form the basis for exercise tests to detect ischemic heart disease.[57] The tachycardia of exercise

normally may be attended by considerable changes in the orientation and potential of the T vector, varying with the severity of exercise. With moderate exercise, the T vector generally swings leftward,[16] but with severe "anaerobic" exercise, the T vector may be directed anteriorly and rightward and show increased potential. The S-T segment is better than the T vector in separating normal from ischemic responses. The "nonischemic" responses to exercise are either no S-T segment shift or a depression of the S-T segment junction with the QRS complex (J depression) without sustained S-T

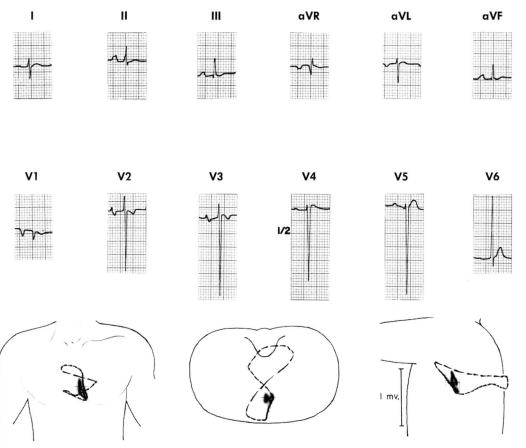

FIGURE 12-47   ANTERIOR MYOCARDIAL INFARCTION PATTERN

Pattern of anterior myocardial infarction in a 3-year-old with endocardial fibroelastosis. (From Guntheroth, *Pediatric Electrocardiography*, W. B. Saunders Co., 1965.)

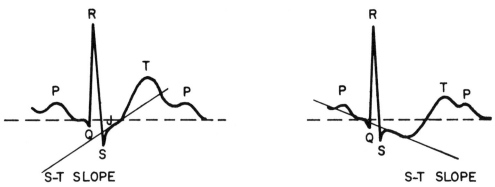

FIGURE 12-48 NON-ISCHEMIC AND ISCHEMIC S-T SEGMENTS

Non-ischemic S-T segment alterations with exercise are represented on the left, with a characteristic J-depression. Ischemic S-T segment shift is seen on the right, with a downward sloping segment and a diphasic T wave. (From Guntheroth, *Pediatric Electrocardiography*, W. B. Saunders Co., 1965.)

depression (Fig. 12–48). The ischemic response is manifested by a depressed S-T segment, which is horizontal for over .08 second, or by a segment that slants downward followed by a diphasic or inverted T wave. The greater the S-T segment depression, the greater is the disorder. Curiously, the subjects with junctional depression have a slightly better prognosis than even the group with no S-T or T wave changes.[58]

Other normal activities such as drinking ice water, eating, posture changes, hyperventilation and breath holding, may change the direction and magnitude of the T vector, but do not produce the pathological changes in the S-T segment as defined. Some of these changes in repolarization may be mediated by autonomic nerves. Although adrenergic and cholinergic nerves have marked effects on heart rate with attendant changes in the S-T and T vector, it is difficult to separate the neural from the humoral effects. It

seems probable, however, that the vagus augments the magnitude of the T vector, and sympathetic stimulation diminishes the magnitude and may change the orientation of the T vector.[59]

HYPOXIC DISORDERS

Myocardial hypoxia may result from respiratory or circulatory disorders. Disorders of repolarization are the earliest manifestations of myocardial hypoxia, but severe hypoxia may produce changes in rhythm, rate and ventricular conduction. Central and peripheral stimulation of both adrenergic and cholinergic systems occur with hypoxia, and tissue hypoxia accentuates the centrally produced adrenergic effects.[59] Hypoxia affects the cell membrane, probably through interference with the ion pump, permitting an increase in intracellular sodium and extracellular potassium. It is probable that a wide range of disorders have this final pathway of expression, explaining in part the nonspecific nature of changes in the S-T and T vectors. Figure 12–49 is a series of ECG's from a dog after respiratory arrest due to pentobarbital. The progression includes peaking of T waves, disappearance of P waves, broadening and distortion of the QRS complex, sinusoidal QRS-T complexes and finally ventricular fibrillation. These changes are indistinguishable from those due to progressive hyperkalemia.

The manifestation of hypoxic effects varies according to the preceding state of the ECG and the severity and duration of hypoxia. It is clear that interpretation of an ECG is assisted greatly by previous records and knowledge of the stage of a particular hypoxic episode (Fig. 12–45). It should be emphasized that in diffuse hypoxic states of some duration, there may be

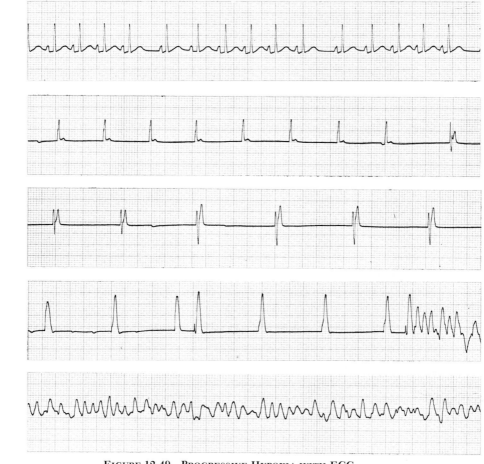

FIGURE 12-49 PROGRESSIVE HYPOXIA WITH ECG

A sequence of ECG's from a dog with progressive hypoxia due to respiratory arrest (pentobarbital induced). Note the similarity of C to the electrocardiographic changes in marked hyperkalemia. The terminal rhythm is ventricular fibrillation. (From Guntheroth, *Pediatric Electrocardiography*, W. B. Saunders Co., 1965.)

no change in the direction of the T vector, but only a decrease in magnitude of the T vector. This may be seen in chronic anemia, shock and numerous metabolic disorders. Some hypoxic states may produce indirect changes in the ECG through effects on the pulmonary vascular resistance, which may result in right heart "strain."

INFLAMMATORY AND FIBROTIC PROCESSES

As with diffuse states of hypoxia, wide-spread inflammation or fibrosis may produce no change in direction of the T vector but may produce a reduction in voltage. Also, in a manner similar to that of hypoxic episodes, there is a characteristic evolution of S-T and T patterns in the disease process. The earliest change in purulent pericarditis is an increase in magnitude of the T vector, with elevated S-T segments in the same leads that present the highest T wave amplitude, suggesting earlier repolarization rather than a true shift of the S-T segment.[60] Generally, in the early stages, the S-T segment will be directed to the left, inferiorly and slightly anteriorly. As the T vector subsides in magnitude in the intermediate stages, the S-T segment may return toward normal. The explanation may be a balancing of forces of early repolarization by the development of a current of injury from the normal cells to the injured cells, which actually elevates the T-Q segment. The coincidence of the two processes may produce an essentially normal ECG in the intermediate process of myocardial injury (Fig. 12–50). There is no question that in the intermediate stages of evolution of purulent pericarditis the S-T and T vectors may appear essentially normal.[61] In the period of resolving peri-

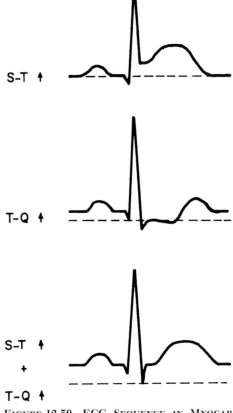

FIGURE 12-50   ECG SEQUENCE IN MYOCARDIAL INJURY

Postulated sequence of ECG changes in myocardial injury. Initially, the S-T segment tends to be elevated. Later, a current of injury causes an elevation of the T-Q (or P-Q) segment, and if these two processes occur simultaneously, a normal appearing ECG is possible during the intermediate stages of injury. In each of the three drawings, the dotted line represents the true isoelectric line. (From Guntheroth. *Pediatric Electrocardiography*. W. B. Saunders Co., 1965.)

carditis, the S-T segment and T vector may be directed oppositely from their direction in the acute state.

In acute, benign pericarditis it is not unusual to see a large volume of pericardial infusion with a completely normal ECG or a simple diminution of all voltages. In order for the ECG to have more significant changes, the epicardial layers of myocardium must be involved. In generalized forms of myocardial disease, such as rheumatic pancarditis, all phases of the cardiac cycle reflect the disorder: A-V conduction is delayed, the electrical axis shifts rightward, the QTc is prolonged and the magnitude of the T vector is diminished.

METABOLIC DISORDERS

Disorders which interfere with the ionic pump or alter directly the ionic concentrations, particularly extracellular potassium, will affect the repolarization process. Myxedema decreases the voltage of the T vector without affecting its orientation. Hypothermia affects the metabolic processes relating to the ionic pump and prolongs all of the intervals in the ECG, but the QTc is much more prolonged than the QRS.[59] The ingestion of glucose may produce a flattening or even inversion of T waves in normal subjects, probably through effects on extracellular potassium. In hypoglycemic shock, on the other hand, the process is more complicated.[59] The QRS complex is increased in amplitude and is prolonged; there is S-T depression, flattening of the T wave, lengthening of the QTc and an increase in prominence of the U wave.

ELECTROLYTE IMBALANCE

Potassium and calcium are the only ions considered to have independent effects upon the ECG. Changes in the sodium ion concentration produce electrocardiographic changes largely through the modification of the effects of potassium. The same indirect role may be ascribed to changes in pH and CO_2 through their effect on the calcium ions. The calcium ion in excess produces few definite changes in either depolarization or repolarization but may have a profound effect on electromechanical coupling.[62] It is through its effects on mechanical systole that hypercalcemia enhances the effects of digitalis. Hypercalcemia shortens the S-T segment somewhat but does not alter the duration of the T wave and produces a shortening of the QTc. Low calcium prolongs the S-T segment and thereby increases the QTc, producing one of the more specific patterns of the ECG (Fig. 12–51B). The S-T segment remains isoelectric and the T vector is not altered.

Low serum potassium on the other hand produces one of the least specific electrocardiographic patterns. Phase 2, the plateau of Figure 12–1, shortens, while Phase 3 is prolonged, manifested peripherally by a shortened S-T segment and an apparently increased QTc due to fusion of the T wave with the U wave.[63] When the serum potassium is below 2.5 mEq/L, S-T segment depression, diphasic T waves and prominent U waves are noted frequently (Fig. 12–51C). When the potassium is above this level, the ECG is not a reliable predictor of hypokalemia. All the ECG features of hypokalemia may be found in the "strain" pattern of LVH, including prominent U waves. With hypokalemia, however, the S-T segment vector is toward the left and posterior, whereas in left ventricular "strain" the opposite direction is common. There is a marked similarity of the ECG pattern of hypokalemia to the effects of digitalis, but the latter produces a shortened QTc and ordinarily no prominence of the U wave. Hypokalemia may have an important indirect effect by enhancing digitalis toxicity.

Hyperkalemia is the most spectac-

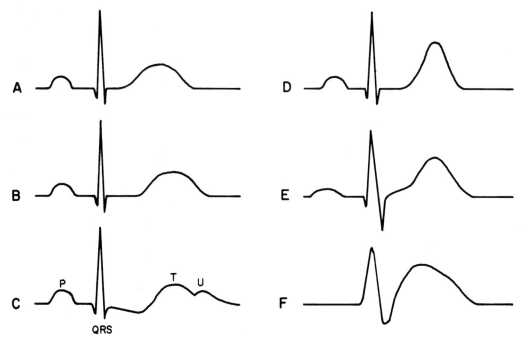

FIGURE 12-51   EFFECTS OF ELECTROLYTE DISORDERS

A, Normal ECG cycle.

B, Hypocalcemia. The T wave is uninvolved, and there is no S-T depression. The essential feature is the prolongation of the S-T segment, accounting for the prolongation of the Q-Tc.

C, Hypokalemia. The S-T segment is depressed ending in a diphasic T wave. The Q-Tc appears to be prolonged due to fusion of the T wave with a prominent U wave.

D, E and F, Progressive hyperkalemia. Earliest changes are a tall, symmetrical T wave (D). Above 7 mEq./L., the P wave is depressed, the P-R interval is prolonged, the QRS widened and right axis shift occurs (E). With levels greater than 9 mEq./L., the P waves are absent, and a sinusoidal QRS-T complex is formed (F). (From Guntheroth, *Pediatric Electrocardiography*, W. B. Saunders Co., 1965.)

ular as well as the most lethal of electrolyte disorders. The recognition from the electrocardiogram is made more urgent by the availability of dialysis and even simpler techniques for reversing the process at least temporarily. Recognition of modest degrees of hyperkalemia is easier, of course, if the ECG is otherwise normal. ECG changes may not occur until the serum potassium level is greater than 7 mEq/L. Above that, there is usually a gradation of effect with increasing levels of serum potassium (Fig. 12-51D, E and F). The characteristic early change of increased magnitude of the T waves are found with fairly modest increases of serum potassium. Higher levels will produce prolongation of the PR interval and the QRS duration, the latter being the most important criterion to watch in relation to dialysis. Prolongation of the QRS by greater than 50 per cent over the normal for that patient is an indication for prompt measures to reduce the serum potassium.

Multiple electrolyte abnormalities are not uncommon clinically and some of the combinations may be recognizable. Low calcium and low potassium will produce a long S-T segment and an abnormal T, followed by a prominent U wave. Low calcium and high potassium will produce a long S-T segment and high, symmetrical T waves.

PHARMACOLOGIC EFFECTS

Digitalis effects are the most important of this group. Short of toxic effects, the alterations are primarily those affecting repolarization. The most reliable evidence of digitalis effect is shortening of the QTc. Frequently, "strain" pattern with mild prolongation of the QTc occurs in the patient prior to digitalization, making a control ECG mandatory before beginning therapy with digitalis. In addition to relative shortening of the QTc, digitalis effect frequently alters the S-T segment and the T vector, particularly with exercise. With exercise, the S-T and T wave changes of digitalis are identical with those of ischemia, making a test such as the Master's impossible to interpret.[16] Digitalis intoxication, as opposed to digitalis effect, will prolong A-V conduction. This is a much more reliable sign of digitalis intoxication than other arrhythmias such as bigeminy, which is a remarkably rare sign of digitalis intoxication in the pediatric age group.[38] Potassium therapy will reduce or abolish most of the effects of digitalis, including the toxic effects. Lowering of serum calcium by a chelating agent is also effective in reversing digitalis toxicity.

Epineohrine and other catecholamines produce a shortening of mechanical systole and a shortening of the QTc. In addition, prominent U waves may appear, although the distinction between a U wave and a positive after-potential is uncertain.[64] Acetylcholine shortens the QTc, but by a different method, the plateau of Phase 2 of the intracellular action potential is shortened, owing to increased permeability of the cell membrane to potassium.

Various poisons and certain widely used drugs alter the cell membrane. The ECG pattern produced by these drugs strongly resembles that produced by excessive extracellular potassium. The cellular toxicity of quinidine, diphenylhydantoin and procaine are used to reduce automaticity of ectopic pacemakers. In using such drugs as quinidine, an increase by 50 per cent in the QRS duration is an important danger sign, as with elevation of serum potassium.

CONCLUSIONS

Drawing final conclusions from a given electrocardiographic record should be done with the full knowledge of the clinical status of the patient. Although the ECG is a precise technique and there are many charts and tables available for definitions of normals, the nonunique nature of these electrical phenomena must be kept in mind. In order to transform these changes into sound clinical inferences, additional information such as previous electrocardiographic records on the same patient, an awareness of the probable disease category of the patient, electrolyte status, age and medications will greatly improve the ability of the physician to make a more definitive conclusion about the meaning of electrocardiographic changes.

REFERENCES

1. GUNTHEROTH, W. G. *Pediatric Electrocardiography.* Philadelphia, W. B. Saunders Co. 1965.
2. WOODBURY, L. A., WOODBURY, J. W., and HECHT, H. H. Membrane resting and

action potentials of single cardiac muscle fibers. *Circulation*, 1:264, 1950.

3. PAGE, E. The electrical potential difference across the cell membrane of the heart muscle. *Circulation*, 26:582, 1962.

4. WEIDMANN, S. Resting and action potentials of cardiac muscle. *Ann. New York Acad. Sci.*, 65:663, 1957.

5. WEST, T. C. Ultramicroelectrode recording from the cardiac pacemaker. *J. Pharmacol. & Exper. Therap.*, 115:283, 1955.

6. HOFFMAN, B. F., PAES DE CARVALHO, A., DE MELLO, W. C., and CRANEFIELD, P. F. Electrical activity of single fibers of the atrioventricular node. *Circulat. Res.*, 7: 11, 1959.

7. SCHER, A. M., RODRIGUEZ, M. I., LIIKANE, J., and YOUNG, A. C. The mechanism of atrioventricular conduction. *Circulat. Res.*, 7:54, 1959.

8. SCHER, A. M., and YOUNG, A. C. The pathway of ventricular depolarization in the dog. *Circulat. Res.*, 4:461, 1956.

9. SCHER, A. M. The sequence of ventricular excitation. *Amer. J. Cardiol.*, 14:287, 1964.

10. SCHMITT, O. H., LEVINE, R. B., and SIMONSON, E. Electrocardiographic mirror pattern studies. *Amer. Heart J.*, 45:416, 500, 655, 1953.

11. FRANK, E., KAY, C. F., SEIDEN, G. E., and KEISMAN, R. A. A new quantitative basis for electrocardiographic theory: the normal QRS complex. *Circulation*, 12:406, 1955.

12. SCHAEFER, H. The general order of excitation and of recovery. *Ann. New York Acad. Sc.*, 65:743, 1957.

13. NELSON, C. V. Human thorax potentials. *Ann. New York Acad. Sc.*, 65:1014, 1957.

14. BOINEAU, J. P., SPACH, M. S., and AYERS, C. R. Genesis of the electrocardiogram in atrial septal defect. *Amer. Heart J.*, 68: 637, 1964.

15. EINTHOVEN, W., FAHR, G., and DEWAART, A. Über die Richtung und die manifeste Grösse der Potentialschwankungen im menschlichen Herzen und über den Einfluss der Herzlage auf die Form des Elektrokardiogramms. *Arch. ges Physiol.*, 150: 275, 1913. Translated by H. E. Hoff and P. Sekelj, *Amer. Heart J.*, 40:163, 1950.

16. GRANT, R. P. *Clinical Electrocardiography.* New York, McGraw-Hill Book Co., 1957.

17. SCHWAN, H. P., and KAY, C. F. The conductivity of living tissues. *Ann. New York Acad. Sci.*, 65:1007, 1957.

18. SCHER, A. M., and YOUNG, A. C. Frequency analysis of the electrocardiogram. *Circulat. Res.*, 8:344, 1960.

19. WILSON, F. N., JOHNSTON, F. D., ROSENBAUM, F. F., ERLANGER, H., KOSSMANN, C. E., HECHT, H., COTRIM, N., DE OLIVEIRA, R. M., SCARSI, R., and BARKER, P. S. The precordial electrocardiogram. *Amer. Heart J.*, 27:19, 1944.

20. MCFEE, R., and JOHNSTON, F. D. Electrocardiographic leads. *Circulation* 9:868, 1954.

21. GOLDBERGER, E. *Unipolar Lead Electrocardiography.* Philadelphia, Lea and Febiger, 1953.

22. WILSON, F. N., JOHNSTON, F. D., and KOSSMAN, C. E. Substitution of the tetrahedron for the Einthoven triangle. *Amer. Heart J.*, 33:594, 1947.

23. FRANK, E. An accurate, clinically practical system for spatial vectorcardiography. *Circulation*, 13:737, 1956.

24. HELM, R. A. An accurate lead system for spatial vectorcardiography. *Amer. Heart J.*, 53:415, 1957.

25. SCHMITT, O. H., and SIMONSON, E. The present status of vectorcardiography. *Arch. Int. Med.*, 96:574, 1955.

26. DOWER, G. E., MOORE, A. D., ZIEGLER, W. G., and OSBORNE, J. A. On QRS amplitude and other errors produced by direct-writing electrocardiographs. *Amer. Heart J.*, 65:307, 1963.

27. COUNCIL ON PHYSICAL MEDICINE AND REHABILITATION. Minimum requirements for acceptable electrocardiographs. *J.A.M.A.*, 143:654, 1950.

28. VALLEY, G. E., and WALLMAN, M. *Vacuum Tube Amplifiers.* New York, McGraw-Hill Book Co., 1948.

29. GUNTHEROTH, W. G. Book review of *Fetal Electrocardiography* by S. D. Larks. *Quart. Rev. Surg.*, 28:236, 1961.

30. BURCHELL, H. B. Electrocution hazards in the hospital or laboratory. *Circulation*, 27:1015, 1963.

31. LANGENDORF, R., and PICK, A. Cardiac arrhythmias in infants and children. *Pediat. Clin. N. Amer.*, 2:215, 1954.

32. MORGAN, B. C., BLOOM, R. S., and GUNTHEROTH, W. G. Cardiac arrhythmias in premature infants. *Pediatrics*, 35:658, 1965.

33. MORGAN, B. C. Cardiac complications of diphtheria. *Pediatrics*, 32:557, 1963.

34. ZIEGLER, R. F. *Electrocardiographic Studies in Normal Infants and Children.* Springfield, Charles C Thomas, 1951.

35. ALIMURUNG, M. M., JOSEPH, L. G., NADAS, A. S., and MASSELL, B. F. Unipolar precordial and extremity electrocardiogram in normal infants and children. *Circulation*, 4:420, 1951.

36. ASHMAN, R., and HULL, E. *Essentials of Electrocardiography for the Student and Practitioner of Medicine* (2nd ed.). New York; The Macmillan Co., 1941.

37. WEINSTEIN, L. Cardiovascular manifestations in some of the common infectious diseases. *Mod. Concepts Cardiovas. Dis.*, 23:229, 1954.

38. GUNTHEROTH, W. G. Digitalis in pediatrics. *Pediat. Digest*, 6:41, 1964.

39. SCHER, A. M. Excitation of the heart, P. 299

in *Handbook of Physiology: Circulation,* Vol. 1, W. F. Hamilton, Ed. Washington, D.C., Amer. Physiol. Soc. 1962.

40. SCHERF, D., and SCHOTT, A. *Extrasystoles and Allied Arrhythmias.* New York, Grune & Stratton, 1953.

41. SCHERF, D., and COHEN, J. *The Atrioventricular Node and Selected Cardiac Arrhythmias.* New York, Grune & Stratton, 1964.

42. SCHERF, D. Versuche zur Theorie des Vorhofflatterns und Vorhofflimmerns. *Ztschr. ges. exper. Med.,* 61:30, 1928.

43. KOUWENHOVEN, W. B., JUDE, J. R., and KNICKERBOCKER, G. G. Closed-chest cardiac massage. *J.A.M.A.,* 173:1064, 1960.

44. BAZETT, H. C. An analysis of the time relationship of the electrocardiogram. *Heart,* 7:353, 1920.

45. LEPESCHKIN, E., and SURAWICZ, B. The measurement of the QT interval of the electrocardiogram. *Circulation,* 6:378, 1952.

46. GRANT, R. P. The relationship of unipolar chest leads to the electrical field of the heart. *Circulation,* 1:878, 1950.

47. YANO, K., and PIPBERGER, H. V. Correlations between radiologic heart size and orthogonal electrocardiograms in patients with left ventricular overload. *Am. Heart J.,* 67:44, 1964.

48. THOMAS, P., and DEJONG, D. The P wave in the electrocardiogram in the diagnosis of heart disease. *Brit. Heart J.,* 16:241, 1954.

49. MILNOR, W. R. Electrocardiogram and vectorcardiogram in right ventricular hypertrophy and right bundle branch block. *Circulation,* 16:348, 1957.

50. PIPBERGER, H. V. The normal orthogonal electrocardiogram and vectorcardiogram. *Circulation,* 17:1102, 1958.

51. KATZ, L. N., and WACHTEL, H. The diphasic QRS type of electrocardiogram in congenital heart disease. *Amer. Heart J.,* 13:202, 1937.

52. ELLIOTT, L. P., TAYLOR, W. J., and SCHIEBLER, G. L. Combined ventricular hypertrophy in infancy. *Amer. J. Cardiol.,* 11: 164, 1963.

53. CABRERA, C. E., and MONROY, J. R. Systolic and diastolic loading of the heart. *Amer. Heart J.,* 43:661, 1952.

54. GRANT, R. P. Left axis deviation. *Mod. Concepts Cardiovas. Dis.,* 27:437, 1958.

55. BAYLEY, R. H. On certain applications of modern electrocardiographic theory to the interpretation of electrocardiograms which indicate myocardial disease. *Amer. Heart J.,* 26:769, 1943.

56. LINTERMANS, J. P., KAPLAN, E., MORGAN, B. C., BAUM, D., and GUNTHEROTH, W. G. Infarction patterns in endocardial fibroelastosis. *Circulation,* 33:202, 1966.

57. MASTER, A. M., and JAFFE, H. L. Electrocardiographic changes after exercise in angina pectoris. *J. Mount Sinai Hosp. N.Y.,* 7:629, 1941.

58. ROBB, G. P., and MARKS, H. H. Exercise electrocardiogram in coronary artery disease. *Mod. Med.,* 32:93, 1964.

59. SCHAEFER, H., and HAAS, H. G. Electrocardiography. P. 323 in *Handbook of Physiology: Circulation,* Vol. 1, W. F. Hamilton, Ed. Washington, D.C., Amer. Physiol. Soc., 1962.

60. SAMSON, W. E., and SCHER, A. M. Mechanism of S-T segment alteration during acute myocardial injury. *Circulat. Res.,* 8:780, 1960.

61. NADAS, A. S. *Pediatric Cardiology* (2nd Ed.). Philadelphia, W. B. Saunders Co., 1963.

62. LÜTTGAU, H. C., and NIEDERGERKE, R. The antagonism between Ca and Na ions on the frog's heart. *J. Physiol.,* 143:486, 1958.

63. SURAWICZ, B. Electrolytes and the electrocardiogram. *Mod. Concepts Cardiovas. Dis.,* 33:875, 1964.

64. CANNON, P., and SJÖSTRAND, T. The occurrence of a positive after-potential in the ECG in different physiological and pathological conditions. *Acta med. scandinav.,* 146:191, 1953.

CHAPTER 13

CONGENITAL MALFORMATIONS OF THE HEART

By Warren G. Guntheroth

I. CIRCULATORY CHANGES AT BIRTH

The early development of the circulatory system is characterized by the formation and regression of various channels to accommodate the growth patterns of the developing structures. By the eleventh week, the heart of a human embryo has been formed into a four-chambered organ with the corresponding arterial trunks. The circulatory pattern established at this time persists throughout the remainder of fetal development.

THE FETAL CIRCULATION

While the fetus remains in the uterus, the basic functions of respiration, digestion and elimination of waste products are carried out by the mother. The circulatory system must perform its logistic function during this parasitic type of existence and yet be capable of rapid accommodation to independent existence immediately after the fetus is delivered to the external world. Since the most critical commodity in both the fetus and the newborn infant is oxygen, the mecha-

nisms required for independent respiratory activity have great importance.

In the fetus, the lungs are collapsed and have no respiratory function. The resistance to the flow of blood through the vessels of atelectatic lung tissue is extremely great. Before birth, the vascular resistance is so much greater in the pulmonary vasculature than in the systemic circulation that most of the flow is diverted around the lungs. The foramen ovale and ductus arteriosus act as bypasses permitting blood from the systemic veins to enter the systemic circulation without passing through the lungs.

If there is no orifice in the interatrial septum, left ventricular output is restricted to the quantity of blood flowing through the lungs. Under these conditions, the left ventricle pumps abnormally small amounts and may not develop normally. For example, Patten[1] illustrated the heart from an infant in whom the foramen ovale was sealed prematurely; the left ven-

418

tricular cavity was very small, and the wall was poorly developed. The fetal circulatory pattern can be viewed in terms of the mechanisms by which the output of the two ventricles can remain comparable in the face of greatly retarded pulmonary flow (Fig. 13–1A).

The flow of blood through the circulatory systems of human fetuses delivered by legal abortion has been studied angiocardiographically by Lind and Wegelius.[2] Blood returning from the placenta flows through the umbilical vein and enters the ductus venosus and vascular networks of the liver. This blood carries oxygen and nutrient materials delivered by the maternal blood in the placenta. Entering the vena cava, this partially oxygenated blood merges with systemic venous blood from the caudal portions of the fetus. Much of the blood flowing from the inferior vena cava into the right atrium streams across the chamber and passes through the foramen ovale into the left atrium. According to Windle and Becker,[3] all or nearly all of the blood from the inferior vena cava passes through the foramen ovale, while blood from the superior vena cava streams through the right atrium into the right ventricle with little mixing of the two streams. On the other hand, Everett and Johnson,[4] who used more sensitive radioisotope techniques, reported that about one fourth of the blood from each of the vena caval streams becomes mixed. Rudolph and Heymann[5], using labeled microspheres in sheep, found that the degree of mixing and the organ distribution were strongly influenced by PO_2 and pH. In the normal state, none of the superior vena cava flow went to the left atrium; with decreasing PO_2 and pH, increasing shunting to the left atrium occurred, and the proportion of left heart output that went to the upper body increased.

Since the pulmonary venous return is relatively sparse, most of the oxygenated blood from the placenta flows directly into the left side of the heart to be pumped into the ascending aorta. Thus, the first branches of the aorta receive blood with maximal oxygen content for delivery to the heart and the rapidly developing brain (Fig. 13–1A). The arterial saturation, at best, is poor compared to adult values, and the ability of the fetus to thrive in a state of chronic hypoxia is still incompletely understood. The blood flow through the pulmonary circulation probably increases as the lungs develop but never even approaches the flow through the systemic circuit. The output of the right and left ventricles is balanced by variations in the quantity of blood bypassing the lungs through the ductus arteriosus and through the orifices which persist in the interatrial septum (Fig. 13–1). The flow of blood from the right into the left atrium and from the pulmonary artery into the aorta provides a functional demonstration of the fact that pressures in the right atrium, right ventricle and pulmonary artery exceed the pressures in the corresponding channels on the left. This condition is the reverse of that seen shortly after birth (Table 13–1).

POSTPARTUM CIRCULATION

Cardiorespiratory Adjustments after Delivery. When the umbilical cord is severed after delivery, the infant's only source of oxygen is eliminated pending the establishment of effective respiratory exchange in the lungs. Not only must air enter the lungs promptly, but blood flow through the pulmonary channels must be quickly augmented as well. Ardran et al.[8] demonstrated that the initial inflation of the lungs in fetal lambs

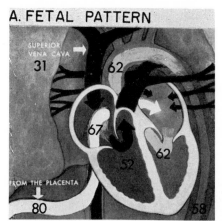
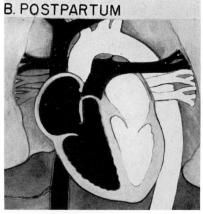
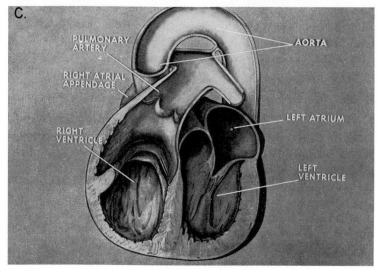

FIGURE 13–1   CIRCULATION ADJUSTMENTS AT BIRTH

A, The fetal circulatory pattern is adapted for intra-uterine existence. Venous blood from the superior vena cava flows into the right atrium and predominantly into the right ventricle. This unsaturated blood is ejected into the pulmonary artery where a major portion continues through the ductus arteriosus into the descending aorta. Resistance to flow through the collapsed lung is so great that only a small quantity of blood enters the pulmonary arteries. A correspondingly small amount of blood returns to the left atrium through the pulmonary veins. Oxygenated blood from the placenta joins the blood flowing through the inferior vena cava and tends to stream across the right atrium through the foramen ovale into the left atrium. This flow of oxygenated blood into the left atrium supplements the scanty venous return from the lungs. The mixture of oxygenated and unsaturated blood enters the left ventricle and is pumped into the aorta, from which the carotid arteries arise to supply the brain. In the descending aorta, this blood is joined by unsaturated blood flowing through the ductus and the mixture is distributed to the lower portions of the body. Numbers indicate average oxygen saturation.[6]

B, Very shortly after birth, the flow of oxygenated blood from the placenta is interrupted. Respiratory function of the lungs must be promptly initiated if the infant is to survive. Pulmonary expansion diminishes pulmonary resistance and the pulmonary blood flow is greatly increased. Constriction of the ductus arteriosus separates the aortic flow from the pulmonary circuit. When the increased pulmonary flow elevates left atrial pressure sufficiently to close the foramen ovale, the adaptation to extra-uterine existence is complete.

C, The components of the fully developed heart are illustrated as viewed from the left anterior oblique position for comparison with drawings portraying various developmental defects.

Table 13–1. *CIRCULATORY FUNCTIONS IN FETAL LAMB BEFORE AND AFTER LUNG EXPANSION*[7]

	CONTROL	30 MIN. AFTER LUNG EXPANSION
Aortic pressure (mm. Hg)	56	60
Pulmonary artery pressure (mm. Hg)	58	34
Right atrial pressure (mm. Hg)	3.5	5.0
Left atrial pressure (mm. Hg)	2.7	7.5
Aortic flow (ml./kg./min.)	97	164
Pulmonary artery flow (ml./kg./min.)	138	189
Effective cardiac output	198	156
Ratio: systemic/pulmonic resistance	.14	2.7

was promptly followed by a precipitous fall in pressure in both the aorta and the pulmonary arteries (as much as 30 per cent of the initial pressure). This change was accompanied by a marked acceleration of flow through the pulmonary vascular tree, as would be expected from a reduced resistance to the flow of blood. Tying the umbilical cord caused both pressures to rise together toward or above their initial level. However, as the ductus arteriosus closed, pressures in the pulmonary artery progressively fell below that in the aorta.

Closure of the Ductus Arteriosus. In the fetus, the tunica media of the ductus arteriosus is loose in structure and composed of elastic fibers and smooth muscle.[9] This histologic pattern is quite different from the compact tunica media of the other arterial trunks. Very shortly after respiratory activity is initiated, the ductus arteriosus closes down. The prompt functional closure of the ductus arteriosus is probably due to contraction of smooth muscle within its walls.[10] Barclay et al.[11] reported angiocardiographic studies indicating that the ductus arteriosus is functionally closed

5 to 7 minutes after respiration begins, although the contrast medium was observed to flow through the channel intermittently for a considerable period. However, Everett and Johnson,[12] employing sensitive radioisotope techniques, found some reduction in ductus arteriosus flow 1 to 2 hours after birth but a greater reduction after 9 hours. A small slit-like lumen in the ductus persisted from about the twelfth hour post partum until the eighteenth day, when anatomic obliteration was usually complete. Eldridge et al.[13] demonstrated that the oxygen content of "arterialized" blood from the hand and from the feet are different immediately after delivery. This difference persisted during observations lasting 3 hours and was still observable in some infants after 3 days. The lower oxygen content of blood from the feet was attributed to shunting of venous blood through the ductus arteriosus into the aorta. The oxygen content of arterialized blood in the upper and lower extremities apparently becomes equal when the ductus arteriosus is closed or the direction of flow through this channel has reversed because pressure in the pulmonary artery was lower than that in the aorta.

In normal infants, with no hypoxia, the ductus closes within one hour, but during that hour a left-to-right shunt of 35 per cent of the cardiac output may be found, and frequently a small right-to-left shunt is found.[14]

Closure of the Foramen Ovale. Soon after birth, the blood flow through the pulmonary circuit increases greatly because of the reduced resistance which follows inflation of the lungs. Functional closure of the ductus arteriosus diverts the entire right ventricular output through the lungs. These factors greatly increase the pulmonary venous flow into the left atrium. As soon as the left atrial pressure exceeds right atrial pressure, the valvula is pressed against the margin of the foramen ovale and partitioning of the heart is finally complete. The closure is facilitated by a reduction in the right atrial pressure secondary to closure of the ductus venosus and reduction in the umbilical venous return. Anatomic obliteration of the potential aperture of the foramen ovale requires many weeks or years. In fact, about 20 per cent of all adults have at least probe patency of this orifice,[15] a phenomenon without functional significance unless pressure in the right atrium becomes higher than that in the left. The interatrial communication will then be restored and may even enlarge until significant quantities of venous blood are shunted into the left atrium.

Changes in Arterial Pressure after Birth. The pulmonary arterial pressure immediately before birth probably ranges around 60/40 mm. Hg and slightly exceeds systemic arterial pressure (Table 13–1). As pulmonary resistance falls and systemic arterial resistance rises, the pressures in the pulmonary artery and aorta diverge progressively. Ultimately, they reach the values typical of adults: systemic arterial pressure 120/80 and pulmonary arterial pressure 25/8.

The marked hemodynamic changes with the first breath, enhanced by umbilical cord clamping, are as drastic as any the organism will experience during its lifetime. Most of the adjustments appear to be directly accomplished, and neural involvement is minimal. Baroreceptor mechanisms, however, are functional shortly after birth.[16] At birth, the two ventricles are accustomed to equal pressures and are very nearly equal in mass. Thus, moderate pressure overload for the right ventricle, whether by virtue of a narrowed pulmonary valve or higher pulmonary resistance, will be easily tolerated in infancy.

II. CONGENITAL MALFORMATIONS OF THE HEART

SIMPLE SHUNTS

The most common developmental defects in the heart and great vessels are incomplete partitioning of the pulmonary from the systemic circulation. During the development of the septa dividing the heart and truncus arteriosus, apertures may persist, leaving orifices at various sites in the walls separating the atria, ventricles and arterial trunks. The foramen ovale and the ductus arteriosus normally remain functional until after delivery, and incomplete closure of these shunts is among the most common developmental defects. The functional effects of the different simple shunts are similar whenever they occur as isolated lesions, uncomplicated by other developmental or acquired pathologic changes. The principal effect of any of these communications between the systemic and pulmonary circuits is the recirculation of oxygenated blood through the lungs, producing abnormally large pulmonary blood flow. The factors determining the direction of blood flow through simple shunts form the basis for any logical approach to the diagnosis of congenital malformations of the heart.

THE DIRECTION OF FLOW THROUGH SIMPLE SHUNTS

In the normal person, the pressures in the right atrium, right ven-

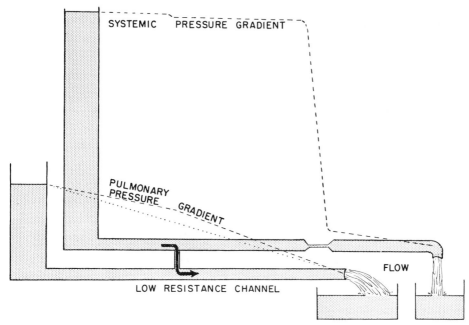

FIGURE 13–2   FLOW THROUGH SHUNTS

Beginning very soon after delivery, the resistance to flow through the pulmonary circuit becomes very low while the total peripheral resistance in the systemic circuit rises. The pressures in the left ventricle and aorta greatly exceed corresponding pressures in the right ventricle and pulmonary artery so long as the pulmonary vascular bed remains a low-resistance channel. These large pressure differences propel oxygenated blood through communicating channels from the systemic system into the pulmonary circuit. So long as pulmonary resistance remains low, pulmonary blood flow can be greatly increased with little change in pulmonary arterial pressure. The flow through abnormal channels connecting the pulmonary and systemic channels depends upon the size of the orifice and the magnitude of the pressure difference.

tricle and pulmonary artery are lower than the corresponding pressures in the left atrium, ventricle and aorta. As indicated in Chapter 1, the very slight resistance to flow through the vascular system in the lungs is the fundamental reason for the low pressures in the pulmonary artery and right ventricle since the flow is the same in both pulmonic and systemic circuits in the normal adult. The pressure in the right atrium is lower than that in the left because the thin-walled right ventricle is more easily distended during diastolic filling. So long as the pulmonary resistance remains low in relation to systemic resistance and the right ventricular

chamber remains normally distensible, the pressures in all the channels leading to the lungs are lower than those in corresponding channels leading to the systemic vascular tree.

Under these conditions, the pressure differences promote the flow of blood from the systemic to the pulmonary circuit through any communication between them as illustrated schematically in Figure 13–2. The quantity of blood passing through such simple shunts depends upon the pressure difference across the shunt and the resistance to flow through it. The resistance to flow is determined primarily by the caliber of the aperture or channel.

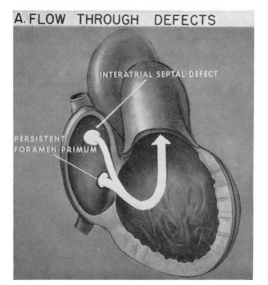
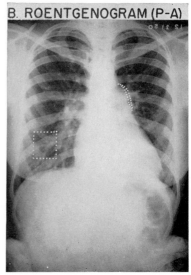

FIGURE 13–3   ATRIAL SEPTAL DEFECTS

A, Interatrial septal defects most commonly occur in the region of the foramen ovale. Occasionally the foramen primum fails to close. In either case, oxygenated blood surges from the left atrium into the right atrium and ventricle to be recirculated through the lungs along with the venous return from the systemic circulation.

B, The increased total pulmonary blood flow produces dilatation of the pulmonary artery, which appears as a vigorously pulsating bulge on the left side of the mediastinum. The pulmonary vascular markings are more prominent than normal. Increased pulsation of the smaller branches of the pulmonary artery is observed by fluoroscopic examination of small areas in the peripheral lung field (e.g., dotted square). Right ventricular enlargement as well as right atrial enlargement can usually be demonstrated. The left ventricle and left atrium are ordinarily not enlarged in the conventional septum secundum defect.

DEFECTS IN THE ATRIAL SEPTUM

The most common congenital malformation of the heart is a functionally significant aperture in some part of the interatrial septum. The large proportion of individuals (20 per cent of the general population) with probe patency of the foramen ovale are not included in this group. Most interatrial defects are located at some distrance from the tricuspid valves, in the general region of the foramen secundum or foramen ovale (Fig. 13–3*A*). Another fairly common site is in the vicinity of the foramen primum. These defects range from simple. apertures less than 1 cm. in diameter through multiple defects of

varying size to virtual absence of the interatrial septum.

Functional Effects of Atrial Septal Defects. As indicated in the preceding section, the pressure in the left atrium generally exceeds right atrial pressure so long as the right ventricle is more distensible than the left. The distensibility of the two ventricles is determined largely by the average systolic pressure required of them by their respective circulations; i.e., by the respective resistances of the systemic and pulmonic circulation. In the adult, the systemic resistance is normally over ten times that of the pulmonary resistance. Consequently, the right ventricle is much more distensible and will fill to a greater extent than the left ventricle for the same filling pressure, for limited filling intervals. The pressure gradient between the left atrium and right is normally 5 mm. Hg. However, in patients with large atrial septal defects, there is no measurable pressure gradient using conventional catheters and pressure transducers. Using special, sensitive techniques[17, 18] left atrial pressure has been shown to exceed slightly the right atrial pressure at all times except for a transient reversal of the pressure gradient at the onset of atrial systole.

The oxygenated blood that flows through the defect enters the right atrium and mingles with the returning systemic venous blood flowing to the lung (Fig. 13–3). Thus, the blood flowing through the shunt recirculates through the lung, increasing the total flow through the lung. The quantity of oxygenated blood flowing into the left ventricle and pumped through the systemic arteries to the tissues is approximately normal, being controlled by complex neural and humoral mechanisms indicated in Chapters 3 and 4.

Hickam[19] measured pulmonary blood flows of 15 to 20 liters per minute in resting patients with simple atrial septal defects. Thus, the right ventricular output was three or four times greater than left ventricular output. These large volumes were propelled through the lungs by a pressure difference of only 12 or 13 mm. Hg from the pulmonary artery to the left atrium. In one patient, blood flow of 15 liters per minute was maintained through the pulmonary circuit by a pressure gradient of only 4 mm. Hg. Such tremendous flow produced by a small pressure gradient signifies that the pulmonary resistance remains very low.

Continuous measurement of pulmonary artery and superior vena cava oxygen saturation with a fiberoptic catheter has demonstrated that the pulmonary blood flow does not increase during exercise in these patients with atrial septal defects.[20] The systemic output increases in a normal fashion, resulting in a relative decrease in the left-to-right shunting during exercise. This may explain the clinical observation that children with large atrial septal defects usually have good exercise tolerance.

Diagnostic Signs of Atrial Septal Defects. Clinical evidence of atrial septal defects stems primarily from the functional effects of greatly increased pulmonary blood flow and its secondary effects.

AUSCULTATION A systolic murmur in the pulmonary area on the precordium is usually the first clue to the presence of heart disease in patients with defects in the interatrial septum. These murmurs are usually absent at birth and may not become audible for months or years. Immediately after birth, the right ventricle has a relatively thick wall and functions under a pressure load similar to that of the left ventricle since the pressures in the pulmonary and systemic arterial systems are similar. Thus, there is little difference in the distensibility of the two ventricles, and insignificant quantities of blood pass through the interatrial shunts. As the pulmonary arterial resistance falls and systemic peripheral resistance rises, the pressure differences between the two systems become greater. The left ventricle becomes thick-walled, and the right ventricle becomes more distensible as its pressure load diminishes. Flow through interatrial communications then increases greatly. The intensity of the murmur appears to bear some relation to the volume flow through the interatrial defect. However, the sounds are actually due to the rush of abnormally large quantities of blood through the pulmonary conus. Thus, this systolic murmur is produced by the same mechanism that causes "functional" murmurs. The pulmonary origin of this murmur was graphically demonstrated by phonocardiograms recorded directly from the surface of a dog's heart in which an interatrial septal defect had been produced surgically. Although a very distinct systolic murmur promptly appeared over the pulmonary conus and pulmonary artery, no murmur was recorded over either the right or the left atrium.[21] In patients, the murmur often attains such intensity that it is widely transmitted over the precordium and is associated with a thrill palpated in the pulmonary area.

Another characteristic auscultatory finding is relatively wide splitting of the second heart sound in the pulmonary area. Although most children exhibit splitting with maximal inspiration, patients with atrial septal defect have splitting with every heart beat, with little change during respiration. Splitting in atrial septal defect indicates that the pulmonary artery pressure is normal, since it disappears with pulmonary hypertension. Presumably, the splitting reflects a large ventricular stroke volume, prolonging right ventricular ejection; the second component of the second sound is the pulmonary closure.

A medium-pitched diastolic murmur beginning with the third heart sound may be heard at the lower left sternal border in patients with moderately large defects. This is sometimes referred to as a shunt murmur or as relative tricuspid stenosis, since it is thought to be produced by increased flow across the tricuspid valve during the rapid filling phase of ventricular diastole.

An apical pansystolic blowing murmur in a patient that otherwise has characteristics of a simple secundum atrial defect strongly suggests mitral regurgitation caused by a çongenital cleft, a combination diagnostic of a primum atrial septal defect. This entity is a partial form of a persistent atrioventricular canal or endocardial cushion defect, depending upon the choice of terminology. The complete form will be discussed subsequently.

ROENTGENOGRAPHY. In most patients with interatrial defects, the right atrium and ventricle become enlarged because of the increased volume load (increased pulmonary blood flow). Roentgenographic evidence of anterior protrusion of the enlarged right ventricle is more easily observed when the patient is in the true lateral or left anterior oblique position. The main pulmonary artery will be quite prominent in patients with large pulmonary flow, and the entire pulmonary vascular bed will be prominent. Although fluoroscopy is not routinely done now, the hilar vessels may be seen to have an intrinsic pulsation if a small area is observed, preferably with an image intensifier.

ELECTROCARDIOGRAPHY. The right atrium is enlarged but not under high pressure in a simple secundum atrial defect, and the P waves are usually normal. However, the P-R interval is commonly increased beyond normal limits, causing first-degree A-V block. The QRS complexes characteristically show right bundle branch block (Fig. 12–40). This electrocardiographic term suggests a delay (block) in conduction, but studies with intramyocardial electrodes revealed no decrease in conduction velocity but a lengthened pathway due to dilatation of the right ventricle.[22] The conventional electrocardiogram presents a broadened QRS complex with the slurred terminal portion directed to the right and anteriorly. Increased voltage to the right and anterior are also common, suggesting right ventricular hypertrophy.

CARDIAC CATHETERIZATION AND ANGIOCARDIOGRAPHY. A patient with the characteristic clinical findings of an atrial septal defect who has definite cardiac enlargement, indicating that he is a candidate for surgical repair, should have cardiac catheterization. The right heart pressures are usually within normal limits, although there may be a slight pressure gradient across the pulmonary valve, particularly if there is a very large pulmonary blood flow. An increase in the blood oxygen will be found at the right atrial level, the magnitude depending on the size of the shunt. The increase in oxygen will be sustained downstream from the right atrium. Pulmonary hypertension is extraordinarily rare in simple atrial septal defects in the first two decades of life but thereafter occurs with increasing frequency.

Angiocardiography provides little additional information in most instances. Selective injection into the main or right pulmonary artery may demonstrate anomalous connection of the right pulmonary veins, which are associated with atrial septal defects in 20 per cent of the operated cases,[23] but this will be apparent to the surgeon anyway. If the left ventricle is entered, an angiocardiogram there may demonstrate mitral regurgitation or the deformity of the left ventricular outflow tract characteristic of an endocardial cushion defect. If this latter deformity is absent, a septum primum atrial defect is very unlikely, but the absence of mitral regurgitation does not rule out a cleft mitral valve of a septum primum defect.

Surgical Correction. Most centers recommend surgical closure of the atrial septal defect utilizing cardio-pulmonary bypass for significant left-to-right shunts, defined as having a pulmonary blood flow at least twice the systemic.[24] For those having a pulmonary blood flow smaller than 1.5 times the systemic, it is difficult to justify the morbidity and mortality of open-heart surgery on the basis of present knowledge of the prognosis of this disease. There is, for example, no appreciable chance of developing bacterial endocarditis in the secundum defect, and pulmonary hypertension has never been proven to be a result of a small atrial septal defect.

ABERRANT RIGHT PULMONARY VEINS

The veins draining the right lung normally empty into the left atrium very near the interatrial septum. It is not surprising that as a result of defective development, the right pulmonary veins occasionally empty into the right atrium. Aberrant right pulmonary veins drain fully oxygenated blood from the right lung into the right atrium. This has precisely the same functional effects as the shunting of the same quantity of oxygenated blood through an interatrial septal defect. For this reason, the clinical signs and symptoms of the two conditions are identical.[25] Furthermore, an interatrial septal defect and aberrant pulmonary veins are frequently seen in the same patient, with functional effects corresponding to those of a very large atrial septal defect. Rarely, all the pulmonary veins drain into the right atrium, a condition producing a quite different set of symptoms and signs which will be considered later.

The presence of right pulmonary veins emptying into the right atrium can often be demonstrated by inserting the tip of a cardiac catheter, under direct fluoroscopic control, into such a

vein and withdrawing fully oxygenated blood from the channel. However,
it is equally likely that the catheter
may have passed through the atrial
defect prior to entering the pulmonary
vein. Only if the vein empties into the
superior vena cava can one be relatively certain of the anomalous connection.

VENTRICULAR SEPTAL DEFECTS

During the last stages of partitioning in the heart, an aperture in the
interventricular septum persists (Fig.
2–2F). Endocardial cushion tissue
proliferates into this aperture and later
thins out to form the membranous portion of the interventricular septum just
below the origin of the aorta and pulmonary arteries (Fig. 13–4). Incomplete closure of this opening is the
most common defect in the interventricular septum although apertures
in the muscular portion of the septum
are occasionally reported.

*Functional Effects of Ventricular
Septal Defects.* Through an aperture
connecting the two ventricular cavities, oxygenated blood is propelled
from the left ventricle into the right
by pressure differences which can be
very large during systole (e.g., 100
mm. Hg) and relatively small during
diastole (0 to 10 mm. Hg). Large flows
through the shunt must result unless
the ventricular septal defects are
small or the pressure difference is
greatly reduced. If the defect is as
large as the aortic valve, the left ventricular pressure will be transmitted
undiminished to the right ventricle,
in which case the ratio of pulmonary
to systemic flow will be determined
entirely by the ratio of pulmonary to
systemic resistance. Maintenance of
normal systemic blood flow will require more pulmonary resistance than
normal, and the very fact of survival

demonstrates that a higher pulmonary
resistance has been present since
birth in these patients with large ventricular septal defects.

An important functional effect of a
large ventricular septal defect is the
pulmonary vascular congestion. This
congestion is in addition to the over-
perfusion that is seen in atrial septal
defects and is due to a high left atrial
pressure, which results in a higher
pulmonary capillary pressure, favoring edema formation in the alveoli.
In addition to increased stiffness of
the lung, these patients have a marked
susceptibility to pneumonia, a common cause of death in infants with
large ventricular septal defects. Patients with large atrial septal defects
usually have larger pulmonary blood
flows than patients with large ventricular septal defects but do not have high
left atrial pressure and rarely are
bothered with pneumonia.

*Diagnostic Signs of Ventricular
Septal Defects.* The clinical evidence of a ventricular septal defect
reflects the increased flow and pressure in the pulmonary circuit and the
actual flow through the defect.

AUSCULTATION. In the smaller
ventricular septal defects, the pressure
gradient across the defect is larger and
the systolic murmur is much louder
than in the patients with large defects.
This systolic murmur, although loud,
is of uniform, high frequency and is
maximal at the third and fourth left
intercostal spaces at the left sternal
border. This murmur does not transmit well to the neck, back or axilla,
relative to its intensity at the sternal
border. The second sound in the pulmonary area is dependent on the pulmonary artery pressure: with high
pressure, the sound becomes unsplit
and accentuated, but if the pressure is
low, the second sound may be normal
in splitting and intensity. In larger

A

B

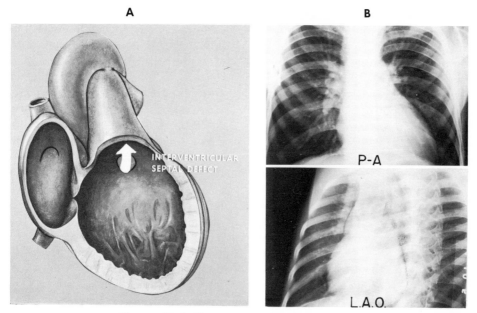

FIGURE 13–4 VENTRICULAR SEPTAL DEFECTS

A, Typical Site of Shunt. Defects in the interventricular septum most frequently occur in the membranous septum just below the roots of the aorta and pulmonary artery. This region corresponds to the interventricular foramen, which is the last portion of the septum to be filled in. Oxygenated blood surges through this orifice from the left ventricle at high velocity during systole because the difference in pressure between the ventricular cavities is very large. Loud coarse systolic murmurs are produced by the rush of blood through the restricted orifice. They have maximum intensity in the third or fourth intercostal spaces along the left sternal border.

B, Roentgenograms. Usually the interventricular defect is small and is not accompanied by symptoms of any kind. The cardiac silhouette is normal in size and configuration, and the principal sign is the loud systolic murmur. This picture conforms to the classic descriptions of Roger's disease. However, if the defect is large enough to be functionally significant, frontal roentgenograms will reveal cardiac enlargement, particularly the left atrium and ventricle, seen in the P-A and left anterior oblique roentgenograms. The dilated, pulsating pulmonary artery is accompanied by increased pulmonary vascular markings.

shunts, there may be an accentuated third sound at the apex, followed by a mid-diastolic, low-pitched murmur. This murmur is believed due to an increased flow across the mitral valve with ventricular filling.

ROENTGENOGRAPHY. The course of the shunt in ventricular septal defects determines the roentgenographic prominence of the various chambers: left ventricle to right ventricle to pulmonary circulation to left atrium to left ventricle and so forth. The degree of enlargement of these chambers will depend primarily on the size of the shunt, and in the smallest defects, the cardiac roentgenograms will be normal. If the shunt is small due to high pulmonary vascular resistance of long duration, then the hilar pulmonary arteries will be quite prominent without chamber enlargement, since ventricular hypertrophy without dilatation of the chamber will not usually be apparent on plain films.

ELECTROCARDIOGRAPHY. In the very small ventricular septal defect the electrocardiogram is normal. In those septal defects permitting a modest left-to-right shunt without a significant increase in right ventricular pressure, left ventricular hypertrophy is found (Fig. 12–31). With larger shunts, combined ventricular hypertrophy is common (Fig. 12–37), reflecting the increased work of both ventricles. In later stages of pulmonary hypertension with vascular obstruction, right ventricular hypertrophy suggests the disappearance of a left-to-right shunt and heralds the occurrence of cyanosis because of right-to-left shunting.

CARDIAC CATHETERIZATION AND ANGIOCARDIOGRAPHY. These special diagnostic procedures are unnecessary for the small ventricular septal defects but are indicated for the surgical candidate. The right ventricular and pulmonary artery pressures range from normal to systemic pressure, depending on the size of the ventricular septal defect. The pulmonary artery wedge, or "pulmonary capillary" pressure is usually slightly elevated and may be definitely elevated in the large shunts associated with heart failure, particularly in infancy. An increase in oxygen content occurs at the ventricular level. The systemic blood flow is usually normal except in the occurrence of congestive failure, and the pulmonary blood flow may be 2 to 3 times the systemic blood flow, depending on the size of the defect and the pulmonary vascular resistance.

Angiocardiography for simple ventricular septal defects, as in other types of simple left-to-right shunts, is infrequently necessary. In the larger defects, particularly in infants, right ventricular injections to demonstrate the relationship of the two great vessels is a wise precaution.

Surgical Correction. Small ventricular septal defects which cause no cardiac enlargement have not been proven to be a significant risk to longevity or health, and the morbidity and small mortality of open-heart surgery are not justified in the opinion of most centers. When the pulmonary blood flow exceeds twice the systemic, surgical closure utilizing cardiopulmonary bypass is recommended at a convenient age, usually four or five years. If severe pulmonary hypertension exists, the size of the shunt may be so small that surgery is not warranted, since the risk of surgery is great and the likelihood of achieving any substantial improvement is slight. The risk of developing inoperable pulmonary vascular obstruction, fortunately, is confied to the larger defects and pulmonary hypertension will be present from infancy.[26] The infant with congestive failure due to a large shunt will frequently require surgical assistance. Some centers prefer a moderate-risk operation, banding of the main pulmonary artery with a fabric ligature creating a local increased resistance to flow through the lungs, reducing the pressure beyond the band to approximately one third of the aortic mean pressure.[27] As the infant grows, the fixed ligature becomes relatively more restrictive, and the child may develop cyanosis in a few years. Ultimately, all banded patients will require open-heart repair with cardiopulmonary bypass. A few centers, ours included, accept the somewhat higher initial risk of complete repair in infancy, particularly if the infant is at least six months old, in preference to the combined risk of the early banding plus the later complete repair.[28]

A few infants with ventricular septal defects, some with large shunts, will have spontaneous closure of the defect with an unknown sequence. Occasionally, the defect closes or narrows in school-age children, not often enough to defer surgery, but often enough to encourage a conservative approach in the smaller defects.

ENDOCARDIAL CUSHION DEFECTS (A-V CANAL)

Septum primum atrial defects, referred to in the section on atrial defects, are a partial form of an atrioventricular canal, with a low atrial septal defect and a cleft in the septal leaflet of the mitral valve. The effect of the shunt has been adequately described, but there is also mitral regurgitation in most patients, resulting in an apical, blowing, pansystolic murmur. The electrocardiogram is distinctive, with a superior axis and right bundle branch block (Fig. 12–43). The precordial leads are unaffected by the congenital conduction disturbance causing the superior axis, and if there are tall R-waves over the right precordium diagnostic of right ventricular hypertrophy, then the right ventricular pressure will nearly always be elevated, due either to an additional anomaly of pulmonic stenosis or to a ventricular defect. In the latter instance, a complete A-V canal is present, and the functional effects will be those of a large ventricular septal defect.

A left ventricular angiocardiogram will demonstrate a characteristic abnormality of the mitral valve. The valve plane orientation is more vertical than normal, and there is usually mitral regurgitation. In the frontal plane a cleft-like filling defect appears in the left ventricular margin under the anterior leaflet of the mitral valve (Fig. 13–5).

Surgical correction of the primum atrial defect requires direct suture of the cleft mitral valve. For the complete canal, the ventricular portion of the defect must be closed and the free-floating common atrioventricular valve must be secured to the upper part of the ventricular septum. Finally, the atrial defect is closed. The chance of damaging the atrioventricular node or the common bundle is considerable, and the overall mortality for complete repair is as high as 50 per cent nationally.

PATENT DUCTUS ARTERIOSUS

If the ductus arteriosus fails to close (Fig. 13–6), part of the oxygenated blood ejected by the left ventricle surges through this shunt into the pulmonary artery and merges with venous blood passing out to the lungs. The pressure difference across the ductus arteriosus can be extremely large, ranging as high as 100 mm. Hg during systole and around 70 mm. Hg during diastole. The signs and symptoms of a small persistent ductus arteriosus are distinctly different from those resulting when this channel has large caliber, just as in the case of ventricular septal defects.

Functional Effects of Patent Ductus Arteriosus. The ductus arteriosus serves as a low-resistance channel through which blood rushes out of the systemic arterial system. The high-velocity flow of blood through the restricted channel into the larger pulmonary artery produces turbulence.

Escape of blood from the systemic arterial system tends to depress the diastolic pressure. Since the oxygenated blood flowing through the ductus does not contribute to perfusion of the tissues, left ventriclar stroke volume is augmented to compensate for the shunted blood.

In a large ductus, one finds the problems of increased pulmonary flow and pressure and higher pulmonary capillary pressure described with large ventricular septal defects.

Clinical Signs of Patent Ductus Arteriosus. The volume of flow through a *small* ductus arteriosus is

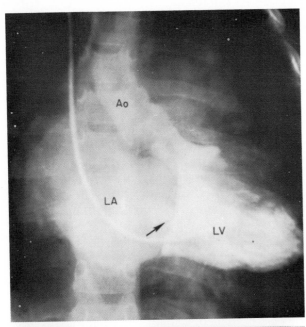

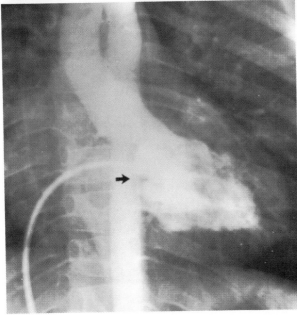

FIGURE 13–5   ENDOCARDIAL CUSH-
ION DEFECT: ANGIOCARDIOGRAPHIC
FEATURES

Angiocardiograms in the frontal
projection of the left ventricle in two
patients with endocardial cushion
defect.

Above, Mitral regurgitation is
present, resulting in opacification of
the left atrium. The plane of the mitral valve (arrow) is almost vertical,
in contrast to the more horizontal
orientation in the normal. LA = left
atrium, LV = left ventricle, and Ao =
aorta.

Below, The irregular margin of
left ventricular contour under the
aortic valve (arrow), characteristic
of endocardial cushion defects, is
due to the deformity of the anterior
leaflet of the mitral valve. In this patient, there was no substantial mitral
regurgitation. (From Morgan, Guntheroth *et al.*[24])

not sufficient to require any compensatory mechanism to maintain normal
blood flow through the systemic circulation. Left ventricular output is readily increased to provide normal
systemic flow plus the small quantity
of blood which escapes through the
shunt. The slight increase in left ventricular dimensions is often not apparent from roentgenographic examination (Figs. 13–6B, C), the electrocardiogram is within normal limits,

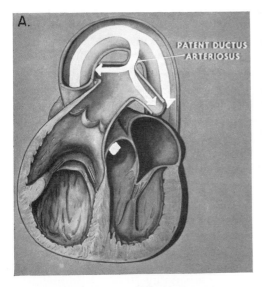

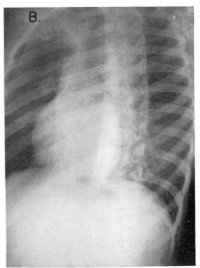

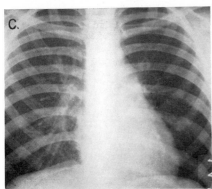

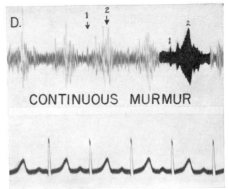

FIGURE 13–6   PATENT DUCTUS ARTERIOSUS

A, If the ductus arteriosus remains patent, the high pressure in the aorta forces oxygenated blood into the pulmonary artery, increasing pulmonary blood flow.

B, The configuration of the cardiac silhouette in the left anterior oblique position conforms to the outline of the schematic drawing in *A.* If the ductus arteriosus is small, the cardiac silhouette may remain within normal limits when viewed from this angle. Since left ventricular stroke volume is generally increased, the left ventricle may be enlarged.

C, In many patients the size and configuration of the cardiac silhouette are entirely normal. Dilatation of the pulmonary artery with normal or increased pulmonary vascular markings can often be demonstrated in the postero-anterior view. Left ventricular enlargement is indicated by elongation of the heart. Definite evidence of cardiac enlargement generally signifies that the ductus arteriosus is large.

D, The most characteristic sign of patent ductus arteriosus is a "continuous" murmur which begins shortly after the first heart sound gains intensity during late systole and diminishes during diastole. This murmur has maximal intensity in the left infraclavicular region.

the arterial blood pressure remains normal and the only obvious sign is the characteristic murmur (Fig. 13–6D).

AUSCULTATION. The most distinctive sign of patent ductus arteriosus is the "continuous" murmur. The pressure difference between the aorta and the pulmonary artery persists throughout the cardiac cycle but is greatest during systole. Thus, the velocity of flow, the degree of turbulence and the intensity of the resulting murmur reach a maximum during late systole and progressively diminish during diastole. In contrast to the systolic and diastolic murmurs associated with semilunar valvular disease, there is neither an interruption of the murmur nor a change in quality of the sound at the transition between systole and diastole. For this reason, the continuous, machinery-like quality of the murmur is quite distinctive. The murmur is best heard high on the left precordium, usually in the left infraclavicular area. In a large proportion of patients, the characteristic murmur is the only definite sign of the lesion. In about 10 per cent of patients, the diastolic component of the murmur is either inaudible or absent. This usually signifies elevated pulmonary pressure, retarding the flow of blood through the ductus during the diastolic interval, and is associated with an accentuated, unsplit second heart sound in the pulmonary area.

ROENTGENOGRAPHY. If the ductus arteriosus is narrow, the size and configuration of the cardiac silhouette are usually normal except for a bulge on the left border which signifies dilatation of the pulmonary artery. A larger ductus will cause enlargement of the left atrium, left ventricle and ascending aorta, all of which are involved in the increased blood flow due to the shunt.

ELECTROCARDIOGRAPHY. The electrocardiograms in patients with a patent ductus arteriosus have a similar range as in patients with a ventricular septal defect: normal with small shunts and normal pressures, left ventricular hypertrophy with moderate shunts but nearly normal pulmonary artery pressure, combined hypertrophy with larger shunts and higher pulmonary pressures and, in the extreme, right ventricular hypertrophy with pulmonary vascular obstruction and little left-to-right shunt.

CARDIAC CATHETERIZATION AND ANGIOCARDIOGRAPHY. These investigations are unnecessary for the patient with a typical continuous, machinery-like murmur, with compatible roentgenography and electrocardiography. If there is uncertainty, catheterization is certainly safer than a thoracotomy. For a small ductus, the right heart pressures will be normal, and the only positive finding will be a step-up in oxygen saturation at the pulmonary artery level. A larger ductus will usually have some increase in right ventricular, pulmonary artery and pulmonary artery wedge pressures. With modest skill, the cardiac catheter can usually be maneuvered into the left pulmonary artery, into the ductus and then down the descending aorta, which allows a specific diagnosis of ductus arteriosus, as opposed to the rare aortic septal defect (aortic-pulmonary window). Aortography to prove the presence of a ductus may rarely be necessary: the contrast material is injected through a catheter in the ascending aorta after introduction by direct arteriotomy, or in larger patients, by the percutaneous Seldinger method.[29]

Surgical Treatment of Patent Ductus Arteriosus. Although a small ductus will produce few or no symptoms, the life-time risk of subacute bacterial endocarditis appears to be greater than the risk of surgical division (less than 1 per cent) in a fully staffed and equipped center. However, a skilled surgeon in a small hospital that does not regularly experience thoracic surgery may have a mortality as high as 10 per cent,[30] and such risks are totally unwarranted for a small ductus. For the ductus with a larger shunt, symptoms will usually require intervention, occasionally even in infancy.[31]

AORTIC SEPTAL DEFECT OR AORTIC-PULMONARY WINDOW

Although the clinical signs and symptoms of patent ductus arteriosus appear distinctive, this lesion cannot be differentiated from a functionally identical communication between the pulmonary artery and the aorta. During the partitioning of the truncus arteriosus by the proliferating spiral aortic-pulmonary septum (see Fig. 2–3), incomplete fusion may leave a residual aperture just above the semilunar valves. Fortunately, this aortic-pulmonary septum (see Fig. occurs, blood from the aorta surges through into the pulmonary artery during both systole and diastole. The resulting continuous murmur is very similar to that heard in a patient with patent ductus arteriosus, although the greatest intensity is heard lower on the precordium (e.g., in the third intercostal space to the left of the sternum) when the murmur results from an aortic septal defect. The shunts are always large, and pulmonary hypertension is present. Confusion of the aortic septal defect with a small ductus is therefore unlikely. An aortogram will differentiate the two lesions, if the course of the catheter has not previously proven the lesion.

Surgical correction has been successful without the use of cardiopulmonary bypass, but the latter is safer with today's techniques.

SIMPLE SHUNTS WITH OBSTRUCTED PULMONARY FLOW

Normally, the pulmonary resistance is so slight that an arteriovenous pressure gradient of 4 to 6 mm. Hg is sufficient to propel not only the normal resting flow through the lungs (4 to 5 liters per minute) but as much as three times this amount with no increase in pulmonary arterial pressure. In the systemic circulation, the same volume flow is propelled from the aorta to the venae cavae by a mean arteriovenous pressure difference of some 90 mm. Hg or more. Thus, the normal resistance to flow through the systemic circuit must be some 10 to 15 times greater than pulmonary vascular resistance.

The consequences, then, of a large communication between the systemic and pulmonary circulation beyond the atrial level are high pressure in the pulmonary circuit and large flow (Fig. 13–7A), unless some obstruction to pulmonary flow has developed (Fig. 13–7B). The obstruction may develop on three main levels, pulmonary arterial, pulmonary venous and pulmonary valvular (including infundibular stenosis), and the obstruction may present sufficient resistance that the shunt becomes right-to-left. If the obstruction is present from birth, a separate form of congenital heart disease is present and will be discussed in a subsequent section, *Developmental Defects with Intrinsic Cyanosis*.

Pulmonary Arteriolar Obstruction

In the fetus, the walls of the pulmonary arteries have thick muscular coats (which normally thin out during early childhood). The pulmonary resistance actually exceeds systemic resistance, and pulmonary blood flow is much less than systemic flow. Immediately after birth, pulmonary resistance normally diminishes progressively and systemic resistance rises. The high pulmonary resistance may persist longer than normal in infants surviving with large shunts, with high pressure. The development of increased pulmonary vascular re-

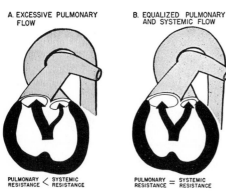

A. EXCESSIVE PULMONARY FLOW

B. EQUALIZED PULMONARY AND SYSTEMIC FLOW

PULMONARY RESISTANCE < SYSTEMIC RESISTANCE

PULMONARY RESISTANCE = SYSTEMIC RESISTANCE

Figure 13–7 The Significance of Pulmonary Resistance

A, The pulmonary vascular resistance is greatly increased when there are large shunts in the partitions of the heart beyond the atrial level. The functional importance of the response is illustrated by an extreme example in which the interventricular septum failed to form. Blood ejected from the single ventricle would tend to flow predominantly into the pulmonary artery, since this circuit offers less resistance. If the pulmonary resistance were only one-tenth that of the systemic circuit, a correspondingly small fraction of the total ventricular ejection would enter the aorta to perfuse the tissues. Usually, pulmonary blood flow exceeds systemic flow by only three- or four-fold, indicating that pulmonary resistance is much higher than normal.

B, The flow through the systemic and pulmonary circuits can be the same only if the pulmonary resistance equals systemic arterial resistance.

sistance is beneficial to the infant with a very large ventricular septal defect (Fig. 13–7), but the cause of this development and the factors that cause it to progress to irreversibility are uncertain and controversial. High pressure in the pulmonary vessels from birth appears to be the most predictable cause of pulmonary arteriolar obstruction. Histologic changes in the walls of pulmonary arterial branches are generally demonstrable in patients with persistent severe pulmonary hypertension. Civin and Edwards[32] have reported finding extensive hypertrophy of the media in the muscular arteries within the lungs of patients with large shunts between the ventricles or arterial trunks. This hypertrophy was often accompanied by intimal hyperplasia. However, the development of pulmonary hypertension in patients with atrial defects is a late occurrence, usually in the third decade or later. This suggests that large flow without hypertension is not as powerful a stimulus to pulmonary vascular obstruction as high transmitted pressures.

The age at which pulmonary hypertension becomes fixed has great significance relative to the age at operation and even to the question of operability on a patient with a shunt. It seems that very high resistance is unlikely to return to normal after the first one or two years of life, and conversely, normal or only moderately increased pulmonary resistance is unlikely to progress rapidly in the first four or five years. Various methods for prediction of regression of high resistance in individual patients to decide upon surgery have included administration of oxygen, acetylcholine and tolazoline, but none of these has been reliable. If there is a significant left-to-right shunt (pulmonary blood flow 1.5 to 2 times systemic, or greater), the patient is usually offered operation, but at high risk.

PULMONARY VENOUS HYPERTENSION

If the pulmonary venous pressure is elevated for an extended period of time, pulmonary arteriolar constriction will occur, increasing the pulmonary vascular resistance, in addition to the total pulmonary resistance which is elevated directly by the increased pulmonary venous pressure. The pulmonary venous hypertension most often is due to left heart failure, but hypoplasia of the left ventricle, mitral stenosis or atresia and cor triatriatum may be the cause also. Rudolph and Nadas[33] even suggest that pulmonary venous hypertension may be *the* cause of progressive pulmonary vascular obstruction, although others have demonstrated that pulmonary hypertension due to pulmonary venous hypertension is more reversible, postoperatively, than that associated with left-to-right shunts.[34] At any rate, pulmonary artery wedge pressures should certainly be obtained before declaring that a patient has inoperable pulmonary vascular obstruction, since the group with pulmonary venous hypertension contains several entities which are correctable.

PULMONARY STENOSIS

Obstruction to pulmonary flow may occur with valvular pulmonary stenosis, either congenital or acquired naturally or surgically. The congenital type of pulmonary stenosis will be discussed in the next section; it is not progressive or acquired naturally. On the other hand, infundibular stenosis may be gradually acquired, particularly in association with ventricular septal defect. In ventricular septal defect there is frequently a displacement of one or both arms of the crista supraventricularis, and with increasing right ventricular hypertrophy, there is a parallel increase in infundibular obstruction.[54] Infants with typical clinical signs of a simple shunt through a ventricular septal defect may reappear in three or four years as a tetralogy of Fallot.

STENOTIC LESIONS WITHOUT SHUNTS

PULMONARY STENOSIS

Three main types of congenital pulmonary stenosis are found: valvular stenosis, infundibular stenosis and arterial stenosis. In the first type, (Fig. 13–8) the pulmonary valvular cusps are fused during embryologic development into a diaphragm or conical membrane with a small central orifice. Infundibular stenosis sometimes develops as a long narrow muscular channel replacing the normally capacious outflow tract of the right ventricle. More commonly, there is a narrow constriction at some level below the pulmonary valve. As an isolated lesion, valvular stenosis is much more common than infundibular stenosis; occasionally they occur together. In contrast, infundibular stenosis is a much more common cause of pulmonary obstruction in the tetralogy of Fallot (see later).

The mainstem of the pulmonary artery is often grossly dilated just beyond the valvular stenosis, and even the right and left branches may be larger than normal in spite of diminished pulmonary blood flow. This poststenotic dilatation is a typical response to many kinds of local obstruction in the vascular system.

Peripheral pulmonary arterial stenosis usually is quite mild and is

A. PULMONARY VALVULAR STENOSIS

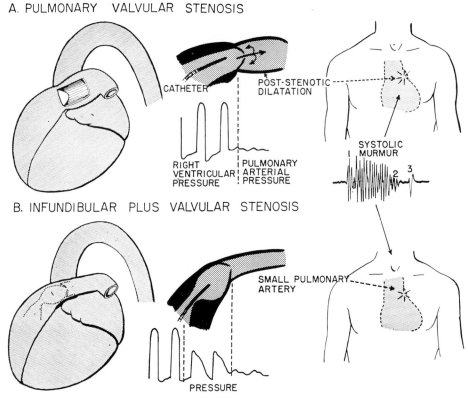

B. INFUNDIBULAR PLUS VALVULAR STENOSIS

FIGURE 13–8   PULMONARY STENOSIS

A, Congenital stenosis of the pulmonary valve may occur as an isolated lesion, or it may be accompanied by defects in either the atrial or the ventricular septum. The pulmonary valve consists of a conical diaphragm with a small aperture at the apex, and the pulmonary artery beyond the valve is usually dilated (post-stenotic dilatation). To overcome the high resistance to flow through the restricted valvular orifice, the right ventricular systolic pressure becomes elevated. The mean pulmonary arterial pressure beyond the constriction is usually normal, but the pulse pressure is greatly reduced. Turbulent flow of blood through the small orifice produces a systolic murmur which is widely transmitted over the precordium, but has maximal intensity in the pulmonary area. Post-stenotic dilatation of the pulmonary artery produces a prominent bulge on the left border of the mediastinal shadows in the posterio-anterior position.

B, A combination of infundibular and valvular stenosis produces signs and symptoms similar to those of isolated pulmonary valvular stenosis. In this condition, the pulmonary artery is generally hypoplastic rather than dilated. Pressure records obtained during slow withdrawal of a catheter usually demonstrate a stepwise change in pressure rather than the abrupt change in pressure patterns observed with isolated pulmonary valvular stenosis.

found as an incidental pressure gradient between the peripheral and main pulmonary arteries on cardiac catheterization. However, if multiple and severe stenotic lesions occur, the picture will be similar to severe pulmonary hypertension.

Functional Effects of Pulmonary Stenosis. Constriction of the outflow

tract of the right ventricle imposes a requirement for a greater systolic ventricular pressure to eject the normal complement of blood into the pulmonary artery. Obviously, the magnitude of the pressure gradient between the right ventricle and the pulmonary artery depends upon the resistance to outflow (caliber of channel) and the velocity of blood flow. The systolic pressure in the right ventricle ranges from high normal values to levels exceeding 200 mm. Hg. A long-continued right ventricular pressure load causes the right ventricle to assume many of the characteristics of the left ventricle. This is particularly true in congenital malformations where the load is present at least from birth. The right ventricular wall is very thick (often exceeding 1 cm.). The chamber is more rounded in contour instead of having a crescentic cross section. So long as myocardial hypertrophy is an adequate compensatory mechanism, right ventricular dilatation is not functionally significant. The rush of blood through the constricted pulmonary outflow tract produces intense turbulence, with loud systolic murmurs occupying most of the systolic interval but often exhibiting maximal intensity in midsystole (such as occurs with aortic stenosis).

Many patients with isolated pulmonary stenosis have no symptoms whatever. Their growth, appearance, exercise tolerance and subjective feeling of well-being are deceptively normal. When the condition is more severe, mild or moderate dyspnea on exertion is noted. If the orifice is small, the principal effect is limitation in the maximum cardiac output which can be maintained by the right ventricle. Very high pressures may be required to provide high-velocity flow through restricted apertures. Right ventricular failure is the principal hazard in these patients.

Diagnostic Signs of Isolated Pulmonary Stenosis

AUSCULTATION. The murmur of pulmonary stenosis is widely transmitted over the precordium, but usually is loudest in the pulmonary area,

the second and third intercostal spaces at the left sternal margin. The murmur is coarse and increases to a peak intensity by the first third or half of systole (Fig. 13–9). The second sound in the pulmonary area will be single, the aortic closure, with an inaudible pulmonary closure. The impression on auscultation is that of diminished intensity of the second sound.

ROENTGENOGRAPHY. The heart size, barring heart failure, is not appreciably increased in isolated pulmonary stenosis. Valvular stenosis with poststenotic dilatation usually can be identified in the anteroposterior position by the local bulge on the left of the mediastinum in the presence of diminished vascular markings in the lung fields (Fig. 13–8). In patients with infundibular stenosis, the midportion of the left border of the cardiac silhouette is normal or concave.

ELECTROCARDIOGRAPHY. The electrocardiogram, unlike the roentgenogram, is an excellent predictor of severity of the pulmonary stenosis. High right ventricular pressures are associated with high amplitude R-waves over the right precordium, and if quite severe, peaked P-waves and wide QRS-T angles producing a "strain" pattern (Fig. 12–35).

CARDIAC CATHETERIZATION AND ANGIOCARDIOGRAPHY. During catheterization, a definitive diagnosis of pulmonary stenosis can be obtained if systolic pressure in the right ventricle is elevated and accompanied by a sharp drop in pressure in the pulmonary artery (Fig. 13–8). The arteriovenous oxygen difference and the cardiac output will be normal until congestive failure occurs. In the latter instance, the end-diastolic pressure of the right ventricle will be quite elevated, as will the a-wave of the right atrium. Infundibular stenosis will

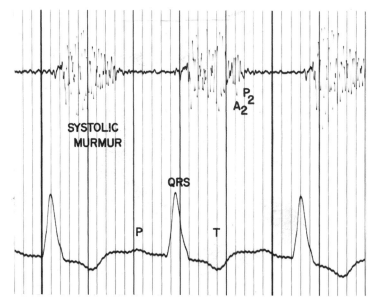

FIGURE 13-9   ISOLATED PULMONARY STENOSIS: PHONOCARDIOGRAM

Phonocardiogram in a patient with valvular pulmonic stenosis. The murmur is diamond-shaped, with the maximal intensity in early to mid-systole. The aortic closure (A_2) is the only audible component of the second heart sound; the pulmonic closure (P_2) is markedly diminished. (From Morgan, Guntheroth et al.[24])

produce a "third chamber" between the body of the right ventricle and the pulmonary artery of intermediate systolic pressure but with the same diastolic pressure as in the body of the right ventricle. Selective angiocardiography, injecting contrast material into the right ventricle, provides essential anatomic information as to the location and nature of the stenosis. If the stenosis is entirely valvular, an incision in the thick right ventricle can be avoided, and the operative approach of choice is through the pulmonary artery. If the infundibulum of the right ventricle is only hypertrophied, this may be expected to regress after relief of the valvular obstruction, whereas discrete obstruction by abnormal muscle bands of the crista supraventricularis will require attack through a ventriculotomy (Fig. 13 – 10).

Surgical Correction. Mild degrees of pulmonary stenosis are well tolerated. Since surgery very rarely restores the valve to completely normal function, bacterial endocarditis is not prevented by early operation. For more severe pulmonary stenosis, with right ventricular pressures over 90 to 100 mm. Hg, surgical opening of the valves is indicated, using cardiopulmonary bypass. In infants with very severe obstruction causing congestive failure relief may be more safely carried out with mild hypothermia and brief inflow occlusion, if the stenosis is simple valvular obstruction.

CONGENITAL AORTIC STENOSIS

Congenital abnormalities of the aortic valve are quite common and very

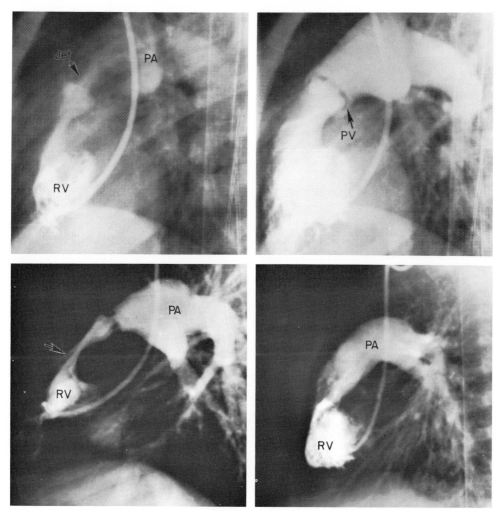

FIGURE 13–10   ISOLATED PULMONARY STENOSIS: ANGIOCARDIOGRAMS

Lateral angiocardiograms follow injection of radiopaque contrast material into the right ventricle in pulmonic stenosis.

Above, Two frames from the same patient. On the left a jet may be seen coming through the stenotic valve. On the right, the relatively thick dome of the pulmonic valve is visualized (PV) between the right ventricle (RV) and the dilated pulmonary artery (PA).

Below, Infundibular hypertrophy is seen in the film on the left, involving all of the outflow tract, whereas the patient on the right demonstrates discrete hypertrophy of muscle bundles in the infundibulum. These bundles are hypertrophied and misplaced components of the crista supraventricularis. (From Morgan, Guntheroth *et al.*[24])

likely many have escaped detection in the past; they appear as "calcific aortic stenosis" in older patients. The deformity is most often a relative underdevelopment of one or two of the three leaflets, with fusion, causing a bicus-pid valve. A bicuspid valve does not open as widely as a valve with three cusps which fold back more completely during ejection. A bicuspid valve also coapts less well, and minor degrees of regurgitation are common.

Congenital aortic stenosis may also occur as a membrane below the valve or as a supravalvular stenosis caused by a narrow annulus from which the aortic cusps are suspended. The subvalvular type is the rarest and may be confused with the more common muscular subaortic stenosis.

Functional Effects of Aortic Stenosis. The functional effects of aortic stenosis are similar to those of pulmonary stenosis. The requirement to maintain a normal cardiac output dictates the degree of hypertension in the left ventricle to overcome the fixed resistance of the aortic stenosis. Symptoms of severe aortic stenosis (fainting and angina pectoris) reflect deficiencies in perfusion of two critical vascular beds downstream from the obstruction.

Diagnostic Signs of Congenital Aortic Stenosis

AUSCULTATION. The murmur of aortic stenosis is identical to that of pulmonary stenosis, grating in quality, with peak intensity in early or midsystole. The murmur is usually loudest at the second right interspace at the sternal border, but it is frequently loudest at the second left interspace, where it may be confused with pulmonary stenosis. In aortic stenosis, the second sound at the second left interspace is normal in intensity and splitting. A systolic click, sounding like a widely split first heart sound, may be heard in both aortic and pulmonary stenoses and is apparently due to rapid distension of the dilated vessel beyond the stenosis. An early, high-pitched diastolic whiff at the mid or lower left sternal border indicates aortic regurgitation and the aortic valve as the cause of stenotic murmur; normal aortic diastolic pressures of 80 mm. Hg are much more apt to produce regurgitation compared to a diastolic pressure in the pulmonary

artery in the normal range of 10 to 15 mm. Hg.

ROENTGENOGRAPHY. The heart size with congenital aortic stenosis is normal unless there is significant aortic regurgitation or failure. Although its detection requires some experience, dilatation of the ascending aorta is common. If there is aortic regurgitation, the left ventricle will be enlarged and the cardiac silhouette will be displaced downward, to the left and posterior.

ELECTROCARDIOGRAPHY. The correlation between electrocardiographic abnormalities and the severity of stenosis is good, although less strong with aortic stenosis than for pulmonary stenosis. Left ventricular hypertrophy, based on voltages greater than normal, is found in moderate aortic stenosis. Severe aortic stenosis will, in most cases, produce marked S-T segment shift and a wide QRS-T angle, or "strain pattern" (Fig. 12–36).

CARDIAC CATHETERIZATION AND ANGIOCARDIOGRAPHY. The possibility of underestimating the severity of aortic stenosis has led some centers to recommend left heart catheterization of all patients with this clinical diagnosis. Unfortunately, access to the left heart is via hazardous routes, either by a transseptal needle[35] or retrograde, via a peripheral artery.[29] The transseptal needle is inserted into the femoral vein and advanced through the inferior vena cava to the right atrium. The interatrial septum is punctured, and a catheter is advanced into the left atrium and ventricle. The orientation of the transseptal needle in three dimensions is obviously crucial to the safe execution of the puncture, and the safety of the procedure is to some extent proportional to the frequency with which the procedure is practiced. The retrograde arterial study requires some degree of trauma to an artery, usually the brachial artery by direct exposure in the upper arm or by percutaneous method in the femoral artery.[29] Complications in children are frequent and sometimes long-lasting. A recent follow-up of children after arterial studies showed a high percentage with significant shortening of the involved leg.[36] Our present policy is to perform left heart catheterization if the patient has either definite cardiovascular symptoms or left ventricular hypertrophy with S-T segment of T-vector shifts. In patients with borderline findings, we may inject contrast material in the main pulmonary artery and after an appropriate delay, obtain biplane films of the left heart. The thickness of the left ventricle, dilatation of the left atrium and ventricle and ascending aorta and reasonably good assessment of the aortic valve may be obtained in this manner. If the changes suggest severe aortic stenosis, the pressure gradient across the aortic valve should be determined by left heart catheterization.

The peak systolic pressure gradient has been used in some publications as an indication of severity, but bicuspid aortic valves appear to require a high pressure to open, and once open, very little pressure gradient is necessary to maintain a normal flow.[37] Therefore, mean ejection pressure gradient or valve area calculated from Gorlin's formula[38] are more reliable indications of severity. The latter takes into account the cardiac output, as well as the period of ejection and gradient.

The site and nature of the obstruction and a general indication of severity may be obtained from angiocardiography (Fig. 13–11).

Surgical Correction. An important consideration as to on whom, and when, surgery should be recommended, is the difficulty—or impossibility—of restoring a congenitally stenotic aortic valve to normal function. Thus, mild and moderate aortic stenosis will frequently have as much stenosis postoperatively as before and may have severe regurgitation.[37] In severe aortic stenosis, with mean ejection gradient of greater than 45 mm. Hg or valve area of 0.6 cm.[2] or less, commissurotomy from the aortic route, utilizing cardiopulmonary bypass is indicated. In severe obstruction in infancy, emergency surgery using inflow occlusion or hypothermia may be necessary. Valve replacement with currently available artificial valves in a child should never be considered except in a desperate situation with no other alternatives.

COARCTATION OF THE AORTA

The site of normal embryonic fusion of the fourth aortic arch with the dorsal aorta at the level of the sixth arch (the precursor of the ductus arteriosus) is the site of the vast majority of coarctations; an abnormality of union at that site was suggested by Abbott as the cause of coarctation.[39] An isthmus at that site can be detected in the normal newborn, for the lesion varies from complete atresia of the aorta to a hemodynamically insignificant angiocardiographic finding. A high percentage of patients with coarctation also have a bicuspid aortic valve, and less frequently, a patent ductus arteriosus. Although anatomic details are of consequence to the surgeon and the physiologic consequences may be profoundly different in the various types of coarctation, the earlier preoccupation with "infantile" and "adult" types of coarctation has given way to an interest in the individual physiology and anatomy of each patient.

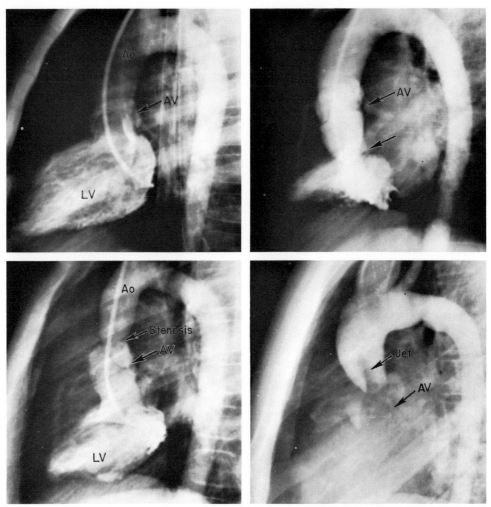

FIGURE 13–11   CONGENITAL AORTIC STENOSIS: ANGIOCARDIOGRAMS

Injections in the left ventricle or aorta (*lower right*); lateral projections show the site of obstruction. AV = aortic valve. (From Morgan, Guntheroth *et al.*[24])

Functional Effects of Coarctation of the Aorta. The major abnormality of function in coarctation is hypertension. The mechanism controlling the hypertension has been debated for years. The suggestion that the hypertension is secondary to mechanical obstruction of the aorta ignores the known receptors involved in control of the cardiovascular system. The only known baroreceptors are in the aortic arch and carotid arteries, *upstream* of the mechanical obstruction. In coarcta-

tion, the baroreceptors are over-ridden by some form of slow-acting, nonneural mechanism. Tetraethylammonium chloride, a ganglionic blocker, does not reduce the blood pressure to normal, as it does in young patients with essential hypertension.[41] After surgical abolition of the obstruction, the hypertension does not disappear for several days.[42] In experimental coarctation, if a kidney is transplanted above the site of coarctation, hypertension does not develop.[42] Thus, the evidence for renal involvement in the hypertension in coarctation is strong, in spite of inability to find increased plasma renin in these patients.[43]

With increased pressure in the ascending aorta and the development of collateral vessels, perfusion of the lower body is quite adequate. However, the pressure overload for the left ventricle may precipitate congestive failure, usually in infancy. In most infants, if the coarctation is an isolated condition, digitalization will tide them over the first year, after which failure is unlikely to occur until much later in life.

If the coarctation is associated with a large patent ductus arteriosus, pulmonary hypertension will be present and a right-to-left shunt may develop, most of which will be into the descending aorta, causing differential cyanosis. The latter signifies that the pulmonary vascular resistance exceeds the systemic resistance in the lower body and is an unfavorable sign in relation to surgical risk and prognosis.

Diagnostic Signs of Coarctation of the Aorta

PHYSICAL FINDINGS. The diagnostic findings of coarctation are hypertension for age[44] in the upper extremities and lower pressure in the lower extremities. There will usually be diminished femoral and posterior tibial pulses, and sometimes these pulses will be delayed in comparison with the upper extremities. There may be a systolic murmur at the upper left sternal border and in the upper left paravertebral area representing flow through the actual coarctation, but considering the frequent coincidence of bicuspid aortic valves, systolic murmurs at the base may suggest a degree of aortic stenosis.

ROENTGENOGRAPHY. The heart size, except for congestive failure, is normal or only slightly increased. The

pulmonary vascular markings will be normal in the absence of a shunt such as a ductus. Rib-notching due to enlargement of intercostal arteries for collateral circulation is rarely of diagnostic help in younger children, because it is rarely present until later. Much more useful is the visualization in the frontal roentgenogram of the left border of the aortic knob, the actual coarctation, and the post-stenotic dilatation, forming a 3-sign (Fig. 13–12). If a barium swallow is filmed, the mirror image of these landmarks leaves an impression on the esophagus, referred to as the E-sign.

ELECTROCARDIOGRAPHY. For obscure reasons, right bundle branch block is common in infants with coarctation, but left ventricular hypertrophy is characteristic after the first six months. If right ventricular hypertrophy is present, pulmonary hypertension is probable, and the presence of a ductus is likely.

CARDIAC CATHETERIZATION AND ANGIOCARDIOGRAPHY. Special studies are ordinarily unnecessary for a straight-forward coarctation. If there are any unusual auscultatory, roentgenographic or electrocardiographic findings, a study is indicated. Right heart catheterization will characteristically show no shunt and normal pressures except for a slight elevation of the pulmonary artery wedge pressure. In children, excellent visualization of the left heart anatomy may be obtained by injecting the contrast material into the pulmonary artery (Fig. 13–13).

Surgical Correction.
The coarctation can be resected without cardiopulmonary bypass and an end-to-end anastomosis performed. The age at which surgery should be performed is subject to some controversy. Considering the excellent response of patients with uncomplicated coarctation to medical management, surgery

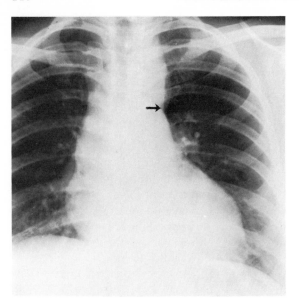

FIGURE 13–12 COARCTATION OF THE AORTA: ROENTGENOGRAM

Roentgenogram of patient with coarctation of the aorta. The arrow points to the site of the coarctation; the bulge above and below the site create the characteristic "3-sign." No rib-notching is seen in this relatively young child. (From Morgan, Guntheroth et al.[24])

is not usually justified in infancy because of the higher operative mortality and the possibility of recurrence of stenosis. On the other extreme, there is no substantial evidence that recurrence of stenosis is greater with correction at age 4 or 5 than at age 10 or 12, and operation at the earlier age spares the vasculature that many years of hypertension.

An infant with a large ductus or ventricular septal defect and coarctation will rarely do well even with vigorous and skillful medical management. Surgical relief of the coarctation, division of the ductus and banding of the pulmonary artery is a reasonable operation to undertake, in spite of the high risk, because of the severity of the disease and the prevention of irreversible pulmonary vascular disease.

DEVELOPMENTAL DEFECTS WITH INTRINSIC CYANOSIS

Cyanosis is such an obvious clinical sign that congenital malformations of the heart are usually divided into a cyanotic and a noncyanotic group. However, under certain conditions, namely increasing obstruction to pulmonary flow, cyanosis develops in patients with simple shunts which are generally classified as noncyanotic. Nevertheless, cyanosis accompanies certain types of developmental defects with sufficient regularity that they can be grouped in the cyanotic category if it is recognized that even these lesions do not always produce cyanosis in all cases or at all times. For example, some patients with these lesions develop cyanosis immediately after birth, while others do not exhibit this sign for some months after delivery. The widely diversified lesions which characteristically produce cyanosis have two features in common: (*a*) defects in the partitions of the heart and (*b*) anatomic obstruction to the flow of systemic venous blood into or through the lungs. The differential diagnosis of these defects is facilitated by always considering the site of the shunt and the nature and location of the obstruction to flow of venous blood

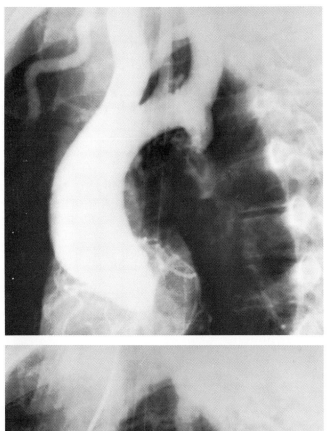

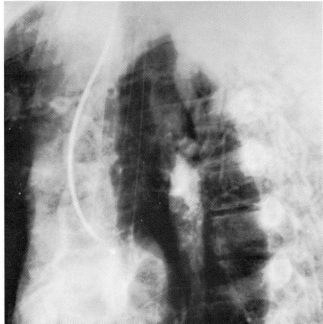

FIGURE 13–13   COARCTATION OF THE AORTA: ANGIOCARDIOGRAMS

Adult coarctation. Injection in the aorta, left oblique projection, shows total aortic occlusion and collateral circulation which begins in the subclavian arteries and, through the internal mammary and intercostal branches, delivers blood to the distal aorta. (From Morgan, Guntheroth et al.[24])

into the lungs. Variations in these two factors produce a spectrum of malformations, many of which are extremely rare. The more common examples will serve to illustrate the basic approach to their diagnosis, but a short discussion of cyanosis and hypoxia will be presented first, since the effects of these may be seen in all of the defects.

CYANOSIS

As used for purposes of classification, cyanosis implies arterial unsaturation; at sea level, this means that arterial hemoglobin is less than 95 per cent saturated with oxygen. However, the clinician must make an inference of arterial saturation based on the skin color which is determined primarily by blood in the subpapillary venous plexus. Although mixed venous blood is only 70 per cent saturated, cutaneous tissues extract very little oxygen, at normal flows, so that the amount of reduced hemoglobin within the cutaneous capillaries is only slightly larger than that in arterial blood. In the normal person, the red oxyhemoglobin in cutaneous capillaries and venules is responsible for pink flesh tones, particularly where dense vascular networks are near the surface (e.g., lips, mucous membranes, nailbeds, cheeks). If the percentage of reduced hemoglobin in these cutaneous vessels rises, the bluish color characteristic of venous blood replaces the pinkish hue in these areas. This bluish tinge, or cyanosis, must be considered in terms of the factors which alter the percentage of hemoglobin saturation in the small cutaneous vessels.

The saturation of the venous blood from any particular tissue depends upon four factors: (a) the total hemoglobin concentration in the blood, (b) the saturation of the arterial blood, (c) the rate of blood flow through the tissue and (d) the rate of oxygen utilization by the tissue. With profound anemia, even marked degrees of arterial unsaturation may not be perceived as cyanosis; the lower limit was found to be 5 gm. of hemoglobin per 100 ml.[45] Conversely, if a patient is polycythemic for any reason, it may be quite difficult to decide whether the patient has arterial unsaturation or is simply plethoric. If the flow to the skin is slow, due to poor cardiac output accompanied by vasoconstriction, the arteriovenous extraction will be increased, even though the oxygen consumption of the cutaneous tissue is small. Consequently, patients with severe heart failure may appear to be cyanotic, even if the arterial saturation is normal. Cold, particularly in children, also causes cutaneous vasoconstriction, and many normal children will have markedly blue lips after swimming in cold water.

The actual arterial saturation is most closely related to the quantity of blood being oxygenated by the lungs. Under some conditions, the entire systemic venous return mixes with the blood returning from the lungs without producing cyanosis. As an oversimplified example, consider a patient in whom the interventricular septum failed to develop (Fig. 13–14). Blood returning from the systemic veins and from the lungs mixes within a single ventricular chamber and is then ejected into both the pulmonary artery and the aorta. In such cases, it is rather common for the pulmonary blood flow to be three times as large as systemic flow. If 5 liters of systemic venous blood (6.7 gm. of reduced hemoglobin per 100 ml.) were completely mixed with 15 liters of fully oxygenated blood from the lungs, the arterial blood would contain only 1.7

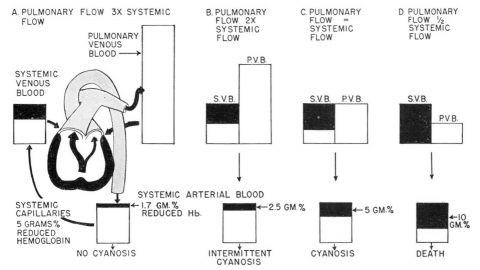

FIGURE 13–14 ETIOLOGY OF CYANOSIS

The conditions under which cyanosis would appear when the systemic and pulmonary venous blood is completely mixed in a single chamber can be evaluated by making certain assumptions which are not always applicable. First, that cyanosis becomes visible when the blood in superficial vessels of the skin contains approximately 5 gm. of reduced hemoglobin per 100 ml. Let us assume that during flow through the skin, 2 gm. of oxyhemoglobin per 100 ml. of blood is converted to reduced hemoglobin by oxygen extraction in the skin capillaries. Under these conditions, the arterial content of reduced hemoglobin must be increased to 3 gm. per 100 ml. to produce a total of 5 gm. per 100 ml. in the skin. To simplify discussion, assume that pulmonary venous blood is fully oxygenated and contains no reduced hemoglobin, and that the total hemoglobin is 15 gm. per 100 ml. blood.

A, Under the conditions outlined, if the pulmonary blood flow is three times the normal systemic flow, the mixture in the arterial blood would contain 1.7 gm. of reduced hemoglobin per 100 ml. The additional 2 gm. of reduced hemoglobin per 100 ml. acquired in the skin brings the level to 3.7 gm. of reduced hemoglobin per 100 ml., a quantity insufficient to produce regularly recognizable cyanosis.

B, If pulmonary blood flow were only twice the systemic flow, the skin vessels would contain about 4.5 gm. per 100 ml. of reduced hemoglobin so that an increase in oxygen consumption (e.g., exercise) or retardation of blood flow (crying) could produce visible cyanosis.

C, Equal flow through the systemic and pulmonary circuits would result in an arterial content of reduced hemoglobin of more than 5 gm. per 100 ml. of blood, which should produce a cyanosis at rest that would become more severe under various conditions. Note that the mixed venous content of oxygen is greatly depressed, indicating that the oxygen tensions in the tissues are probably depressed.

D, If pulmonary resistance increased so much that pulmonary flow was reduced to one-half the systemic flow, the arterial blood would contain 10 gm. of reduced hemoglobin (only 5 gm. of oxyhemoglobin) per 100 ml. and mixed venous blood would be completely unsaturated. Obviously, this situation could not be survived.

gm. of reduced hemoglobin of a total of 15 gm., a saturation of 89 per cent. During flow through the cutaneous vessels, extraction of 1 or 2 gm. more of hemoglobin per 100 ml. of blood would be insufficient to produce cyanosis (see Fig. 13–14A) of a degree that could be detected by most observers. The threshold varies with the observer, as well as with the patient.

In a carefully controlled experiment with normal subjects breathing various gas mixtures, Comroe and Botelho[46] found that in some patients most observers could detect cyanosis at 85 per cent arterial saturation, but with other patients the majority of observers could detect desaturation only below 75 per cent. Similarly, if pulmonary blood flow were just twice systemic flow (Fig. 13–14B), the mixed blood leaving the single ventricle would be 83 per cent saturated (2.5 gm. of reduced hemoglobin), barely detectable by most observers under resting conditions; a patient with this degree of arterial unsaturation would develop cyanosis more easily during retarded blood flow in the skin (cold) or during greater oxygen consumption and unsaturation of the systemic venous blood (e.g., exercise). Furthermore, cyanosis would be more readily visible if the cutaneous vessels were engorged with blood. If pulmonary and systemic flows were equal (pulmonary resistance = systemic resistance), the mixed blood in the arteries would contain 5 gm. of reduced hemoglobin per 100 ml. and cyanosis would surely be detected with an arterial saturation of 67 per cent (Fig. 13–14C). If pulmonary blood flow were diminished to one half of the systemic flow, the arterial and venous blood would contain 10 and 15 gm. of reduced hemoglobin per 100 ml., respectively (Fig. 13–14D). In other words, the arterial blood would contain little oxygen and venous blood would contain none, a condition which would not support life unless cardiac output and the oxygen carrying capacity of the blood were greatly increased.

In summary, arterial unsaturation may be considerable before it is detected, and cyanosis may appear with peripheral factors and a normal arterial saturation. Help in detecting true arterial unsaturation may come from corollary findings. If a patient has unsaturation of any degree, he will have an elevated hemoglobin or hematocrit for age. At birth, normal values are 17 gm. per 100 ml., and 52 per cent, respectively, dropping in 2 months to levels that remain lower than adult values for the next 10 years, namely

11.5 gm. of hemoglobin per 100 ml. and 38 per cent hematocrit.[47] Additional help is obtained from observation of the toes and fingers. If arterial unsaturation with cyanosis persists for long, a bulbous enlargement of the terminal phalanges of the fingers and toes develops. In this condition, called clubbing, the configuration of the distal phalanges changes from a roughly cylindrical to a more spherical shape. The nails develop a pronounced longitudinal curvature. The cause of clubbing is not known, but is associated with an increase in the number of arteriovenous glomeruli; the flow through the clubbed digit is considerably increased.[48] A bichromatic ear piece oximeter will give a reliable indication of unsaturation, and, of course, an arterial blood sample analyzed for gas content, PO_2 or saturation will settle the issue.

In patients with pulmonary blood flow considerably reduced below normal such as indicated in Figure 13–14D, the maximum amount of oxygen picked up in the lungs may not meet the metabolic needs of the patient, particularly with exertion. This is, by definition, generalized hypoxia. Hypoxia is much more threatening to life and health than mere cyanosis. If it continues, anaerobic metabolic pathways are used, and there may be an accumulation of lactic acid to the point of serious acidosis. In some forms of congenital heart disease with severely restricted pulmonary blood flow, the patient may be in aerobic balance only when asleep.

TETRALOGY OF FALLOT

The most familiar congenital defect typically accompanied by cyanosis is the tetralogy of Fallot, so named because four main items were included in the original description: (a) a defect in the membranous portion of the interventricular septum, (b) an overriding aorta in which the aortic orifice lies over the interventricular septum, (c) pulmonary stenosis (valvular or infundibular) and (d) right ventricular hypertrophy. Two of these four features are redundant. An overriding aorta cannot occur without an interventricular septal defect, and pulmonary stenosis regularly causes right ventricular hypertrophy. The basic defects are interventricular septal defect and pulmonary stenosis, which acts to obstruct the flow of unsaturated systemic venous blood into the lungs (Figs. 13–15).

Although the exact embryologic origin of this type of defect is not established, its location suggests abnormal partitioning of the conus region by the spiral aortic pulmonary septum (see Fig. 13–15A). If the ridges which ultimately form this spiral septum deviated toward the right during their original development, the caliber of the outflow tract from the right ventricle would be reduced and the aortic orifice would be relatively large. The spiral aortic septum could not fuse with the proliferating interventricular septum, and an interventricular septal defect would be left directly below the origin of the aorta (an overriding aorta). This explanation is probably oversimplified, but it gives some insight into the possible mechanisms underlying this defect. It seems significant that most patients with tetralogy of Fallot have an infundibular type of stenosis, probably related to the displacement of the bands of the crista supraventricularis.[54]

Functional Effects of Tetralogy of Fallot. The pulmonary stenosis impedes the flow of blood into the pulmonary artery. Because of the large interventricular septal defect, the right ventricular systolic pressure equals the left ventricular pressure which is controlled by the baroreceptors. Whereas the patient with pulmonary stenosis and an intact septum may develop very high right ventricular pressures and right heart failure, the limitation to the systemic pressure in tetralogy makes failure, and even cardiac enlargement, very rare in children. This limitation also will usually result in a reduction in pulmonary blood flow in tetralogy, whereas in isolated pulmonary stenosis there is no reduction until failure occurs. If resistance to flow through the stenotic region into the pulmonary artery is greater than the systemic vascular resistance, unsaturated blood from the right ventricle joins the oxygenated blood from the left ventricle, entering the aorta for distribution throughout the systemic circulation. The arterial blood therefore contains increased quantities of reduced hemoglobin, producing visible cyanosis.

If the pulmonary blood flow is sufficiently reduced, the maximal oxygen uptake may be inadequate for even resting metabolism and hypoxia may develop. Paroxysmal hyperpnea consists of increased rate and depth of respiration in an attempt to correct the hypoxia, but with the physically restricted pulmonary blood flow, the hyperpnea actually worsens the right-to-left shunting and a vicious cycle may develop.[49] Any method of improving the blood flow to the lung will be beneficial. Thus, the effect of a patent ductus arteriosus on pulmonary and systemic flow is beneficial even though the arterial blood passing into the pulmonary artery is only slightly unsaturated and can take up only limited quantities of oxygen during passage through the lungs. Unfortunately, the

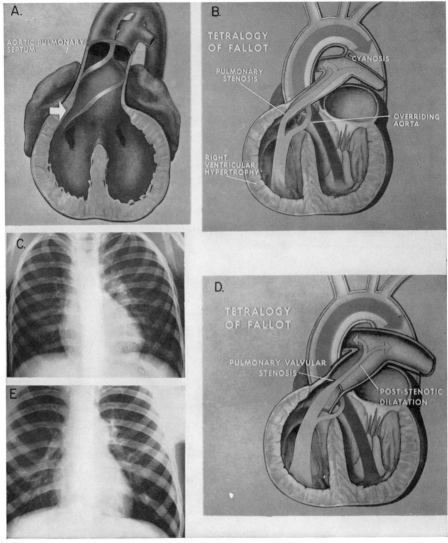

FIGURE 13–15   TETRALOGY OF FALLOT

A, If the lower portion of the spiral aortic-pulmonary septum deviated toward the right during its development, the infundibular portion of the right ventricle would be constricted and the aorta would override the interventricular septum. This schematic diagram is probably oversimplified, but it illustrates a mechanism by which the tetralogy of Fallot could develop.

B, The tetralogy of Fallot is characterized by an infundibular type of pulmonary stenosis, over-riding of the aorta, a large interventricular septal defect, and right ventricular hypertrophy. Because of the increased resistance to flow past the infundibular obstruction into the lungs, cyanosis generally develops during the first weeks or months of life.

C, The outflow tract of the right ventricle and the pulmonary trunk are usually diminished in size, so the left border of the cardiac silhouette is concave in the frontal view. The vascular markings in the peripheral lung fields are greatly reduced. There is a right aortic arch frequently present in tetralogy.

D, In a small proportion of patients with tetralogy of Fallot, the pulmonary valve is stenotic, with or without an accompanying infundibular type of stenosis. The functional effects of valvular and in-fundibular stenosis are the same, so the clinical pictures are correspondingly similar. Surgical considerations require careful distinction, however.

E, Pulmonary valvular stenosis is often accompanied by post-stenotic dilatation of the pulmonary artery which appears as a prominent bulge on the left side of the mediastinum. Note the similarity of the findings to those of pulmonary hypertension.

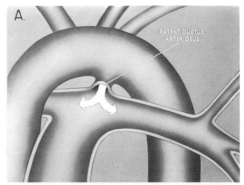

FIGURE 13–16 SURGICAL THERAPY OF IN-SUFFICIENT PULMONARY FLOW

A, In patients with tetralogy of Fallot or other congenital deformities including obstruction of flow into the pulmonary artery, the pulmonary blood flow is supplemented by blood flowing through a patent ductus arteriosus. When the ductus arteriosus closes spontaneously, total pulmonary blood flow is diminished, cyanosis becomes worse and exercise tolerance is further reduced.

B, By joining a subclavian artery to a branch of the pulmonary artery, Blalock produced an artificial ductus arteriosus to supplement pulmonary blood flow.

C, A direct anastomosis of the descending left aorta to the pulmonary artery was developed by Potts as an alternative method for producing an artificial ductus arteriosus.

An anastomosis between the posterior wall of the ascending aorta and the anterior wall of the right pulmonary artery, introduced by Waterston (not illustrated), has almost entirely replaced the Potts' procedure as a palliative operation to improve the pulmonary blood flow.

These surgical procedures often produce dramatic improvement in the condition of patients with scanty pulmonary blood flow, even though systemic arterial blood is used to supplement pulmonary flow.

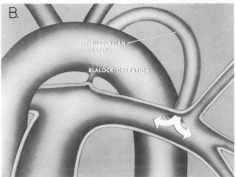

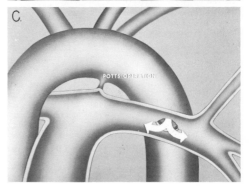

ductus arteriosus closes shortly after birth and it rarely remains patent in tetralogy. A re-creation of a ductus-like situation is the basis for surgical therapy aimed at increasing the flow to the lungs and therefore the maximal oxygen uptake (Fig. 13–16).

Clinical Signs of Tetralogy of Fallot. The typical roentgenographic changes in patients with tetralogy of Fallot include diminished pulmonary vascular markings in the peripheral lung fields on roentgenograms. The shadows in the hilar region may be prominent in those patients with predominantly valvular pulmonary stenosis (Fig. 13–15E). Infundibular stenosis is generally associated with a small main pulmonary artery which leaves a prominent convexity in the midportion of the left border of the cardiac silhouette. Right ventricular hypertrophy tends to elevate the apex of the heart. The resulting cardiac

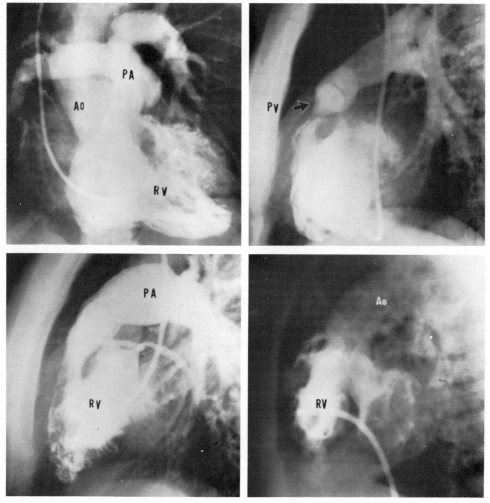

FIGURE 13–17 TETRALOGY OF FALLOT: ANGIOCARDIOGRAMS

Above, Injection in the right ventricle demonstrates valvular and infundibular pulmonic stenosis and a ventricular septal defect with right-to-left shunting into the aorta. Arrow points to the pulmonary valve (PV).

Below, Injection in the right ventricle in an "acyanotic" tetralogy with pulmonary valve stenosis (left) and in "pseudotruncus" type with pulmonary atresia (right). (From Morgan, Guntheroth *et al.*[24])

silhouette is shaped like a wooden shoe, the *coeur en sabot.* However, right ventricular hypertrophy is more easily demonstrated with the patient in the left anterior oblique position. The enlarged right ventricle protrudes anteriorly toward the sternum and increases the angulation at the junction of the right ventricle and the ascending aorta.

Right ventricular hypertrophy produces the characteristic changes in the electrocardiographic pattern, with the electrical forces deviated to the right and anterior. The P waves are generally tall and peaked in leads I and II, indicating right atrial hypertrophy.

Loud coarse systolic murmurs are widely transmitted over the precordium, but have maximum intensity in the third left intercostal space. The second sound in the "pulmonary" area (second left intercostal space) may sound normal in intensity but will be unsplit—the pulmonary component will be inaudible. These findings, plus right ventricular hypertrophy on ECG and a normal-sized heart with diminished pulmonary vascular markings on roentgenograms, allow a clinical diagnosis of tetralogy of Fallot. Definitive diagnosis, with precise definition of the anatomic details, requires cardiac catheterization and selective angiocardiography (Fig. 13–17).

Treatment of Tetralogy of Fallot. The severe limitation of pulmonary blood flow in patients with tetralogy of Fallot led to the development of the Blalock-Taussig operation. Anastomosing a subclavian artery to a pulmonary artery produces an artificial ductus arteriosus and increased pulmonary blood flow (Fig. 13–16B). Potts' modification of this procedure involves a direct anastomosis between the pulmonary artery and descending aorta (Fig. 13–16C). This procedure was introduced for infants in whom the vessels were too small to permit a successful Blalock-Taussig anastomosis. The Potts' anastomosis has proved to be difficult to take down at the time of total repair of the child at an older age, using cardiopulmonary bypass. The most popular shunt procedure for infants currently is that introduced by Waterston, an anastomosis between the ascending aorta and the right pulmonary artery. Definite improvement followed these procedures because pulmonary blood flow was supplemented even though the artificial shunts carried partially oxygenated blood from the systemic system. The pulmonary venous return, which is fully saturated with oxygen, will be increased and therefore the total amount of oxygen for metabolism will be increased toward normal. The inefficiency of the augmentation is less crucial than the relief of hypoxia. Definitive repair of the ventricular septal defect and the pulmonary stenosis is usually postponed until 3 to 5 years of age.

TRICUSPID ATRESIA

If the tricuspid orifice is blocked during embryologic development, the right ventricle fails to develop normally and persists as a small rudimentary chamber usually as the outflow tract below the pulmonary artery. Since venous blood from the systemic circuit cannot enter the right ventricle directly, it must flow through a defect in the interatrial septum (Fig. 13–18A). In the left atrium this unsaturated blood mixes with the oxygenated blood returning from the lungs. The mixed blood then enters a large left ventricular cavity. Blood ejected from this functionally single ventricle flows readily into the aorta but must pass through an interventricular septal defect into the rudimentary right ventricle and then into the pulmonary artery which is usually small (Fig. 13–18B). The high resistance to flow past these various obstructions restricts pulmonary blood flow and results in cyanosis and sometimes hypoxia.

The severity of the cyanosis and diminished exercise tolerance is related to the degree of resistance to flow into the pulmonary artery. Most patients have severe pulmonary stenosis and correspondingly severe cyanosis. If the single ventricle is not accompanied by some obstruction to pulmonary blood flow, pulmonary hypertension may be present. Some patients achieve an excellent degree of

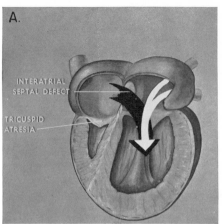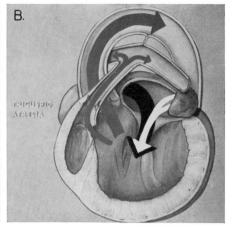

FIGURE 13-18   TRICUSPID ATRESIA

A, Tricuspid atresia blocks the channel between the right atrium and right ventricle so the entire systemic venous return must pass through an atrial septal defect and mix with pulmonary venous blood in the left atrium.

B, The mixed blood enters the left ventricle. Blood ejected from this single chamber flows readily into the aorta, but must pass through an interventricular septal defect into a rudimentary right ventricular chamber. Flow into the pulmonary artery is usually restricted by either infundibular or pulmonary valvular stenosis, so pulmonary blood flow is less than systemic flow. This condition often leads to severe cyanosis. However, if the channel to the lungs offers slight resistance and pulmonary flow exceeds systemic flow, cyanosis can be slight.

hindrance to pulmonary blood flow which keeps the pulmonary pressure near normal but permits them good color and surprising exercise tolerance.

Diagnosis of Tricuspid Atresia. Because of the small pulmonary outflow tract and pulmonary artery, the left border of the heart is concave, closely resembling tetralogy of Fallot in the frontal projection. The pulmonary vascular markings are diminished in the peripheral lung fields, and the hilar shadows generally appear disorganized from dilatation of the bronchial vessels (Fig. 13-19). The cardiac silhouette is usually flattened anteriorly. The right atrium may be prominent. Evidence of left ventricular enlargement appears on both roentgenograms and electrocardiograms. Thus, cyanosis associated with diminished pulmonary blood flow and left ventricular enlargement are the characteristic features of this condition.

Definition of the anatomy requires angiocardiography (Fig. 13-20). Transposition of the great vessels frequently accompanies this anomaly, and the location of the great vessels and particularly the size of the pulmonary arteries may determine the need and feasibility of palliative surgery. Short of successful cardiac transplantation, there is no cure for tricuspid atresia. Nevertheless, improvement of pulmonary blood flow is possible by shunting from a systemic artery to the pulmonary artery, or, in the Glenn procedure, from the superior vena cava directly to the right pulmonary artery. The latter procedure will work only if the pulmonary vascular resistance is low and the two vessels are reasonably matched in size.

TRUNCUS ARTERIOSUS

A persistent truncus arteriosus with a large pulmonary artery branch-

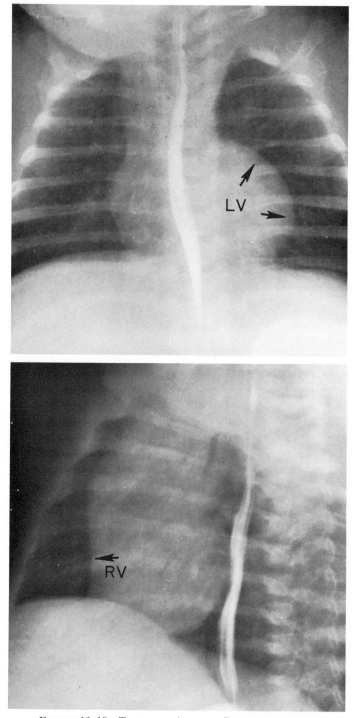

FIGURE 13–19   TRICUSPID ATRESIA: ROENTGENOGRAMS

Frontal (above) and oblique (below) roentgenograms of a patient with tricuspid atresia. The pulmonary blood flow is less than normal, suggested by the sparse pulmonary vascular markings. The frontal view is compatible with the appearance of tetralogy of Fallot, but the left anterior oblique projection reveals an underdeveloped right ventricle (RV). (From Morgan, Guntheroth et al.[24])

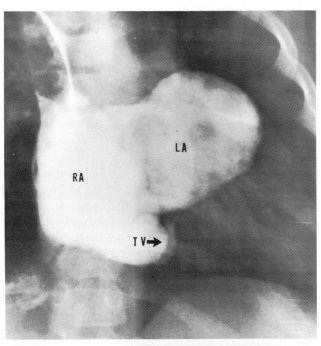

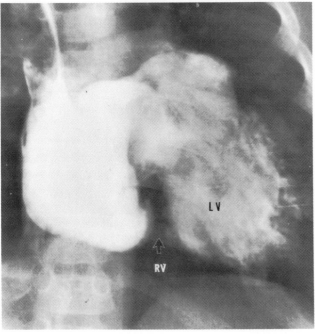

FIGURE 13-20   TRICUSPID ATRESIA: ANGIOCARDIO-GRAMS

Injection in the right atrium, frontal projection, demonstrates the flow through the atrial septum and none through the atretic tricuspid valve (TV). The origin of pulmonary flow is not shown. (From Morgan, Guntheroth et al.[24])

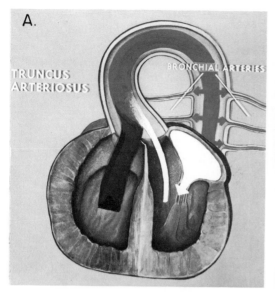
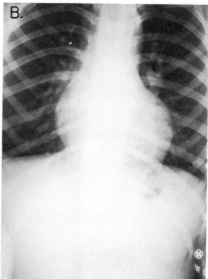

FIGURE 13–21   TRUNCUS ARTERIOSUS

A, If the pulmonary arteries fail to develop, the truncus arteriosus persists and the lungs are served solely by dilated bronchial arteries (see Fig. 1–22). The blood flow through the lungs is scanty, so the oxygenated blood is mixed with larger volumes of highly unsaturated systemic venous blood and cyanosis is very intense. Most patients with this condition usually succumb during the first few weeks of life.

B, On roentgenograms exposed in the postero-anterior position the left border of the cardiac silhouette is concave and the mediastinum is very narrow because the pulmonary artery is missing. The lung fields are abnormally clear and the pulmonary vascular shadows are spotty and lack continuity. In the left anterior oblique view, the heart shadow resembles an apple suspended from a curved stem, as suggested by the contours of the schematic drawing in *A.* The right ventricle forms an angle of almost 90 degrees with the ascending aorta, a condition known as shelving.

ing off is very similar in function to an aortic-pulmonary window, and some classifications include the latter as one type of truncus. These patients will have equal pressures in the systemic and pulmonary circuit and very large pulmonary flows, with subsequent reduction due to pulmonary vascular obstruction. Surgical cure with cardiopulmonary bypass is feasible prior to the vascular obstructive phase.

If the truncus arteriosus persists because the pulmonary artery is absent, the lungs are served only by dilated bronchial arteries (Fig. 13–21A). Under these conditions, pulmonary blood flow is extremely sparse and cyanosis is severe immediately after birth. Most patients with this type

of lesion expire during the first few weeks of life. No surgical therapy for the condition has been devised. Since the pulmonary artery is missing, the cardiac silhouette has a concave left border in the frontal view (Fig. 13–21B). The ventricular shadow often appears rounded, and the mediastinal shadow is often narrow. In the left anterior oblique position, the heart shadow is reminiscent of a large apple suspended on a stem, the truncus arteriosus (Fig. 13–21A).

COMPLETE TRANSPOSITION OF THE ARTERIAL TRUNKS

If the truncus arteriosus is divided by a straight septum rather than the normal spiral septum, the right ventricle pumps systemic venous blood into the aorta and the left ventricle ejects oxygenated blood back through the pulmonary artery (Fig. 13–22A, C). When the arterial trunks are transposed in this manner (Fig. 13–22B), all the normal partitions dividing the heart act to obstruct the flow of systemic venous blood into the lungs. If no defects in the partitions remain, none of the oxygenated blood from the lungs can be distributed to the tissues of the body and the patient promptly expires (Fig. 13–22C). On the other hand, any patient with a large atrial septal defect and a large patent ductus arteriosus has a chance of surviving at least for some years (Fig. 13–22D). If only one shunt persists between the pulmonary and systemic circuits, flow through the shunt must periodically reverse its direction. This means that the pressures on the two sides of the communication must fluctuate in opposite directions.

Paradoxically, the patients with transposition that do better in infancy, those with a large ventricular septal defect, are least amenable to surgical repair at a later date due to pulmonary vascular obstruction. The combination of high pressure and chronic hypoxia seems to be a potent stimulus to an early progression of the process of medial hypertrophy and intimal hyperplasia of the pulmonary arterioles.

Clinical Signs of Transposition of the Great Arteries. A loud systolic murmur in transposition usually indicates the presence of a ventricular septal defect, although if the murmur is grating in quality, it may represent pulmonary stenosis. Transposition, *per se*, produces no murmurs. The second sound in the pulmonary area will usually represent the aortic closure.

Roentgenograms demonstrate varying degrees of cardiac enlarge-ment with characteristically narrow supracardiac silhouette (Fig. 13–23). This narrowing of the cardiac "waist" is due to a greater degree of overlap of the ascending aorta and pulmonary artery in the frontal projection, abetted in infants by the shrinkage of the thymus secondary to hypoxic stress. Depending on the presence and degree of shunts or pulmonary stenosis, the pulmonary vascular markings may be increased, normal or diminished. The electrocardiogram will show right ventricular hypertrophy in the young patient with uncomplicated form of transposition since the right ventricle supports the systemic circulation. If the pulmonary ventricle, the left, is hypertensive, combined ventricular hypertrophy may develop. If there are serious septational defects, a single ventricle may produce a peculiar electrocardiogram diagnostic of neither right nor left nor combined hypertrophy, most often a vector directed rightward but posterior, producing an rS pattern throughout the precordial leads.

Catheterization may be confusing unless the position of the catheter is checked in lateral view. The right ventricle in transposition of the great arteries will be at systemic pressure, and there may or may not be shunts at the atrial or ventricular level. There will almost always be an interatrial communication, at least a patent foramen ovale, and the left (pulmonary) ventricular pressure should be determined. If the pressure is high, it indicates pulmonary hypertension unless pulmonary stenosis exists. Angiocardiography requires lateral views for the definition of the anterior position of the aorta, coming off the right ventricle (Fig. 13–24).

Treatment of Transposition of the Great Arteries. Cardiac catheterization offers an unusual therapeutic

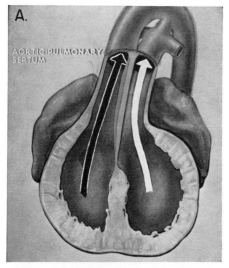
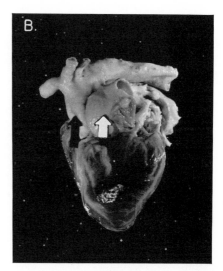
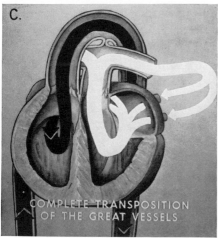
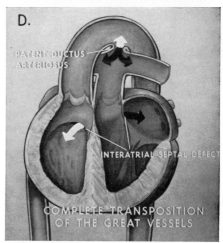

FIGURE 13–22   COMPLETE TRANSPOSITION OF THE ARTERIAL TRUNKS

A, The spiral form of the aortic pulmonary septum accounts for the manner in which the aorta and the pulmonary arteries are entwined in the fully developed heart. If the aortic pulmonary septum were straight, the arterial trunks would be parallel and the right ventricle would empty into the aorta and the pulmonary artery would arise from the left ventricle.

B, A specimen from a patient with complete transposition of the great vessels demonstrates the parallel courses of the aorta and pulmonary artery suggested in *A.* The arterial trunks arise from the wrong ventricles, and the aorta is anterior to the pulmonary artery.

C, When the arterial trunks are completely transposed, systemic venous blood enters the right ventricle and is pumped directly back into the aorta. Oxygenated blood from the pulmonary veins enters the left ventricle and is recirculated right back through the lungs. All the partitions of the heart serve to obstruct the flow of systemic venous blood to the lungs.

D, Complete transposition of the great vessels would be fatal immediately after birth unless there are communications between these two independent circulatory systems. Through defects in the atrial or ventricular septa or through a patent ductus arteriosus sufficient exchange of blood may occur to support life. In this case, larger defects in the partitions of the heart are most advantageous, and may be induced surgically in the atrial septum.

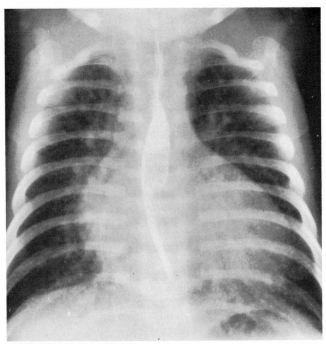

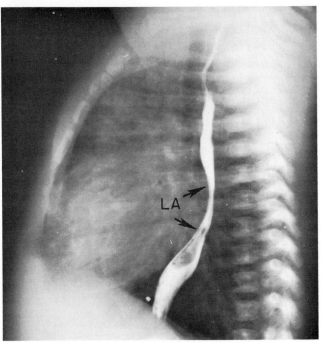

FIGURE 13–23 TRANSPOSITION OF THE GREAT VESSELS: ROENTGENOGRAMS

Frontal (above) and lateral (below) roentgenograms of a patient with transposition of the great arteries. The pulmonary vascular markings are increased. The heart is enlarged, but the supracardiac shadow is narrow. The left atrium (LA) is prominent. (From Morgan, Guntheroth *et al.*[24])

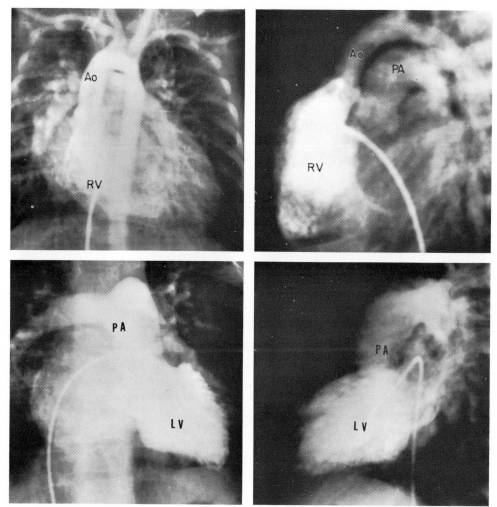

FIGURE 13–24   TRANSPOSITION OF THE GREAT VESSELS: ANGIOCARDIOGRAMS

Above, Injection in the right ventricle shows the aorta arising from this chamber anterior to the pulmonary artery.

Below, Injection in the left ventricle demonstrates the pulmonary artery arising posteriorly. The catheter has passed through an atrial septal defect. (From Morgan, Guntheroth *et al.*[24])

opportunity through the introduction by Rashkind of balloon rupture of the atrial septum.[50]

A balloon-tipped catheter is advanced under fluoroscopic control to the left atrium, inflated with 1 to 3 ml. of contrast material and pulled back to the inferior vena cava, tearing the atrial septum starting at the foramen. The improved mixing of the two circu-lations may be life-saving. The increase in arterial saturation will frequently be 20 to 30 per cent saturation in successful cases. The alternative is the creation of an atrial defect surgically, called a Blalock-Hanlon procedure. This procedure usually gives a longer period of relief, allowing postponement of corrective surgery to 3 or 4 years of age, whereas the

Rashkind procedure, which produces a smaller opening, may not permit as long a delay. If there is a sizable atrial or ventricular communication, neither type of atrial septostomy will produce substantial benefits.

Complete repair of transposition of the great arteries is now possible in many centers, at a reasonable mortality if the child is 3 or 4 years of age and has no pulmonary hypertension. The first technically successful correction by interatrial venous transposition was performed by Merendino[51] in 1957. Currently, our center has had success in total correction in infants, using profound hyperthermia.

COMPLETE TRANSPOSITION OF THE PULMONARY VEINS

If the common pulmonary vein fails to join the posterior wall of the left atrium, one of several pre-existing connections with the systemic venous system will persist and enlarge. The anomalous connection can be above the heart, at the atrial level or infradiaphragmatic. Unless there is pulmonary vascular obstruction, arteriolar or venous, these patients have a very large pulmonary blood flow with complete mixing similar to the situation in Figure 13–14A, except the mixing is at the atrial level. The cyanosis is usually mild, reflecting the high ratio of pulmonary venous return to systemic return.[52] The infradiaphragmatic group constitutes a rather distinct group. The veins drain into the ductus venosus and must traverse the liver. Death in this group occurs very early due to the high venous pressure, producing a large liver, a small heart and pulmonary venous congestion. The groups draining into the heart or superior vena cava may do well for many years.

Clinical Signs of Transposition of the Pulmonary Veins. The patient usually does not have loud murmurs, but may have a venous hum type of murmur at the base, and frequently a prominent fourth heart sound, due to the increased force of contraction of the enlarged right atrium. In the group surviving the first few days of life, cyanosis and clubbing are moderate. The second sound at the pulmonary area is usually mildly to moderately accentuated, and splitting varies inversely with the degree of pulmonary hypertension.

Roentgenograms may be diagnostic (Fig. 13–25). In the supracardiac type, the anomalous drainage pattern creates a "snowman" configuration or "figure-of-eight." The pulmonary vascular markings are increased. If there is pulmonary venous hypertension, a picture resembling pulmonary edema may be seen. The electrocardiogram demonstrates marked right ventricular hypertrophy, and p-pulmonale is common.

Catheterization indicates the level of the drainage by the level at which the oxygen saturation rises sharply; the saturation in the right atrium and in all chambers and vessels downstream will have approximately the same saturation. A selective angiocardiogram, injecting into the main pulmonary artery and programmed so that the pulmonary venous channels are filmed will show the detailed anatomy of the anomalous connection (Fig. 13–26).

Treatment of Transposition of the Pulmonary Veins. If the patient is older than 3 years and has no pulmonary hypertension, surgical repair is attended by a modest risk. The common pulmonary vein is anastomosed to the left atrium, which may have to be enlarged by repositioning the atrial

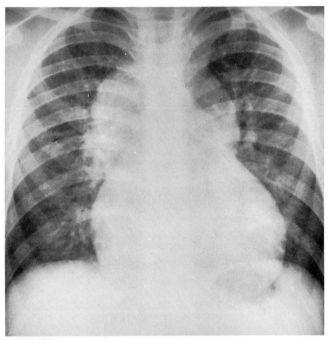

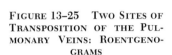

FIGURE 13–25   TWO SITES OF
TRANSPOSITION OF THE PUL-
MONARY VEINS: ROENTGENO-
GRAMS

Frontal roentgenograms of
two patients with different sites
of transposition of the pulmonary veins.

Above, The pulmonary
veins drain into the left superior
vena cava and from there into
the right superior vena cava,
creating a prominent supracardiac shadow and an overall silhouette resembling a snowman
or a figure 8. The pulmonary
vasculature is engorged, and the
right heart is enlarged.

Below, The pulmonary
veins connect to the coronary
sinus. The right heart is quite
enlarged, and the pulmonary
vasculature is engorged. (From
Morgan, Guntheroth *et al.*[24])

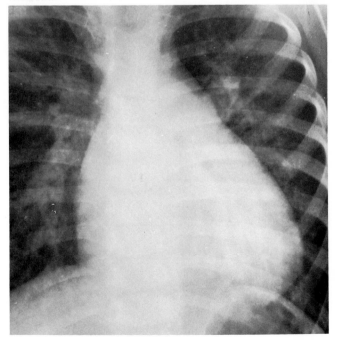

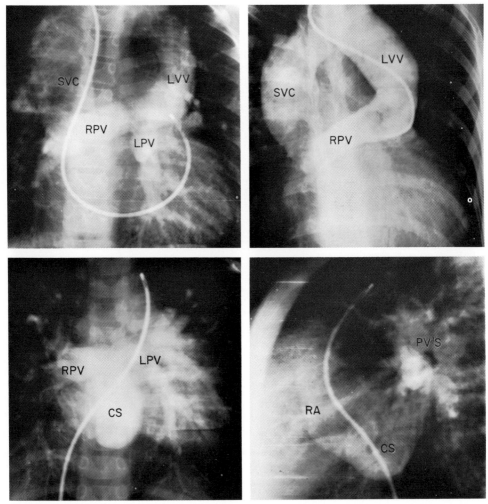

FIGURE 13–26   COMPLETE TRANSPOSITION OF PULMONARY VEINS: ANGIOCARDIOGRAMS

Angiocardiograms of patients with complete transposition of the pulmonary veins.

Above, Connection to the left vertical vein (LVV) or left superior vena cava (SVC), an alternate term. The frame on the right was produced by injecting contrast material into the common right pulmonary vein (RPV); the opacified blood flows vertically to join the superior vena cava and then to the right atrium.

Below, Frontal and lateral angiocardiograms which demonstrate pulmonary venous return into the coronary sinus (CS) and from there into the right atrium (RA). (From Morgan, Guntheroth *et al.*[24])

septum. The former anomalous channel is then tied off, monitoring the pulmonary venous pressure to ascertain that the new connections and channels are adequate to handle the flow. Infants in severe congestive failure present a serious problem: they are too young for safe perfusion with cardiopulmonary bypass, and no palliative procedure is available to carry them through infancy. Our center has very encouraging results using profound hypothermia in infants with transposition of the pulmonary veins.[53]

REFERENCES

1. PATTEN, B. M. *Human Embryology.* Philadelphia, The Blakiston Co., 1948.
2. LIND, J., and WEGELIUS, C. Angiocardiographic studies on the human fetal circulation. A preliminary report. *Pediatrics*, 4:391–400, 1949.
3. WINDLE, W. F., and BECKER, R. J. The course of the blood through the fetal heart: an experimental study in the cat and guinea pig. *Anat. Rec.*, 77:417–426, 1940.
4. EVERETT, N. B., and JOHNSON, R. J. Use of radioactive phosphorus in studies of fetal circulation. *Amer. J. Physiol.*, 162:147–152, 1950.
5. RUDOLPH, A. M., and HEYMANN, M. A. The circulation of the fetus in utero: Methods for studying distribution of blood flow, cardiac output and organ blood flow. *Circulat. Res.*, 21:163–184, 1967.
6. DAWES, G. S., MOTT, J. C., and WIDDICOMBE, J. The foetal circulation in the lamb. *J. Physiol.*, 126:563–587, 1954.
7. ASSALI, N. S., MORRIS, J. A., and BECK, R. Cardiovascular hemodynamics in the fetal lamb before and after lung expansion. *Amer. J. Physiol.*, 208:122–129, 1965.
8. ARDRAN, G. M., DAWES, G. S., PRICHARD, M. M. L., REYNOLDS, S. M. R., and WYATT, D. G. The effect of ventilation of the foetal lungs upon the pulmonary circulation. *J. Physiol.*, 118:12–22, 1952.
9. JAGER, B. V., and WOLLENMAN, O. J., JR. An anatomical study of the closure of the ductus arteriosus. *Amer. J. Path.*, 18:595–613, 1942.
10. KENNEDY, J. A., and CLARK, S. L. Observations on the ductus arteriosus of the guinea pig in relation to its method of closure. *Anat. Rec.*, 79:349–371, 1941.
11. BARCLAY, A. E., BARCROFT, J., BARRON, D. H., FRANKLIN, K. J., and PRICHARD, M. M. L. Studies of the foetal circulation and of certain changes that take place after birth. *Amer. J. Anat.*, 69:383–406, 1941.
12. EVERETT, N. B., and JOHNSON, R. J. A physiological and anatomical study of the closure of the ductus arteriosus in the dog. *Anat. Rec.*, 110:103–112, 1951.
13. ELDRIDGE, F. L., HULTGREN, H. N., and WIGMORE, M. E. The physiological closure of the ductus arteriosus in newborn infants: a preliminary report. *Science*, 119:731–732, 1954.
14. GESSNER, I., KROVETZ, L. J., BENSON, R. W., PRYSTOWSKY, H., STENGER, V., and EITZMAN, D. V. Hemodynamic adaptations in the newborn infant. *Pediatrics*, 36:752–762, 1965.
15. PATTEN, B. M. The changes in circulation following birth. *Amer. Heart J.*, 6:192–205, 1930.
16. DOWNING, S. E., GARDNER, T. H., and SOLIS, R. T. Autonomic influences on cardiac function in the newborn lamb. *Circulat. Res.*, 19:947–959, 1966.
17. SHAFFER, A. B., SILBER, E. N., and KATZ, L. N. Observations on the interatrial pressure gradients in man. *Circulation*, 10:527–535, 1954.
18. LITTLE, R. C., OPDYKE, D. F., and HAWLEY, J. G. Dynamics of experimental atrial septal defects. *Amer. J. Physiol.*, 158:241–250, 1949.
19. HICKAM, J. B. Atrial septal defect. A study of intracardiac shunts, ventricular outputs and pulmonary pressure gradient. *Amer. Heart J.*, 38:801–812, 1949.
20. GAMBLE, W. J., HUGENHOLTZ, P. G., MONROE, R. G., POLANYI, M., and NADAS, A. S. The use of fiberoptics in clinical cardiac catheterization. *Circulation*, 31:328–343, 1965.
21. SCHUELER, L. A., JR. The mechanisms of origin and transmission of heart sounds and murmurs. Medical thesis. University of Washington School of Medicine, 1952.
22. BOINEAU, J. P., SPACH, M. S., and AYERS, C. R. Genesis of the electrocardiogram in atrial septal defect. *Amer. Heart J.*, 68:637–651, 1964.
23. GUNTHEROTH, W. G., NADAS, A. S., and GROSS, R. E. Transposition of the pulmonary veins. *Circulation*, 18:117–137, 1958.
24. MORGAN, B. C., GUNTHEROTH, W. G., FIGLEY, M. M., DILLARD, D. H., and MERENDINO, K. A. Operable congenital heart disease. *Ped. Clin. North Amer.*, 13:105–219, 1966.
25. SNELLEN, H. A., and ALBERS, F. H. The clinical diagnosis of anomalous pulmonary venous drainage. *Circulation*, 6:801–816, 1952.
26. STANTON, R. R., and FYLER, D. C. The natural history of pulmonary hypertension in children with ventricular septal defects assessed by serial right-heart catheterization. *Pediatrics*, 27:621–626, 1961.
27. MULLER, W. H., JR., and DAMMANN, J. F., JR. The treatment of certain congenital malformations of the heart by the creation of pulmonic stenosis to reduce pulmonary hypertension and excessive pulmonary blood flow. *Surg. Gynec. Obstet.*, 95:213–219, 1952.
28. KIRKLIN, J. W., and DUSHANE, J. W. Repair of ventricular septal defect in infancy. *Pediatrics*, 27:961–966, 1961.
29. SELDINGER, S. I. Catheter replacement of the needle in percutaneous arteriography. *Acta Radiol.*, 39:368–376, 1953.
30. HOTCHKISS, W. S. Patent ductus arteriosus and the occasional cardiac surgeon. *J.A.M.A.*, 173:244–247, 1960.
31. GROSS, R. E., and LONGINO, L. A. The patent ductus arteriosus. Observations from 412 surgically treated cases. *Circulation*, 3:125–137, 1951.

32. CIVIN, W. H., and EDWARDS, J. E. Pathology of the pulmonary vascular tree. I. A comparison of the intrapulmonary arteries in the Eisenmenger complex and in stenosis of ostium infundibuli associated with biventricular origin of the aorta. *Circulation*, 2:545–552, 1950.

33. RUDOLPH, A. M., and NADAS, A. S. The pulmonary circulation and congenital heart disease. *New England J. Med.*, 267: 968–974, 1022–1029, 1962.

34. REEVE, R., *et al.* Reversibility of pulmonary hypertension following cardiac surgery. *Circulation*, 33:I-107–114, 1966.

35. BROCKENBROUGH, E. C., BRAUNWALD, E., and ROSS, J. Transseptal left heart catheterization. *Circulation*, 25:15–21, 1962.

36. BASSETT, F. H., III. Quoted in *Medical World News*, Oct. 25, 1968.

37. MORGAN, B. C., GUNTHEROTH, W. G., BAUM, D., and MERENDINO, K. A. Reassessment of operative indications for moderate congenital aortic stenosis. *J. Thoracic & Cardiovas. Surg.*, 43:150–158, 1965.

38. GORLIN, R., and GORLIN, S. G. Hydraulic formula for calculation of the area of the stenotic mitral valve, other cardiac valves, and central circulatory shunts. *Amer. Heart J.*, 41:1–29, 1951.

39. ABBOTT, M. E. Coarctation of the aorta of the adult type. *Amer. Heart J.*, 3:392–421, 574–618, 1928.

40. PATTEN, B. M. The development of the heart. p. 24 in *Pathology of the Heart* (2nd ed.), S. E. Gould, Ed. Springfield, Ill., Charles C Thomas, 1960.

41. GUNTHEROTH, W. G., HOWRY, C., and ANSELL, J. S. Renal hypertension. A review. *Pediatrics*, 31:767–779, 1963.

42. SCOTT, H. W., JR., and BAHNSON, H. T. Evidence for a renal factor in the hypertension of experimental coarctation of the aorta. *Surgery*, 30:206–217, 1951.

43. AMSTERDAM, E. A., *et al.* Plasma renin activity in hypertension with aortic coarctation and renal artery stenosis. *Clin. Res.*, 15:195, 1967.

44. GUNTHEROTH, W. G., and NADAS, A. S. Blood pressure measurement in infants and children. *Pediat. Clin. North Amer.*, 2:257–263, 1955.

45. LUNDSGAARD, C. Primary causes of cyanosis. *J. Exper. Med.*, 30:259–269, 1919.

46. COMROE, J. H., and BOTELHO, S. The unreliability of cyanosis in the recognition of arterial anoxemia. *Amer. Med. Sci.*, 214:1–6, 1947.

47. MOE, P. J. Normal red blood picture during the first three years of life. *Acta Paediat. Scand.*, 54:69–80, 1965.

48. MENDLOWITZ, M. Clubbing and hypertrophic osteoarthropathy. *Medicine*, 21: 269–306, 1942.

49. GUNTHEROTH, W. G., MORGAN, B. C., and MULLINS, G. L. Physiologic studies of paroxysmal hyperpnea in cyanotic congenital heart disease. *Circulation*, 31: 70–76, 1965.

50. RASHKIND, W. J., and MILLER, W. W. Creation of an atrial septal defect without thoracotomy. *J.A.M.A.*, 196:991–992, 1966.

51. MERENDINO, K. A., JESSEPH, J. E., HERRON, P. W., THOMAS, G. I., and VETTO, R. R. Interatrial venous transposition. *Surgery*, 42:898–909, 1957.

52. GUNTHEROTH, W. G., NADAS, A. S., and GROSS, R. E. Transposition of the pulmonary veins. *Circulation*, 18:117–137, 1958.

53. DILLARD, D. H., *et al.* Correction of total anomalous pulmonary venous drainage in infants utilizing deep hypothermia with total circulatory arrest. *Circulation*, 35: 105–110, 1967.

54. GUNTHEROTH, W. G. Tetralogy of Fallot. P. 432 in *Heart Disease in Infants, Children and Adolescents*, F. H. Adams and A. J. Moss, Ed. Baltimore, Williams and Wilkins, 1968.

CHAPTER 14

VALVULAR HEART DISEASE

By J. R. Blackmon and John A. Murray

ETIOLOGY

In the past, valvular heart disease was almost synonymous with rheumatic heart disease. Rheumatic heart disease is still the most common cause of valvular heart disease, however, other types are being recognized more commonly (Table 14–1). Since the prognosis and therapy varies with the cause of the valvular lesion, careful consideration as to etiology is essential in the evaluation of each patient.

A detailed account of all the causes of valvular heart disease is not possible in this chapter; however, acute rheumatic fever will be reviewed in light of recent studies. For the other less common entities, recent references are provided.

I. ACUTE RHEUMATIC FEVER

Definition. Acute rheumatic fever is a systemic disease characterized by inflammatory lesions of connective tissue and endothelial tissue. While acute rheumatic lesions are most commonly noted in the heart,[1-4] lungs,[5] skin[6] and brain,[7] changes in many other tissues have been described.

ETIOLOGY

The etiology of acute rheumatic fever is as yet incompletely defined. It has been well demonstrated that infection with Group A streptococci is the initiating factor[8,9]; however, host susceptibility plays a major modifying role. Host factors of importance are heredity,[10] immunologic response,[11] climate,[12] season[13] and living conditions.[14] While many of the host factors are nonspecific and overlapping, they seem to have a definite effect on the incidence and severity of acute rheumatic fever.

IMMUNOLOGIC ASPECTS OF ACUTE RHEUMATIC FEVER

Initiation of antibody formation is the initial step in acute rheumatic fever. Two theories have been formulated to describe this phase of pathogenesis.[15-17]

(1) The *hypersensitivity theory* is based on the fact that acute rheumatic fever follows streptococcal pharyngitis

469

Table 14-1.   ETIOLOGY OF
VALVULAR HEART DISEASE

1. Rheumatic Fever
2. Congenital
3. Ischemic Heart Disease
4. Infection
   a. Bacterial
   b. Fungal
   c. Spirochaetal
5. Connective Tissue Disorders
   a. Marfan's Syndrome
   b. Cystic Medial Necrosis
   c. Rheumatoid Disease
   d. Takayasu's Arteritis
   e. Mucopolysaccharidoses
   f. Ehlers-Danlos Syndrome
6. Trauma
7. Malignant Carcinoid

by an average time lapse of 18 days and superficially resembles a serum sickness type of reaction. It is also true that individuals who develop acute rheumatic fever have exaggerated antibody response and that the peak antibody levels are found 2 to 3 weeks following infection. In repeated attacks, this interval is shorter. However, these individuals do not produce excessive antibody levels to nonstreptococcal antigens.

(2) *Autoantibodies* have been postulated to cause acute rheumatic fever.[16,17] However, the evidence from immunofluorescent studies is indirect and became unconvincing when it was shown that nonrheumatic injury produced similar antibodies.

At the present time, there is reasonable evidence that antibodies are involved in the pathogenesis of acute rheumatic fever; however, the precise mechanism remains obscure.

MANIFESTATIONS OF ACUTE RHEUMATIC FEVER

A definitive diagnosis of rheumatic fever can be made with confidence only when a particular patient displays a number of the systemic manifestations of the disease. Until a specific test becomes universally accepted, the exact diagnosis of many patients will remain controversial. Without specific criteria for the diagnosis, data on the incidence of the disease and on the effectiveness of various therapeutic programs is difficult to evaluate. For this reason, Jones[18] grouped the various common signs of the disease into major and minor manifestations for the purpose of standardizing the diagnosis for statistical purposes (Fig. 14–1). Patients exhibiting various combinations of these manifestations can be regarded as having acute rheumatic fever. These relatively rigid criteria for controlled investigation have demonstrable value when applied to groups of patients, but they are no substitute for clinical judgment in the care of an individual patient. The classification of signs and symptoms proposed by Jones originally in 1944 and modified in 1955[19] forms a convenient organization for a discussion of this complex disease entity.

MAJOR MANIFESTATIONS

Carditis. Inflammation of the heart is termed carditis and is manifested clinically by appearance of (1) significant heart murmurs, such as any diastolic murmur or systolic murmurs which are pansystolic and show little change during respiratory and cardiac cycles, (2) signs of pericarditis, such as pericardial friction rub or proven increases in pericardial fluid, (3) cardiac enlargement and (4) congestive heart failure.

Polyarthritis. The development of painful, swollen, warm and red joints is definite evidence of arthritis. In acute rheumatic fever, the typical

A. MAJOR MANIFESTATIONS   B. MINOR MANIFESTATIONS

1. CARDITIS   1. ARTHRALGIA

2. CHOREA   2. FEVER

                                           3. PREVIOUS HISTORY ARF

                                           4. LABORATORY TEST
                                              a. elevated ASO titer
3. SUBCUTANEOUS   b. increased ESR
   NODULES   c. leukocytosis
                                              d. prolonged PR interval

4. POLYARTHRITIS

5. ERYTHEMA MARGINATUM

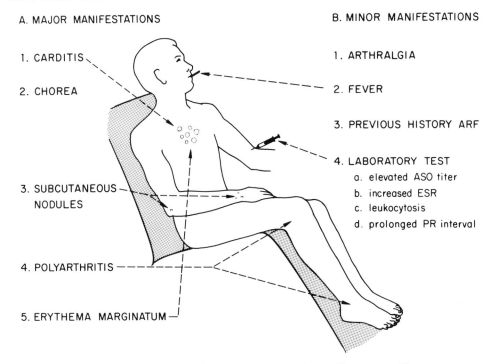

FIGURE 14-1   CLINICAL MANIFESTATIONS OF ACUTE RHEUMATIC FEVER

The principal signs of acute rheumatic fever are illustrated schematically. According to Jones, a diagnosis of acute rheumatic fever is made if a patient has two major manifestations or one major and two minor manifestations. These criteria are particularly valuable in gathering statistics for various types of research problems, but may not be applicable to an individual patient. The above criteria are enhanced by evidence of previous streptococcal infection such as positive throat culture or known scarlet fever.

pattern of involvement is that the arthritis migrates from one joint to another; it may or may not be symmetrical. Nonspecific polyarthralgia (joint discomfort without physical signs) should not be considered a major manifestation of acute rheumatic fever but is considered a minor manifestation.

Chorea. Irregular, jerky, purposeless movements are the hallmarks of chorea; however, signs of personality change usually precede the choreiform movements. This manifestation is usually only seen in children and predominately females. Carditis is frequently associated; however, it may be mild and completely gone by the time the patient presents with

typical chorea, which is a late symptom in acute rheumatic fever.

Subcutaneous Nodules. These nodulations develop on or near bony prominences on extensor surfaces of hands, wrists, knees, ankles, feet and skull. Subcutaneous nodules in themselves are of no prognostic significance since they almost always occur in combination with carditis, polyarthritis and chorea.

Erythema Marginatum. This manifestation is characterized by reddish macules originating on the trunk. These lesions spread in area and clear centrally. The shape of the lesions varies, hence the various descriptive terms, such as circinatum, anulare and gyratum. While the lesion is felt to be specific for acute rheumatic fever, it always occurs in association with other major manifestations and is of no prognostic value.

MINOR MANIFESTATIONS OF ACUTE RHEUMATIC FEVER

These manifestations represent the reaction to a systemic disease and are generally nonspecific (Fig. 14–1). They do, however, indicate inflammation and are frequently responsible for the patient seeking medical help.

Arthralgia. Arthralgia is the joint pain without the classic physical findings characteristic of arthritis. This joint discomfort may also be migratory in nature.

Fever. An elevated body temperature although not specific is a constant feature of acute rheumatic fever with the exceptions of the patient with chorea or the patient on suppressive therapy.

Previous History of Acute Rheumatic Fever or Rheumatic Heart Disease. It appears that at least a certain proportion of individuals are highly susceptible to acute rheumatic fever, although it is not known whether this is an inherited trait or an environmental factor. Because of the high recurrence rate, this is an important historical fact. In fact, Jones' original classification[18] has a previous history as a major criteria. It was taken out primarily because of studies aimed at gathering initial cases of acute rheumatic fever. Although at the present time it is not considered a major manifestation, it is important in dealing with individual patients.

Laboratory Tests. The acute phase antibody titer is extremely helpful in proving a previous streptococcal infection. The most commonly used titer is the antistreptolysin O (ASO) titer. The value should exceed 250 units in acute rheumatic fever; however, serial determination with a significant increase in titer is also diagnostic of a recent streptococcal infection. Other antibodies are available. Antihyaluronidase and antistreptokinase titers can be obtained. In acute rheumatic fever, the combination of these antibodies shows a significant rise in 95 per cent of cases.

The erythrocyte sedimentation rate although nonspecific is always elevated. There is usually a leucocytosis of greater than 10,000 per cubic millimeter with a shift of the polymorphonuclear leucocytes to the left. C-reactive protein is also another nonspecific but sensitive index of inflammation and is elevated in acute rheumatic fever.

A prolonged PR interval on the electrocardiogram is also considered to be a minor manifestation but is influenced by so many factors that it is probably not reliable and should not be used.

Most of the major and minor manifestations represent changes in tissue other than the heart. Although the diagnosis of acute rheumatic fever depends largely upon extracardiac signs, their severity is not a reliable index to the subsequent valvular damage. Special attention should be directed toward the signs of acute carditis.

OTHER MANIFESTATIONS OF ACUTE RHEUMATIC FEVER

Acute rheumatic fever is a protean systemic disease which has the capacity to involve many organs, so it should not be surprising that it includes some bizarre and unusual manifestations.

Perhaps one of the more important is that of abdominal pain which at times is mistaken for an acute surgical abdomen. This is due to vascular involvement of peritoneum. Another cause of abdominal discomfort in children is congestion of the liver due to right heart failure.

Pleurisy has been reported to occur in 10 to 15 per cent of cases; however, this appears to be an overestimate based on the type of disease seen at this time.

Epistaxis may at times herald the onset of acute rheumatic fever as well as so-called growing pains of a myositis or tenosynovitis. Nonspecific fatigue, weight loss and anorexia may be prodromal symptoms. Perhaps the most common atypical presentation is the finding of a valvular lesion in an adult without symptoms or a history of acute rheumatic fever. It is estimated that this occurs in 30 to 40 per cent of individuals.

CHANGING PATTERN OF ACUTE RHEUMATIC FEVER

The pattern of acute rheumatic fever in the United States has been changing over the past 70 years. The mortality from rheumatic fever has decreased from 5 per 100,000 in 1900 to 0.3 per 100,000 in 1953.[20] This decline began prior to the era of antibiotics. Not only has the mortality changed but also the prevalence of rheumatic heart disease. The decline in the incidence of rheumatic fever has paralleled the development of antibiotics and the improvement in nutrition and living standards in this country.

Ten to twenty years ago it was common to have several patients with acute rheumatic fever on the wards in any large hospital. At the present time, a patient with acute rheumatic fever is unusual and one with severe carditis is a rarity.

Figure 14–2 contrasts the data of Bland and Jones in 1951[21] with that of Feinstein et al., in 1964.[22] Two striking differences are noted. Twenty per cent of the 1000 patients with acute rheumatic fever in the first group were dead within 10 years contrasted to 2.7 per cent of 441 patients in the second group who were dead within 7.8 years. The other striking difference is the number free of rheumatic heart disease, 26 per cent in the earlier series compared to 64 per cent in the later report.

Recent data contradicts the previous information that 3 per cent of individuals with streptococcal pharyngitis develop acute rheumatic fever. This higher percentage may still be valid in epidemic situations with a particularly virulent organism, but, in endemic streptococcal infections, only 0.3 per cent of patients afflicted with streptococcal pharyngitis developed acute rheumatic fever.[23] It is also apparent that the incidence of rheumatic heart disease and death following acute rheumatic fever has changed drastically.

Two prognostic features inherent in the preceding statistics are worth emphasis. Those patients with proven streptococcal pharyngitis in whom there is little antibody rise are unlikely to develop acute rheumatic fever. Those patients with acute rheumatic fever who do not exhibit carditis are unlikely to develop rheumatic heart disease.[22]

PATHOLOGIC MANIFESTATIONS

The initial phases of myocarditis consist of inflammation and edema of the connective tissue stroma and intense eosin staining of the gelatinous ground substance between the collagenous fibers. Later, a homogeneous, waxy appearance of the collagen

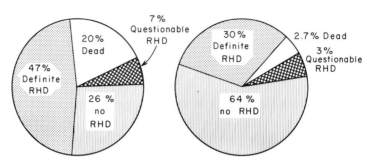

BLAND and JONES 1951   FEINSTEIN et.al. 1964
10year follow up   7.8 year follow up
1000 patients   441 patients

FIGURE 14–2   CHANGING PATTERNS OF ACUTE RHEUMATIC FEVER

The data of Bland and Jones represents 1000 patients with acute rheumatic fever followed for ten years. Data was obtained in 1930's and 1940's. This is contrasted with data from Feinstein's group approximately twenty years later and reflects changing pattern of acute rheumatic fever in the past decade. Each study is divided into four wedges: definite rheumatic heart disease (RHD), no rheumatic heart disease, questionable rheumatic heart disease and deaths. The most striking differences are in percentage of deaths and those patients without residual heart disease.

bundles becomes so marked that individual fibers cannot be identified. This modified collagenous material superficially resembles fibrin. A "proliferative" reaction ensues, consisting of either diffuse accumulations of cells, particularly in the vicinity of blood vessels or localized "granulomata" (Aschoff bodies) (Fig. 14–3D). Round cells, macrophages, fibroblasts and multinucleated giant cells accumulate in focal lesions. Typical giant cells have irregular outlines, slight basophilic staining of the cytoplasm and 2 to 7 round or oval nuclei near the center of the cell, often arranged like a fan (Fig. 14–3). Around the periphery of such lesions is an investment of polymorphonuclear leukocytes, lymphocytes, plasma cells, fibroblasts and occasional eosinophils. As healing progresses, this inflammatory process is replaced by spindle-shaped or triangular scars located between muscle layers and near blood vessels.

Inflammatory reactions also occur in other tissues. Subcutaneous nodules, varying in size from 1 mm. to 2 cm. in diameter, develop predominantly over bony prominences. They develop rapidly, usually disappear quickly and may be overlooked. Microscopically these nodules are not identical with the focal processes in the myocardium. Subcutaneous lesions consist of aggregations of similar cells, but necrosis often develops in the center of the lesion. Similar diffuse and local inflammatory reactions occur in many tissues including tendons, skeletal muscle, joints, serous cavities in general and the adventitia of arteries. Histologic evidence of meningoencephalitis in patients with chorea has been reported. During any particular attack, the pathologic changes may be localized in virtually any combination of the sites previously indicated. Thus, acute rheumatic fever is truly a systemic disease. It affects primarily the supporting structures of the body, collagen and elastica. Despite the widespread

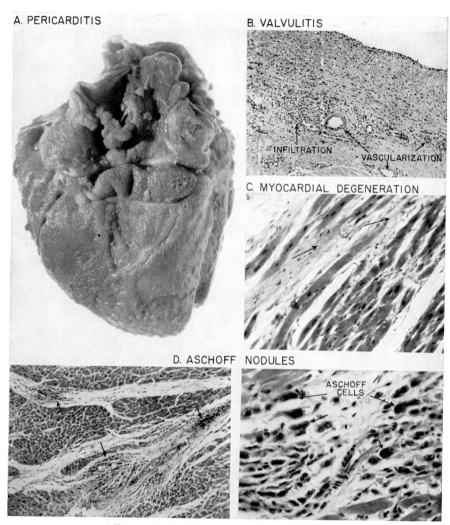

A. PERICARDITIS

B. VALVULITIS

INFILTRATION · VASCULARIZATION

C. MYOCARDIAL DEGENERATION

D. ASCHOFF NODULES

ASCHOFF CELLS

FIGURE 14–3   ACUTE RHEUMATIC CARDITIS

A, Pericarditis of extremely severe degree is illustrated by a specimen from a patient with fatal acute pancarditis. In the average attack of acute rheumatic fever, pericarditis appears to be a transient phenomenon as evidenced by evanescent friction rubs and precordial pain.

B, The valve cusps exhibit inflammatory reactions as evidenced by infiltrated leukocytes and vascularization by the proliferation of blood vessels.

C, Degeneration of myocardial fibers is generally postulated but is rarely demonstrable as clearly as indicated in the photomicrograph above. No doubt functional changes in the myocardium occur without such obvious histologic evidence.

D, Aschoff nodules in the myocardium are generally regarded as a pathognomonic sign of rheumatic fever. The typical nodule consists of a perivascular infiltration with leukocytes, including multinucleated giant cells (Aschoff cells). Healing of such a nodule usually produces triangular fibrous scars surrounding blood vessels in various portions of the heart walls. (These photomicrographs were obtained through the courtesy of Professor Stuart Lippincott.)

distribution of the lesions, most patients recover and little residual damage to vital organs persists, except in the valves of the heart. If valvular damage were not so frequent, this condition would be of no greater concern to cardiologists than is the nonspecific myocarditis associated with a number of other acute and chronic diseases.

ACUTE RHEUMATIC VALVULITIS

Since the first attack of acute rheumatic fever is rarely fatal, pathologic changes during the typical initial attacks are not well established. Available descriptions of the initial pathology in rheumatic endocarditis and valvulitis are based on postmortem studies of patients overwhelmed by rheumatic attacks or of fortuitously discovered endocardial inflammatory processes in accident victims. In neither instance can one be certain that the individuals would have ultimately developed typical rheumatic valvular heart disease. Until rheumatic valvular lesions can be reproduced experimentally, the reconstructed sequence of events must be accepted with some reservations.

Gross and Friedberg[3] concluded that the valve rings were the first portion of the valves to be involved in the rheumatic process. In patients who were believed to have succumbed during their first attack, the valve rings were the most common site of the inflammatory reactions, and, in most cases, all four valve rings were involved. It is postulated that the mitral and aortic valves more frequently become deformed because of the greater "functional trauma" to which they are subjected. In the initial stages, the valves are edematous and infiltrated with mononuclear cells. At later stages,

the valve leaflets become thickened and are no longer transparent. Rows of gray or yellow wart-like vegetations develop along the line of closure of the aortic and mitral valves (Fig. 14–4). The valve edges become thick, and newly formed blood vessels grow into the leaflets from the periphery. The structure and function of the valves frequently become essentially normal after initial attacks of rheumatic fever. Valvular deformities usually occur after repeated inflammatory assaults or protracted severe attacks of rheumatic fever.

During the healing process, the inflammatory lesions are replaced by fibrous tissue. Shrinkage of the collagen fibers usually causes shortening and retraction of the affected cusps. The chordae tendineae of the atrioventricular valves become shortened and fused, drawing the valve edges toward the papillary muscles. Fusion between the valve leaflets begins at the commissures and extends toward the center of the valve ring. As a result, the flexible mitral valve leaflets are finally converted into a rigid funnel with a narrow orifice held deep within the left ventricular cavity by the shortened, fused chordae tendineae (Fig. 14–4). The semilunar valve leaflets are also thickened and shortened, with their edges rolled outward, and fusion of the commissures between the valve cusps restricts the valve orifices. Various types of valvular deformities and their functional effects are discussed later.

THERAPY OF ACUTE RHEUMATIC FEVER

Bed Rest. The traditional approach to the patient with acute rheumatic fever is to put the patient to bed for months. There is little evidence that this is necessary partic-

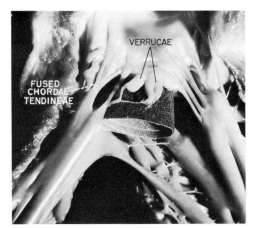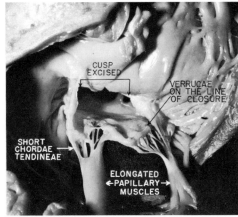

FIGURE 14-4 ACUTE RHEUMATIC VALVULITIS

Some effects of acute rheumatic valvulitis on the mitral and tricuspid valves are indicated by a specimen from a patient who expired in the course of her initial attack.

A, The mitral valve edges are greatly thickened with verrucae extending along filamentous chordae tendineae. Some of the chordae tendineae are fused together. All the chordae tendineae appear shorter and thicker than normal and the papillary muscles are unusually long, but at least part of this relation could have antedated the inflammatory process. The mitral orifice was only slightly diminished in area.

B, In the same patient a row of verrucae, up to 3 mm. thick, developed along the line of valve closure on all tricuspid valve cusps. The short, thick chordae tendineae are also associated with elongated papillary muscles. (This specimen is presented through the courtesy of Dr. S. A. Creighton, pathologist, Children's Orthopedic Hospital, Seattle, Washington.)

ularly in patients who do not exhibit carditis. Lendrum *et al.*[24] in a comparative study of prolonged bed rest versus early ambulation noted no differences. The duration and strictness of bed rest should be governed by symptoms, laboratory signs and good judgment until more facts are available.

Drug Therapy. Salicylates although nonspecific are an effective form of therapy in acute rheumatic fever. The clinical signs (fever, arthritis, elevated sedimentation rate) of inflammation usually show prompt defervescence and a state of well being is established. Although the point is still debated, it is doubtful that salicylates alter the incidence of rheumatic heart disease in later life. The dose of salicylates should be adequate to suppress the clinical signs of inflammation yet produce no toxic-

ity. Salicylates are continued until the inflammatory signs subside, and then they are tapered. On withdrawal, if inflammatory signs reappear, the drug should be restarted in adequate doses.

Steroids work as nonspecific anti-inflammatory agents but are more potent than salicylates. Evidence to date from several large studies[25, 26, 27] however, show no advantage of steroids over salicylates in preventing residual rheumatic heart disease. In a retrospective, nonrandomized study by Czoniczer and colleagues,[28] there was an impressive decrease in mortality in patients with severe carditis who were treated with steroids. Absolute conclusions regarding choice of drugs in acute rheumatic fever cannot be reached at this time; however, it appears that steroids offer a therapeutic advantage in patients with severe carditis and heart failure but do not provide an advantage over salicylates in decreasing residual rheumatic heart disease.

As with salicylates, steroids should be administered in doses sufficient to suppress the clinical and laboratory signs of inflammation. As the inflammatory signs subside, the dose should be tapered. If, during the tapering, there is a rebound, the dosage should be increased until inflammatory manifestations subside.

Antibiotics. Penicillin should be administered for 10 days to 2 weeks to eradicate the streptococcal infection; thereafter, prophylaxis with penicillin or sulfa drugs should be continued.

Prevention and Prophylaxis. It is well established that acute rheumatic fever can be prevented by the administration of antibiotics. Catanzaro[8] and colleagues have shown that treatment with penicillin even 9 days after the onset of the streptococcal pharyngitis will prevent acute rheumatic fever. Denny et al.[9] have shown

that adequate treatment of streptococcal pharyngitis will prevent acute rheumatic fever 95 per cent of the time. Penicillin therapy for a period of 10 days is necessary.

Prophylaxis against recurrent streptococcal infection has made a significant contribution to the therapy of recurrent acute rheumatic fever and rheumatic heart disease. And, at the present time, it is recommended that prophylaxis be maintained indefinitely in all patients with rheumatic heart disease.[29]

Prophylaxis has been shown to reduce recurrences of acute rheumatic fever by 80 to 90 per cent. Effective prophylaxis can be obtained by oral penicillin, 250,000 units twice daily, oral sulfa, 1 gm daily, or by depot penicillin, 1.2 million units per month. The latter method is most successful because the oral preparations are not always taken daily and the injection gives higher tissue concentration of penicillin capable of eradicating the streptococcus.

II. DIAGNOSIS OF VALVULAR DISEASE

The ventricles can function as efficient pumps only if the inflow and outflow valves open adequately and close effectively. Deformities of the valves produce two main types of functional disturbance: stenosis and regurgitation. Valvular stenosis produces a restricted orifice through the valve. Valvular incompetence or insufficiency implies that the valves fail to close and seal allowing blood to flow in a retrograde direction. Identifying the affected valve is important, particularly now that palliative surgery for valvular deformities is available. Each valve functions under different conditions and is more likely to be affected by one cause of deformities than

another. The mitral valve is the most common site of rheumatic valvular heart disease, followed by aortic, tricuspid and pulmonary valves, in that order. Combined mitral and aortic disease is more common than pure aortic lesions of rheumatic etiology. However, nonrheumatic lesions have their highest incidence in the aortic valve. The tricuspid valve is rarely the only valve involved but is involved 5 to 10 per cent of the time when mitral disease is present. The pulmonic valve is rarely involved in rheumatic heart disease. Congenital valvular disease is discussed in Chapter 13 and will not be considered here.

The clinical signs and symptoms

of valvular disease should be considered in terms of the functional stresses imposed by the deformed valves and the compensatory mechanisms evoked in response to the load imposed on the circulatory system. Although these lesions frequently occur together, analysis is simplified by discussing them individually.

MITRAL STENOSIS

Mitral stenosis is caused primarily by acute rheumatic fever and affects females more frequently than males.

PATHOPHYSIOLOGY

The initial problem in mitral stenosis is the increased resistance to the flow of blood at the mitral valve. Because of increased resistance at the stenotic valve orifice, left atrial pressure rises, producing a pressure gradient, to fill the left ventricle. The rise in left atrial pressure is transmitted to the pulmonary veins, pulmonary capillary bed and pulmonary arteries. With the passage of time, anatomic changes (medial hypertrophy and intimal sclerosis) take place in the pulmonary arterioles causing a second area of increased resistance. As the duration of the mitral obstruction increases, pulmonary vascular resistance increases, the right ventricle fails and systemic venous congestion develops.

COMPENSATORY MECHANISMS

During the sequence of events just described, a number of compensatory mechanisms develop. Many of the symptoms and signs of mitral stenosis are due to these compensatory changes.

Left Atrium. In mitral stenosis, left atrial pressure is increased and hypertrophy and dilatation of the atrium occur.[30] In the normal subject, the atrium functions mainly as a reservoir or conduit for blood passing from the lungs to the left ventricle.[31] In patients with mitral stenosis or left ventricular disease, atrial contraction causes significant augmentation to left ventricular filling and function.[32] With further dilatation, atrial fibrillation ensues and causes decreased cardiac output due to the loss of atrial contraction. With extreme atrial dilatation, compression of the esophagus and bronchus may occur.

Pulmonary Vasculature. The high pressure in the left atrium due to mitral stenosis is transmitted to pulmonary veins which act as a conduit, and the pressure is transmitted to the pulmonary capillaries and arterioles with a resultant rise in pressure and resistance (Fig. 14–5). When the pressure in the pulmonary capillary bed reaches 25 to 30 mm. Hg, it exceeds the oncotic pressure of blood and transudation of fluid into the alveoli occurs giving rise to pulmonary congestion.

Because man has a long thorax and lungs, the pressure and flow are greatest in the most dependent portions of the lungs, and, with the greatest pathologic change in the lower lobe pulmonary vessels, there is a shift of the blood flow to the upper lobes (Fig. 14–6).

The increased resistance in the pulmonary arterioles provides a chronic and eventually overwhelming load on the right ventricle. It has also been postulated to act as a buffer to the pulmonary capillary bed, preventing sudden pressure rises and therefore preventing pulmonary edema.

The central blood volume in mitral stenosis has been a much debated issue. Early workers reported extremely large central blood volumes with some values being greater than 50 per cent of the cardiac output. This was

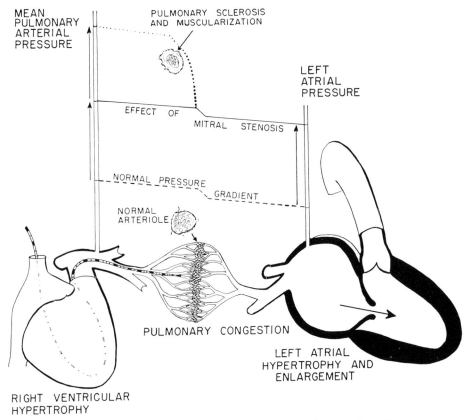

MEAN PULMONARY ARTERIAL PRESSURE

PULMONARY SCLEROSIS AND MUSCULARIZATION

LEFT ATRIAL PRESSURE

EFFECT OF MITRAL STENOSIS

NORMAL PRESSURE GRADIENT

NORMAL ARTERIOLE

PULMONARY CONGESTION

LEFT ATRIAL HYPERTROPHY AND ENLARGEMENT

RIGHT VENTRICULAR HYPERTROPHY

FIGURE 14–5   PULMONARY HYPERTENSION WITH MITRAL STENOSIS

The resistance to flow through the normal pulmonary vascular tree is so slight that the gradient in mean pressures from pulmonary artery to left atrium ranges around 4 to 6 mm. Hg even at flow rates as high as 10 or 12 liters per minute. Mitral stenosis produces an elevation in left atrial pressure (see Fig. 14–9) which is reflected back along the entire pulmonary vascular bed. When pulmonary vascular pressure increases, pulmonary congestion usually follows. Sustained pulmonary hypertension appears to stimulate sclerosis and muscularization of the terminal pulmonary arteries and arterioles in about 40 per cent of patients with mitral stenosis, and greatly increases the resistance to flow through these narrowed channels in 12 to 20 per cent of such patients. The increased pulmonary arterial resistance produces severe hypertension in the pulmonary arteries, which imposes an even greater pressure load on the right ventricle. Under these conditions pressures recorded through a catheter wedged in a terminal pulmonary artery are much lower than in the main arterial trunk.

pointed out to be an artifact of a peripheral injection and sampling site by Marshall and Shepard.[33] Using central injection and sampling sites, McGaff et al.[34] showed an increase in central blood volume in severe mitral stenosis but normal values in mild mitral stenosis. As was mentioned earlier, there is a shift of blood flow from the bases to the apices of the lungs as the severity

of the pulmonary vascular disease increases.

Right Ventricle. The right ventricle hypertrophies due to the chronic pressure load but is poorly adapted for working as a pressure pump and eventually fails, another factor causing a decrease in cardiac output. The right ventricular end-diastolic pressure rises and is transmitted to the right atrium.

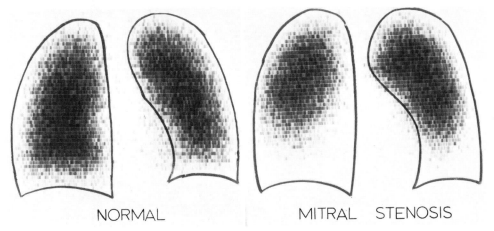

NORMAL   MITRAL STENOSIS

FIGURE 14-6   ABNORMAL PULMONARY BLOOD FLOW IN MITRAL STENOSIS

A radioactive iodine tagged albumen macroaggregate lung scan from a healthy person demonstrates pulmonary blood flow (radioactive counts) to be evenly distributed between upper and lower lobes. In the patient with mitral stenosis the lower lobes of the lungs are not well perfused due to pulmonary vascular changes following abnormal pressure-flow relationships in the lower lobes which have been produced by mitral stenosis.

Systemic venous hypertension occurs with edema formation and cardiac cirrhosis with all its attendant problems.

Cardiac Output and Regional Blood Flow. The cardiac output is variable in mitral stenosis in the resting state[35] but restricted during exertion.[36] During upright exercise to maximal oxygen intake, patients with mitral stenosis were shown to exhibit normal increases in heart rate and oxygen extraction but a restricted stroke volume.[36] It has often been stated that patients with mitral stenosis compensate for a reduced cardiac output by increased oxygen extraction, but this is not true when the per cent of maximal oxygen consumption is used as the frame of reference (Fig. 14-7).

It is well known that a redistribution of left ventricular output from visceral organs to working muscle occurs during increased metabolic demands. This has been thought by some workers[35] to be excessive in patients with mitral stenosis. However, Blackmon and colleagues[36] found the hepatic clearance of indocyanine green in patients with mitral stenosis during maximal exercise to be similar to that of normal subjects when expressed as a percentage of maximal oxygen intake.

Arterial saturation is maintained in mitral stenosis until severe pulmonary congestion develops. Chronic hyperventilation is possibly the compensatory mechanism partly explaining the normal oxygen tension (Fig. 14-8). Ralston and colleagues[37] noted a significant correlation between elevated pulmonary artery pressure and minute ventilation.

CLINICAL PRESENTATION

Symptoms. The major symptoms of mitral stenosis are *dyspnea* (orthopnea and paroxysmal nocturnal dyspnea) due to pulmonary venous congestion and *fatigue* due to a reduced and restricted cardiac output (Fig. 14-9).

Palpitations due to paroxysmal and eventually chronic atrial fibrilla-

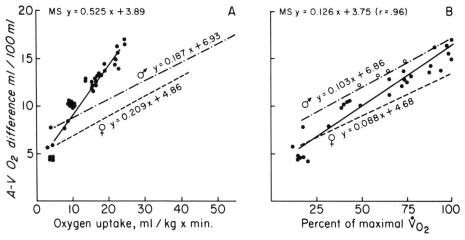

FIGURE 14–7   PERIPHERAL OXYGEN EXTRACTION IN MITRAL STENOSIS

Total body arteriovenous oxygen difference at rest and during exercise is shown for seven patients with mitral stenosis (solid circles) and contrasted with regression lines (dashed lines) for 11 normal young women (♀) and 12 normal young men (♂). These data are plotted with respect to absolute oxygen uptake (ml./kg. × min.) (A) and relative oxygen uptake (B).

tion or flutter are common and frequently precipitate an episode of pulmonary edema since tachycardia reduces diastolic filling period and increases the left atrial pressure.

Arterial emboli are a frequent complication of mitral stenosis and are particularly prone to occur after the development of atrial fibrillation. Symptoms are related to the site of lodgment of the embolus.

Hemoptysis occurs in about 10 per cent of patients with mitral stenosis. This symptom is alarming to the patient but is rarely massive or fatal. The postulated mecanism is that the high pulmonary venous pressure is transmitted to the bronchial vessels in the mucosa causing rupture.

Cough is usually a late symptom in mitral stenosis. The cough is generally dry, occurring at night or following exertion. Pulmonary congestion or bronchial compression due to the large left atrium are the probable mechanisms.

The symptoms of *edema, ascites*

and *right upper quadrant discomfort* are due to right heart failure. These occur late in the course of mitral stenosis.

Other less common symptoms are *hoarseness* and *paralysis of vocal cords* due to compression of the left recurrent laryngeal nerve between the aorta and dilated pulmonary artery;[38] *dysphagia* due to compression of the esophagus by the large left atrium; and *syncope* due to the ball valve action of a pedunculated left atrial thrombus.

Signs. If right ventricular hypertrophy is present, pulsation along the left sternal border or in the epigastrium may be noted. An active pulmonary artery may reveal a slight pulsation, and, in a thin-chested patient in normal sinus rhythm, pulsation of a dilated left atrial appendage can be detected. The neck veins will be normal unless right heart failure or tricuspid disease is present. Peripheral cyanosis may be present in severe cases.

FIGURE 14-8 ARTERIAL BLOOD GASES AND ACID-BASE RELATIONSHIPS DURING EXERCISE IN MITRAL STENOSIS

Arterial blood gases and acid-base at rest and during three intensities of work. Results from a single subject reflecting the hyperventilation in mitral stenosis with low pCO_2 and HCO_3^-, and high pH during rest and exercise.

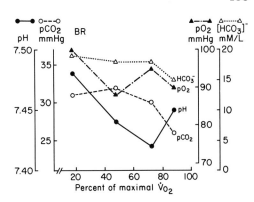

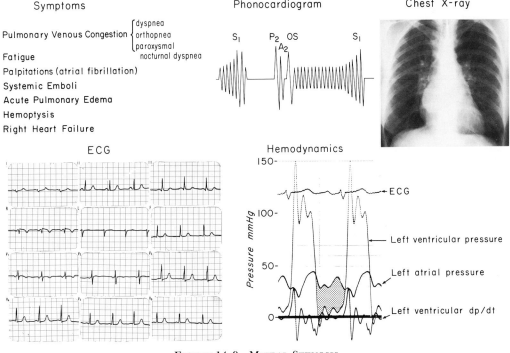

Symptoms

Pulmonary Venous Congestion { dyspnea orthopnea paroxysmal nocturnal dyspnea }

Fatigue

Palpitations (atrial fibrillation)

Systemic Emboli

Acute Pulmonary Edema

Hemoptysis

Right Heart Failure

Phonocardiogram

S_I P_2 OS S_I
A_2

Chest X-ray

ECG

Hemodynamics

ECG

Left ventricular pressure

Left atrial pressure

Left ventricular dp/dt

Pressure mmHg

FIGURE 14-9 MITRAL STENOSIS

Prominant *symptoms* are those of pulmonary venous hypertension, low cardiac output and arrhythmia. Typical *auscultatory findings* in mitral stenosis are a 1st heart sound (S_1) and 2nd pulmonic heart sound (P_2) of increased intensity an opening snap (OS) .06 to .12 sec after P_2 and a low frequency, low amplitude, diastolic murmur (rumble) with a presystolic accentuation if atrial contraction occurs.

Chest x-ray in the frontal plane demonstrates an enlarged left atrium (double density behind right atrium) and pulmonary artery.

Electrocardiographic findings of right axis deviation (QRS axis greater than 90 degrees due to right ventricular hypertrophy) and left atrial enlargement are common.

Hemodynamic features include left atrial-left ventricular pressure gradients during diastole (shaded area), elevated atrial pressures and normal left ventricular pressures.

Palpation usually confirms the findings of inspection, a right ventricular heave and active pulmonary artery or atrial appendage. In addition, a presystolic or diastolic thrill, sometimes an opening snap and an increased M_1 (mitral first sound) and P_2 (pulmonary second sound) can be felt.

The pulmonary second sound is accentuated and may be delayed due to the increased pulmonary artery pressure causing prolonged right ventricular systole. The mitral first sound is increased in intensity and delayed presumably due to the pathologic changes in the valve and chordae.

An *opening snap* (O.S.) is usually best heard between the apex and left sternal border. The 2-O.S. interval (that time between the second heart sound and the opening snap) ranges between 0.5 and 0.12 seconds. A narrow 2-O.S. interval correlates with a higher degree of stenosis. The pathogenesis of the opening snap is thought to be an abrupt halt in the downward excursion of the mitral cusps due to their pathologic fusion. With a rigid, heavily calcified mitral valve, the opening snap is faint or not heard. Recognition of the opening snap is clinically important since it may be the most obvious auscultatory clue to mitral stenosis when the characteristic diastolic rumble is faint or absent.

The *diastolic rumbling murmur* located at or near the apex is the hallmark of mitral stenosis. When the patient is in normal sinus rhythm, the rumble may be presystolic and crescendo ending in the loud M_1. The presystolic accentuation is due to atrial contraction and is lost with the advent of atrial fibrillation. Probably the most common presentation of the diastolic rumble is its appearance after the opening snap and continuing through diastole. The murmur is produced by the turbulence caused by blood forced through a small opening by the pressure gradient (Fig. 14–9).

Other murmurs associated but rarely due to mitral stenosis are the so-called Graham Steele murmurs of pulmonic regurgitation due to longstanding pulmonary hypertension. While a decrescendo, early diastolic murmur is frequently present, it is most commonly due to aortic regurgitation. A systolic murmur at the apex is common and due to mitral regurgitation.

X-Ray. The full-blown x-ray appearance of the heart in mitral stenosis is quite characteristic (Fig. 14–9). The PA and lateral views are adequate. In the PA view, the left border of the cardiac silhouette is straightened, the pulmonary artery is enlarged, there is a double density of the large left atrium. The left main stem bronchus is elevated. The lung fields show increased pulmonary venous markings in the upper lobes and Kerley's B lines in the lower lung fields. If the valve is heavily calcified, it may be seen in the conventional x-ray. In the lateral projection, the enlarged left atrium and right ventricle can be seen (Fig. 11–14).

Electrocardiogram. The electrocardiographic features of mitral stenosis are typical. When the patient is in normal sinus rhythm, the P-wave is bifid and prolonged, the so-called P-mitrale. The electrical axis is usually vertical and right ventricular hypertrophy may be present. Atrial fibrillation in an electrically vertical heart without hypertrophy is common. (Fig. 14–9).

Exercise Testing. Assessment of functional capacity is an essential part of evaluating cardiac patients. It is well known that historical classification is in error in at least 20 per cent of patients. Treadmill testing to symp-

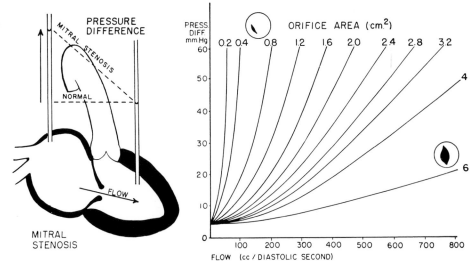

FIGURE 14–10   PRESSURE DROP ACROSS STENOTIC MITRAL VALVES

Mitral stenosis necessitates a steep pressure gradient to force the normal increments of blood past the restricted orifice between the left atrium and ventricle. The magnitude of the pressure difference is related to the area of the effective mitral orifice, as indicated by the graph. If the mitral orifice is large, very rapid ventricular filling can result from a relatively slight increase in left atrial pressure. In contrast, the flow through extremely small orifices (0.2 or 0.4 cm.²) increases only slightly even when the pressure gradient reaches very high levels (after Gorlin and Gorlin[40]). This graph illustrates the important roles played by valvular orifice area and rate of blood flow in the production of pulmonary hypertension and congestion.

tomatic maximal exertion as described by Bruce and colleagues[39] has been shown to be safe and informative in determining functional impairment.

Hemodynamics. The classical finding in mitral stenosis is a diastolic pressure gradient between the left atrium and left ventricle. (Fig. 14–9). Although a gradient confirms the diagnosis of mitral stenosis, it does not accurately quantitate the severity of the stenosis and frequent clinical errors are made by relying on the gradient alone.

Gorlin and Gorlin[40] put the estimation of valvular stenosis on a quantitative basis by adapting a hydraulic formula to clinical usage. Pressure in the left atrium is influenced by the amount of diastolic blood flow through the stenotic valve (Fig. 14–10). As the area of the mitral valve decreases, assuming flow is maintained, the left atrial pressure rises; or, if the orifice

of the mitral valve is held constant, left atrial pressure will rise or fall with increases or decreases in flow across the restricted valve orifice, thus the gradient is dependent upon flow.

The formula for calculating mitral valve orifice is as follows:

$$MVO = \frac{F}{HR \cdot DFP \cdot K \cdot \sqrt{P_1 - P_2}}$$

where

MVO = mitral valve orifice (sq. cm.)

F   = flow

K   = empirical constant (includes corrections for coefficient of orifice contraction, coefficient of velocity, gravitational acceleration)

HR = heart rate in beats per minute

DFP = diastolic filling period (diastolic time per beat)

$P_1 - P_2$ = mitral valve gradient

Example:
Cardiac output 5000 cc./min.
  (forward and
  regurgitant flow)
Heart rate 72 beats/min.
Diastolic filling period 0.56 sec./beat
Planimetered mean gradient
  (LA-LV) 16 mm.
Hg. (Fig. 14–9)
K 41
by substitution (numbers are rounded off)

$$MVO = \frac{5000}{72 \cdot 0.56 \cdot 41 \cdot \sqrt{16}}$$

$$= \frac{5000}{1650 \cdot 4}$$

$$= \frac{5000}{6600} = 0.76 \text{ cm.}^2$$

Criticism of the application of the Gorlin formula comes from theoretical considerations which are that blood is not a homogenous fluid, that the valve orifice is not round or necessarily short and that flow is pulsatile rather than constant. These objections are valid in the sense that they are true but from a clinical point of view they are not germane. A second source of criticism comes from comparison of pathologic and hemodynamic measurements of the mitral valve area.[42] In these studies, either filling pressure was ignored during pathologic study or assessment of mitral regurgitation was not made clinically. Probably the most valid criticism is the use of the Gorlin formula when the pressure gradient is small; since large errors are known to occur.

Angiocardiography. Angiocardiography has become an important part of the clinical assessment of mitral stenosis. The contrast material is injected into the left atrium and cineangiocardiograms or biplane angiocardiograms taken. These films provide information about atrial size, presence of filling defects (thrombus or tumor), thickness and mobility of the mitral valve and size of the left ventricle. In addition to providing anatomic confirmation of mitral stenosis, the films aid in predicting the type of surgery preoperatively.

NATURAL HISTORY

The natural history of mitral stenosis is for many reasons imperfectly known. There is no doubt that as a group, patients with mitral stenosis live significantly shortened life spans whether the average age at death is forty-five or fifty-five years. Of 250 patients followed by Rowe and colleagues[43] for 20 years including 138 patients less than 30 years of age, 39 per cent were dead in 10 years. Of the 115 patients followed 20 years, 43 per cent of them grade 1 and 45 per cent grade 2, 79 per cent were dead. Oleson[44] found an 83 per cent mortality in 271 patients with mitral stenosis (who averaged 41 years of age when first entered in the study) followed for an average of 12 years.

The most common causes of death in mitral stenosis are congestive heart failure, systemic emboli, pulmonary emboli and bacterial endocarditis.[43] Cardiac surgery is also a significant cause of death.

MITRAL REGURGITATION

In contrast to mitral stenosis, mitral regurgitation has many causes. While acute rheumatic fever is still the most common, papillary muscle rupture,[45] papillary muscle dysfunction[46] and ruptured chordae tendineae[47, 48] are not uncommon. Marfans syndrome[49] is a rare cause of mitral regurgitation.

PATHOPHYSIOLOGY

The initiating problem in mitral regurgitation is the backward flow of blood from the left ventricle into the left atrium during ventricular systole. It takes only a small aperture in the mitral valve to permit significant regurgitation to occur since the systolic pressure gradient from the left ventricle to the left atrium is extremely high.

Chronic Mitral Regurgitation. In chronic mitral regurgitation, high pressures in the left atrium, pulmonary capillary bed and pulmonary arteries eventually develop leading to the same sequence of events as in mitral stenosis, however, the time course is delayed.

Acute Mitral Regurgitation. In acute mitral regurgitation due to ruptured chordae tendineae or papillary muscle rupture, the magnitude of the regurgitation is so great that the left atrium and left ventricle become essentially a common chamber (Fig. 14–11). The acute change in pressure-volume relationships overwhelm the compensatory mechanism of increased compliance in both the atrium and ventricle. Since this buffering mechanism does not develop, extremely high systolic and diastolic pressures are transmitted to the pulmonary vasculature with rapid development of pulmonary hypertension. The right ventricle does not have adequate time to develop right ventricular hypertrophy due to this rapid pressure overload with resulting right ventricular failure and systemic venous congestion.

COMPENSATORY MECHANISMS

During the sequence of events in mitral regurgitation, compensatory mechanisms are called into play accounting for some of the symptoms and signs of mitral regurgitation.

Left Atrium. Due to the increased volume of blood under elevated pressure in atrial diastole, the left atrium dilates to a greater degree than in mitral stenosis. The precise mechanism by which volume overload causes dilatation and pressure overload hypertrophy is not known. Dilatation of the left atrium is a compensatory mechanism which protects the pulmonary capillary bed from increased pressure. In many cases of chronic mitral regurgitation, the left atrium is huge but the pressure only slightly elevated.[50, 51] The increased compliance of the left atrium is probably the most significant factor in the longer clinical course of mitral regurgitation.

Left Ventricle. The left ventricle is also burdened by a volume load which causes both dilatation and hypertrophy. The end-diastolic volume increases markedly with little or no increase in left ventricular end-diastolic pressure until heart failure ensues or unless left ventricular restriction or constriction is present from previous injury. The left ventricle by its increase in end-diastolic volume and compensatory hypertrophy is able to maintain a normal cardiac output at rest, but cardiac output is restricted during exertion.

CLINICAL PRESENTATION

Symptoms. *Fatigue* and *weakness*[52] are probably the initial symptoms in chronic mitral regurgitation, although most patients on seeing a physician will have the combination of fatigue, *dyspnea* and *palpitations*. The mechanisms of symptoms are the same as for mitral stenosis. In acute mitral regurgitation, the overwhelming symptoms are those of acute pulmo-

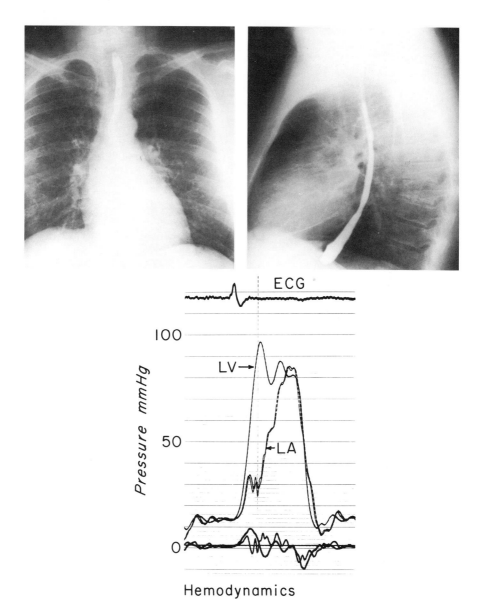

Hemodynamics

FIGURE 14–11   RADIOGRAPHIC AND HEMODYNAMIC FINDINGS IN ACUTE MITRAL INSUFFICIENCY

Anteroposterior and lateral chest x-rays in acute mitral regurgitation demonstrate that neither the left ventricle nor left atrium are grossly enlarged but there is marked pulmonary venous congestion. The hemodynamics in the lower panel show a ventricularized left atrium. The large V-wave in the left atrial tracing is consistently seen in acute mitral regurgitation and represents a failure of the compensatory dilatation of the left atrium. The left ventricular end-diastolic pressure is also elevated and the rate of rise of the left ventricular pressure (dp/dt) is reduced.

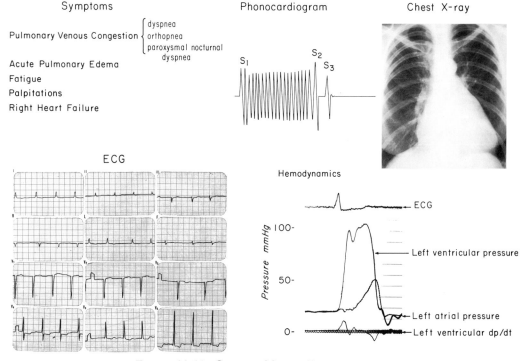

| Symptoms | Phonocardiogram | Chest X-ray |

Pulmonary Venous Congestion { dyspnea / orthopnea / paroxysmal nocturnal dyspnea

Acute Pulmonary Edema

Fatigue

Palpitations

Right Heart Failure

ECG

Hemodynamics

FIGURE 14–12   CHRONIC MITRAL REGURGITATION

The most common *symptoms* are noted in upper left panel. The typical *murmur* is described as a pansystolic, blowing murmur and is heard best at the cardiac apex with typical radiation into the left axilla and back. The first heart sound (S_1) is frequently obscured by the murmur. A diastolic ventricular gallop (S_3) is shown.

The *chest x-ray* demonstrates enlargement of left ventricle, left atrium, left atrial appendage (convex shadow on left heart border) in the frontal projection. A typical *electrocardiogram* shows atrial fibrillation, left ventricular hypertrophy and "strain".

The major *hemodynamic* features are prominent "V" waves in the left atrium, an elevated left ventricular end-diastolic pressure and a reduced rate of left ventricular pressure change (dp/dt).

nary venous congestion, *dyspnea at rest, orthopnea, paroxysmal nocturnal dyspnea* and *acute*, frequently refractory, *pulmonary edema* (Fig. 14-12).

Systemic emboli are infrequently seen in mitral regurgitation. With blood entering from four pulmonary veins, a regurgitant flow from the left ventricle and no obstruction at the mitral valve, there is little reason for emboli to occur except during atrial fibrillation.

Cough and *hemoptysis* are seen in mitral regurgitation but appear later in the course of the disease than in mitral stenosis. *Pulmonary edema* occurs in the course of mitral regurgitation and is due to left ventricular failure. Edema, ascites and right upper quadrant discomfort are due to *right heart failure* and are late manifestations of mitral regurgitation.

Signs. The left ventricle in mitral regurgitation enlarges and causes a large pulsation on the chest wall sometimes rippling in nature. The pulmonary artery and left atrial appendage may be seen as in mitral stenosis.

Palpation confirms inspection – a

left ventricular heave with fairly wide distribution is felt. A systolic thrill may be present and an S₃ gallop may be palpable.

Auscultation reveals a pansystolic or holosystolic murmur best heard at the apex with radiation into the left axilla (Fig. 14-12). The murmur of mitral regurgitation may be heard over the trachea, cervical spine, cranium, and into the carotids. These unusual locations are due to jet lesions striking the bronchus, spine and great arteries. A higher pitched musical murmur may be present with ruptured chordae tendineae.

The first heart sound at the apex is reduced since rapid changes in intraventricular pressure are modified by mitral regurgitation. An S_3 gallop or ventricular filling sound is frequently present. The timing of this third heart sound is 0.12 to 0.16 seconds after the second heart sound.

A diastolic filling murmur may be present when the regurgitant volume is large and is due to relative mitral stenosis. This murmur is usually of higher frequency than that of organic mitral stenosis.

X-Ray. The x-ray appearance of the heart in mitral regurgitation is again characteristic. The left ventricle is enlarged; the left atrium is enlarged usually more so than in mitral stenosis. These changes are seen in PA projection by the left ventricle protruding downward and to the left (Fig. 14–12). The left atrium is seen as a double density. If extremely large, it may form the right border of the heart. In the lateral view, the left atrium impinges on the esophagus; and, if right ventricular hypertrophy is present, the retrosternal space is filled. The changes in pulmonary vasculature previously described may be present.

Electrocardiogram. The major electrocardiographic difference be-

tween mitral stenosis and regurgitation is the influence of the enlarged left ventricle. In mitral regurgitation, left ventricular hypertrophy is usually present. In chronic mitral regurgitation, combined ventricular hypertrophy may be present. P-mitrale or atrial fibrillation are common (Fig. 14–12).

Hemodynamic-Angiocardiographic Findings. The major hemodynamic finding in mitral regurgitation is the presence of an increased V-wave in the left atrium. This, however, is not always present even in significant regurgitation. In addition, prominent V-waves occur in a noncompliant left atrium from right ventricular systole. Attempts at quantitation and clinical correlations have not been helpful (Fig. 14–12).

The best method of assessing mitral regurgitation, both qualitatively and quantitatively is by angiocardiography.

The angiocardiographic assessment of mitral regurgitation necessitates injection of contrast material into the left ventricle. The rapidity of left atrial opacification, visualization of pulmonary veins during ventricular systole and persistence of left atrial opacification are major features in estimating mitral regurgitation.

Quantitative angiocardiographic measurement of mitral regurgitation necessitates measurement of left ventricular volume (Chapter 11, p. 351). In addition, forward cardiac output is determined by the Fick principle. The amount of regurgitation is determined by subtracting the Fick output from the angiocardiographic output.

Examples of chronic and acute mitral regurgitation are seen in Table 14-2.

The preceding hemodynamic-angiocardiographic examples show the differences in pressure volume relationship in acute and chronic mitral

Table 14-2.   *MITRAL REGURGITATION*

PRESSURE (mm Hg)	CHRONIC	ACUTE
RA	8 mean	9 mean
RV	55/10	74/12
PA	55/25	74/35
LA	38/10 v=38	65/9 v=65
LV	90/14	95/20
AO	90/68	95/62
VOLUME (cc)		
LA max.	530	176
LV EDV	316	236
LV ESV	84	66
LV SV	234	170
HR (beats/min.)	60	77
Angiographic		
CO L/min.	14.0	13.1
Fick CO L/min.	3.9	2.3
Regurgitant		
Flow L/min.	10.1	10.8

RA = right atrial
RV = right ventricular
PA = pulmonary arterial
LA = left atrial
LV = left ventricular
AO = aortic
EDV = end diastolic volume
ESV = end systolic volume
SV = stroke volume
CO = cardiac output

regurgitation. In chronic regurgitation, left atrial volume is high and pressure normal or moderately elevated. In acute mitral regurgitation; the left atrial volume is normal or moderately increased and pressure high. The implication of these marked differences will be discussed further under *Therapy of Valvular Heart Disease.*

NATURAL HISTORY

The natural history of mitral regurgitation is essentially unknown. Since the etiology is variable, the prognosis is dependent to a large extent on cause. Thus, acute mitral regurgitation without surgical therapy has a poor

prognosis. It is the general impression that chronic mitral regurgitation has a more prolonged course than that of mitral stenosis, but this impression is not quantitated.

TRICUSPID VALVULAR DISEASE

The etiology of tricuspid regurgitation varies as does mitral regurgitation. The most common form is "functional" regurgitation, due to right ventricular dilatation and failure from other primary lesions. Organic tricuspid regurgitation may be caused by rheumatic fever, bacterial endocarditis, trauma and metastatic malignant carcinoid.[53] In most cases, the cause is rheumatic, and there is concomitant mitral disease.[3]

Tricuspid stenosis is almost always due to rheumatic fever but can be mimicked by tumors or thrombi as in mitral disease. Tricuspid stenosis of clinical significance probably occurs in about 5 per cent of patients with rheumatic heart disease but rarely as an isolated lesion.

Both tricuspid lesions cause an increased volume and pressure in the right atrium thus causing systemic venous hypertension and congestion.

CLINICAL PRESENTATION

Symptoms.   The major symptoms of both tricuspid regurgitation and stenosis, from a theoretical point of view, would be *fatigue, edema* and *ascites.* Since tricuspid disease is rarely an isolated lesion, symptoms from other valvular lesions predominate. The formation of edema and ascites early in the course of a patient with valvular heart disease suggests a tricuspid lesion.

Signs.   The most valuable sign in either regurgitation or stenosis is obtained from observation of the jugular venous pulse. When normal sinus rhythm is present, a large V-wave is seen in tricuspid regurgitation and a large A-wave in tricuspid stenosis. The A-wave is lost if atrial fibrillation is present.

Increased dullness to percussion is noted to the right of the sternum due to right atrial enlargement. Auscultation in tricuspid regurgitation reveals a pansystolic murmur located along the left lower sternal border. The murmur increases in intensity with inspiration (Corvallo's sign) and with long diastolic pauses in atrial fibrillation. An S_3 gallop may be present.

Auscultation in triscuspid stenosis reveals a diastolic rumbling murmur best heard in the left fourth or fifth intercostal space. The murmur is usually of higher frequency than the mitral diastolic rumble; on occasion it is of decrescendo quality and mimics aortic or pulmonic regurgitation. The murmur increases in intensity with inspiration. An opening snap may be present 0.06 to 0.08 seconds following the pulmonic second sound. Since mitral stenosis and/or regurgitation are almost inevitably present, the auscultatory findings of tricuspid disease may be missed, thus careful observation of the jugular venous pulse is the most helpful physical sign in tricuspid disease.

X-Ray. The most striking change in both tricuspid stenosis and regurgitation is right atrial enlargement. In regurgitation, the right ventricle is also enlarged and best seen in the lateral projection (Chapter 11, Figure 11–13).

Electrocardiogram. The most distinctive finding is tall, peaked or bifid P-waves if normal sinus rhythm is present. The electrocardiogram is largely influenced by the associated valvular lesions.

Hemodynamic-Angiocardiographic Findings. As in mitral regurgitation, a prominent V-wave may be present and the mean right atrial pressure is usually greater than 10 mm. Hg. Demonstration of regurgitation is accomplished by injection of contrast material into the right ventricle and noting the amount of reflux into the right atrium. Practical quantitative methods are not available.

Tricuspid stenosis like mitral stenosis is characterized by a pressure gradient across the stenotic valve. An orifice of 1.5 sq. cm. is considered significant restriction.

Angiocardiography in tricuspid stenosis reveals thickening and doming of the tricuspid valve.

AORTIC STENOSIS

ETIOLOGY

Obstruction to blood flow from the left ventricle by the aortic valve has the same anatomic and physiologic sequela regardless of the cause of aortic valve abnormality. Rheumatic damage to the valve, with subsequent fibrosis and calcification, is most frequent and is often seen in conjunction with mitral valve disease,[54] while isolated aortic stenosis appears to result from these same changes in a congenitally abnormal valve.[55] Calcification occurs in all damaged aortic valves and is not diagnostically helpful *per se.*

If aortic stenosis is present prior to age 30, it is most likely due to a congenital valvular deformity, usually a bicuspid valve. In patients over 50 with aortic stenosis the etiology remains obscure, but these also may represent congenitally abnormal valves with calcification or the calcifica-

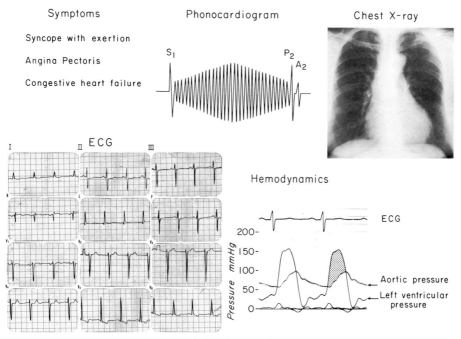

FIGURE 14–13   AORTIC STENOSIS

Symptoms in aortic stenosis include syncope, angina and heart failure. The typical *murmur* is a harsh, systolic crescendo-decrescendo (diamond shaped, ejection type) sound heard best in the right 2nd or 3rd intercostal space with radiation into the neck and carotid arteries.

Frontal *chest x-ray* demonstrates concentric left ventricular enlargement and post stenotic aortic dilatation. On the *electrocardiogram* left axis deviation (mean QRS axis $> -30°$) with left ventricular hypertrophy and strain are seen.

Hemodynamic study demonstrates a significant pressure gradient between left ventricle and aorta (shaded area) and an elevated left ventricular end-diastolic pressure.

tion may be associated with tissue aging.

Several syndromes may mimic valvular aortic stenosis. These include (1) idiopathic hypertrophic subaortic stenosis, where a functional muscular obstruction in the left ventricular outflow tract is present;[56, 57] (2) supravalvular aortic stenosis which is of interest in its association with mental retardation, hypercalcemia and dental anomalies[58, 59, 60] and (3) subvalvular anatomic stenosis with deformity of outflow tract and valve.[61]

PATHOPHYSIOLOGY

The physiologic changes of aortic stenosis result from the gradual re-

striction of the orifice of the aortic valve from its normal 2.5 to 3.5 sq. cm. to a critical range of 0.5 to 1.0 sq. cm. where compensatory mechanisms fail and clinical symptoms develop. Recent description of the impedance to blood flow in aortic stenosis have provided instantaneous details of this hemodynamic lesion.[62] Marked pressure gradients develop across the aortic valve in the advanced forms. These peak to peak pressure differences between left ventricle and aorta may exceed 100 mm. Hg (Fig. 14–13). The slow rising nature of the aortic pulse wave (reduced dp/dt) is characteristic of aortic stenosis.

Cardiac output remains nearly normal at rest but may be markedly restricted during exercise in severe aortic stenosis. Myocardial work is increased by the pressure load, but mechanical efficiency is maintained until decompensation occurs.[63]

Thus, the major functional effect of aortic stenosis is that the pressure developed by the contracting left ventricle must exceed the pressure in the aorta by an amount sufficient to maintain a normal stroke volume in spite of the increased resistance to ejection.

Left Ventricular Response. The myocardial response to increased systolic pressure (afterload) is hypertrophy. Increased left ventricular wall thickness and mass have been demonstrated by quantitative angiocardiography in all degrees of aortic stenosis.[64] During the initial period of hypertrophy, end-systolic volume, end-diastolic volume and the ventricular stress radii are reduced, as a result, only mild increases in wall stress and Young's modulus occur.[65] With temporal progression of the disease, volumes and stress radii increase which would imply decompensation, even though the patient remains asymptomatic.[64] The mechanics of left ventricular ejection also deteriorate under the influence of increased afterload and uncompensated wall tension with a reduction in ejection fraction (stroke volume/end-diastolic volume).

The increased muscle mass and wall tension greatly increase the myocardial oxygen consumption. When the oxygen demand exceeds the ability of the coronary blood flow to provide oxygen, myocardial ischemia and angina pectoris result. The amount of blood perfusing the coronary arteries depends upon (1) the mean pressure gradient from aortic root to coronary veins and (2) the resistance through these vessels. Coronary flow may be markedly impaired by both the relatively low aortic pressure generated during systole and by the high, prolonged intramural pressure during ventricular systole, however, reductions in blood flow per unit mass have not been found.[66] This suggests that insufficient perfusion may exist at the cellular level.

Further increases in afterload, left ventricular end-diastolic volume, left ventricular end-diastolic pressure and decreases in the contractile capacity of the myocardium result in pulmonary capillary congestion with pulmonary edema and a fixed forward blood flow with syncope and poor tissue perfusion.

CLINICAL PRESENTATION

The natural history of aortic stenosis is remarkable in its malignancy once symptoms begin.[55, 61, 67] Patients frequently have known of a heart murmur for some years and then develop congestive heart failure, syncope or angina pectoris. At this point in their history, survival averages 2, 3 and 5 years respectively for each symptom complex. Of those with symptoms, 10 to 15 per cent die suddenly.[55] The clinical findings have been reported in detail.[67, 68, 69, 70]

Symptoms. Clinical symptoms do not occur until the aortic valve orifice is less than 50 per cent of normal, unless atherosclerotic coronary artery disease, anemia or other superimposed cardiac insults occur.

Fatigue and *dyspnea* appear to be the most common presenting symptoms in the younger age group, while *syncope, angina pectoris* and *heart failure* afflict the older individuals. *Syncope during exertion* is a symptom very suggestive of aortic stenosis.

Signs. The presence of left ventricular hypertrophy without ventricular dilatation may be difficult to detect by inspection and percussion, but almost always the ventricular apical impulse is more vigorous and thrusting in nature even if not displaced on the thoracic wall.

The harsh, high-pitched, crescendo-decrescendo murmur heard over the second and third intercostal spaces at the right sternal border and neck during systole is characteristic of aortic stenosis (Fig. 14–13). This murmur may appear with minimal impedance to flow and does not necessarily mean significant physiologic obstruction. A thrill will frequently accompany the murmur. An ejection click may occur 0.04 to 0.08 seconds following the first heart sound, during the murmur. The second heart sound may be single if the aortic valve excursion is limited.

Pulse and blood pressures measurements may demonstrate the slow rising anacrotic pulse (Fig. 14–13). Often aortic stenosis is accompanied by aortic insufficiency, and the features of these two lesions may be mixed.

X-Ray. The cardiac silhouette may be normal on the plain chest roentgenogram if only concentric hypertrophy of the left ventricle is present. Post stenotic aortic dilatation due to the local trauma of a valvular jet lesion is often present, and easily demonstrable aortic valvular calcification is a frequent finding.[71] Selective opacification of the left ventricle reveals characteristic changes by quantitative angiocardiography (Chapter 11, Figure 11–16).[64]

Electrocardiogram. Significant aortic stenosis is almost always associated with the increased QRS amplitude produced by an increased myocardial mass. Sinus rhythm persists if atrial pressures and volumes are normal. ST and T wave changes of myocardial ischemia may be interrup-

ted as the electrical "strain" pattern (Fig. 14–13).

AORTIC INSUFFICIENCY (AORTIC REGURGITATION)

ETIOLOGY

Aortic insufficiency is most commonly caused by rheumatic valvular damage, which produces a chronic lesion[73] and bacterial valvular damage which is associated with an acute hemodynamic lesion. Other less common conditions which damage the aortic root or valves include syphilis, trauma,[73] dissecting aortic aneurysm,[74, 75] Marfan's syndrome,[76] rheumatoid spondylitis,[77] Reiter syndrome[78] and aortic dilatation.[79]

A recent series of over 100 cases reported aortic insufficiency to be due to rheumatic damage in 54 per cent, unknown in 23 per cent, aortic dilatation in 5 per cent, luetic in 3 per cent, congenital in 2 per cent, associated with calcific aortic stenosis in 7 per cent and other causes in 6 per cent.[80]

PATHOPHYSIOLOGY

In all these conditions, insufficiency of the aortic valve during diastole allows regurgitation of blood from the aorta into the left ventricle. Because of the high pressure gradient between aorta and ventricle at end-systole, large regurgitant flows can occur through small regurgitant orifices (Fig. 14–14). These flows may range from less than 1 to 15 liters per minute in patients studied at rest and may constitute over 50 per cent of the left ventricular stroke volume.[64] In an anesthetized, open-chested man, the percentage of regurgitation did not change although the volume with each beat fell, over a wide range of heart rates in the physiologic range, 50 to 170 beats per minute. Increased end-diastolic pressure (and volume) increased forward blood flow, but an increase in ventricular afterload during aortic constriction reduced the net forward blood flow.[81]

Patients with aortic insufficiency increase cardiac output in response to exercise by the positive inotropic effect of exercise, which dominates the other factors as long as the myocardium is able to respond.

In chronic volume overload with aortic regurgitation, the hemodynamic and mechanical pathology results initially in an increased end-diastolic volume and pressure, with a resulting increase in the end-diastolic ventricular wall stress. With progressive impairment and decompensation of the ventricular myocardium, left ventricular weight, systolic and diastolic wall stress and total work load increase and systolic ejection is impaired.[82, 83] The increase in oxygen demands by the myocardium, increase in diastolic filling pressure and dilatation of the left ventricle, all contribute to the eventual decompensation of the myocardium. Reduction in the velocity of contractile element shortening occurs as myocardial failure occurs.[84] In acute valvular damage due to trauma or bacterial infection, these pathologic changes are accelerated and the compensatory mechanisms fail; therefore, the clinical features are telescoped in time.

CLINICAL PRESENTATION

Symptoms. The patient with aortic insufficiency is often a young male, who first learned of a heart murmur following a physical examination for military induction or an insurance policy. Symptoms follow an asymptomatic period of several years and consist of *palpitations, light-headedness, dyspnea on exertion, chest pain or congestive heart failure* (Fig. 14–14).

Signs. The constellation of remarkable physical findings in classical aortic insufficiency suggests long-standing hermodynamic changes. The peripheral arterial signs of widened pulse pressure; collapsing, "waterhammer" or Corrigan pulse; head nodding of de Musset's sign; capillary pulsations of Quincke's pulse and the systolic and diastolic femoral murmur of Duroziez's sign are all associated with "free" aortic regurgitation.

Cardiac examination demonstrates a remarkable enlargement of the left ventricle which presents itself as a diffuse, heaving, apical impulse in the fifth to sixth intercostal space, lateral to the midclavicular line. A soft, high-pitched, diastolic murmur along the left sternal border with diminishing amplitude during diastole is characteristic of aortic insufficiency (Fig. 14–14). Commonly associated with this murmur is a loud, harsh, systolic murmur of crescendo-decrescendo intensity, which is best heard in the second or third right intercostal space near the sternum. This sound represents flow through the diseased aortic valve, but a significant systolic pressure gradient is not necessarily present. These physical findings do not correlate well with the degree of aortic insufficiency demonstrated angiographically.[85]

Two other murmurs may also be present. The first is that of mitral regurgitation. As the left ventricle dilates, the mitral annulus stretches and the valve may become incompetent. The second is the Austin Flint murmur. This low pitched, diastolic flow murmur probably originates from turbul-

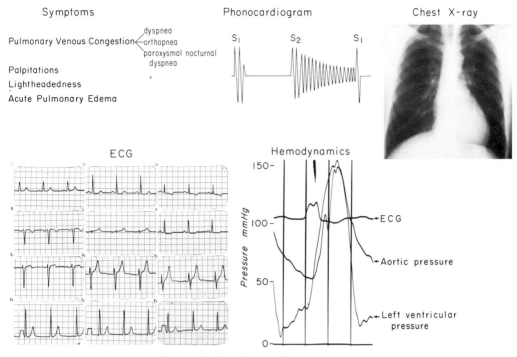

FIGURE 14–14   AORTIC REGURGITATION

Symptoms of aortic regurgitation usually develop late in the natural history. The *murmurs* of aortic regurgitation is a high frequency, low amplitude sound in early systole, heard best in the 3rd-4th ICS at the left sternal margin as a "whiff" immediately following the second heart sound.

Chest x-ray demonstrates left ventricular enlargement with both dilatation and hypertrophy. The *electrocardiogram* is compatible with left ventricular hypertrophy.

Hemodynamics include a widened aortic pulse pressure and an elevated left ventricular end-diastolic pressure.

ence near the anterior leaflet of the mitral valve, which is between the regurgitant jet from the aortic valve and the incoming blood from the left atrium. This murmur and ventricular and atrial filling sounds (gallops) are more apt to be present with heart failure.

X-Ray. On chest x-ray, selective left ventricular enlargement of a moderate or marked degree is present. Dilatation of the ascending aorta is common.[71]

Electrocardiogram. Electrocardiographic findings are those of left ventricular hypertrophy with an increase in QRS voltage and ST and T wave abnormalities, which accompany this increase, the "strain" pattern.

Hemodynamic Findings. At cardiac catheterization, widened pulse pressure, increased diastolic pulse slope, normal cardiac output and increased left ventricular end-diastolic pressure and volume are present hemodynamically. Supravalvular aortic injection of radio-opaque contrast material demonstrates reflux from aorta to the left ventricle during cinefluoroscopic filming.[79] Quantitation of the regurgitant volume may be done by subtracting the forward or net cardiac output (Fick) from the output determined angiocardiographically.[64]

III. THERAPY OF VALVULAR HEART DISEASE

MEDICAL THERAPY

PREVENTION

Medical management of patients with valvular heart disease is directed toward the prevention of rheumatic fever recurrences, bacterial endocarditis, control of arrhythmias, compensation of heart failure and treatment of complications.

The optimal therapy of valvular disease would be prevention. Prompt therapy and prophylaxis of streptococcal infection has had a clear effect in decreasing acute rheumatic fever and rheumatic heart disease.[86]

Additional prophylaxis against bacterial endocarditis should be provided those with rheumatic or other valvular deformities during dental and surgical procedures. Therapeutic dosages of either penicillin or other antibiotics should be used.

Attempts should be made to prevent influenza infections in patients with symptomatic valvular disease, as respiratory illness is particularly debilitiating in these patients.

ARRHYTHMIAS

Atrial arrhythmias occur when atrial pressures and volumes are elevated. Atrial fibrillation with an uncontrolled ventricular response is the most common arrhythmia in valvular heart disease. Prevention by quinidine therapy; control of the rapid ventricular rate by digitalis and reversion to normal sinus rhythm by electric cardioversion are all effective.

Conduction delays in the AV node and ventricular conduction system are common in aortic stenosis but uncommonly require treatment.

Many arrhythmias in valvular dis-

ease are related to excessive digitalis therapy in the presence of reduced intracellular potassium associated with diuretic therapy.

CONGESTIVE HEART FAILURE

Treatment of congestive heart failure is directed toward restoration of a compensated hemodynamic state which provides relief of symptoms and improvement in function but usually no change in the underlying anatomic lesion. The major implements of treatment are digitalis, which improves myocardial contractile function, and diuretics, which reduce blood volume and, hence, ventricular volumes and pressure with restoration of contractile and geometric integrity of the cardiac chambers. Potent oral diuretic agents, furosemide and ethacrynic acid have made treatment of congestive heart failure more effective. Hazards of digitalis therapy include cardiac arrhythmias and gastrointestinal disturbances. Hazards of diuretic therapy include hypovolemia, hypokalemia and drug idiosyncrasies.

COMPLICATIONS OF VALVULAR DISEASE

Systemic arterial emboli occur with significant frequency in patients with mitral valvular disease. Left atrial thrombi are present in one half of those with mitral stenosis and atrial fibrillation.[87] Anticoagulant therapy should be considered in patients who have suffered an arterial embolus.

Pulmonary embolus is a frequent complication in patients with right ventricular failure and elevated venous pressures. Physical inactivity and peripheral venous stasis predispose to this complication. Pulmonary embolus may be a cause of cardiac decompensation in a previously stable patient. Anticoagulant therapy should be considered following pulmonary emboli in patients with valvular heart disease.

Bacterial endocarditis occurs almost exclusively in the presence of previous valvular damage. Treatment should be based upon specific antibiotic sensitivities, with high dose parenteral therapy given. Emergent surgical replacement of the affected valve may be necessary if the hemodynamic lesion is sudden, massive and poorly tolerated.

Hemolytic anemia due to red blood cell destruction provoked by the trauma of the blood turbulence of a valvular lesion may be present. This complication is most prevalent with aortic disease but is more evident with prosthetic cardia valves.[88] Treatment with folic acid and iron may allow compensation for the red cell loss by the bone marrow.

SURGICAL THERAPY[89]

Successful palliative correction of congenital and acquired valvular lesions was initiated by Bailey and Harken.[90, 91] With the development of a clinically useful pump oxygenator (heart-lung machine) by Gibbon and De Wall, intracardiac lesions were approached by various surgical techniques.[92]

In summary, surgical correction of valvular lesions is recommended when the possibility of improvement warrants the risk of the surgical procedure. It is essential to take into consideration the late complications of valvular surgery because deaths resulting from this appear to equal or exceed in number the early and operative deaths (see Table 14-3).

"Closed" procedures are done primarily on the mitral valve and do not involve the use of cardiopulmonary bypass. "Open" procedures are done with full exposure of the intracardiac structure while the patient is supported by cardiopulmonary bypass.

MITRAL STENOSIS

Operations for mitral stenosis include closed commissurotomy,[93, 94] open commissurotomy and valve replacement.[95]

Closed commissurotomy is currently recommended for patients with mitral stenosis who have no or insignificant mitral regurgitation, a mobile mitral valve and no demonstrable valvular calcification. Fracture of the fused mitral commissures is accomplished by a metal dilator introduced through the left ventricle and guided into position by a finger placed in the left atrial appendage. This therapy is recommended for patients with American Heart Association Class II limitation. It has been found to be a safe and effective procedure for the prevention of disability, emboli and arrhythmias due to mitral stenosis.

Recurrence or re-stenosis may occur in 5 to 15 years and requires further operative therapy.

Prosthetic replacement of the mitral valve during cardiopulmonary bypass is now offered to patients who have Class III or IV symptoms by American Heart Association criteria.[96, 97, 98] Technical indications for replacement include immobility and destruction of the valve tissue, significant calcification and associated mitral regurgitation. The surgical mortality rate is 25 per cent if both early and late deaths are included.

MITRAL REGURGITATION

Mitral insufficiency of a degree to produce clinical Class III status may

Table 14-3.   *CURRENT STATUS OF VALVULAR SURGERY*

VALVULAR LESION	AHA CLINICAL CLASS	OPERATIVE PROCEDURE	MORTALITY EARLY AND LATE (PER CENT)
Simple MS	II-III	Open or Closed Commissurotomy	5
Simple MS	IV	Open or Closed Commissurotomy	15
Complex MS	III-IV	Open Commissurotomy	10
Complex MS	III-IV	Open Replacement	25
Simple MR	II-III	Open Repair or Replacement	10
Complex MR	III-IV	Open Replacement	25
Aortic Stenosis	III-IV	Open Replacement	25
Aortic Insufficiency	III-IV	Open Replacement	25
Combined aortic and mitral	III-IV	Open Replacement	40
Combined aortic, mitral and tricuspid	III-IV	Open Replacement	40

Simple MS	— Isolated mitral stenosis without significant valve immobility or calcification.
Complex MS	— Mitral stenosis with associated regurgitation, valvular immobility or calcification.
Simple MR	— Isolated mitral regurgitation due to torn valve, ruptured chordae tendineae or papillary muscle.
Complex MR	— Mitral regurgitation with associated valve deformity.
Combined aortic and mitral	— Replacement and/or repair of aortic and mitral valves.
Combined aortic, mitral and tricuspid	— Replacement and/or repair of aortic and mitral and tricuspid valves.

be repaired by annuloplasty or prosthetic valve replacement during cardiopulmonary bypass. Those patients with acute mitral regurgitation due to ruptured chordae tendinae have an excellent prognosis whether treated by valve replacement[99] or annuloplasty[100] and may be offered operative treatment at an earlier clinical stage.

Valve replacement in chronic mitral insufficiency appears to have operative results similar to valve replacement in mitral stenosis.[96, 97, 98]

AORTIC STENOSIS

The operation of choice for aortic stenosis is prosthetic replacement of the diseased valve by either a synthetic valve[55, 69] or a homograft transplant.[101] Operative therapy is generally offered to any patient with angina pectoris, syncope or congestive heart failure thought due to aortic stenosis.

Operative mortality for isolated aortic valve replacement is about 30 per cent if both early and late deaths in large series are considered.[55, 97, 98]

AORTIC INSUFFICIENCY

Replacement of the aortic valve by a prosthetic valve or homograft transplant is also the surgical method of choice in treatment of aortic insufficiency. The appropriate timing of this operation is difficult. Many patients with this disorder do well for many years, however, a down hill clinical course is heralded by the onset of mitral regurgitation due to annular dilatation or of atrial fibrillation usually associated with distention of the left atrium.

Emergent valve replacement in aortic insufficiency due to bacterial infection, aortic dissection or trauma is clearly the treatment of choice in those patients whose heart failure cannot be managed by medical therapy.

COMPLICATIONS OF CARDIAC SURGERY[92, 102]

Preoperatively, accurate anatomic and physiologic diagnosis is essential if the surgeon is to improve cardiac function the necessary 30 per cent required for the patient to survive surgical treatment. Aggressive management of heart failure, potassium depletion, infection and pulmonary disorders are included in the preoperative preparation.

Intraoperative errors in surgical and anesthetic techniques produce prolongation of the cardiopulmonary bypass time which produces morbidity and mortality. Systemic air or foreign body emboli also complicate recovery from open heart surgery. High profile prosthetic valves placed in the mitral area may obstruct the left ventricular outflow tract and produce an undesired result.

Early postoperative complications include (1) the low cardiac output syndrome with poor perfusion of brain, cardiac, hepatic, and renal tissue; (2) postoperative respiratory compromise and (3) acid-base abnormalities. Poor tissue perfusion leads to loss of cerebral function with prolonged coma, acute brain syndrome, localizing neurological deficits or psychiatric abnormalities as the presenting patient state. Poor hepatic perfusion produces serum enzyme elevations, bleeding tendencies, jaundice and hepatic coma. Renal ischemia may be associated with acute tubular necrosis and renal failure. Treatment of the low perfusion syndrome by cardiotonic agents (digitalis and isoproterenol) and vasodilators (steroids and alpha adrenergic blocking agents) may prevent or reverse these changes.

The incidence of postoperative pulmonary insufficiency has been reduced by the use of hemodilution priming for cardiopulmonary bypass, reduction of bypass time and improved anesthetic management. Mechanical respirators and blood gas monitoring are essential to recovery.

Acid base abnormalities are usually due to the metabolic acidosis (elevated lactic and other organic acids) due to poor tissue perfusion or to a respiratory alkalosis associated with injudicious use of the artificial respirator. Congestive heart failure and cardiac arrhythmias are treated rigorously if present during the postoperative period.

Late complications of valvular surgery include (1) infections of the operative site and blood stream, (2) nonspecific febrile illnesses including postpericardiotomy syndrome[103] and postperfusion syndrome which is due to infection by cytomegalovirus given to the patients in blood transfusions,[104, 105] (3) serum hepatitis, (4) hemolytic anemia due to red blood cell trauma from the prosthetic valve,[88] (5) postoperative leaks around or through the prosthetic devise,[95, 97] (6) systemic emboli originating from a prosthetic valve and (7) structural deterioration of the prosthetic replacement.[106, 107]

All these complications necessarily add to the hazard of valvular surgery and should be taken into account prior to embarking on this type of treatment for valvular heart disease.

REFERENCES

1. GROSS, L. Lesions in the roots of the pulmonary artery and aorta in rheumatic fever. *Amer. J. Path.*, 11:631–646, 1935.
2. GROSS, L. Lesions of the left auricle in rheumatic fever. *Amer. J. Path.*, 11:711–735, 1935.
3. GROSS, L., and FRIEDBERG, C. K. Lesions of the cardiac valve rings in rheumatic fever. *Amer. J. Path.*, 12:469–493, 855–909, 1936.
4. WAGNER, B. M., and TEDESCHI, C. G. Studies in rheumatic fever. *Arch. Path.*, 60:423–430, 1955.

5. Lustok, M., and Kuzma, J. P. Rheumatic fever pneumonitis: A clinical and pathologic study of 35 cases. *Ann. Int. Med.*, 44:337–357, 1956.

6. McEwen, C. Cytologic studies on rheumatic fever. III. A comparison of cells of subcutaneous nodules from patients with rheumatic fever, rheumatoid arthritis and syphilis. *Arch. Path.*, 25:303–314, 1938.

7. Greenfield, J. G., and Wolfsohn, J. M. The pathology of Sydenham's chorea. *Lancet*, 2:603–606, 1922.

8. Catanzaro, F. J., Stetson, C. A., Morris, A. J., Chamovitz, R., Rammelkamp, C. H., Stolzer, B. L., and Perry, W. D. The role of the streptococcus in the pathogenesis of rheumatic fever. *Amer. J. Med.*, 17:749–756, 1954.

9. Denny, F. W., Wannamaker, L. W., Brink, W. R., Rammelkamp, C. H., and Custer, E. A. Prevention of rheumatic fever—treatment of the preceding streptococci infection. *J.A.M.A.*, 143:151–153, 1951.

10. Massell, B. F., and Jones, T. D. Some practical aspects of the rheumatic fever problem which have an important bearing in military service. *Amer. Heart J.*, 27:575–587, 1924.

11. Swift, H. F. Rheumatic heart disease–pathogenesis and etiology in their relation to therapy and prophylaxis. *Medicine*, 19:417–440, 1940.

12. Paul, J. R., and Dixon, G. L. Climate and rheumatic heart disease. *J.A.M.A.*, 108: 2096–2100, 1937.

13. Paul, J. R. *The Epidemiology of Rheumatic Fever and Some of Its Public Health Aspects*. 2nd Edition. New York, Am. Heart Assn., 1943.

14. Wheeler, S. M., and Jones, T. D. Factors in the control of the spread of acute respiratory infections with reference to streptococcal illness and acute rheumatic fever. *Amer. J. Med. Sci.*, 209:58–64, 1945.

15. Anderson, H. C., Kunkel, H. G., and McCarty, M. Quantitative antistreptokinase studies in patients infected with group A hemolytic streptococci: A comparison with serum antistreptolysin and gamma globulin levels with special reference to the occurrence of rheumatic fever. *J. Clin. Invest.*, 27:425–434, 1948.

16. Davelti, Philip, A. Autoimmunologic disease. *J. Allergy*, 26:95–106, 1955.

17. Kaplan, M. H., and Svec, K. Immunologic relation of streptococcal and tissue agents. III. Presence in human sera of streptococcal antibody cross-reactive with heart tissue. Association with streptococcal infection, rheumatic fever, and glomerulonephritis. *J. Exper. Med.*, 119:651–666, 1964.

18. Jones, T. D. The diagnosis of rheumatic fever. *J.A.M.A.*, 126:481–484, 1944.

19. American Heart Association: Report of Committee on Standards and Criteria for Programs of Care of the Council on Rheumatic Fever: Jones criteria (modified) for guidance in diagnosis of rheumatic fever. *Mod. Concepts Cardiovas. Dis.*, 24:291–293, 1955.

20. Stamler, J. Cardiovascular diseases in the United States. *Amer. J. Cardio.*, 10:319–340, 1962.

21. Bland, E. F., Jones, J. D. Rheumatic fever and rheumatic heart disease. *Circulation*, 4:836–843, 1951.

22. Feinstein, A. R., Stern, E. K., and Spagnuolo, J. The prognosis of acute rheumatic fever. *Amer. Heart J.*, 68:817–834, 1964.

23. Stollerman, G. H. Factors determining the attack rate of rheumatic fever. *J.A.M.A.*, 177:823–828, 1961.

24. Lendrum, B. L., Simon, A. J., Mack, I. Relation of duration of bed rest in acute rheumatic fever to heart disease present 2 to 14 years later. *Pediatrics*, 24:389–394, 1959.

25. Combined Rheumatic Fever Study Group: A comparison of the effect of prednisone and acetylsalicylic acid on the incidence of residual rheumatic heart disease. *New Eng. J. Med.*, 262:895–902, 1960.

26. Combined Rheumatic Fever Study Group, 1965: A comparison of short-term intensive prednisone and acetylsalicylic acid therapy in the treatment of acute rheumatic fever. *New Eng. J. Med.*, 272:63–70, 1965.

27. Joint Report of United Kingdom and United States: The natural history of rheumatic fever and rheumatic heart disease. Ten-year report of a cooperative clinical trial of ACTH, Cortisone, and aspirin. *Circulation*, 32:457–476, 1965.

28. Czoniczer, G., Amezcua, F., Pelargonio, S., and Massell, B. F.: Therapy of severe rheumatic carditis. Comparison of adrenocortical steroids and aspirin. *Circulation*, 29:813–819, 1964.

29. Committee Reports: Prevention of rheumatic fever. *Circulation*, 31:948–952, 1965.

30. Hawley, R., Dodge, H. T., and Graham, T. P. Left atrial volume and its changes in heart disease. *Circulation*, 34:989–996, 1966.

31. Murray, John A., Kennedy, J. Ward, and Figley, Melvin M. Quantitative angiocardiography II. The normal left atrial volume in man. *Circulation*, 37:800–804, 1968.

32. BRAUNWALD, E., and FRAKAM, C. J. Studies on Starlings law of the heart IV. Observations on the hemodynamic functions of the left atrium in man. *Circulation*, 24:633–642, 1961.

33. MARSHALL, R. J., and SHEPARD, J. T. Interpretation of changes in "central" blood volume and slope volume during exercise in man. *J. Clin. Invest.*, 40:375–385, 1961.

34. McGAFF, C. J., ROUETI, G. C., GLOSSMAN, E., and MILNAR, W. R. The pulmonary blood volume in rheumatic heart disease and its alteration by isoproterenol. *Circulation*, 27:77–84, 1963.

35. WADE, O. L., and BISHOP, J. M. *Cardiac Output and Regional Blood Flow*. Oxford, Blackwell Scientific Publications, 1962.

36. BLACKMON, J. R., ROWELL, LORING B., KENNEDY, J. WARD, TWISS, RICHARD D., and CONN, ROBERT D. Physiologic significance of maximal oxygen intake in "pure" mitral stenosis. *Circulation*, 36:497–510, 1967.

37. RALSTON, L. A., COBB, L. A., and BRUCE, R. A. Acute circulatory effects of arterial bleeding as determined by indicator-dilution curves in normal human subjects. *Amer. Heart J.*, 61:770–776, 1961.

38. CAMISHION, R. C. Paralysis of left recurrent laryngeal nerve secondary to mitral valve disease. *Ann. Surg.*, 163:818, 1966.

39. BRUCE, R. A., BLACKMON, J. R., JONES, J. W., and STRAIT, G. Exercise testing in adult normal subjects and cardiac patients. *Pediatrics*, 32:742, 1963.

40. GORLIN, R., and GORLIN, S. G. Hydraulic formula for calculation of the area of the stenotic mitral valve, other cardiac valves, and central circulatory shunts. *Amer. Heart J.*, 41:1–29, 1951.

41. BLACKMON, J. R. Unpublished Data.

42. RICHTER, H. S. Mitral valve area: Measurement soon after catheterization. *Circulation*, 28:451–454, 1963.

43. ROWE, J. C., BLAND, E. F., SPRAGUE, H. B., and WHITE, P. D. The course of mitral stenosis without surgery: Ten- and twenty-year perspectives. *Ann. Int. Med.*, 52:741–749, 1960.

44. OLESON, K. H. The natural history of 271 patients with mitral stenosis under medical treatment. *Brit. Heart J.*, 24:349–357, 1962.

45. BRENEMAN, G. M., and DRAKE, E. H. Ruptured papillary muscle following myocardial infarction with long survival. *Circulation*, 25:862–868, 1962.

46. PHILLIPS, J. H., BUICH, G. E., and DE PASQUALE, N. P. The syndrome of papillary muscle dysfunction: Its clinical recognition. *Ann. Int. Med.*, 59:508–520, 1963.

47. ROBERTS, W. C., BRAUNWALD, E., and MORROW, A. Acute severe mitral regurgitation secondary to ruptured chordae tendineae: Clinical, hemodynamic, and pathologic considerations. *Circulation*, 33:58–77, 1966.

48. MENGES, H., ANKENEY, J. L., and HELLERSTEIN, H. K. Clinical diagnosis and surgical management of ruptured mitral chordae tendineae. *Circulation*, 30:8–16, 1964.

49. WOOLEY, C. F., MOLNAR, W., HOSIER, D. M., SIRAK, H. D., and RYAN, J. M. Etiology of mitral regurgitation: Marfan's syndrome. *Circulation*, 32 (Suppl. II): 221–222, 1965.

50. BRAUNWALD, E., and AWE, W. C. The syndrome of severe mitral regurgitation with normal left atrial pressure. *Circulation*, 27:29–35, 1963.

51. LIU, C. K., PICCIRILLO, R. T., and ELLESTAD, M. Distensibility of the postmortem human left atrium in nonrheumatic and rheumatic heart disease. *Amer. J. Cardiol.*, 13:232–238, 1964.

52. GORLIN, R., LEWIS, B. M., HAYNES, F. W., and DEXTER, L. Studies of the circulatory dynamics at rest in mitral valvular regurgitation with and without stenosis. *Amer. Heart J.*, 43:357–394, 1952.

53. ROBERTS, W. C., and SJOERDSMA, A. The cardiac disease associated with the carcinoid syndrome (carcinoid heart disease). *Amer. J. Med.*, 36:5–34, 1964.

54. KARSNER, H. T., and KOLETSKY, S. *Calcific Disease of the Aortic Valve*. Philadelphia, J. B. Lippincott Co., 1947.

55. MORROW, A. G., ROBERTS, W. C., ROSS, J. JR., FISHER, R. D., BEHRENDT, D. M., MASON, D. T., and BRAUNWALD, E. Obstruction of left ventricular outflow. *Ann. Intern. Med.*, 69:1255–1286, 1968.

56. BRAUNWALD, E., LAMBREAU, C. T., ROCKOFF, S. D., ROSS, J. JR., MORROW, A. G., and PIERCE, G. E. Idiopathic hypertrophic subaortic stenosis. *Circulation*, 30 (Suppl. IV):63–119, 1964.

57. COHEN, J., EFFAT, H., GOODWIN, J. F., OAKLEY, C. M., and STEINER, R. E. Hypertrophic obstructive cardiomyopathy. *Brit. Heart J.*, 26:16–32, 1964.

58. BEUREN, A. J., SCHULZE, C., EBERLE, P., HARMJANZ, D., and APITZ, J. The syndrome of supravalvular aortic stenosis, peripheral pulmonary stenosis, mental retardation and similar facial appearance. *Amer. J. Cardiol.*, 13:471–483, 1964.

59. BLACK, J. A., and CARTER, R. E. B. Association between aortic stenosis and facies of severe infantile hypercalcemia. *Lancet*, 2:745–758, 1963.

60. LOGAN, W. F. W. E., JONES, E., WYN, W. E., COULSHED, N., and EPSTEIN, E. J.

Familial supravalvar aortic stenosis. *Brit. Heart J.*, 27:547–559, 1965.

61. HASTREITER, A. R., OSHIMA, M., MILLER, R. A., LEV, M., and PAUL, M. H. Congenital aortic stenosis syndrome in infancy. *Circulation*, 28:1084–1095, 1963.

62. SPENCER, M., and EDMUNDS, L. H., JR. Evaluation of operative left ventricular outflow tract lesions with a fluid impedance plot. *Circulation*, 37:912–921, 1968.

63. KENNEDY, J. W., TWISS, R. D., BLACKMON, J. R., and MERENDINO, K. A. Hemodynamic studies one year after homograft aortic valve replacement. *Circulation*, 37–38 (Suppl. II): 110–118, 1968.

64. KENNEDY, J. W., TWISS, R. D., BLACKMON, J. R., and DODGE, H. T. Quantitative angiocardiography III: Relationships of left ventricular pressure, volume, and mass in aortic valve disease. *Circulation*, 38:838–845, 1968.

65. WAGNER, H. R., HUGENHOLTZ, P. G., and SANDLER, H. Congenital aortic stenosis compensating mechanisms in pure pressure overload. *Circulation*, 37–38 (Suppl. VI):199, 1968.

66. ROWE, G. C., AFONSO, S., LUGO, J. E., CASTILLO, C. A., BOAKE, W. C., and CRUMPTON, C. W. Coronary blood flow and myocardial oxidative metabolism at rest and during exercise in subjects with severe aortic valve disease. *Circulation*, 32:251–257, 1965.

67. OLESON, K. H., and WARBURG, E. Isolated aortic stenosis — The late prognosis. *Acta Med. Scan.*, 160:437, 1958.

68. MITCHELL, A. M., SACKETT, C. H., HUNZICKER, W. J., and LEVINE, S. A. The clinical features of aortic stenosis. *Amer. Heart J.*, 48:684, 1954.

69. CULLHED, I. *Aortic Stenosis*. Upsula, Almquist and Wiksell, 1964.

70. BRAUNWALD, E., BOLDBLATT, A., AYGEN, M. M., ROCKOFF, S. D., and MORROW, A. G. Congenital aortic stenosis. *Circulation*, 27:426–462, 1963.

71. KLATTE, E. D., TAPAS, J. P., CAMPBELL, J. A., and LURIE, P. R. The roentgenographic manifestations of aortic stenosis and aortic valvular insufficiency *Amer. J. Roent.*, 88:57–69, 1962.

72. EDWARDS, J. E. Pathologic aspects of cardiac valvular insufficiencies. *A.M.A. Arch. Surg.*, 77:634–649, 1958.

73. LEVINE, R. J., ROBERTS, W. C., and MORROW, A. G. Traumatic aortic regurgitation. *Amer. J. Cardiol.*, 10:752–763, 1962.

74. LEVY, M. J., SIEGAL, D. L., WANY, Y., and EDWARDS, J. E. Rupture of aortic valve secondary to aneurysm of ascending aorta. *Circulation*, 27:422–425, 1963.

75. LEWIS, M. G. Idiopathic medionecrosis causing aortic incompetence. *Brit. Med. J.*, 1:1478, 1965.

76. SINCLAIR, R. J. G., KITVHIN, A. H., and TURNER, R. W. D. The Marfan syndrome. *Quart. J. Med.*, 29:19–46, 1960.

77. CLARK, W. S., KULKA, J. P., and BAUER, W. Rheumatoid aortitis with aortic regurgitation. *Amer. J. Med.*, 22:580–592, 1957.

78. CSONKA, G. W., LITCHFIELD, J. W., OATES, J. K., and WILLCOX, R. R. Cardiac lesions in Reiter's disease. *Brit. Med. J.*, 1:243, 1961.

79. BARRETT, J. S., HELWIG, J., JR., KAY, C. F., and JOHNSON, J. Cine-aortographic evaluation of aortic insufficiency. *Ann. Int. Med.*, 61:1071–1083, 1964.

80. STAPLETON, J. F., and HARVEY, W. P. Aortic incompetence — A clinical analysis. *Postgrad. Medicine*, 46:156–165, 1969.

81. BRAWLEY, R. K., and MORROW, A. G. Direct determinations of aortic blood flow in patients with aortic regurgitation: Effects of alterations in heart rate, increased ventricular preload or afterload, and isoproterenol. *Circulation*, 35:32–45, 1967.

82. SANDLER, H., and DODGE, H. T. Left ventricular tension and stress in man. *Circulat. Res.*, 13:91–104, 1963.

83. HOOD, W. P., RACKLEY, C. E., and ROLETT, E. L. Wall stress in the normal and hypertrophied human left ventricle. *Amer. J. Cardiol.* 22:550–558, 1968.

84. BRAUNWALD, E., ROSS, J. JR., GAULT, J. H., MASON, D. T., MILLS, C., GABE, I. T., and EPSTEIN, S. E. Assessment of cardiac function. *Ann. Int. Med.*, 70:369–399, 1969.

85. FRANK, M. J., CASANEGRA, P. M., ANGELO, J., and LEVINSON, G. E. The clinical evaluation of aortic regurgitation. *Arch. Int. Med.*, 116:357–365, 1965.

86. FEINSTEIN, A. R., WOOD, H. F., SPAGNUOLO, M., TARANTA, A., JONAS, S., KLEINBERG, E., and TURSKY, E. Rheumatic fever in children and adolescents. *Ann. Int. Med.*, 60 (Suppl. V):87–123, 1964.

87. FISHER, D. L., BRENT, L. B., KENT, E. M., and MAGOVERN, G. J. Preoperative detection of atrial thrombi by selective left atriography. *J. Thor. Cardiov. Surg.*, 50: 473–481, 1965.

88. BRODEUR, M. T. H., SUTHERLAND, D. W., KOLER, R. D., STARR, A., KIMSEY, J. A., and GRISWOLD, H. E. Red blood cell survival in patients with aortic valvular disease and ball-valve prostheses. *Circulation*, 32:570–581, 1965.

89. DEXTER, L., and WERKO, L. (Eds.). Evaluation of results of cardiac surgery. *Circulation*, 37–38 (Suppl. V), 1968.

90. BAILEY, C. P., GLOVER, R. P., and O'NEILL, T. J. E. The surgery of mitral stenosis. *J. Thor. Surg.*, 19:16–49, 1950.

91. HARKEN, D. E., ELLIS, L. B., WARE, P.

F., and NORMAN, L. R. Surgical treatment of mitral stenosis I. Valvuloplasty.
New Eng. J. Med., 239:801–809, 1948.

92. NORMAN, J. C. *Cardiac Surgery.* New York,
Meredith Publishing Co., 1967.

93. ELLIS, L. B., and HARKEN, D. E. Closed
valvuloplasty for mitral stenosis. *New
Eng. J. Med.*, 270:643–650, 1964.

94. HOEKSEMA, T., WALLACE, R. B., and
KIRKLIN, J. W. Closed mitral commissurotomy. *Amer. J. Cardiol.* 17:825–828,
1966.

95. MORROW, A. G., HARRISON, D. C., ROSS,
J., JR., BRAUNWALD, N. S., CLARK, W. D.,
and ROSS, R. S. The surgical management of mitral valve disease: A symposium on diagnostic methods, operative
techniques and results. *Ann. Int. Med.*,
60:1073–1100, 1964.

96. MORROW, A. G., OLDHAM, H. N., ELKINS,
R. C., and BRAUNWALD, E. Prosthetic replacement of the mitral valve. *Circulation*, 35:962–989, 1967.

97. BIGELOW, J. C., HERR, R. H., WOOD, J. A.,
and STARR, A. Multiple valve replacement. *Circulation*, 38:656–663, 1968.

98. BEALL, A. C., JR., BLOODWELL, R. D.,
BRICKER, D. L., OKIES, J. E., COOLEY,
D. A., and DEBAKEY, M. E. Prosthetic
replacement of cardiac valves. *Amer. J.
Cardiol.* 23:250–257, 1969.

99. KLUGHAUPT, M., FLAMM, M. D., HAN-
COCK, E. W., and HARRISON, D. C. Non-

rheumatic mitral insufficiency. *Circulation*, 39:307–316, 1969.

100. HESSEL, E. A., II, KENNEDY, J. W., and
MERENDINO, K. A. A reappraisal of non-
prosthetic reconstructive surgery of mitral regurgitation based on an analysis of
early and late results. *J. Thor. Cardiov.
Surg.*, 52:193–206, 1966.

101. BARRATT-BOYES, B. G. Homograft replacement for aortic valve disease. *Mod. Conc.
Cardiovascu. Dis.*, 36:1–6, 1967.

102. ROSKY, L. P., and RODMAN, T. Medical
aspects of open heart surgery. *New Eng.
J. Med.*, 274:833–893, 1966.

103. URICCHIO, J. F. Postcommissurotomy
(postpericardiotomy) syndrome. *Amer. J.
Cardiol.*, 12:436–438, 1963.

104. REYMAN, T. A. Postperfusion syndrome.
Amer. Heart J., 72:116–123, 1966.

105. LANG, D. J., and HANSHAW, J. B. Cytomegalovirus infection and the postperfusion syndrome. *New Eng. J. Med.*, 280:
1145–1149, 1969.

106. DUVOISIN, G. E., WALLACE, R. B., ELLIS,
F. H., ANDERSON, M. W., and MCGOON,
D. C. Late results of cardiac valve re-
placement. *Circulation*, 37–38 (Suppl.
II):75, 1968.

107. HYLEN, J. C., KLOSTER, F. E., HERR, R. H.,
STARR, A., and GRISWOLD, H. Sound
spectrographic diagnosis of aortic ball
variance. *Circulation*, 37–38 (Suppl. VI):
105, 1968.

CHAPTER 15

THE CARDIAC RESERVE AND CONGESTIVE HEART FAILURE

The cardiovascular system is designed to meet the widely varying metabolic requirements of the body, shifting blood flow patterns to favor one set of tissues or another as they serve various bodily activities. However, the total sustained blood flow through the system in normal individuals can be increased by three- to five-fold above the resting values, depending on the state of physical fitness. When an individual develops heart disease, the maximal cardiac output he can sustain is usually curtailed, because reserve capacity of his cardiovascular system is being utilized to make up the deficit imposed by disease even during routine activity. Thus, the attributes of the various components of the cardiovascular reserve are very important in understanding the functional response to heart disease.

The cardiac reserve will be considered in terms of six factors: (a) the venous oxygen reserve, (b) the maximum effective heart rate, (c) the stroke volume reserve, (d) the work of the heart, (e) the coronary vascular reserve and (f) cardiac enlargement. Particular attention will be directed to the limitations in each factor.

I. THE CARDIOVASCULAR RESERVE CAPACITY

The reserve capacity of the cardiovascular system is most sorely taxed during physical exercise. The severity of the exercise that can be performed over any extended period of time apparently is limited by the maximal capacity of the cardiovascular system to deliver oxygen to the tissues because it is this substance which is stored in the least quantity in relation to its utilization rate. The quantity of oxygen consumed by the tissues is limited by the cardiac output and the amount of oxygen extracted from each increment of blood. In other words, the oxygen available to the tissues depends upon the cardiac output (blood flow per unit time) and magni-

506

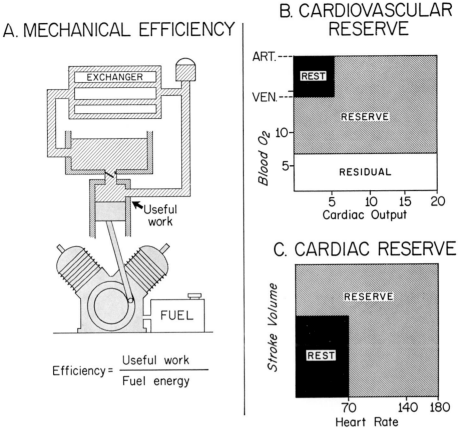

FIGURE 15-1   PUMPING INSUFFICIENCY AND RESERVE

A, The useful mechanical work of a pump in a hydraulic system takes the form of propelling fluid onward against a pressure head. The efficiency is determined by the useful work per unit of fuel consumption.

B, The oxygen delivery to the tissues at rest is determined by the product of the A-V oxygen difference and the cardiac output (black area). The maximum oxygen delivery is achieved by greater oxygen extraction and increased cardiac output (hatched area), corresponding to the cardiovascular reserve for oxygen delivery. Residual oxygen remains in the mixed venous blood even at maximal levels of oxygen transport.

C, Cardiac reserve refers to the extent to which cardiac output can be increased by greater stroke volume and acceleration of the heart rate (hatched area). Note that the heart rate is increased to greater extent than the stroke volume (see Figure 15-2).

tude of the arteriovenous oxygen difference.

The manner in which these factors are related can be represented by a mechanical pumping system (Fig. 15-1A). Under basal conditions, the quantity of fluid pumped through the system is determined by the stroke volume and the number of strokes per minute (rate). A mechanical pump generally ejects a fixed volume during each cycle, but the stroke volume of the ventricles may be increased over a two-fold range. The total quantity of material delivered from the exchanger in the mechanical system is determined by the total flow each minute and the amount extracted from each unit of fluid passing through the exchanger. Similarly, the oxygen delivery to the tissues at rest is represented by a rectangular area, which is the product of the blood flow (cardiac output) and the oxygen extracted from each increment of blood. Thus, 250 cc. of oxygen would be delivered by a systemic flow of 5 liters of blood with each liter giving up 50 cc. of oxygen. This is equivalent to an arteriovenous oxygen difference of 5 cc. per 100 cc. of blood or 5 volumes per cent (Fig. 15–1B). Theoretically, extraction of a large quantity of oxygen from the blood and a simultaneous five-fold increase in the cardiac output can increase the maximum oxygen delivery by as much as ten-fold (cross-hatched area).

In traditional concepts, the increased oxygen consumption during strenuous exercise was attributed to almost equal contributions by each of the three major mechanisms: stroke volume, heart rate and oxygen extraction. However, in dogs exercising on a treadmill, only a slight change in stroke volume was indicated by direct recordings of left ventricular length, circumference or diameter. This observation led to a re-examination of the relative contributions of these three factors,[1, 2] by compiling data reported by various investigators as collected during various levels of exercise by normal human subjects participating in ten series of experiments (Fig. 15–2).

The results of this compilation (Fig. 15–2) confirmed the impressions derived from the studies on dogs that stroke volume changed but little over a wide range of exercise from minimal to fairly heavy, but the magnitude of the change in stroke volume was highly dependent upon whether supine or erect control values were utilized in the comparison. It also set off a controversy based on different interpretations of similar data. As noted in Chap-

ter 7, the ventricular dimensions are at or near maximal when dogs or men are relaxed and recumbent. When the subject stands at rest, the stroke volume is diminished by some 20 to 30 per cent and the reduction in cardiac output is determined by the degree of tachycardia which may appear. It has been demonstrated[4] that absolutely minimal activity in the erect position (i.e., alternately lifting the feet a couple of inches off the floor) was accompanied by prompt increase in stroke volume from the lower erect resting control to a level approximating the recumbent control. An increase in the level of exercise above that level was accompanied by either slight increase or slight decrease in stroke volume, dependent largely upon the degree of tachycardia in the different subjects. The heart rate increases progressively with increasing exertion and oxygen consumption (Fig. 15–2D) up to levels ranging between 180 and 200 beats/ min. At extremely severe exertion, which may be sustained only for a few minutes by healthy subjects, the heart rate levels off and the stroke volume may show a substantial increase. The rise in stroke volume to the peak values at maximal exercise may represent an increase of 2 to 2½ times over the erect control values. Chapman et al.[3] laid particular emphasis on these more extreme values and concluded that increasing exertion was associated with progressively increasing stroke volume. However, over a wide range of exertion from minimal to heavy, the stroke volume tends to be surprisingly constant and highly dependent upon the compensatory changes in heart rate.[4]

The relationships displayed in Figure 15–2 are applicable to average normal persons. Among patients in whom the increase in heart rate is

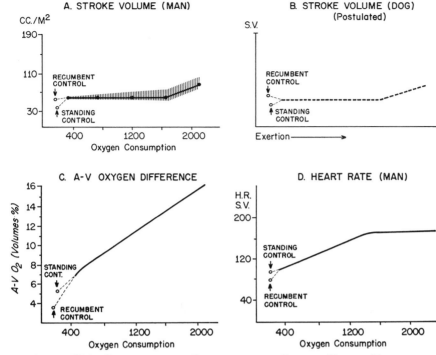

FIGURE 15-2 UTILIZATION OF CARDIOVASCULAR RESERVE DURING EXERTION

A, In normal human subjects, the mean values for stroke volume remain remarkably constant over a very wide range of exertion, from marking time to running on a treadmill. In some series the stroke volume appears to remain constant over an extended range of exertion and, in others, the stroke volume increases on the average about 10 per cent. Included in these data are individuals whose stroke volume actually diminished as exercise became more severe. At maximum levels of exertion the stroke volume unquestionably tends to increase as the heart rate levels off.

B, Available evidence suggests that the stroke volume increases little or not at all in dogs over wide ranges of exertion. It is postulated that stroke volume increases at the maximum levels of exertion as in man.

C, The oxygen extraction increases progressively during exertion up to the maximum that can be sustained for even brief periods (i.e., 2½ minutes).

D, The heart accelerates progressively up to about 180/min. where it tends to level off as the oxygen consumption continues to rise.

limited during exertion, the stroke volume unquestionably contributes more to the greater cardiac output during exercise. Thus, patients with abnormal conduction and atrioventricular block have a slow, constant heart rate and unquestionably achieve a greater cardiac output by greater stroke volume. When Warner et al.[5] controlled the heart rate of exercising dogs, the cardiac output was increased to a nor-

mal degree by increased stroke volume. Many trained athletes have slow heart rates at rest (as low as 50 to 60 beats a minute) and display much less tachycardia during exertion than do untrained individuals under the same conditions. This bradycardia is more commonly associated with training for long distance events than that for sprints and appears to be a response to long-sustained demands for increased cardiac output. In the same way, increased stroke volume is the typical response to sustained volume loads induced by various disease states (see later discussion).

The arteriovenous oxygen difference apparently increased progressively over the full range of oxygen consumption in Figure 15–2C. This results from a greater oxygen extraction from blood flowing rapidly through actively contracting muscle and also from blood flowing slowly through other inactive tissues where compensatory vasoconstriction has occurred (see Chapter 4). The oxygen extraction increases progressively with greater work loads, and at maximal levels of exertion some 75 per cent of the oxygen is removed from the blood passing through the systemic capillaries. The venous oxygen reserve can be depleted this completely only if oxygen extraction increases in both active and inactive tissues.

Venous Oxygen Reserve

It was pointed out in Chapter 1 that delivery of oxygen from the blood to the tissues depends upon a diffusion gradient determined by the differences in the partial pressures of oxygen in the blood and in the cell. If the cells become more active and take up oxygen at a more rapid rate, the lower end of this diffusion gradient will fall, the transfer of oxygen to the cells will be accelerated and more oxygen will be removed from the blood.

Each 100 cc. of arterial blood entering the capillary network contains approximately 19 cc. of oxygen. Different tissues extract different amounts of oxygen from the capillary blood. The amount of oxygen extracted from each increment of blood during its passage through the capillary networks

is determined by the relation between the oxygen consumption of a particular tissue and the volume flow of blood.

The oxygen consumption and blood flow in cerebral vessels is normally quite constant, so the oxygen extraction remains relatively fixed. The blood flow through the kidneys, skin and inactive muscle is so great in relation to oxygen consumption that large quantities of oxygen remain in the venous blood leaving these tissues. Indeed, most inactive tissues extract relatively little of the oxygen available in the arterial blood. In contrast, active skeletal muscle and the myocardium extract more than 75 per cent of the oxygen from the capillary blood. In fact the oxygen content of blood collected from the coronary sinus or from veins draining contracting skeletal muscle may have less than 1 ml. of oxygen in 100 ml. of blood and may even be too low to measure accurately. Vasoconstriction in inactive tissues would tend to shunt blood through the dilated capillary networks in the active muscles. During muscular exertion, blood flow may be diverted into active muscles from the skin, kidneys, gastrointestinal tract, spleen and so forth. These tissues then utilize more oxygen from the remaining blood flow at the expense of a moderate reduction in the oxygen tensions within the tissues. Thus, increased oxygen consumption characteristically causes an increased arteriovenous oxygen difference in both active and inactive tissues.

Maximum Effective Heart Rate

During sustained exercise, the heart responds to an increase in volume flow through the circulation with an acceleration of the heart rate, tachycardia. Tachycardia encroaches mainly

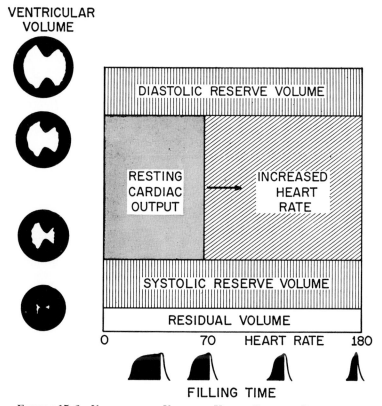

FIGURE 15–3   VENTRICULAR VOLUMES UNDER VARIOUS CONDITIONS

The normal resting cardiac output, about 5 liters per minute (dark stippled area) is the product of stroke volume (about 70 cc.) and heart rate (about 70 beats per minute). The cardiac output can increase maximally to about six times the resting value (total cross-hatched area) if heart rate and stroke volume increase simultaneously. Heart rate can increase to about 180 beats per minute, which would increase cardiac output two and a half times if the reduced filling time did not diminish stroke volume. Stroke volume can also increase through utilization of the systolic reserve and diastolic reserve volumes. The residual volume is the quantity of blood remaining in the ventricle after a maximal systolic ejection.

upon the interval of diastasis during which little or no filling occurs (see Fig. 15–3). The maximal effective increase in heart rate is approximately two and a half times (i.e., from a resting rate of about 70 beats per minute to levels of 170 to 180 beats per minute).[6] At faster heart rates, the rapid filling period is curtailed and the stroke volume tends to diminish. Tachycardia is very effective in rapidly increasing cardiac output in response to increased systemic blood flow, but it involves a sacrifice of efficiency in

both ventricular contraction and the diastolic filling. Further, an increase in cardiac output by extreme tachycardia probably interferes with coronary blood flow.

STROKE VOLUME RESERVE

The left ventricle functions at or near its maximal dimensions in relaxed, reclining dogs, and the stroke volume also approaches maximal levels under these conditions. However, in the change from the recum-

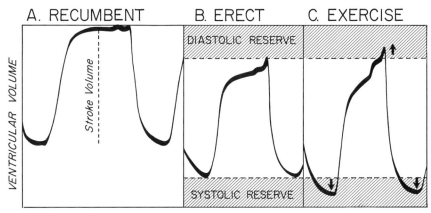

FIGURE 15–4   RESERVE STROKE VOLUME

Changes in ventricular volume are represented schematically. In the supine position, the diastolic volume is approximately maximal and the stroke volume is relatively large. On standing, diastolic ventricular volume and stroke volume diminish to provide potential diastolic and systolic reserve capacity. During exertion, any increase in stroke volume may be attained by either greater diastolic filling, more complete systolic ejection or both.

bent to the standing position, the ventricular dimensions diminish and the stroke deflection is also smaller (Fig. 15–4). Under these conditions, an increase in stroke volume can theoretically be achieved by an increase in diastolic distention, by greater systolic ejection or by augmentation of both.[7] In other words, the extent to which the ventricles can distend further represents a diastolic reserve capacity. The ability to increase the degree of ejection constitutes a systolic reserve capacity. These two reserves may be utilized to varying degrees in different animals or in the same animal on various occasions. Examples can be easily distinguished among the illustrations in Chapter 7.

At rest in the erect position, a stroke volume of about 80 cc. at a heart rate of 70 beats a minute will provide a cardiac output of 5600 cc. per minute. The heart rate may increase to about 180 beats a minute, and the stroke volume can increase by utilizing the diastolic and systolic reserve capacities. By these mechanisms, the cardiac output can be increased by five or six fold.

Systolic Reserve Volume. At the end of normal systolic ejections, considerable quantities of blood remain within the cardiac chambers. Attainment of increased stroke volume by utilization of the systolic reserve volume ordinarily implies an increased shortening of the myocardium.

Diastolic Reserve Volume. The magnitude of the diastolic filling is determined by the effective filling pressure in relation to the resistance to distention offered by the ventricular walls. Ventricular contraction beginning at a large diastolic size is favorably influenced by (a) a greater energy release (the Frank-Starling mechanism), (b) the large volume of blood ejected per unit of myocardial shortening and (c) reduced internal friction (viscosity) within the myocardium. On the other hand, the radii of the circles described by the myocardial fibers are increased and much greater myocardial tension is required to produce equivalent elevation of intraventricular pressure during ejection (according to the formula $P = T/R$). (The factors which determine the extent of diastolic distention have been discussed in detail in Chapter 3.) The heart appears to function with greater efficiency at a larger diastolic (and systolic) size. However, the question of efficiency must be considered in terms of the quantity of useful work performed in relation to the quantity of fuel consumed by the myocardium (oxygen utilization).

THE WORK OF THE HEART

In a mechanical pump, the useful work performed can be easily visualized in terms of the energy expended in propelling fluid through pipes (see Fig. 15–1A). It is common knowledge that only part of the energy released in a combustion engine is delivered as useful work. The remainder is wasted as heat, which is dissipated in many different ways. Thus, we speak of the efficiency of such an engine in terms of the relation between the energy supplied (fuel burned) and the useful external work accomplished. In such a hydraulic analogue, the work produced by the pump is directly limited by the rate at which fuel is supplied to the engine. Certain features of such a mechanical device are applicable to the functioning of the heart as a pump.

Energy produced by the oxidation of organic fuels such as glucose, glycogen or lactic acid is partly converted to mechanical energy during myocardial contraction. For purposes of discussion, the avenues of energy dissipation will be divided into two main categories: (a) useful work, expressed as the energy expended for ejection of blood under pressure into the arterial trunks, and (b) wasted energy, including all other avenues of energy dissipation.

Useful Work of the Heart. This work occurs during active ejection of blood from the ventricular chambers. No external work is accomplished by the ventricles during isovolumic contraction, isovolumic relaxation or diastole. During the ejection phase of ventricular contraction, blood is propelled into the root of the aorta. A major portion of the potential energy is stored as tension in the arterial walls. The kinetic energy imparted to the moving blood has been generally ignored on the basis of the widely quoted statement by Prec et al.[8] that it represents only about 0.25 to 2.0 per cent of the total useful work. Chapman[9] found that these estimates, based on average values, could be greatly underestimated. The kinetic energy is a greater proportion of the total useful work of the right ventricle because the potential energy is much less than in the left ventricle. The distinction between potential and kinetic energy is somewhat artificial because most of the potential energy is converted to kinetic energy in producing flow through the vascular elements. In other words, the arterial blood pressure produces flow through the circulatory bed, so the potential energy is converted into kinetic energy and then into heat due to friction. The total quantity of useful work accomplished by the heart is ultimately dissipated by frictional losses as the blood circulates except for the potential energy at the point of venous inflow into the next ventricle in the circuit. This energy is utilized to distend the ventricle during diastole.

Energy Waste During Ventricular Contraction. Such waste takes many forms. The metabolic activity required to maintain and repair the myocardial cells is essential for myocardial integrity but does not contribute to the circulation of the blood. The energy expended in the wave of excitation is in a similar category. However, these two processes dissipate negligible amounts of energy in comparison to other forms of energy waste associated with chemical reactions, the frictional heat produced by myocardial viscosity, turbulence in the blood and energy stored as interfascicular tension (Chapter 3). A major portion of both useful work and energy waste occurs during ventricular systole, illustrated schematically in Figure 15–5. As the useful work of the heart increases, the amount of energy waste usually increases simultaneously. Since the useful work of the heart is the only external evidence of energy dissipation, the large quantities of wasted energy are frequently overlooked, although they have considerable functional importance. The myocardium must release energy equal to both the "wasted energy" and the useful work. Enough oxygen must be delivered to the heart through coronary blood flow to meet this total energy expenditure. Some disease processes interfere with oxygen delivery to the myocardium (diseases of the coronary arteries, ventricular hypertrophy). Other types of heart disease reduce the efficiency with which the myocardium converts chemical energy into the mechanical energy of contraction.

Efficiency of Ventricular Energy Release. The efficiency of the ventricular myocardium may be defined as the relation of the quantity of useful work performed to the total energy expended. The total energy release can be estimated from the oxygen consumption of the myocardium by assuming that 2 kg.-m. of work are performed in the process of utilizing 1 cc. of oxygen. Coronary sinus catheterization is providing information on the efficiency of the left ventricular myocardium.[10, 11] Measurements of coronary blood flow, myocardial oxygen consumption and useful work of the left ventricle provide the necessary data for computing the efficiency of the left ventricular myocardium as indicated by the formula:

$$\text{Efficiency (\%)} = \frac{\text{Ventricular work}}{\text{(kg.-m./min.)}} \Big/ \frac{\text{Energy uptake}}{\text{(kg.-m./min.)}}$$

The efficiency of the normal left ventricle may improve during exercise when the increase in its useful work is more than the increase in myocardial oxygen consumption. On the other hand, in patients with congestive heart failure, the efficiency of left ventricular energy conversion is reduced at rest[10] and declines even further during exercise.

Energy Restoration in the Heart. Since cardiac activity cannot be interrupted for long intervals, the delivery of oxygen and metabolic fuels must be continuously maintained at levels commensurate with the energy released by the myocardium. The total energy released during systole must be restored during the succeeding diastolic interval. Oxygen and metabolic fuels are delivered to the myocardium by the coronary blood flow. After passing through the capillaries of the coronary system, the coronary venous blood of normal humans contains only about 3.9 to 6.9 cc. of oxygen per 100 cc. of blood. Such complete extraction of oxygen from coronary blood signifies that oxygen tension in the myocardial fibers is very low. In other words, the myocardium continuously operates in an environment with a very low partial pressure of oxygen. During exercise and other forms of stress, the oxygen extraction

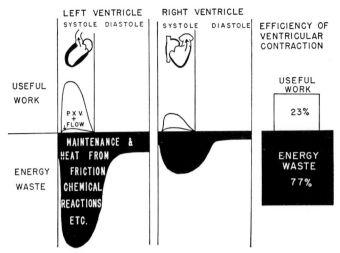

FIGURE 15-5   THE TOTAL WORK OF THE HEART

The useful work of the heart is the potential and kinetic energy imparted to the blood during the ejection phase of systole. The quantity of wasted energy exceeds the useful work by about fourfold, and is probably dissipated largely during systole. However, the exact time relations of this energy waste have never been described. The efficiency of myocardial contraction (useful work/total energy release) varies widely, but averages about 23 per cent.

is even more complete, so the oxygen tension immediately around the myocardial cells must be extremely low. Since the oxygen extraction from blood in the coronary vessels is so complete, the myocardium has little coronary venous oxygen reserve and must depend primarily upon an increase in coronary blood flow to supply increased demands. In this sense, the maximum sustained cardiac output is limited by the cardiac efficiency and the coronary blood supply.

CORONARY RESERVE CAPACITY

The total quantity of oxygen presented to the myocardium can be represented as a rectangular figure obtained as the product of coronary flow per unit time and the oxygen content of the arterial blood. The oxygen extraction at rest is the product of the coronary flow per unit time and the arteriovenous oxygen difference (black area in Fig. 15-6). An increase in oxygen delivery to the myocardium is attained primarily by greater coronary blood flow with little contribution by the venous oxygen reserve (see Fig. 15-6).

As in other tissues of the body, blood flow through the coronary vessels is increased primarily by reducing the resistance to flow through the small vessels. Diminished oxygen tension has a very powerful dilatory effect on the coronary vessels, which may automatically adjust coronary flow in relation to requirements. Other factors influencing coronary flow are presented in Chapter 9.

Acute changes in metabolism are accompanied by greater cardiac output, cardiac work and coronary oxygen delivery through the mechanisms indicated in Figures 15-1, 15-3, 15-5 and 15-6. Various disease states impose chronic loads on the heart for

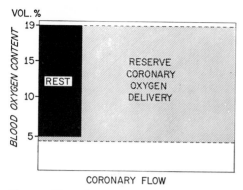

VOL. %

FIGURE 15-6   CORONARY RESERVE CAPACITY

Oxygen transport to the myocardium depends upon the coronary flow and the oxygen extraction from coronary blood (A-V oxygen difference). The coronary venous blood contains very little residual oxygen and increased oxygen delivery must be attained in direct proportion to the increase in coronary flow.

which the characteristic compensations are changes in the size of the ventricular chambers and the thickness of their walls.

CARDIAC ENLARGEMENT

As indicated in Chapter 2, the architecture of the right and left ventricles reflects the nature of the normal load which they sustain. The left ventricle is a roughly cylindrical cavity enclosed by a thick wall of myocardium, encircling the ventricle like a clenched fist. Such a chamber is ideally suited to develop high pressure for ejecting blood against high outflow pressure. In contrast, the right ventricular cavity is a relatively narrow crescentic space between two broad surfaces—the free wall and the interventricular septum. This chamber has a very large surface area which would necessitate great myocardial tension to develop high intraventricular pressures but which can readily

eject large volumes of blood against low outflow resistance. In the course of various disease processes, the right or left ventricle may be individually taxed by having to overcome higher outflow pressure or resistance (increased pressure load) or to pump larger volumes of blood continuously (increased volume load). Compensation to such chronic loads involves gross changes in the size and shape of the ventricles (Fig. 15–7).

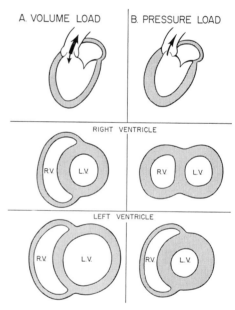

FIGURE 15–7   VENTRICULAR RESPONSES TO LOADS

A, The right ventricle is such an efficient volume pump that it can accommodate to an abnormal volume load with little change in chamber size or wall thickness, so long as the outflow pressure remains low. In contrast, the left ventricle accommodates to an increased volume load by distending to greater diastolic and systolic ventricular dimensions.

B, In response to a chronic pressure load, the right ventricle develops thick walls and a rounded contour; it assumes some of the characteristics of the normal left ventricle as it becomes a pressure pump. The left ventricle adjusts to a chronic pressure load by greater wall thickness, usually without much increase in diastolic ventricular volume.

II. VENTRICULAR VOLUMES AND MYOCARDIAL MASS IN PATIENTS WITH HEART DISEASE

by ROBERT D. CONN

In patients with heart disease clinicians have attempted to evaluate cardiac function using a variety of direct and indirect measurements acquired during cardiac catheterization. Cardiac enlargement, a reduced cardiac output, elevated arteriovenous oxygen difference, increased ventricular end diastolic pressure and alterations in the contractile state as measured by the rate of pressure rise (dp/dt) and ejection times have been used to characterize the hemodynamic alterations in patients with advanced heart disease. Basic to the understanding of many of these physiologic principles is accurate determinations of ventricular volumes. Until recently methods were not available for the determination of cardiac volumes either in the experimental situation or in patients, and assumptions regarding ventricular volumes were frequently drawn from the cardiac filling pressures. The development of angiographic techniques for the determination of ventricular volumes has permitted many correlations to be made between previously acquired physiologic data and the clinical physiology of patients with heart disease.

Left ventricular volumes have been determined by quantitative angiography in many forms of clinical heart disease.[12, 13, 14] Although there is still some argument as to the absolute validity of the method, the correlations between left ventricular volumes determined by angiographic methods and the volumes at postmortem examination are of enough similarity to permit physiological interpretation.[15-17]

Furthermore, this method permits the clinician to evaluate the functional derangements in valvular and congenital heart disease through the determination of total left ventricular stroke volume. By calculating the total ventricular stroke volume and comparing it with the forward cardiac output from the left ventricle as determined by the Fick or dye dilution methods, regurgitant volumes can be measured. In addition, the mass of the left ventricle can be determined by extrapolating wall thickness from the method for determining the end diastolic volume of that chamber.[16] The determination of left ventricular mass has in part clarified the relationship between hypertrophy and pressure and volume relationships in the left ventricle. Using the angiographic method the end diastolic volume, end systolic volume and mass of the left ventricle can be measured. From these relationships the total stroke volume of the left ventricle and ejection fraction (stroke volume/end diastolic volume) can be determined. Table 15–1 lists the typical values determined for each of these measurements for the normal left ventricle and for the left ventricle in patients with diseases primarily affecting that chamber.

In man with chronic disease of the left ventricle, the pathophysiologic processes usually involve alterations in the pressure-volume relationships of the chamber, abnormalities of the properties of contractility of the muscle or both. Cardiac dilatation (Frank-Starling mechanism) and cardiac hypertrophy may compensate for de-

Table 15-1.   VENTRICULAR VOLUMES DETERMINED BY QUANTITATIVE VOLUME ANGIOGRAPHY IN PATIENTS WITH HEART DISEASE

	END DIASTOLIC VOLUME M¹/M²	END SYSTOLIC VOLUME M¹/M²	LV STROKE VOLUME M¹/M²	LV EJECTION FRACTION SV/EDV	LV MASS (LVM) GM/M²	MASS-VOLUME RATIO LVM/EDV	END DIASTOLIC PRESSURE MM. HG
Normal	70	24	45	0.67	92	1.3	5–12
Aortic Regurgitation	Increased ×3	Increased ×3	Increased ×3	Normal	Increased ×3	Low ×0.8	Increased ×1.8
Aortic Stenosis	Normal	Normal	Normal	Normal	Increased ×2	Increased ×1.5	Increased ×1.5
Hypertrophic Subaortic Stenosis	Normal	Low ×0.8	Normal	Normal	Increased ×3	Increased ×2	Increased ×2
Mitral Regurgitation	Increased ×2	Increased ×2	Increased ×2	Normal	Increased ×2	Low ×0.8	Increased ×1.2
Mitral Stenosis	Normal	Normal	Normal	Normal	Normal	Normal	Normal
Myocardial Disease Primary or Secondary	Increased ×2	Increased ×2	Decreased	Decreased	Increased ×2	Variable	Variable
Constrictive Pericarditis	Decreased ×0.8	Decreased ×0.7	Normal	Normal or High ×1.2	Indeterminate	Indeterminate	High ×2

creased contractile force and increased mechanical loads. When these compensatory mechanisms are unable to sustain an adequate forward cardiac output, congestive heart failure may occur (see Part IV). On the other hand it is difficult to tell clinically when cardiac dilatation and ventricular hypertrophy are inappropriate as compensatory mechanisms. The inferences regarding ventricular function derived from indirect parameters, such as forward cardiac output, end diastolic pressure and dp/dt, can only be confirmed and corroborated by a knowledge of the volume and mass changes occurring in the diseased state in man.[18] Figure 15–8A shows the relationship between end diastolic volume and stroke volume. The close correlation between these parameters supports the Frank-Starling mechanism in the adjustment of ventricular function to volume overload. Figure 15–8B shows the relative unreliability of end diastolic pressure as an index of end diastolic volume. Figure 15–8C shows that dilatation of the heart is associated with ventricular hypertrophy and implies that chronic enlargement of ventricular volumes is probably always associated with hypertrophy.[18] However, in clinical circumstances of impedance to the flow from the left ventricle (aortic stenosis and IHSS) the degree of hypertrophy, as represented by the LV mass/end diastolic volume relationship differs from that of patients in whom volume alterations have occurred primarily (Table 15–1). Furthermore, the functional state (contractility) of the left ventricle can in general be related to the ejection fraction which represents the adequacy of the left ventricle as a pump. Although many other factors are involved in evaluating the muscle function of the left ventricle the con-

cept of the ejection fraction can be related to pump function in many clinical circumstances. Examples of the use of these data in patients with chronic heart disease are as follows.

LEFT VENTRICULAR VOLUME OVERLOAD

Patients with chronic aortic and mitral valve regurgitation have enlargement of end diastolic and end systolic volume proportionate to the degree of regurgitation, and compensatory mechanisms involve an increase in total left ventricular stroke volume and left ventricular hypertrophy as represented in Figures 15–9A and 15–9B. In the majority of patients with regurgitant lesions the systolic ejection fraction remains normal.[18] However, often only a fraction of the total left ventricular stroke volume is derived as useful cardiac output while the other fraction regurgitates into the left ventricle or left atrium. In Figures 15–9A and 15–9B the patients have all the usual parameters of heart failure: large volumes, some elevation of the end diastolic pressure, a low forward cardiac output and a widened arteriovenous oxygen difference. On the other hand, the contractility function of the ventricles is not grossly impaired since the ejection fraction continues to be in the normal range. Therefore the enlargement of the ventricular volumes cannot be interpreted per se as myocardial failure although the pathological state has resulted in alterations that clinically characterize heart failure.

Figure 15–9C indicates the typical hemodynamic and angiographic findings of a patient with valvular aortic stenosis. There is significant ventricular hypertrophy, and the left ventricular and diastolic pressures are ele-

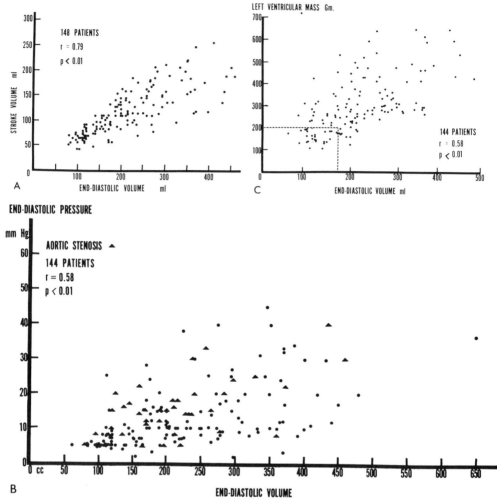

FIGURE 15–8 VENTRICULAR VOLUMES

From ventricular volumes calculated from biplane angiocardiograms the following graphs were constructed.

A, The stroke volume appears to be closely related to end-diastolic volume over a very wide range of values in patients with various forms of heart disease.

B, The end-diastolic volume is quite independent of end-diastolic pressure even when the ventricles are greatly dilated.

C, The end-diastolic volume and left ventricular mass (computed) are somewhat related as might be expected from the Laplace relation.

(After Dodge and Baxley.[18])

vated. The ventricle is hypertrophied without volume alterations giving a remarkably high mass-volume ratio. In spite of the hypertrophy, the ejection fraction remains normal and cardiac output is not compromised. End diastolic pressure in this instance does not accurately reflect end diastolic volume. The hypertrophy can best be considered as an appropriate compensatory mechanism, although at a later point in time "failure" might

A. Aortic regurgitation

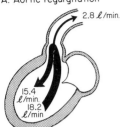

EDV   350 ml (234 ml/m²)
ESV   122 ml (81 ml/m²)
SV   228 ml (152 ml/m²)
Ejection fraction 65%

AVO difference 7.5 vol. %
End diastolic pressure 14 mm Hg
LV Mass 368 gm (245 gm/m)
Mass-Volume ratio 1.05

C. Aortic stenosis

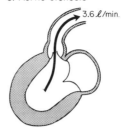

EDV   112 ml (75 ml/m²)
ESV   45 ml (30 ml/m²)
SV   68 ml (45 ml/m²)
Forward output 3.6 L/min

AVO difference 3.9 vol. %
End diastolic pressure 15 mm Hg
LV mass 246 gm (164 gm/m²)
Mass-Volume ratio 2.2

B. Mitral regurgitation

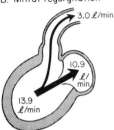

EDV   290 ml (194 ml/m²)
ESV   116 ml (77 ml/m²)
SV   174 ml (116 ml/m²)
Ejection fraction 60%

AVO difference 7.0 vol. %
End diastolic pressure 16 mm Hg
LV Mass 323 gm (215 gm/m²)
Mass-Volume ratio 0.9

D. Myocardial failure

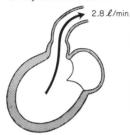

EDV   500 ml (333 ml/m²)
ESV   465 ml (310 ml/m²)
SV   35 ml (23 ml/m²)
Ejection fraction 11%

AVO difference 7.5 vol. %
End diastolic pressure 25 mm Hg
LV Mass 550 gm (367 gm/m²)
Mass-Volume ratio 1.1

FIGURE 15-9   LEFT VENTRICULAR VOLUME OVERLOAD

Representative cardiac catheterization and quantitative left ventricular angiographic data from typical patients with aortic regurgitation, mitral regurgitation, aortic stenosis and nonspecified myocardial failure. Heart rate is assumed to be 80 beats/min. and body surface area as 1.5 m². EDV–end diastolic volume, ESV–end systolic volume, SV–stroke volume, LV–left ventricular.

occur and be reflected by an increase in volume and mass and reduction in ejection fraction and cardiac output. Similar relationships have been noted in patients with idiopathic hypertrophic subaortic stenosis (IHSS), but the degree of hypertrophy of the left ventricular muscle is even greater in relation to the normal ventricular volumes, and the end diastolic pressure is elevated remarkably indicating significant alterations in the compliance of the left ventricle.[19]

LEFT VENTRICULAR MYOCARDIAL DISEASE

Figure 15-9D is representative of patients in whom the pump function of the left ventricle is impaired. Such alterations might be seen in patients with coronary artery disease, myo-

carditis or idiopathic myocardial hypertrophy or at the end stages of valvular heart disease. In addition to a reduced forward cardiac output and elevated filling pressures, the left ventricle is markedly dilated, and the ejection fraction significantly reduced. The low ejection fraction indicates excessive left ventricular dilatation relative to the stroke volume and signifies that the left ventricle has dilated to the point where the stroke volume is maintained primarily through the Frank-Starling mechanism. Thus, heart failure can be defined in patients with any form of left ventricular disease in terms of the useful work as evidenced by an adequate forward stroke volume and forward cardiac output and to some extent by the pressure-volume relationships. On the other hand, ventricular function can be further defined by relating the ejection fraction to the other hemodynamic alterations.

Oxygen Delivery to Hypertrophied Myocardial Fibers. Normal myocardial fibers range from 13 to 16 μ in diameter. Hypertrophied myocardial fibers may reach 25 to 32 μ in diameter but rarely exceed that value. The apparent limitation on hypertrophy of myocardial fibers has been attributed to retardation of oxygen delivery because of the greater diffusion distance to the center of the fibers.

The rate of diffusion through tissues varies as the square of the distance, which accounts for the prolongation of the time required for saturation of fibers with larger diameters. Harrison[20] reasoned that slower diffusion of oxygen to the center of hypertrophied myocardial fiber would prolong the recovery time required for the fiber to fully regain its energy-rich state. On this basis, the heart rate should be much slower when the ventricle is hypertrophied than when it is in the normal state. However, the heart rates in such patients are either normal or elevated, so the hypertrophic myocardium is probably suffering some degree of oxygen deficiency. This type of analysis indicates that the diameter of myocardial fibers rarely exceeds a value of 32 μ because the central core of larger myocardial fibers would not receive adequate oxygen (Fig. 15–10). At every turn we encounter examples which indicate that the rate of oxygen delivery to the myocardium limits the cardiac output while the maximum cardiac output limits the amount of physical exertion which can be sustained.

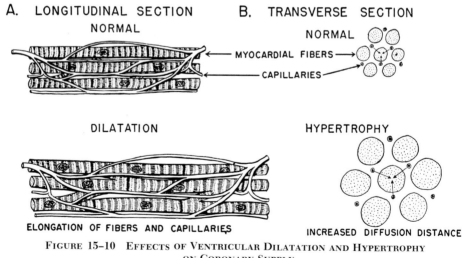

FIGURE 15–10   EFFECTS OF VENTRICULAR DILATATION AND HYPERTROPHY
ON CORONARY SUPPLY

A, Chronic ventricular dilatation involves elongation of both the myocardial fibers and the coronary capillaries. The mass of myocardial contractile units being supplied is greater and the distance traversed by the blood is increased. A greater proportion of oxygen in the blood is probably extracted under these conditions.

B, Ventricular hypertrophy is accomplished by proliferation of contractile units within the individual myocardial fibers. The distance of diffusion from the capillaries to the center of adjacent fibers is increased, retarding the exchange of various substances, particularly oxygen. The diameter of myocardial fibers rarely exceeds 32 μ even in extreme degrees of hypertrophy.

SUMMARY

In the normal individual, the cardiovascular reserve mechanism provides a prompt and effective response to widely varying demands for blood flow to provide oxygen and metabolic fuels, to dissipate heat, for digestion of food, for proper function of glands and excretory organs and for other essential functions. The maximum oxygen delivery to tissues depends upon four principal components of cardiovascular reserve: the venous oxygen reserve, the maximum cardiac output which can be sustained, the efficiency of myocardial energy release and the oxygen delivery to the myocardium. Depletion of any one of these components diminishes the total reserve, deleteriously affecting all other reserve factors. The various types of cardiac disease affect total cardiovascular reserve in different ways, but the end result is always some reduction in the total oxygen delivery to tissues which can be sustained during physical exertion. Thus, diminished exercise tolerance is a common denominator of cardiac disease.

III. COMPENSATION TO HEART DISEASE

Many patients with various forms of heart disease continue to lead relatively normal, moderately active lives for many years. Often individuals with functionally significant valvular disease live a normal life span. Their exercise tolerance may be reduced, but the average person rarely utilizes his maximal exertion capacity. Thus, patients can frequently live fairly normal lives in spite of restrictive forms of heart disease so long as they retain cardiovascular reserve capacity at rest. Under these conditions they can increase their level of activity by utilizing whatever reserve remains for them. Although a particular form of heart disease may directly deplete only one form of the cardiovascular reserve capacity, other reserve factors are generally affected to some degree. For this reason, all portions of the cardiovascular reserve should be kept in mind in evaluating the status of any patient with heart disease (see Fig. 15–11). These can be summarized as follows.

MAXIMUM OXYGEN TRANSPORT

The total oxygen delivery to the tissues of the body is determined by the average quantity of oxygen extracted from each increment of blood (mean arteriovenous oxygen difference) and the systemic blood flow (cardiac output). Thus, the total oxygen delivery can be represented by an area determined by the product of the cardiac output and the average oxygen extraction from the blood (Fig. 15–11A). The total oxygen delivery at rest amounts to about 250 cc. per minute (5 liters of blood per minute times 50 cc. of oxygen per liter). Tissues may be supplied with increased oxygen by greater cardiac output or by greater oxygen extraction from the blood. Since a number of vital tissues must be supplied with blood even though their oxygen extraction is relatively slight (kidneys, central nervous system and so forth), the mixed venous oxygen content rarely falls below some critical value. Thus, there is a

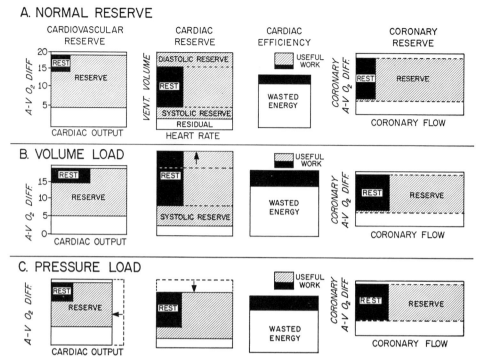

FIGURE 15–11   EFFECTS OF LOADS ON THE COMPONENTS OF CARDIOVASCULAR RESERVE

A, The components of cardiovascular reserve are dependent upon one another since cardiac reserve affects cardiovascular reserve. Cardiac efficiency and coronary reserve influence cardiac reserve.

B, In response to a volume load, the cardiac output at rest is increased leading to diminished efficiency. The coronary flow at rest is greater than normal so the reserve is reduced.

C, A pressure load ultimately tends to diminish the maximum cardiac output and stroke volume reserve. The work is increased without a corresponding increase in oxygen delivery. The coronary flow is increased to deliver the greater oxygen requirements.

minimal residual oxygen content of blood which is rarely encroached upon except in certain persons with severe cyanosis from congenital malformations of the heart (see Chapter 13). In such instances the tissues apparently accommodate to existence in an environment of very low oxygen tensions.

CARDIAC OUTPUT

The cardiac output is determined by the product of the stroke volume and the heart rate. At rest, a heart rate of slightly more than 70 beats per minute and a stroke volume of about

70 cc. of blood accounts for a cardiac output of about 5 liters per minute. The stroke volume may be increased by greater diastolic distention or by more complete systolic ejection (Figs. 15–3 and 15–11).

EFFICIENCY OF THE HEART AS A PUMP

The cardiac output represents only about 20 per cent of the total energy release, the remainder of the energy being wasted in the form of friction, lost in chemical reactions and so forth (Figs. 15–5 and 15–11). When cardiac output increases, the energy waste is also greater and may reach very large values during maximal effort.

Myocardial contraction represents the conversion of chemical energy into mechanical energy. During each cardiac cycle the contractile mechanisms must be restored to the high-energy, resting state. Obviously the total energy restoration must equal the total energy release over a period of time. In these circumstances the rate at which oxygen reaches the contractile units is a limiting factor in the process of attaining the high energy state.

TOTAL OXYGEN DELIVERY TO THE MYOCARDIUM

The oxygen delivery to the myocardium depends upon the same factors which determine oxygen delivery to the other tissues of the body, namely, the blood flow and the average quantity of oxygen removed from each increment of blood. The oxygen extraction from coronary blood is so great that little oxygen remains after the blood passes through the capillaries. For this reason, the principal mechanism for increasing oxygen delivery to the heart is increased coronary flow.

COMPENSATION FOR CHRONIC VOLUME AND PRESSURE LOADS

In response to a *chronic volume load*, the amounts of oxygen in the arterial and venous blood are normal, indicating that the venous oxygen reserve is not utilized at rest so long as the heart remains capable of fully compensating for the increased demands placed upon it (Fig. 15–11B). The quantity of blood ejected each minute is increased, so the cardiac reserve capacity is utilized to some extent

at rest. The heart rate is normal at rest indicating that the stroke volume at rest is greater than normal. In many cases, the discrepancy becomes larger with exercise. The increased stroke volume is associated with a distention of the heart such that the diastolic volume is larger than normal. The systolic ejection is greater, and there is a larger residual volume which cannot be utilized as a systolic reserve capacity. In this manner, a significant portion of the cardiac reserve is utilized at rest, but the ability to increase cardiac output through tachycardia tends to remain as a reserve to be employed during exertion.

In a purely physical sense, the quantity of blood being moved by the ventricle is increased so the useful work is augmented. From a functional point of view, the normal quantity of oxygen is delivered by an increased quantity of cardiac work. In this sense the efficiency of the cardiovascular system is diminished and the oxygen requirements of the myocardium are increased at rest and at all levels of exercise. The coronary oxygen delivery at rest must be increased to support this greater energy release. The coronary flow must be greater than normal at all times: thus, the coronary flow reserve capacity must be diminished. In this example, the reserve capacity of all components are adversely affected by the chronic volume load. The cardiovascular system cannot support the normal maximal oxygen delivery, and the exercise tolerance is less than normal.

Under the influence of a *chronic pressure load* (e.g., systemic arterial hypertension or aortic stenosis), cardiac output and the overall arteriovenous oxygen difference are both normal at rest. Superficially, the cardiac reserve appears to be entirely normal (Fig. 15–11C). However, the myocardium must develop a great deal more systolic tension to raise the intraventricular pressure to eject the normal complement of blood into the aorta. On this basis, the useful work of the heart is greatly increased at rest and the total energy expenditure much greater than normal at all levels of exercise. The mass of myocardial fibers is increased, so the oxygen delivery by coronary flow must be accelerated. Since the coronary flow reserve is partially utilized at rest, some decrease in exercise tolerance might well be expected. In the early stages of hypertension, the left ventricular cavity is not greatly enlarged so long as the coronary oxygen delivery is adequate to maintain function. In more advanced stages of hypertension, the left ventricle tends to distend and the myocardial fibers display patchy degeneration[22] as though the coronary supply were inadequate. Coronary insufficiency is probably the major factor in converting a fully compensated ventricle into a failing ventricle as described in Part IV.

SOME CONDITIONS WHICH LIMIT MAXIMAL OXYGEN TRANSPORT

A few specific clinical conditions have been selected to illustrate the relations between these various components of cardiovascular reserve. The primary effects are schematically illustrated in Figure 15–12 by altering the configuration of the graphs in Figure 15–11.

Anemia. If the hemoglobin concentration of the blood is diminished, the oxygen content of blood may be reduced from 20 volumes per cent to 12 volumes per cent. In the systemic capillaries, a smaller amount of oxygen is extracted from each 100 ml. increment of blood since the mixed venous oxygen content is not decreased be-

low some critical value. Thus, the principal adjustment to a reduced arteriovenous oxygen difference caused by anemia is an increase in the cardiac output (Fig. 15–12A). Since the cardiac output is increased at rest, the reserve is diminished and the maximal sustained increase in cardiac output is less than normal. The increased systemic flow is not as effective as normal oxygen extraction in supplying the tissue because of the reduced oxygen capacity of the blood. The arterial blood entering the coronary capillaries also carries a reduced quantity of oxygen, impairing the oxygenation of the myocardium. Further, cardiac acceleration is more pronounced with moderate exercise than normal. Thus, significant anemia deleteriously affects a number of components of cardiovascular reserve: oxygen transport, total energy release and total oxygen delivery to the myocardium.

Complete Atrioventricular Block. When the atrioventricular node blocks all impulses of atrial origin, a site in the ventricle usually assumes the role of pacemaker. It emits impulses at a slow but fairly constant rate of about 40 to 50 per minute even during exertion. Thus, the cardiac reserve is limited because the normal cardioacceleration does not occur in response to increased requirements for greater peripheral blood flow (Fig. 15–12B). As the heart rate is slower than normal, the stroke volume is excessive even with normal resting cardiac output. Thus, the stroke volume reserve is diminished and compensatory acceleration is abolished. With such extreme limitation in cardiac reserve, compensation to exertion must produce an abnormally increased arteriovenous oxygen difference in the peripheral blood. If the atrioventricular block persists, the ventricles often dilate

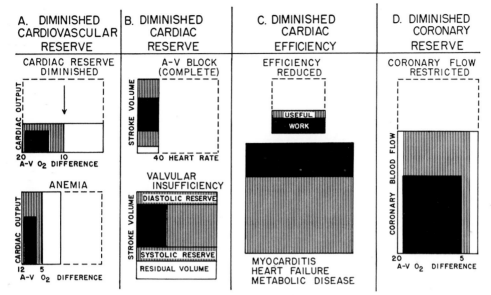

FIGURE 15-12   EFFECTS OF DISEASE ON CARDIOVASCULAR RESERVE

The effects of various cardiac abnormalities on the cardiovascular reserve are schematically illustrated by appropriate modifications of Figure 15-11.

A, Diminished cardiac reserve limits the maximal amount of oxygen which can be delivered to the tissues. More complete utilization of venous oxygen reserve and restricted tolerance to exertion are obvious sequelae to this condition. Most forms of heart disease diminish cardiac reserve in one way or another. The cardiovascular reserve is also depleted by conditions which interfere with the transport of oxygen by the blood, such as occur in anemia. Some of the cardiac reserve capacity is used at rest and a smaller increment is therefore available during increased activity.

B, Cardiac reserve can be diminished in many ways. However, complete A-V block with the heart rate fixed at 40 beats per minute is a rather pure form of restriction of the heart rate response. Under these conditions, cardiac output can be increased only through augmented stroke volume. Valvular insufficiency is a common source of diminished stroke volume reserve. The affected ventricle must pump a quantity of blood equal to flow through the vessels plus the amount which regurgitates through the valve. The stroke volume is greatly increased and the reserve is depleted. Constrictive pericarditis tends to limit stroke volume in a very direct way.

C, The conditions which deleteriously affect mechanical efficiency of the heart have not been completely tabulated. It seems clear that myocarditis, heart failure and certain metabolic diseases may diminish all the other components of cardiovascular reserve by reducing cardiac efficiency. This places an added load on the coronary oxygen delivery as well as restricting the maximal stroke volume and oxygen transport.

D, Restricted coronary flow limits oxygen delivery to the myocardium. In this way it diminishes total energy release by the ventricles and reduces reserve cardiac output and the maximal sustained oxygen transport by the blood.

because increased stroke volume is constantly required. Dilatation produces elongation of the coronary capillaries and may produce extraction of more oxygen from the coronary blood. Unfortunately, atrioventricular block is commonly caused by coronary insufficiency or occlusion. Impeded oxygen delivery to the myocardium may well limit the energy restoration and here, again, several components of cardiac reserve may be affected.

Adhesive Pericarditis. Diastolic distention of the ventricles may be seriously restricted by the thickened, adherent pericardium produced by chronic pericarditis. Under these conditions, the diastolic reserve volume is extremely limited and the principal mechanism for increasing stroke volume is a greater ejection fraction. The effective filling pressure is markedly elevated in most instances, even though this is of little avail. Marked venous congestion is a characteristic sign of the condition. Furthermore, the stroke volume reserve is so depleted that the principal adjustment in cardiac output is cardio-acceleration. Thus, the heart rate is very labile, reflecting every change in output. Tachycardia interferes with coronary flow and oxygen delivery to the myocardium. Since cardiac efficiency is considerably reduced when a particular level of cardiac output is attained, predominantly by tachycardia, the energy waste is greater and the total energy expenditure must be increased.

Reduced Cardiac Efficiency. Although the normal heart may operate with 20 per cent efficiency, certain disease processes reduce the efficiency of cardiac contraction by means other than the effects of tachycardia previously mentioned. This means that energy wastage and total energy expenditure must be greater, that the energy restoration and oxygen delivery in the myocardium must be accelerated and that the cardiac reserve is curtailed (Fig. 15–12C). For example, some young patients with apparently normal hearts may develop myocarditis and, in a short space of time, develop the classic signs and symptoms of heart failure, including severe cardiac enlargement, venous congestion and edema. Patients with serious degrees of heart disease may compensate for long periods of time before signs of heart failure appear. One alteration which may precipitate an attack of heart failure is a reduction in the efficiency of cardiac contraction, as has been indicated in direct measurements of myocardial oxygen utilization in relation to the work of the heart.

Diminished Coronary Oxygen Delivery. Obstruction or occlusion of the coronary arteries impedes blood flow to the myocardium and restricts the quantity of oxygen which can reach the contractile units (Fig. 15–12D). In addition to direct mechanical interference with coronary flow, oxygen delivery may be retarded by a number of other circumstances, such as hypertrophy of the myocardial fibers, diminished pressure gradient along the coronary arteries (aortic stenosis and aortic insufficiency), myocarditis with interstitial edema and tachycardia. Indeed, inadequate myocardial oxygenation may be the prime limitation on the cardiac output in many pathologic conditions of the heart and circulation.

IV. CONGESTIVE HEART FAILURE

Patients with heart disease may have neither symptoms nor external signs of it during routine activity so long as they remain "compensated." This term actually means that the cardiovascular reserve capacity is sufficient for the range of activity usually encountered by a particular patient. The diminished cardiac reserves become manifest during more intense exertion by the appearance of breathlessness, perceptibly forceful heart beat and fatigue at levels of exercise which could previously be tolerated with ease. As the cardiovascular reserves become further depleted, the maximal sustained cardiac output is seriously curtailed and a greater proportion of oxygen transport is attained by oxygen extraction which widens the arteriovenous oxygen difference. The final stages are reached when the cardiac output is barely adequate for the metabolic requirements at rest. As various components of the cardiac reserve are progressively depleted, diminished exercise tolerance is the most obvious symptom. In many patients with advanced heart disease, the heart remains compensated for a long time and the signs and symptoms of congestive heart failure appear abruptly without any obvious precipitating cause. Some patients with moderately advanced heart disease may display severe signs of congestive heart failure while other individuals with apparently more serious cardiac impairment remain compensated.

The factors involved in the transition from compensation to decompensation have not been clearly elucidated. The failing ventricle has been described[23] as having a slower pressure rise during isometric contraction, a lower systolic peak pressure, a larger diastolic size, a higher filling pressure and diminished efficiency. This description is consistent with a reduction in dynamic performance as illustrated in Figure 3–17 and 3–18. The reduction in the mechanical efficiency of myocardial contraction is an important factor in heart failure. Detailed investigation of the changes in myocardial metabolism should clarify the nature and significance of ventricular failure.

LEFT VENTRICULAR FAILURE

Depletion of the left ventricular reserve capacity should curtail the maximum sustained cardiac output in accordance with the principles discussed previously. This fact has been clearly established by several studies utilizing cardiac catheterization to measure cardiac output in normal individuals and in patients with heart disease.

Hickam, Cargill and Golden[24] studied the cardiovascular responses of patients with heart disease and normal subjects and arrived at the following conclusions: "(1) In normal persons during exercise there is an increase in both cardiac output and arteriovenous oxygen difference, but the increase in cardiac output predominates; (2) in persons with congestive heart failure, there is little or no increase in the cardiac output during exercise, but there is a large increase in arteriovenous oxygen difference . . . (3) in frank chronic congestive heart failure the resting output is the greatest that can be consistently maintained, but even at rest this output may not be great enough to supply the tissues with blood at a rate normally commensurate with their metabolic needs." Briggs et al.[25] measured many variables including cardiac output, blood volume, thiocyanate space and filling pressures of the heart. They found that the oxygen saturation of mixed venous blood correlates best with the clinical status in compensated and uncompensated patients.

OXYGEN EXTRACTION IN PATIENTS WITH HEART FAILURE

As cardiac function is impaired by disease, the maximum sustained increase in cardiac output is curtailed. Under these conditions, increased oxygen needs are met by a more complete oxygen extraction than normal. In patients with seriously limited cardiac performance, the resting cardiac output may be significantly diminished

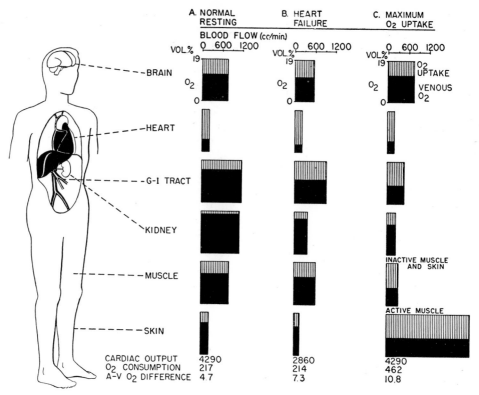

FIGURE 15–13   THE UTILIZATION OF VENOUS OXYGEN RESERVE

The rectangular area, delimited by plotting oxygen content against blood flow, represents the quantity of oxygen per minute delivered to each tissue by the arterial blood. The area covered by vertical lines indicates the quantity of oxygen extracted by each tissue. The black areas represent the venous oxygen reserve, the quantity of oxygen remaining in the blood when it leaves the tissue.

A, The normal distribution of blood flow and oxygen extraction.

B, In patients with advanced congestive heart failure, the resting cardiac output may be abnormally low (2860 cc. per minute). A greater proportion of the venous oxygen reserve is utilized because flow is diminished and greater oxygen extraction occurs in all the tissues except the myocardium. Even cerebral blood flow is diminished.

C, A normal individual with an average resting cardiac output (4290 cc. per minute) could theoretically double his oxygen consumption by maximal utilization of the venous oxygen reserve. If the cerebral and coronary flow remain normal, the oxygen extraction from the blood in the splanchnic bed, skin and inactive muscle could be increased to about 12 volumes per cent and in the kidney to 5.5 volumes per cent. These are the maximal arteriovenous oxygen differences reported in the literature. If blood flow is conserved by this means, one-half of the cardiac output can be diverted to active muscles, greatly augmenting their supply of oxygen without an increase in cardiac output. Neither the normal individual nor the patient with acquired heart disease utilizes venous oxygen reserve to this extent. (Data compiled from the literature[24, 25] and organized in this form by Dr. Loren D. Carlson, University of Kentucky.)

even though the oxygen uptake remains normal. For example, a normal resting subject with a mean cardiac output of 4290 cc. per minute and an oxygen consumption of 217 cc. per minute has an average arteriovenous oxygen difference of 4.7 volumes per cent (Fig. 15–13A). Patients with heart failure have about the same resting oxygen uptake (214 cc. per minute) even though the cardiac output is significantly diminished (2860 cc.

per minute), but the arteriovenous oxygen difference is increased (7.3 volumes per cent) (Fig. 15–13*B*). The increased oxygen extraction in the various tissues is accomplished by reduced blood flow through the skin, kidney, gastrointestinal tract, skeletal muscle and even through the brain. When patients with such advanced heart disease exert themselves even mildly, the oxygen consumption increases largely by further reduction in venous oxygen content from various tissues. However, a further diminution in blood flow through the cerebral circulation, kidneys and splanchnic bed is not well tolerated and unpleasant symptoms discourage any form of physical exertion.

A greatly increased oxygen consumption can theoretically be attained solely through utilization of the venous reserve oxygen without any increase in cardiac output. If the blood flow and oxygen extraction in the brain and heart remained normal and if the maximum tolerable oxygen extraction in splanchnic bed, skin and muscle was 12 volumes per cent and in the kidney was 5.5 volumes per cent, the total oxygen consumption could be doubled without any change in total systemic blood flow (Fig. 15–13*C*). Note the tremendous potential increase in oxygen delivery to active muscle by more complete utilization of venous oxygen reserve through redistribution of blood flow. Neither normal individuals nor patients with advanced heart disease utilize these mechanisms to the fullest extent. Such a marked reduction in renal blood flow could probably be tolerated only briefly before it interfered with renal function. Indeed, such an extreme reduction in renal blood flow is rarely encountered even in patients with advanced congestive failure and extensive edema. Reduced renal blood flow resulting from restricted cardiac output may produce serious impairment of kidney function.

PULMONARY CONGESTION

The reservoir capacity of the pulmonary vascular tree is generally believed to be smaller than that of the systemic venous system. Pulmonary congestion can theoretically be caused by a transfer of blood from the systemic venous system into the pulmonary vascular tree (Fig. 15–14). If right ventricular output exceeds left ventricular output, a large quantity of blood would be quickly transferred to the lungs from the systemic venous reservoirs. The right ventricle is so well adapted as a volume pump that transient imbalance between right and left ventricular output could produce some degree of pulmonary congestion under many circumstances. Accumulation of blood within the pulmonary vascular tree is probably more extensive in patients having increased total blood volume (i.e., right ventricular failure). Congestion of the lungs could also result from any factor that displaced blood from the systemic to the pulmonary vascular bed. One such mechanism would be a generalized constriction of veins in the systemic circulation. Shuman et al.[26] found that blockade of the sympathetic nervous system reduced the elevated venous pressure in patients with congestive heart failure. Such changes have been ascribed to redistribution of blood volume by the release of constrictor reflexes that may produce the increased venous and atrial pressures in patients with congestive heart failure.[27, 28] Under these conditions, a reduction in constrictor tone in veins may provide symptomatic relief without any alteration in cardiac function.

Pulmonary edema can be pro-

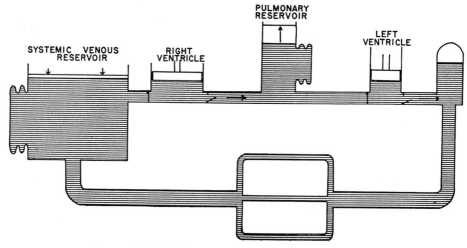

FIGURE 15–14   ETIOLOGY OF PULMONARY CONGESTION

According to current theory, the capacity of the systemic venous reservoir is much larger than that of the pulmonary venous reservoir. Under these conditions, transfer of small quantities of blood from the systemic circulation would produce a relatively large increase in pulmonary vascular volume and pressure. Very slight imbalance between the output of the right ventricular chamber (volume pump) and the left ventricle (pressure pump) could theoretically produce significant pulmonary congestion. A sustained increase in left ventricular filling pressure could theoretically produce chronic pulmonary congestion without appreciable increase in total blood volume.

duced by a wide variety of experimental procedures involving the central nervous system: increasing the intracranial pressure, injecting fibrinogen[29] or veratrine[30] intracisternally or making discrete lesions in the preoptic region of the hypothalamus.[31] The mechanisms by which these neural factors become expressed as pulmonary congestion and edema have not been clarified.

Normal lungs are delicate, spongy, crepitant and resilient. Their color is uniformly salmon pink in young individuals, but with advancing age, accumulation of carbonaceous substances produces a tinge of slate gray. Microscopic sections of inflated pulmonary parenchyma show the delicate alveolar membranes partitioning the alveolar ducts and air sacs (Fig. 15-15A). The blood in the alveolar capillaries comes very close to the alveolar air, so the distance of diffusion for gaseous exchange is extremely short (Fig. 15-15B).

The lungs of patients who have died after chronic left ventricular failure are engorged with blood and are heavy, discolored, tough and indurated. The normal resilience is diminished because connective tissue has proliferated within the parenchyma. The alveolar membranes are thickened and edematous, increasing the distance between the alveolar air and capillary blood (Fig. 15-15C). Many alveoli are partially or completely filled with edema fluid, which would seriously impair respiratory exchange. Scattered throughout the alveolar spaces are phagocytes containing a yellow brown pigment (hemosiderin) derived from erythrocytes extravasated into the alveolar spaces. The caliber of the small bronchial airways may be diminished by congestion and edema of the mucosa and by increased excre-

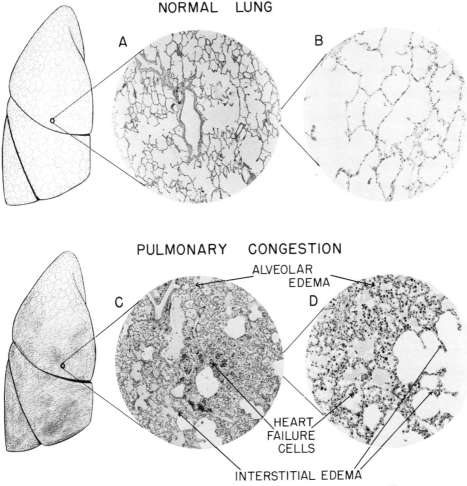

FIGURE 15–15 PULMONARY CONGESTION FROM LEFT VENTRICULAR FAILURE

A, The normal lung is partitioned by delicate alveolar membranes into microscopic air sacs. This structural oganization provides a tremendous surface area for gas exchange.

B, The alveolar membranes are exceedingly thin and blood in capillaries coursing through them comes into almost direct contact with the alveolar air.

C, Pulmonary congestion and edema seriously impede aeration of the alveolar sacs and gas exchange between alveolar air and blood. The presence of edema fluid in alveolar sacs renders them almost functionless and the foaming effect of the fluid impedes respiratory gas movement.

D, Accumulation of fluid within the alveolar walls (interstitial edema) produces an increase in the distance of diffusion, so that gas exchange between alveolar air and blood is slowed even in alveoli which contain no fluid. (Microscopic slides were obtained through courtesy of Dr. Theodore Thorson.)

tion of mucus. Thus, gas exchange in lungs of patients with chronic left ventricular failure is impeded in three ways: (a) by increased resistance to the flow of air in and out of the alveoli, (b) by alveolar flooding with edema fluid and (c) by retarded diffusion of gases from alveolar air to capillary blood by interstitial edema (Fig. 15-15D).

Accumulation of blood within the pulmonary vessels is associated with increased pressure in these channels. Since the lungs function as a blood

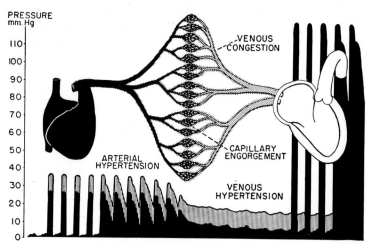

FIGURE 15–16   PULMONARY HYPERTENSION FROM LEFT VENTRICULAR FAILURE

The pressure gradient from pulmonary arteries to left atrium is very slight (about 6 mm. Hg), so any increase in left ventricular filling pressure is immediately reflected throughout the pulmonary vascular tree. Increased pressure in distensible pulmonary veins and capillaries produces marked distention and engorgement. Thus, pulmonary venous and capillary hypertension produces pulmonary congestion and pulmonary edema if the pressures reach sufficient height.

reservoir, the pulmonary vasculature, particularly capillaries and veins, is highly distensible. The pressure in the capillaries and veins must exceed the diastolic pressure in the left ventricle, which is the point of outflow from the pulmonary vessels. The pressure gradient from pulmonary artery to left ventricle is so shallow (6 mm. Hg) that any increase in left ventricular filling pressure produces a generalized increase in pulmonary vascular pressures (Fig. 15–16).

Symptoms from Pulmonary Congestion. The most common presenting symptom of left ventricular insufficiency is dyspnea on exertion. This shortness of breath is characterized by rapid, shallow respiration in contrast to the deep, full inspiration which is the normal respiratory response to exercise. After varying periods of time, the amount of exercise required to induce dyspnea progressively decreases. Eventually the individual may develop respiratory distress when he lies down (orthopnea). Then the patient can breathe comfortably only with his head and trunk erect, even during sleep. For unknown reasons, orthopnea is the initial symptom in many patients with left ventricular insufficiency, particularly that caused by hypertension or coronary insufficiency. Such patients are apt to develop attacks of respiratory distress, similar to asthma, with forced inspiratory and expiratory movements (cardiac asthma), and associated with coughing or choking and expectoration of blood-tinged sputum. Thus, the fundamental symptoms of left ventricular failure are those of respiratory dysfunction associated with pulmonary congestion.

EFFECTS OF PULMONARY CONGESTION ON GAS EXCHANGE. Blood in the pulmonary capillaries can become oxygenated only if oxygen can diffuse rapidly from the alveolar spaces through the intervening membranes to reach the blood. Rapid diffusion of dissolved gases occurs over very short distances in response to steep concentration gradients. An increased distance of diffusion across the alveolar walls theoretically retards the rate of oxygen transfer. For this reason, relatively thin layers of extravascular fluid interposed between the capillaries and the alveolar air should seriously reduce the efficiency with which the blood is oxygenated (Fig. 15–16C). Pulmonary edema results from excessive filtration of fluid through the pulmonary capillaries in accordance with Starling's hypothesis of capillary fluid balance. Flooding of alveolar spaces interferes with aeration of both the alveolar air cells and the blood.

Interference with gas exchange between the alveolar air and the pulmonary capillary blood may well contribute to cyanosis appearing in the terminal stages of left ventricular failure. Since cyanosis is neither a common nor a prominent feature of pulmonary congestion, the extreme degree of pulmonary edema found at postmortem examination (Fig. 15–15C) may not necessarily be typical of most cardiac patients during life.

The presence of fluid in the airways of the lungs is detected clinically by auscultation of the chest. The presence and distribution of râles is generally considered a reliable indication that pulmonary edema is present.

DYSPNEA. In the past, dyspnea was attributed to diminished oxygen and increased carbon dioxide content of the arterial blood reaching the respiratory centers. There is no doubt that inhalation of gas mixtures with either low oxygen tension or increased carbon dioxide concentration results in stimulated respiratory activity. However, under these conditions, increased pulmonary ventilation is accomplished by deep inspiratory excursions rather than by rapid shallow breathing, which

typifies dyspnea. Further, dyspnea occurs in patients with left ventricular decompensation without any evidence of pulmonary edema and with normal arterial oxygen and carbon dioxide levels. Thus, dyspnea cannot be ascribed solely to interference with the primary function of the pulmonary circulation, namely, gaseous exchange between the blood and the alveolar air.

Harrison et al.[32, 33] demonstrated that artificially induced pulmonary congestion in dogs produced rapid shallow breathing which disappeared after section of the vagi. They postulated that such dyspnea resulted from reflex stimulation of respiratory activity initiated by stretch receptors responding to distention of vascular channels within the thorax. Mechanical factors may also be invoked to explain the rapid shallow breathing in response to pulmonary congestion. Congested lungs resemble erectile tissue in that they became rigid and inelastic when engorged with blood. Further, the lungs of patients with chronic pulmonary congestion often become indurated by a proliferation of supporting connective tissue. While the fibrotic reaction may supply additional external support to the pulmonary vessels, it also tends to reduce the mobility and elasticity of the lungs. Under these conditions, increased effort is required to inflate and deflate the lungs.

The underlying connection between congestion of the lungs and the rapid shallow breathing typical of dyspnea in such patients is illustrated in Figure 15–17. Relatively little muscular tension is required to expand a normal lung, and it might be compared with a bellows with a weak spring, as in Figure 15–17A. In contrast, much more muscle tension is needed to overcome the resistance to expansion of the

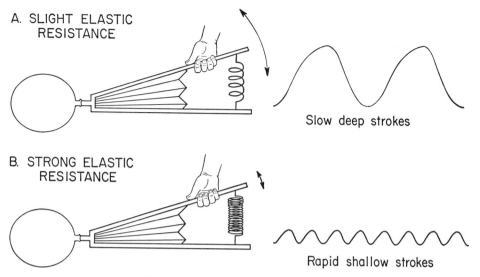

FIGURE 15-17   WORK OF BREATHING

To pump equal volumes of air per unit time, a spring loaded bellows should be operated with short rapid strokes to achieve greatest efficiency and reduce the total work. Congested lungs tend to resist inspiratory distention with greater force than normal so that rapid shallow breathing tends to reduce the work of breathing, particularly when respiratory minute volume must be greatly increased as during exertion. This observation suggests that the dyspnea observed in patients with congestive heart failure may actually diminish the excess work of breathing imposed by the rigidity of the lungs.

congested lung, because it has stiffened. Greater expansion involves even greater tension, and, in general, the congested lung resembles a bellows with a stiff spring (Fig. 15-17B). To pump equal volumes rapidly, the bellows with the weak spring functions most effectively by increasing both rate and stroke volume. Because the work involved in increasing distention and compression is relatively great, the bellows with the stiff spring functions most effectively with rapid shallow strokes. Similarly, the work of breathing is minimized in patients with congested lungs by increasing the respiratory minute volume through rapid shallow breaths. Asked to breathe in and out as rapidly and deeply as possible for some 15 seconds (maximal breathing capacity), patients with left ventricular failure manifest a reduced

ability to increase their respiratory minute volume.

ORTHOPNEA. When the body is erect, blood tends to accumulate in the dependent extremities. The veins are distended by the high hydrostatic pressures. During the day, fluid filters from the capillaries into the tissue spaces in the dependent parts in response to the high intravascular pressures. When a person lies down, the pressure in these vessels diminishes and the excess fluid is reabsorbed, expanding the blood volume at night. At the same time, the blood which had distended the peripheral veins is redistributed and much of it accumulates in the pulmonary tree. In normal individuals, this shift of blood into the lungs produces no disturbance. However, in patients with antecedent pulmonary congestion due to left ventricular failure, the added load induces dyspnea in the reclining position. The patients prop themselves up in bed to avoid the unpleasant consequences of reclining.

Symptoms from Bronchial Congestion. The pulmonary and bronchial arteries serve independent capillary networks except at the respiratory bronchioles and alveolar ducts. However, all the alveolar capillaries and most of the bronchial capillaries drain into the pulmonary veins. Elevation of the left ventricular diastolic pressure and the pulmonary venous pressure is accompanied by congestion in those bronchial vessels which drain by this route. Engorgement of the mucous membranes produces edema and encroachment on the airways. These

events tend to impede movement of air in and out of the lungs (Fig. 15–18). Greater muscular effort is required for respiratory ventilation, and the maximum breathing capacity may be impaired. The result may be a contribution to the shortness of breath closely resembling the asthma produced by allergic reactions.

A productive cough is a prominent symptom in congestive heart failure. The increased production of mucus by congested bronchial mucosa is a logical explanation for this complaint. Although coughing is not a particularly effective mechanism for removing fluid from the alveoli, edema fluid transported to bronchial airways may be eliminated by this mechanism. Blood-tinged sputum is frequently noted and

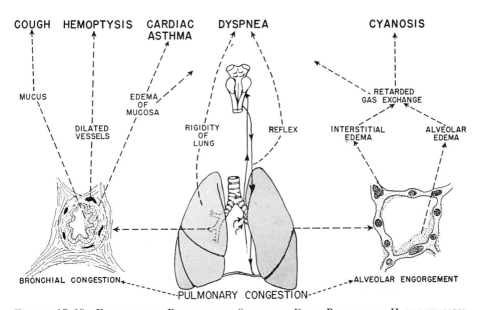

FIGURE 15–18   ETIOLOGY OF RESPIRATORY SYMPTOMS FROM PULMONARY HYPERTENSION

Since most bronchial capillaries drain by way of the pulmonary veins, congestion develops simultaneously in alveolar and bronchial vascular networks. Bronchial congestion tends to stimulate production of mucus, leading to a productive cough. The distended bronchial capillaries may rupture so the patient coughs up blood-tinged sputum (hemoptysis). Edema of the bronchial mucosa increases resistance to air flow, producing respiratory distress similar to asthma. Dyspnea results primarily from reflexes initiated by vascular distention, but may be supplemented by increased rigidity of the lungs and by impaired gas exchange resulting from interstitial edema and accumulation of fluid in alveolar sacs (see Fig. 15–15). Cyanosis is not consistently observed even in patients with severe pulmonary edema (see text).

was formerly explained on the basis of extravasation of erythrocytes into the alveolar sacs. Hemoptysis is now more frequently attributed to small hemorrhages from the congested bronchial mucosa.

Symptoms from Restricted Cardiac Output. Although the classic symptoms of left ventricular failure result from pulmonary dysfunction, restricted cardiac output reserve is an essential feature of this condition. When the resting cardiac output is diminished, the blood flow through nearly all regions of the body is curtailed to some extent and the oxygen extraction is correspondingly increased (see Fig. 15–13). Such depletion of the venous oxygen reserve means that the oxygen tension in these tissues must be subnormal. One would certainly expect evidences of dysfunction to result from such a state. For example, restricted blood flow through skeletal muscle should lead to weakness and fatigability. Richards[34] directed attention to the fact that patients' exercise tolerance may be limited by fatigue or exhaustion as well as by the accompanying dyspnea, from which it must be distinguished. Fatigue is difficult to define or describe and is very easily prevented by voluntary restriction in activity to avoid the unpleasant sensation. For this reason, relief from weakness or fatigability is most readily recognized by patients whose cardiac condition has been rather suddenly improved, e.g., by mitral valvulotomy. The sensation of fatigue subjectively stems directly from exercising muscle and is generally ascribed to oxygen debt and local deficiency in blood flow.

Diminished blood flow through the splanchnic bed might also interfere with gastrointestinal activity. Actually, indigestion is a fairly common complaint in older patients with heart disease, but it is neither distinctive nor consistently observed. Most older patients with advanced heart disease might well have similar gastrointestinal complaints without any heart disease.

The kidney is one tissue in which the blood flow always remains very large in relation to the oxygen extraction. It seems significant that the renal arteriovenous oxygen difference rarely exceeds 3 to 4 cc. per 100 cc. of blood, even in patients with full-blown congestive heart failure (Fig. 15–13). Although renal dysfunction leads to retention of salt and water and the production of generalized venous congestion and peripheral edema, the cause is probably not insufficient oxygenation of the tissue since the kidney must actually work excessively during abnormally great reabsorption of salt and water (see *Peripheral Edema*).

RIGHT VENTRICULAR FAILURE

The right ventricular chamber is so well adapted as a volume pump that it rarely fails as a result of a pure volume load. Certain congenital anomalies produce recirculation of blood through the lungs so that the right ventricular output consistently remains two or three times that of the left ventricle. Such patients may have an essentially normal exercise tolerance and, in them, right heart failure is brought about by the pulmonary hypertension which frequently develops in response to excessive pulmonary blood flow. Thus, the principal cause of right ventricular failure is a chronic pressure load which may result from a number of conditions, including (*a*) left ventricular failure with pulmonary congestion and hypertension, (*b*) mitral stenosis, (*c*) primary disease of the lung with pulmonary hypertension and (*d*) pulmonary valvular stenosis.

PATHOLOGIC EVIDENCE OF RIGHT VENTRICULAR FAILURE

In contrast to left ventricular incompetence, right ventricular failure is manifested in external signs rather than in subjective symptoms. Fully developed right ventricular failure can be recognized from evidence of generalized systemic venous congestion and the development of peripheral edema.

Venous Congestion. Since blood tends to accumulate in those portions of the systemic venous system with the greatest distensibility in relation to the venous pressure, the most obvious engorgement occurs in the systemic venous reservoirs: the liver, spleen, splanchnic bed, skin and the central and peripheral venous channels.

The liver characteristically enlarges in right ventricular failure. It extends well below the right costal border and may descend below the level of the umbilicus. Often the engorged liver is tender on palpation and occasionally is the site of spontaneous abdominal pain. The periportal sinusoids of the liver are engorged with blood. The degree of congestion tends to diminish from the periphery of the lobules toward the hepatic veins (Fig. 15–19). Chronic hepatic congestion may produce proliferation of the connective tissue stroma with a reduction in the size of the liver. The organization of the liver may be seriously disrupted by diffuse necrosis and scarring, which produce the pathologic picture of cirrhosis. It is often difficult to distinguish from cirrhosis with another cause. Chronic congestion of the liver is occasionally associated with evidence of dysfunction in the form of increased bilirubin in the blood or even perceptible jaundice.

Sulfobromophthalein may not be as rapidly extracted from the blood under these conditions. A seriously engorged liver may contain such large quantities of blood that pressure over the organ may significantly distend the superficial cervical veins even when the patient is semi-erect.

The spleen tends to become enlarged during the development of hepatomegaly, presumably because both organs have a reservoir function and a common venous drainage system. However, an enlarged spleen is not as obvious as an enlarged liver.

The kidneys are enlarged, firm dark red. The capillaries in the glomeruli and around the tubules tend to be engorged (Fig. 15–19). Histologic demonstration of such engorgement is difficult because the kidney frequently becomes congested at the time of death from many causes.

The capacious splanchnic bed tends to become engorged in association with hepatomegaly and splenomegaly because blood from the mesenteric veins passes through the liver. Such splanchnic engorgement generally produces neither symptoms nor external signs.

Distention of the superficial veins is an early sign of venous congestion. Since the level of zero effective venous pressure is normally within the thorax, the cervical veins are collapsed when the individual is erect. Generalized engorgement of the venous channels is accompanied by elevated central venous pressure, so the level of zero effective venous pressure is higher. Under these circumstances, the jugular vein remains distended even when the patient is erect. The earliest sign of central engorgement may be elicited by gradually elevating the patient from the supine to the sit-

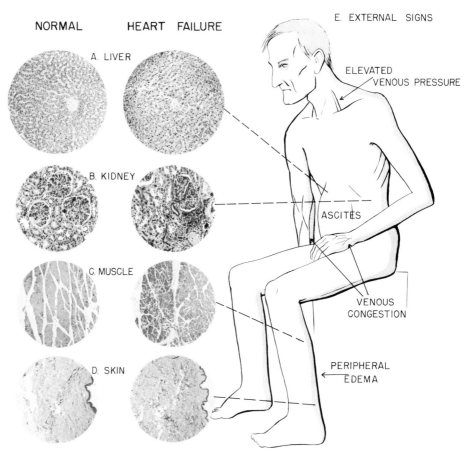

NORMAL HEART FAILURE

E. EXTERNAL SIGNS

A. LIVER

ELEVATED VENOUS PRESSURE

B. KIDNEY

ASCITES

C. MUSCLE

VENOUS CONGESTION

D. SKIN

PERIPHERAL EDEMA

FIGURE 15–19   THE EFFECTS OF RIGHT VENTRICULAR FAILURE

Microscopic sections from a patient who died during an attack of congestive heart failure are compared with those from a young adult killed in an automobile accident.

A, The liver is engorged with blood, distending the liver sinusoids in the periportal regions (around the periphery of the photomicrograph).

B, The congested kidney is characterized by engorgement of both the glomerular and the peritubular capillaries.

C, Normally, the skeletal muscle fibers are packed so tightly that the cell borders cannot be readily distinguished with low power magnification. Edema fluid may force the fibers apart so they stand out individually.

D, Edematous skin becomes greatly thickened and waterlogged. The organization of the connective tissue appears to be disrupted.

E, External signs of advanced congestive heart failure are obvious on superficial inspection. Elevated venous pressure is evidenced by distention of the jugular vein in the erect position and prominence of peripheral veins. Ascites produces increased abdominal girth. Pitting edema tends to be localized in dependent parts. (The slides for this illustration were obtained through the courtesy of Dr. Theodore Thorson and Dr. E. C. Roosen-Runge.)

ting position and observing the level of the transition between collapse and distention of the jugular vein above the sternal notch. Alternatively, the hand can be held dependent until the dorsal veins are distended, then elevated gradually so that the level at which the veins become emptied can be observed. Abnormal distention of veins may be detected before there is any obvious liver enlargement or peripheral edema.

Cyanosis. Cyanosis is severe in certain patients and imperceptible in others for no obvious reason. Since the skin is a major venous reservoir, its blood flow may be curtailed as part of the general conservation of flow, particularly if the cardiac output is diminished. Slow cutaneous flow produces the so-called "stagnant" anoxia, with more complete oxygen extraction and diminished oxygen content of the venous blood.

Peripheral Edema. Swelling of the ankles appearing during the day and subsiding during the night is a characteristic feature of right ventricular decompensation. A considerable quantity of fluid must accumulate in the interstitial spaces before it becomes manifest as edema. The edema accompanying congestive heart failure is generally most severe in dependent regions, particularly the lower extremities. Digital pressure over such edematous regions displaces fluid and leaves a depression which persists for a few minutes (pitting edema). The skin becomes thickened and waterlogged, as illustrated by a specimen from a patient who died with severe congestive heart failure (Fig. 15–19). The soft tissues of the genitalia are particularly prone to develop edema. Skeletal muscle fibers which are normally packed closely together are forced apart by the accumulation of edema fluid in the connective tissue stroma (Fig. 15–19). In bedridden patients with advanced right ventricular failure, edema is often most prominent over the sacrum, which is the most dependent region in the supine position.

Effusion into Serous Cavities. Advanced stages of right ventricular failure in some patients are associated with the accumulation of fluid within the peritoneal cavity (ascites), within the pleural cavity (hydrothorax) and within the pericardium (hydropericardium).

Ascites may produce no signs or symptoms other than an increased abdominal girth and may pass unnoticed. The extent of ascites apparently correlates more with the pressures in the portal circulation than with the cardiac status. A large proportion of patients with severe heart disease develop peripheral edema without demonstrable peritoneal effusion. In contrast, patients with stenosis of the tricuspid valve or constrictive pericarditis often have severe ascites and mild peripheral edema. No satisfactory explanation has been offered for the poor correlation between the severity of edema and of ascites. Perhaps the mechanisms underlying the two conditions are different, since subcutaneous edema fluid usually contains less than 0.5 per cent protein while ascitic fluid contains protein in concentrations approaching that of plasma (5 to 6 per cent).

Pleural effusion occurs most commonly in patients with combined right and left ventricular failure. Bedford and Lovibond[35] cited cases with isolated left ventricular failure and pleural effusion to support their concept that the transudation comes from the capillaries in the visceral pleura which drain into the pulmonary veins. They expressed their belief that elevated pressure in pulmonary veins is a major cause of hydrothorax in such patients. The observation that hydrothorax occurs more frequently in the right pleural space than in the left has never been satisfactorily explained.

Pericardial effusion from congestive heart failure is rarely extensive or significant.

Peripheral edema and effusion into serous cavities represent the accumulation of extravascular fluid, which has previously been attributed to a number of factors, including : (a) increased effective capillary pressure, associated with elevated venous pressure, (b) reduced effective colloid osmotic pressure of the blood from abnormally increased capillary permeability, (c) interference with lymphatic drainage and (d) selective retention of water and electrolytes by the kidneys. Theories based on each of these factors have been discarded or criticized. For example, capillary and venous pressures normally become greatly elevated in dependent extremities without edema formation, evidence for increased capillary permeability has not been convincing, causes of impaired lymphatic drainage have not been elucidated and mechanisms underlying renal retention of salt and water have been controversial. A most unfortunate controversy has existed between proponents of two theories concerning the development of congestive heart failure: the backward failure and forward failure theories. Mention of these two concepts has been studiously avoided on the basis that they have channeled thought and investigative effort along relatively fruitless lines. This controversy is comparable to a debate among police officers concerning the relative seriousness of embezzlement and burglary, sustained to the point that effective investigation of suspects is neglected.

THE CONCEPT OF BACKWARD FAILURE

According to the backward failure theory, the failing ventricle becomes distended and loses contractile power. To maintain the required cardiac output the diastolic filling pressure rises, increasing the stroke volume in accordance with the Frank-Starling mechanism. If the ventricular distention exceeds some critical value, further increase in ventricular filling pressure reduces ventricular output. The increased diastolic pressure in the left ventricle elevates the pressures throughout the venous and capillary channels upstream from the failing chamber. The increased venous pressure is attained by venous engorgement as though the blood were dammed up behind an obstruction in a flowing stream. This idea is sometimes expressed as "the ventricle is unable to eject the quantity of blood which comes to it," although it is not clear what that phrase means in a closed circuit. The generalized increase in venous and capillary pressures augments filtration through the capillary walls so that fluid tends to collect in the interstitial spaces. Fluid lost into the interstitial spaces is replaced by increased fluid intake or by adjustment in renal output so edema and effusion continue until a new equilibrium is established. In response to recent emphasis on the importance of renal retention of salt and water, proponents of this idea have presented evidence that elevation of renal venous pressure produces a diminution in urine output.

Both the strength and the weakness of this concept lie in the fact that it is a functional interpretation of the pathologic changes in patients dying from heart failure. Certainly, the pathologic picture of congestion "looks" like the result of a damming of blood behind a failing chamber. However, a number of discordant factors can be marshalled against this concept.

If blood is dammed up behind the right ventricle, where does all this blood come from? From reference to the hydraulic model in Figure 15–14, it seems clear that a failure of the pump on the left would accumulate fluid in the large reservoir upstream only by evacuating the blood from the smaller (pulmonary) reservoir. Generalized systemic and pulmonary congestion implies a marked increase in total blood volume (renal retention of fluids). If increased renal venous pressure produces renal retention of salt and water, how did the renal venous pressure become elevated in the first place?

Venous hypertension is known to exist in clinical states with little or no edema, e.g., therapeutic ligation of the inferior vena cava. The capillary pressures in the dependent extremities of normal individuals are much higher than the elevated central venous pressure during congestive heart failure. Systemic venous congestion and edema do not appear even after destruction of practically all the right ventricular musculature either in experimental animals or in patients with extensive right ventricular infarction.

Therapeutic procedures, such as a low salt diet or the administration of mercurial diuretics, promote disappearance of edema, decline in venous pressure and reduction in the size of the liver but have no known direct effect on the heart. A syndrome very similar to congestive heart failure can be produced by excessive administration of desoxycorticosterone acetate, which is not supposed to affect the heart significantly. A similar syndrome occurs when large amounts of water and electrolytes are administered to patients with anuria due to renal dis-

ease. Recognition of such deficiencies has led many investigators to favor the forward failure theory.

THE CONCEPT OF FORWARD FAILURE

Advocates of this theory attribute the formation of edema to diminished cardiac output. The forward failure theory antedated the backward failure theory but was not widely accepted for many years. Originally, the diminished cardiac output was believed to produce peripheral constriction and anoxia, which increased capillary permeability and thus produced transudation of fluid into the tissue spaces. However, the capillary endothelium is in direct contact with the blood. If these cells are sufficiently anoxic to increase capillary permeability, what must be the state of the cells at some distance from the capillaries? Neither venous congestion nor edema is characteristically produced by severe anoxia resulting from pulmonary disease, cyanotic congenital heart disease or living at high altitude. However, more recently cardiac catheterization has provided direct evidence of abnormally low cardiac output in many patients with advanced heart failure. Reduction in the renal blood flow of such patients has also been demonstrated. Thus, the diminished cardiac output is now supposed to lead to a diminished renal blood flow and the retention of salt and water. Particularly damaging arguments result from observations that urinary output does not correlate well with renal blood flow and that control of urine volume is vested primarily in the extent of tubular reabsorption. The kidney actually expends more energy in reabsorbing salt and water than in excreting large urine volumes with a specific gravity of about 1.010. The connection between cardiac output and renal tubular function has not been established.

For these reasons, I would like to see both the forward and the backward failure theories discarded to avoid the semantics and the emotional connotations involved.

RENAL RETENTION OF SALT AND WATER

One common omission from discussions of edema is a suggestion of the source of the accumulated extracellular fluid. Patients developing congestive failure and peripheral edema gain weight because the amount of body fluid increases. Similarly, a generalized systemic venous congestion implies an increased total blood volume. This additional fluid in the form of blood, edema and effusion must accumulate as a result of either greater fluid intake or incomplete excretion. Ample evidence now indicates changes in the control of blood and fluid volumes of the body which are very important in promoting this condition.

As Elkington and Squires[36] have stated: "The absolute level of cardiac output does not correlate with the degree of edema, and cannot explain it on either a 'backward' or 'forward failure' theory. An output of the heart which is inadequate in relation to metabolic demands would appear to be a primary factor leading to secondary changes in circulatory dynamics in several regions of the body. Renal retention of salt and water results from more than circulatory disturbance causing a diminished glomerular filtration; tubular transfers are involved and these are conditioned by humoral and cellular, as well as by circulatory factors. . . . In short, the homeostatic mechanisms which control body fluid volume unknown in part, may be functioning in an abnormal way in congestive failure."

Complex control mechanisms are required to maintain both total blood volume and total body fluid volume within a relatively narrow range over long periods in spite of wide variations in food and fluid intake and in excretions and losses of water through various routes. The osmotic pressure in body fluids is also regulated by mechanisms which involve the electrolyte balance. The mechanisms which regulate these exchanges must be very extensive, but they are poorly understood. For example, neural receptors in the left atrium have been described as monitoring the total blood volume and influencing the pituitary gland to excrete varying amounts of antidiuretic hormone to control the output of urine. Osmoreceptors in the diencephalon are believed to adjust urine flow by the same mechanism in response to changes in osmolarity in the body fluids. These are the only mechanisms for control of water balance which appear to have substantial experimental support. In view of the complexity of the problem, these mechanisms constitute only a small step toward an understanding of the whole system that regulates the intake of food, water and electrolytes and the output of these substances as required to maintain the quantity and composition of the blood and other body fluids. The regulation of blood volume is one part of this total picture, but our understanding of this process is also very sketchy.

SUMMARY

Left ventricular failure is characterized by symptoms resulting from pulmonary congestion induced by elevated pressures in the pulmonary vascular bed. The most prominent symptom is dyspnea, which apparently results from increased respiratory effort due to rigidity of a congested and indurated pulmonary parenchyma, perhaps supplemented by reflexes associated with distention of pulmonary veins and the left atrium. Congestion of the bronchial mucosa is associated with pulmonary congestion because the capillary networks of both systems drain by way of the pulmonary veins. Congestion and edema of the membranous lining of the airways increases the resistance to the airflow in and out of the alveoli. Secretion of mucus causes a productive cough. Extravasation of blood from the bronchial capillaries, and possibly into alveolar sacs, may produce blood-tinged sputum (hemoptysis). Vague symptoms such as fatigue, gastrointestinal disturbance and renal dysfunction may be attributed in part to restricted cardiac output.

Right ventricular failure produces generalized systemic venous congestion associated with increased central venous pressure. Peripheral edema consists of accumulation of fluid in the interstitial spaces, first appearing in dependent extremities (ankles) and later advancing up the legs and frequently involving the genitalia. Such subcutaneous fluid contains protein in concentrations less than 0.5 per cent. Effusions in the serous cavities (ascites, pleural and pericardial effusions) represent extravasation of fluid containing protein in considerable quantities (3 to 6 per cent). Generalized venous congestion, peripheral edema and effusion into serous cavities cannot occur unless the total quantity of body fluids increases. In this sense, the renal retention of salt and water must play an important role in the development of congestive failure.

In the past, two concepts have been employed to explain the origin of congestive failure. Advocates of the backward failure theory suggest that blood is dammed up behind the failing ventricle, elevating venous pressure, promoting venous congestion and producing peripheral edema through elevated capillary pressure. The same changes were originally attributed to diminished cardiac output (forward failure), anoxia of peripheral vessels, increased capillary permeability and escape of fluids into the tissues. More recently restricted cardiac output has been assigned a role in causing abnormal retention of salt and water which expands blood volume as well as promoting edema. Serious discrepancies are apparent in both theories. It would seem profitable to investigate the normal mechanisms for monitoring and controlling both the total blood volume and total body fluids. On this basis the aberrations produced by cardiac disease might be more clearly understood.

REFERENCES

1. RUSHMER, R. F. Constancy of stroke volume in ventricular responses to exertion. *Amer. J. Physiol.*, 196:745–750, 1959.
2. RUSHMER, R. F. Postural effects of the baselines of ventricular performance. *Circulation*, 20:897–905, 1959.
3. CHAPMAN, C. B., FISHER, J. N., and SPROULE, B. J. Behavior of stroke volume at rest and during exercise in human beings. *J. Clin. Invest.*, 39:1208–1213, 1960.
4. MARSHALL, R. J., and SHEPHERD, J. T. *Cardiac Function in Health and Disease.* Philadelphia, W. B. Saunders Co. 1968, 409 pp.
5. WARNER, H. R., and TORONTO, A. F. Regulation of cardiac output through stroke volume. *Circulat. Res.*, 8:549–552, 1960.
6. REMINGTON, J. W. Relation between length of diastole and stroke index in intact dog. *Amer. J. Physiol.*, 162:273–279, 1950.
7. RUSHMER, R. F. Work of the heart. *Mod. Conc. Cardiov. Dis.*, 27:473–477, 1958.
8. PREC, O., KATZ, L. N., SENNETT, L., ROSENMAN, R. H., FISHMAN, A. P., and

HWANG, H. Determination of kinetic energy of the heart in man. *Amer. J. Physiol.*, 159:483–491, 1949.

9. CHAPMAN, C. B., BAKER, O., and MITCHELL, J. H. Left ventricular function at rest and during exercise. *J. Clin. Invest.*, 38:1202–1213, 1959.

10. BING, R. J., HAMMOND, M. M., HANDELS-MAN, J. C., POWERS, S. R., SPENCER, F. C., ECKENHOFF, J. E., GOODALE, W. T., HAFKENSCHIEL, J. H., and KETY, S. S. The measurement of coronary blood flow, oxygen consumption, and efficiency of the left ventricle in man. *Amer. Heart J.*, 38:1–24, 1949.

11. CULBERTSON, J. W., HALPERIN, M. H., and WILKINS, R. W. Catherization of the coronary sinus in man. *Amer. Heart J.*, 37:942–951, 1949.

12. JONES, J. W., RACKLEY, C. E., BRUCE, R. A., DODGE, H. T., COBB, L., and SANDLER, H. Left ventricular volumes in valvular heart disease. *Circulation*, 29:887, 1964.

13. MILLER, G. A. H., KIRKLIN, J. W., and SWAN, H. J. C. Myocardial function and left ventricular volumes in acquired valvular insufficiency. *Circulation*, 31:374, 1965.

14. MILLER, G. A. H., and SWAN, H. J. C. Effect of chronic pressure and volume overload on the left ventricular volumes in subjects with congenital heart disease. *Circulation*, 30:205, 1964.

15. DODGE, H. T., SANDLER, H., BALLEW, D. W., and LORD, J. D., JR. The use of biplane angiocardiography for the measurement of left ventricular volume in man. *Amer. Heart J.*, 60:762, 1960.

16. RACKLEY, C. E., DODGE, H. T., CABLE, Y. D., and HAY, R. E. A method for determining left ventricular mass in man. *Circulation*, 29:666, 1964.

17. KENNEDY, J. W., REICHENBACH, D., BAX-LEY, W. A., and DODGE, H. T. Left ventricular mass. A comparison of angiographic measurements with autopsy weight. *Amer. J. Cardiol.*, 19:221, 1967.

18. DODGE, H. T., and BAXLEY, W. A. Hemodynamic aspects of heart failure. *Amer. J. Cardiol.*, 22:24, 1968.

19. CONN, R. D., BLACKMON, J. R., FIGLEY, M. M., PAULSON, P. S., and KENNEDY, J. W. Quantitative left ventricular angiography in idiopathic subaortic stenosis. *Clin. Res.*, 14:123, 1966.

20. HARRISON, T. R. *Failure of the Circulation.* Baltimore, Williams & Wilkins Co., 1939, 502 pp.

21. JONES, R. S. The weight of the heart and its chambers in hypertensive cardiovascular disease with and without failure. *Circulation*, 7:357–369, 1953.

22. BUSCH, V. W. Neue Ergebnisse der Messung und Wägung der Herzkammern bei den verschieden Hypertrophieformen mit besonderer Berücksichtigung der Histologie. *Arch. Kreislaufforsch.*, 22: 267–288, 1955.

23. WIGGERS, C. J. Dynamics of ventricular contraction under abnormal conditions. (The Henry Jackson Memoral Lecture.) *Circulation*, 5:321–348, 1952.

24. HICKAM, J. B., CARGILL, W. H., and GOLDEN, A. Cardiovascular reactions to emotional stimuli. Effect on the cardiac output, arteriovenous oxygen difference, arterial pressure, and peripheral resistance. *J. Clin. Invest.*, 27:290–298, 1948.

25. BRIGGS, A. P., FOWELL, D. M., HAMILTON, W. F., REMINGTON, J. W., WHEELER, N. C., and WINSLOW, J. A. Renal and circulatory factors in the edema formation of congestive heart failure. *J. Clin. Invest.*, 27:810–817, 1948.

26. SHUMAN, C. R., LEARNER, N., and DOANE, J. H., JR. The effect of ganglion blocking agents in congestive heart failure. *Amer. Heart J.*, 47:737–744, 1954.

27. FEJFAR, S., and BROD, J. The mechanism of general haemodynamic changes in heart failure. *Acta med. scand.*, 148:247–272, 1954.

28. BURCH, G. E. Evidence for increased venous tone in chronic congestive heart failure. *Arch. Int. Med.*, 98:750–766, 1956.

29. CAMERON, G. R., and DE, S. N. Experimental pulmonary œdema of nervous origin. *J. Path. Bact.*, 61:375–387, pl. 86, 1949.

30. JARISCH, A., RICHTER, H., and THOMA, H. Zentrogenes Lungenödem. *Klin. Wchnschr.*, 18:1440–1443, 1939.

31. GAMBLE, J. E., and PATTON, H. D. Pulmonary edema and hemorrhage from preoptic lesions in rats. *Amer. J. Physiol.*, 172:623–631, 1953.

32. HARRISON, T. R., CALHOUN, J. A., CULLEN, G. E., WILKINS, W. E., and PILCHER, C. Studies in congestive heart failure. XV. Reflex versus chemical factors in the production of rapid breathing. *J. Clin. Invest.*, 11:133–154, 1932.

33. HARRISON, W. G., JR., CALHOUN, J. A., MARSH, J. P., and HARRISON, T. R. Congestive heart failure. XIX. Reflex stimulation of respiration as the cause of evening dyspnea. *Arch. Intern. Med.*, 53:724–740, 1934.

34. RICHARDS, D. W. The nature of cardiac and of pulmonary dyspnea. (The Lewis A. Conner Memorial Lecture.) *Circulation*, 7:15–29, 1953.

35. BEDFORD, D. E., and LOVIBOND, J. L. Hydrothorax in heart failure. *Brit. Heart J.*, 3:93–111, 1941.

36. ELKINTON, J. R., and SQUIRES, R. D. The distribution of body fluids in congestive heart failure. I. Theoretic considerations. *Circulation*, 4:679–696, 1951.

INDEX

Numbers in *italics* refer to illustrations; (t) refers to tables.

547